OKU 4

Orthopaedic Knowledge Update

Pediatrics

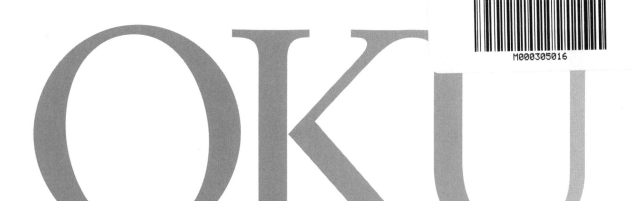

AAOS

AMERICAN ACADEMY OF
ORTHOPAEDIC SURGEONS

OKU
4

Orthopaedic
Knowledge
Update
Pediatrics

EDITOR
Kit M. Song, MD, MHA
Assistant Director of Pediatric Orthopedics
Seattle Children's Hospital
Associate Professor, Department of Orthopedics
University of Washington
Seattle, Washington

DEVELOPED BY THE
PEDIATRIC ORTHOPAEDIC SOCIETY
OF NORTH AMERICA

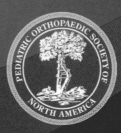

AAOS
AMERICAN ACADEMY OF
ORTHOPAEDIC SURGEONS

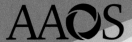

AAOS
AMERICAN ACADEMY OF
ORTHOPAEDIC SURGEONS

Published 2011 by the
American Academy of Orthopaedic Surgeons
6300 North River Road
Rosemont, IL 60018

Copyright 2011
by the American Academy of Orthopaedic Surgeons

ISBN 978-0-89203-643-1
Printed in the USA

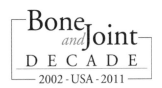

Acknowledgments

Contributors

Benjamin A. Alman, MD
A.J. Lather Professor and Chair of Orthopaedics
Division Head of Orthopaedic Surgery
University of Toronto, Hospital for Sick
  Children
Toronto, Ontario, Canada

Derek F. Amanatullah, MD, PhD
Dr. Denny and Jeanene Dickenson Orthopaedic
  Research Fellow
Department of Orthopaedic Surgery
University of California, Davis
Sacramento, California

Allen F. Anderson, MD
Tennessee Orthopaedic Alliance
Nashville, Tennessee

David D. Aronsson, MD
Department of Orthopaedics and Rehabilitation
University of Vermont College of Medicine
Burlington, Vermont

Wagner A.R. Baratela, MD
Fellow
Department of Orthopaedics
A.I. DuPont Hospital for Children
Wilmington, Delaware

Scott C. Borinstein, MD, PhD
Assistant Professor
Department of Pediatrics
Division of Pediatric Hematology-Oncology
Vanderbilt University
Nashville, Tennessee

Michael T. Busch, MD
Fellowship Director
Children's Healthcare of Atlanta
Children's Orthopaedics of Atlanta
Atlanta, Georgia

Lawson A.B. Copley, MD
Assistant Professor of Orthopaedic Surgery
University of Texas Southwestern
  Medical Center
Children's Medical Center–Texas Scottish Rite
  Hospital for Children
Dallas, Texas

Roger Cornwall, MD
Codirector
Hand and Upper Extremity Center
Assistant Professor of Orthopaedics
Department of Orthopaedic Surgery
Cincinnati Children's Hospital
Cincinnati, Ohio

Donald R. Cummings, CP(LP)
Director of Prosthetics
Department of Prosthetics and Orthotics
Texas Scottish Rite Hospital for Children
Dallas, Texas

Jon R. Davids, MD
Chief of Staff
Shriners Hospital for Children
Greenville, South Carolina

Sean H. Flack, MB ChB, DA, FCA
Assistant Professor
Department of Anesthesiology and
  Pain Medicine
University of Washington School of Medicine
Seattle, Washington

Jeremy S. Frank, MD
Division of Pediatric Orthopaedic Surgery
Joe DiMaggio Children's Hospital
Hollywood, Florida

Peter L. Gambacorta, DO
Fellow
Department of Orthopaedic Surgery and
  Sports Medicine
Children's Hospital Boston
Boston, Massachusetts

Theodore J. Ganley, MD
Director of Sports Medicine
Attending Surgeon
Department of Orthopaedic Surgery
Children's Hospital of Philadelphia
Associate Professor of Orthopaedic Surgery
University of Pennsylvania School of Medicine
Philadelphia, Pennsylvania

Sumeet Garg, MD
Pediatric Orthopaedic Surgeon
Department of Orthopaedics
The Children's Hospital
Assistant Professor of Orthopaedic Surgery
University of Colorado Health Sciences Center
Aurora, Colorado

Gaia Georgopoulos, MD
Associate Professor of Orthopedic Surgery
Department of Orthopaedic Surgery
University of Colorado Health Sciences Center
Denver, Colorado

Charles A. Goldfarb, MD
Associate Professor
Department of Orthopaedic Surgery
Washington University School of Medicine
St. Louis, Missouri

Douglas S. Hawkins, MD
Professor of Pediatrics
Department of Pediatrics
Seattle Children's Hospital
Seattle, Washington

William L. Hennrikus, MD
Professor
Department of Orthopaedics and Pediatrics
Penn State Medical School
Hershey, Pennsylvania

Martin J. Herman, MD
Associate Professor of Orthopedic Surgery
and Pediatrics
Drexel University College of Medicine
St. Christopher's Hospital for Children
Philadelphia, Pennsylvania

John A. Herring, MD
Chief of Staff
Texas Scottish Rite Hospital for Children
Dallas, Texas

Christine Ho, MD
Assistant Professor
University of Texas Southwestern
  Medical Center
Children's Medical Center–Texas Scottish Rite
  Hospital for Children
Dallas, Texas

Steven Hwang, MD
Fellow
Shriners Hospital Philadelphia
Philadelphia, Pennsylvania

Christopher R. Hydorn, MD
Fellow
Department of Orthopaedics
Children's Hospital of Philadelphia
Philadelphia, Pennsylvania

Michelle A. James, MD
Chief of Orthopaedic Surgery
Hand and Upper Extremity Surgeon
Department of Orthopaedic Surgery
Shriners Hospital for Children
  Northern California
Chief, Division of Pediatric Orthopaedics
University of California, Davis School
  of Medicine
Sacramento, California

Charles E. Johnston, MD
Professor of Orthopaedic Surgery
University of Texas Southwestern
  Medical Center
Assistant Chief of Staff
Department of Orthopaedics
Texas Scottish Rite Hospital for Children
Dallas, Texas

Lori A. Karol, MD
Professor
Department of Orthopaedics
University of Texas Southwestern
  Medical Center
Texas Scottish Rite Hospital for Children
Dallas, Texas

Young-Jo Kim, MD, PhD
Assistant Professor of Orthopaedic Surgery
Department of Orthopaedic Surgery
Children's Hospital Boston
Boston, Massachusetts

Mininder S. Kocher, MD, MPH
Associate Director
Division of Sports Medicine
Department of Orthopaedic Surgery
Children's Hospital Boston
Associate Professor of Orthopaedic Surgery
Harvard Medical School
Boston, Massachusetts

Scott H. Kozin, MD
Clinical Professor
Department of Orthopaedics
Temple University
Hand Surgeon
Shriners Hospital for Children
Philadelphia, Pennsylvania

Dennis E. Kramer, MD
Instructor
Division of Sports Medicine
Department of Orthopaedic Surgery
Children's Hospital Boston
Boston, Massachusetts

A. Noelle Larson, MD
Orthopaedic Fellow
Texas Scottish Rite Hospital for Children
Dallas, Texas

Jennifer Lisle, MD
Department of Orthopaedics and Rehabilitation
University of Vermont College of Medicine
Burlington, Vermont

David G. Little, PhD, FRACS(Orth)
Unit Head
Department of Orthopaedic Research and
  Biotechnology
The Children's Hospital at Westmead
Sydney, New South Wales, Australia

William G. Mackenzie, MD
Chair, Department of Orthopaedics
A.I. DuPont Hospital for Children
Wilmington, Delaware

Travis Matheney, MD
Department of Orthopaedic Surgery
Children's Hospital Boston
Boston, Massachusetts

Jordan D. Metzl, MD
Sports Medicine Physician
Hospital for Special Surgery
New York, New York

Lyle Micheli, MD
Director
Division of Sports Medicine
O'Donnell Family Professor of Orthopaedic
  Sports Medicine
Department of Orthopaedic Surgery
Harvard Medical School
Boston, Massachusetts

Firoz Miyanji, MD, FRCSC
Pediatric Orthopedic Surgeon
Department of Orthopedics
British Columbia Children's Hospital
Vancouver, British Columbia, Canada

Jon Oda, MD
Department of Orthopaedic Surgery
Children's Hospital Central California
Madera, California

David A. Podeszwa, MD
Assistant Professor of Orthopaedic Surgery
University of Texas Southwestern
  Medical Center
Texas Scottish Rite Hospital for Children
Dallas, Texas

John D. Polousky, MD
Assistant Professor
Department of Orthopaedic Surgery
University of Colorado School of Medicine
Aurora, Colorado

Maya E. Pring, MD
Associate Clinical Professor
University of California, San Diego
Department of Orthopedic Surgery
Rady Children's Hospital
San Diego, California

Frank Rauch, MD
Shriners Hospital
Montreal, Quebec, Canada

B. Stephens Richards, MD
Assistant Chief of Staff
Texas Scottish Rite Hospital for Children
Dallas, Texas

Amer Samdani, MD
Director of Pediatric Spine
Shriners Hospital for Children
Philadelphia, Pennsylvania

David M. Scher, MD
Associate Professor of Orthopaedic Surgery
Associate Attending Orthopaedic Surgeon
Department of Orthopaedic Surgery
Hospital for Special Surgery
Weill Cornell Medical College
New York, New York

Susan A. Scherl, MD
Associate Professor of Pediatric Orthopaedics
Department of Orthopaedics and Rehabilitation
The University of Nebraska
Children's Hospital and Medical Center
Omaha, Nebraska

Aaron Schindeler, PhD
Research Scientist
Department of Orthopaedic Research and
*   Biotechnology*
The Children's Hospital at Westmead
Sydney, New South Wales, Australia

Suken A. Shah, MD
Codirector
Spine and Scoliosis Service
Attending Pediatric Orthopaedic Surgeon
Department of Orthopaedics
Nemours–A.I. DuPont Hospital for Children
Wilmington, Delaware

Swarkar Sharma, PhD
Postdoctoral Fellow, Molecular Genetics
Seay Center for Musculoskeletal Research
Texas Scottish Rite Hospital for Children
Dallas, Texas

Angela D. Smith, MD
Sports Medicine and Performance Center
Children's Hospital of Philadelphia
Philadelphia, Pennsylvania

Samantha A. Spencer, MD
Instructor in Orthopaedic Surgery
Harvard Medical School
Department of Orthopaedics
Children's Hospital Boston
Boston, Massachusetts

Paul D. Sponseller, MD
Professor of Orthopaedics
Department of Orthopaedic Surgery
Johns Hopkins Medical Institutions
Baltimore, Maryland

Ian A.F. Stokes, PhD
Research Professor
Department of Orthopaedics and Rehabilitation
University of Vermont
Burlington, Vermont

Daniel J. Sucato, MD, MS
Associate Professor of Orthopaedic Surgery
University of Texas Southwestern
*   Medical Center*
Texas Scottish Rite Hospital for Children
Dallas, Texas

Ann E. Van Heest, MD
Professor
Department of Orthopaedic Surgery
University of Minnesota
Minneapolis, Minnesota

C. Douglas Wallace, MD
Clinical Professor
University of California, San Diego
Orthopedic Trauma Director
Department of Orthopedic Surgery
Rady Children's Hospital
San Diego, California

Drew E. Warnick, MD
Pediatric Orthopaedic Surgeon
Children's Orthopaedic and Scoliosis Surgery
*   Associates*
St. Petersburg and Tampa, Florida

Jennifer M. Weiss, MD
Director, Sports Medicine Program
Assistant Professor of Clinical Orthopaedic
  Surgery
Children's Orthopaedic Center
Children's Hospital Los Angeles
Los Angeles, California

David E. Westberry, MD
Medical Staff
Shriners Hospital for Children
Greenville, South Carolina

Roger F. Widmann, MD
Associate Professor of Clinical Orthopaedics
Division of Pediatric Orthopaedic Surgery
Hospital for Special Surgery
New York, New York

Carol A. Wise, PhD
Director of Molecular Genetics
Seay Center for Musculoskeletal Research
Texas Scottish Rite Hospital for Children
Dallas, Texas

Burt Yaszay, MD
Pediatric Orthopedic and Scoliosis Center
Rady Children's Hospital
San Diego, California

Ira Zaltz, MD
Head of Pediatric Orthopaedics
Department of Orthopaedic Surgery
William Beaumont Hospital
Royal Oak, Michigan

Dan A. Zlotolow, MD
Attending Physician
Department of Pediatric Hand Surgery
Shriners Hospital for Children
Philadelphia, Pennsylvania

Preface

It has been a privilege to participate in the creation of this fourth edition of the American Academy of Orthopaedic Surgeons' *Orthopaedic Knowledge Update: Pediatrics*. The number of sections has been expanded in this edition to include basic science, sports medicine, and upper extremity conditions. These topics are a reflection of the rapidly expanding body of knowledge surrounding musculoskeletal conditions in children and the increased sophistication and complexity of care.

With increasing knowledge comes a great responsibility that is highlighted in our current national debate about health care. Safe and appropriate delivery of health care in a cost-effective manner is an increasing challenge. There is a rising demand that we return to a culture of no complications and to the original basic principle of medicine: "First, do no harm." There is tension between our ability and desire to do more and the reality of limited resources and higher risks, with more complex treatments creating a greater potential for error.

The authors and editors of this edition have attempted to place into perspective the large volume of information that has been generated since *OKU: Pediatrics 3* was published. Although we now have more powerful and complex diagnostic and treatment modalities, research into appropriate-use criteria and true patient-centered outcomes should remain our focus. We need to close the gaps between our patients' perceptions of what they want, our understanding of what we intend to do for them, and our analysis of what we have done.

Although this edition focuses on new developments in orthopaedic surgery, the general orthopaedic chapters on infection, anesthesia, and oncology remind us that interdisciplinary care and knowledge of advances in other areas of medicine are essential to better outcomes in patients with complex conditions. Not all surgeons and not all centers can master the myriad new knowledge or should attempt to deliver new, complex treatments. Many of the advances highlighted in these chapters work because of systems created within institutions to coordinate care in a reliable and reproducible manner.

OKU: Pediatrics 4 is not intended to be a comprehensive text, but it is hoped by all of us who have contributed to this work that it will provide useful, up-to-date information leading to the best possible patient care. I am particularly indebted to Steve Richards and the leadership of the Pediatric Orthopaedic Society of North America for asking me to oversee this work. I thank Don Bae, Harry Kim, Min Kocher, Jim McCarthy, Peter Newton, and Ernie Sink for their thoughtful oversight as section editors, as well as Deborah Williams, Michelle Bruno, and Lisa Moore from the AAOS for their contributions to the creation of *OKU: Pediatrics 4*. I am grateful to the many authors who have taken their precious personal time to contribute to this work. Most of all, I am thankful to the wonderful children and families I've had the opportunity to care for and from whom I have learned so much.

Kit M. Song, MD, MHA

Table of Contents

Section 5: Spine

Section 6: Musculoskeletal Trauma

Section 7: Sports-Related Topics

General Topics

SECTION EDITOR:
KIT M. SONG, MD, MHA

Chapter 1

Pediatric Musculoskeletal Infections

Lawson A.B. Copley, MD

Introduction

The spectrum of pediatric musculoskeletal infections ranges from a simple infection that responds to a brief course of antibiotic drugs and resolves quickly without complication to a severe infection that requires intensive inpatient care, aggressive surgical débridement, prolonged hospitalization, and lengthy intravenous and oral antibiotic treatment. A child with a severe infection may have serious adverse effects and lasting consequences.

A pediatric musculoskeletal infection should be evaluated and treated in light of local epidemiologic patterns. Endemic organisms and the antibiotic resistance profiles of the most common causative organisms vary by geographic location. Disease severity also can substantially vary from region to region. In particular, the incidence of community-acquired methicillin-resistant *Staphylococcus aureus* (CA-MRSA) infection is increasing in many geographic areas, and there is greater morbidity among children with infection caused by this organism. The empiric antibiotic therapy recommendations of infectious disease specialists generally are tailored to the local epidemiology.

General Principles

Diagnosis

A child who may have a deep musculoskeletal infection (osteomyelitis, septic arthritis, or pyomyositis) should be evaluated with laboratory studies including complete blood count with differential, erythrocyte sedimentation rate (ESR), C-reactive protein (CRP) level, and blood cultures. The radiographic evaluation should include plain radiographs supplemented by bone scintigraphy or MRI. The focal physical findings usually confirm the area of interest identified by the child or

family. Occasionally, however, the signs and symptoms are subtle, and imaging of a more extensive area is required for diagnosis. Biopsy and culturing of the inflamed area also can be useful in the diagnosis. It is important to be aware that infection can be mimicked by some neoplastic conditions, including leukemia, lymphoma, Ewing sarcoma, metastatic neuroblastoma, and Langerhans cell histiocytosis.

Treatment

An early, comprehensive diagnosis facilitates prompt and effective intervention, which appears to lead to a favorable outcome. Surgical intervention is recommended if a gross abscess is present or if appropriate empiric antibiotic therapy leads to only minimal clinical or laboratory improvement during an observation period. The possibility of residual or recurrent disease can be minimized by selecting the correct empiric antibiotic, the best route of administration, and an adequate dosage and duration of therapy, while ensuring patient compliance until laboratory indices of infection are completely normal. Long-term follow-up sometimes is necessary to ensure a severe infection does not lead to deformity, functional limitation, or limb-length inequality. Many providers and resources are involved in the complex care of children with musculoskeletal infection, and often it is helpful to build collaborative clinical processes and pathways to support multidisciplinary care.

Osteomyelitis

Imaging

Supplemental imaging, usually bone scintigraphy or MRI, is useful for differentiating osteomyelitis from other forms of deep infection with similar signs and symptoms. Bone scintigraphy has been effective in decreasing reliance on MRI for diagnosing uncomplicated osteomyelitis.[1] Bone scintigraphy can be misinterpreted if septic arthritis is present, however; false-positive and negative results are common. MRI with or without intravenous contrast has certain advantages over bone scintigraphy, although it may not be necessary for diag-

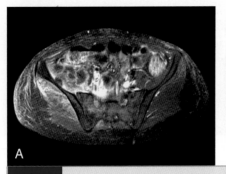
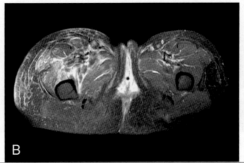
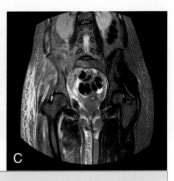

Figure 1	MRI showing the anatomic and spatial extent of pelvic infection in a 16-year-old girl. **A**, A postcontrast axial short-tau inversion recovery (STIR) image of the pelvis shows osteomyelitis of the right ilium and sacral ala, with adjacent pyomyositis of the iliacus muscle and a multiloculated abscess. **B**, A postcontrast axial STIR image of the right hip shows pyomyositis of the adductors with a multiloculated abscess. **C**, A coronal T2-weighted image shows the inflammatory response to infection. MRI guided the surgical decision making; an iliac crest approach was used for the iliac osteomyelitis, pyomyositis, and abscess, and a separate adductor approach was used for the adductor pyomyositis and abscess.

nosing mild osteomyelitis.[2,3] MRI can define the anatomic and spatial extent of an infection; reveal intraosseous, subperiosteal, subfascial, or intramuscular abscesses; guide the choice of surgical procedure and the extent of débridement; and suggest a comprehensive diagnosis by identifying primary and contiguous infected tissues (Figure 1). MRI offers substantial advantages for imaging the pelvis, shoulder, spine, and other anatomic areas that are difficult to see using other modalities.[3,4] Interventions such as aspiration and biopsy do not appear to substantially impair the interpretation of MRI.[2] MRI early in the child's hospitalization usually requires close collaboration among radiology, anesthesiology, orthopaedic surgery, and the primary pediatric service, but it can be very helpful in reducing diagnostic uncertainty and expediting any necessary surgical intervention, thereby limiting the length of hospitalization.[2,5]

Surgical Treatment

Osteomyelitis formerly was believed to respond to antibiotic therapy, without the need for surgery. However, CA-MRSA infection appears to be associated with greater disease severity and a higher rate of surgical intervention.[5-9] The fundamental indications for surgery are an abscess identified through diagnostic imaging and the absence of clinical and laboratory improvement after appropriate empiric antibiotic treatment. No evidence-based guidelines are available to help in determining whether a microabscess is best treated with antibiotics alone or, if surgery is elected, the extent of surgical débridement required to eradicate the infection. Thorough surgical débridement optimizes the local environment for antibiotics, reduces the likelihood that further surgery will be required, and minimizes the possibility of long-term morbidity. Repeated surgical débridement may be necessary for a severe infection.

The epicenter of infection generally is the metaphyseal bone adjacent to the growth plate. Surgery commonly involves exposing the metaphyseal cortex near the focus of infection and incising the periosteum to drain any superiosteal fluid collection. A cortical window of adequate size is created for curettage of the metaphyseal cancellous bone adjacent to the physis. Fluoroscopy is helpful to ensure that the physis is spared during curettage. After adequate irrigation, drains can be placed and the wound approximated.

The cancellous débridement, metaphyseal cortical window, and architectural compromise caused by the infection create a predisposition to pathologic fracture, particularly in a weight-bearing extremity. It is important to guard against fracturing with appropriate activity modification, the use of assistive devices, and supplemental external immobilization with braces, splints, or casts until the bone has healed and remodeled. The time required for healing depends on the extent of infection, the extent of débridement, and the ability of the child to cooperate with activity limitations. Radiographic resolution of the cortical window and cancellous bone may require 12 to 16 weeks, but there may be enough structural integrity for weight bearing after 6 to 8 weeks. Chronic osteomyelitis, with the classic sequestrum and draining sinuses, is extremely rare in a child whose acute hematogenous osteomyelitis was recognized early and was expeditiously and appropriately treated.

Antibiotic Treatment

The selection of antibiotics for empiric therapy generally is based on the most probable causative organism. In communities where CA-MRSA is frequently isolated, clindamycin is the drug of choice.[5,7,8] If the local incidence of MRSA is low, empiric treatment with a first-generation cephalosporin or semisynthetic penicillin may be appropriate.

The adaptive potential of *S aureus* may lead to changes in its antibiotic resistance profile that may further complicate treatment decision making. Clindamycin resistance has been reported in some communities.[7] The commonly used alternatives to clindamycin include vancomycin, rifampin, trimethoprim-sulfamethoxazole, and linezolid.[8] Vancomycin use requires prolonged intravenous access as well as monitoring of renal function and creatinine clearance. Vancomycin is relatively ineffective against intraosseous and intracellular organisms, and the use of synergistic antibiotics such as rifampin should be considered.

When an organism is identified, its sensitivities determine the selection of antibiotics. Only poorly defined guidance is available for determining the route and duration of antibiotic therapy for osteomyelitis, but most clinical investigators recommend 4 to 6 weeks of treatment for an uncomplicated bone or joint infection.[10-12] Sequential parenteral-to-oral antibiotic therapy was found to be effective for most children.[13] The duration of antibiotic therapy generally was based on clinical improvement and on laboratory resolution of the ESR and CRP level. No single treatment can be generally recommended.

Risk Factors for Deep Venous Thrombosis

Several studies found an association between severe deep musculoskeletal infection and deep venous thrombosis (DVT) in children.[7,14-16] The underlying pathophysiology has not been delineated, although bacterial genetics may play a role. One study found that the Panton-Valentine leukocidin (PVL) genetic determinant was disproportionately present in children with DVT.[7]

Children identified as having DVT generally are older than 8 years. They are severely ill and often have an initial CRP level higher than 6 mg/dL.[14] Septic pulmonary emboli and disseminated disease often are discovered, and intensive care with intubation and respiratory support may be required.[14,16] Usually, the musculoskeletal infection is focused in the lower extremity, particularly in the distal femur or proximal tibia, with the DVT in the adjacent popliteal or femoral vein. A child who has such symptoms and clinical findings should undergo ultrasonic or MRI venographic assessment. If DVT is identified, anticoagulation therapy is required.[14]

Septic Arthritis and Related Conditions

Diagnostic Criteria and Differential Diagnosis

An acute onset of joint irritability with associated joint effusion can be caused by several conditions, including septic arthritis, transient synovitis, reactive arthritis (after a streptococcal or enteric infection), or juvenile idiopathic arthritis. For any of these conditions, the best course of action may be aspiration of the joint fluid to assess for a bacterial infection and, sometimes, a formal joint débridement. The adverse consequences of a delay in diagnosis or inadequate preliminary treatment of septic arthritis can be severe, particularly if an immature hip or shoulder is affected.[17-19] The threshold should be low for aspiration and possibly for arthrotomy with lavage of the joint. Clinical prediction guidelines and risk factors can be helpful but may be misleading. The best

treatment decision making for the individual patient requires evaluation of all available clinical and laboratory data. The circumstances of the family also should be considered, particularly the ability to comply with follow-up instructions and to return promptly if the signs or symptoms of infection progress.

Kingella kingae increasingly is being identified in the joint fluid cultures of children age 6 months to 4 years who have septic arthritis.[20,21] This organism is fastidious and difficult to grow in routine laboratory processes. To increase the likelihood of positive identification, the joint fluid should be sent to the laboratory in an aerobic blood culture bottle. The relatively new use of real-time polymerase chain reaction suggests that *K kingae* is one of the most common causes of septic arthritis in young children.[20,21]

Transient synovitis can masquerade as septic arthritis, but it is much less common than septic arthritis in children younger than 3 years or older than 9 years. Observation and nonsteroidal anti-inflammatory medication can be considered if the child is able to ambulate, has minimal pain with a full arc of hip motion, and has moderate relief of symptoms relatively soon after ibuprofen administration. However, the family must be able and willing to completely comply with outpatient clinic follow-up. The family should be carefully instructed to return immediately if the child's condition worsens.

Reactive arthritis has symptoms similar to those of septic arthritis, but they can be more severe and longer lasting. Poststreptococcal reactive arthritis is the most common type in pediatric patients. Recognizing reactive arthritis requires a high index of suspicion. Often, but not always, the child has a remote or recent history of streptococcal infection (such as strep throat). The clinical manifestations of reactive arthritis and the severity of the joint inflammation generally are less than those of a joint infection. Obtaining a serum antistreptolysin O titer often is helpful in making the correct diagnosis. Because reactive arthritis is in the rheumatic fever spectrum and carries a risk of rheumatic heart disease, antibiotic therapy and prolonged antibiotic prophylaxis are appropriate.

Some forms of reactive arthritis occur after an enteric infection. The triggering organism may be *Salmonella, Shigella, Klebsiella, Campylobacter*, or *Chlamydia*. Focal joint inflammation in a child with a recent gastrointestinal infection suggests postenteric reactive arthritis.

Surgical Treatment

Joint arthrocentesis is the most important invasive diagnostic tool used for a joint infection. Joint fluid cell counts can provide useful guidance in deciding whether surgical drainage of the infected joint is necessary. Counts lower than 15,000 cells/mL suggest noninfectious inflammation, and counts higher than 50,000 cells/mL suggest bacterial infection. Good clinical judgment is indispensable in diagnosis and surgical decision making related to septic arthritis.

Both arthroscopic and open surgical drainage have

well-established safety and efficacy, with no significant difference in clinical outcomes.[22-25] The knee is the joint most amenable to arthroscopic procedures in children of almost any age, even when a standard-size arthroscopic cannula is used. Arthroscopy has been used in less accessible joints, such as the shoulder and hip, but is technically demanding.[22-24]

Antibiotic Therapy

Sequential parenteral-to-oral antibiotic therapy is increasingly used for pediatric bone and joint infections. The necessary duration of parenteral therapy before conversion to oral therapy has not been clearly defined for children with septic arthritis. The outcomes of patients treated at a tertiary pediatric center with an average 7.4 days of parenteral antibiotic therapy were compared with the outcomes of patients treated at a different tertiary pediatric center with an average 18.6 days of parenteral antibiotic therapy.[26] No differences in outcomes were found. At another center, children with septic arthritis of the hip were successfully converted to oral antibiotic therapy after an average 3.9 days, using multidisciplinary clinical practice guidelines.[27] The goal of parenteral-to-oral conversion is to shorten the hospital stay by decreasing the duration of parenteral therapy and to avoid hospital readmission because of the failure of home-administered oral antibiotics to resolve the infection. The clinical and laboratory responses to surgery and initial parenteral antibiotic treatment must be considered in determining whether oral antibiotics are appropriate.

Pyomyositis

Diagnosis and Imaging

Nontropical pyomyositis has been reported in otherwise healthy children with increasing frequency during the past 5 years.[5,28,29] The explanation may be the greater invasiveness of *S aureus*, particularly CA-MRSA.[5] Part of the increase may be attributable to the greater use of MRI, which reveals the anatomic and spatial extent of musculoskeletal infection and has led to more frequent diagnosis of the primary and secondary forms of pyomyositis.

The diagnosis can be challenging if striated muscle is a primary site of infection, particularly in the pelvis. The overt clinical manifestations of the infection can be misleading, and a high index of suspicion should be maintained if the child's symptoms are vague, with subtle physical findings in the lower abdomen, pelvis, hip, buttock, or thigh.[28] For example, pyomyositis involving the piriformis or the short external rotators can cause radiating symptoms in the sciatic distribution. Whenever a deep infection involving the pelvis is possible, MRI with and without contrast should be obtained as soon as possible after hospital admission.[30]

Treatment

Pyomyositis is identified in the earliest stage of development, before gross abscess formation, in approximately 10% of patients. Sometimes the disease can be resolved with empiric antibiotic therapy, typically directed against CA-MRSA. More often, surgical or minimally invasive decompression of the abscess is necessary to allow the antibiotic to penetrate the infection epicenter. Surgical decompression and appropriate antibiotic selection usually are followed by fairly rapid improvement, with normal laboratory indices and restoration of full function after a 3- to 4-week course of antibiotic therapy.

Pyomyositis is associated with serious complications including DVT, septic pulmonary embolism, compartment syndrome, and toxic shock syndrome.[14,31,32] Infection with a group A β-hemolytic streptococcus can lead to a rapid clinical decline, and prompt, aggressive débridement of all foci of infection may be required.[26]

Multidisciplinary Management of Pediatric Musculoskeletal Infection

Clinical Practice Guidelines

The broad array of clinical specialties and hospital ancillary services involved in the acute and follow-up care of a child with a musculoskeletal infection includes orthopaedics, pediatrics (hospital and primary care), infectious disease, intensive care, radiology, anesthesiology, hematology, rheumatology, emergency medicine, laboratory, pathology, nursing, physical therapy, and social services. Accurate and reliable communication between services is necessary for optimal care. Ideally, a well-organized multidisciplinary process should be developed to ensure that resources are used effectively, care is based on evidence, and diagnostic studies are obtained in a timely manner. A multidisciplinary clinical practice guideline specific to each type of musculoskeletal infection, such as septic arthritis of the hip, may be useful in improving the process of care. A recent retrospective study found that children treated according to consensus-derived guidelines had a shorter hospital stay, greater compliance with recommended antibiotics, and lower rates of presumptive surgical drainage and bone scintigraphy compared with children who were not treated using such guidelines.[27] The treatment of pediatric musculoskeletal infection varies from region to region and institution to institution because of differences in bacterial epidemiology, experience, and resources. Therefore, clinical practice guidelines usually must be tailored to the facility in which they will be used.

Outpatient Treatment

The transition from hospital-based care to outpatient care is an important but ill-defined threshold. Several factors influence the decision, the most important of which are the patient's clinical condition and laboratory indices. Home health care needs, antibiotic administration requirements, and the family's ability to take responsibility for treatment and follow-up also can influence the timing of hospital discharge. The oral bioavailability of the most commonly used antibiotics is approximately the same as their parenteral availability and usually is sufficient for resolving the infection. If the child cannot make the transition from parenteral to oral antibiotics or requires an intravenous drug such as vancomycin, a peripherally inserted central catheter can be safely and effectively used for home-based intravenous therapy.

Careful outpatient monitoring is necessary to ensure antibiotic compliance, avoid adverse drug effects, confirm that the infection has been completely resolved (as indicated by a normal ESR and CRP level), and recognize any long-term complications such as osteonecrosis, growth disturbance, pathologic fracture, deformity, or joint contracture. A child who has osteomyelitis and contiguous septic arthritis of the hip or shoulder before age 18 months is at increased risk for long-term complications, especially if initial recognition and treatment of the disease were delayed.[17-19] It is important that one person be responsible for the outpatient management of a child with musculoskeletal infection, and a plan for communication among team members is recommended.

Unusual Risk Factors

Orthopaedic surgeons must be particularly aware of the risks associated with certain pathogens and patient factors, such as virulent pathophysiology, immunocompromise, and increased susceptibility to a specific organism. *Salmonella* is more likely to be identified as the cause of a musculoskeletal infection in children with sickle cell disease than in other children. Children who are immunocompromised as a result of chemotherapy or acquired immunodeficiency syndrome are at risk for opportunistic infection from an atypical organism. Neonates are vulnerable to group B streptococci, which can be transmitted from the birth canal and appear as a unifocal decrease in limb movement at age 6 to 8 weeks. An infant with multiple invasive lines placed while in the neonatal intensive care unit is at risk for multifocal infection by multidrug-resistant *S aureus* or *Candida*. A high index of suspicion should be maintained for neonatal bone or joint infection because neonates often do not develop a fever or an elevated ESR or CRP level as an inflammatory response. Children with an infection caused by *Neisseria meningitides* or *Streptococcus pneumoniae* may be at risk for purpura fulminans. Children with a varicella infection are predisposed to streptococcal deep soft-tissue infection. A group A β-hemolytic streptococcal infection can become multifocal and life threatening as a consequence of a toxic shock phenomenon. A nail-puncture wound in the foot can inoculate the deep tissues with *Pseudomonas aeruginosa*, which has a particular affinity for articular cartilage.

Trends in Managing Pediatric Musculoskeletal Infection

The trend toward more severe infections is of concern. Advances in imaging and bacterial subtyping have revealed more complex and extensive mechanisms of injury than was suggested by the older classifications of osteomyelitis and septic arthritis.[5] Human-host genetic factors may have a yet-to-be-defined role in disease susceptibility or severity, particularly with the *PVL* gene;[7,15,33-35] for example, 39 putative bacterial virulence factors have been identified in the genome of *S aureus*.[7,36] Several candidate genes, including *NOS3*, *BAX*, *PTPN22*, interleukin-1α, and Toll-like receptor, may contribute to osteomyelitis susceptibility in humans,[37-41] but the prevalence of these candidate genes has not been studied in a large group of children with musculoskeletal infection.

Summary

The increasing incidence of musculoskeletal infection caused by CA-MRSA appears to be associated with greater invasiveness and clinical severity, which may require surgical intervention. CA-MRSA infections also appear to be associated with an increase in the incidence of DVT and septic pulmonary emboli. Bacterial genetics may be a factor in bacterial virulence, although the genetic association is not clearly defined. The optimal care of children with a musculoskeletal infection appears to require multidisciplinary, disease-specific treatment that takes these complex factors into account.

Annotated References

1. Connolly LP, Connolly SA, Drubach LA, Jaramillo D, Treves ST: Acute hematogenous osteomyelitis of children: Assessment of skeletal scintigraphy-based diagnosis in the era of MRI. *J Nucl Med* 2002;43(10):1310-1316.

2. Kan JH, Hilmes MA, Martus JE, Yu C, Hernanz-Schulman M: Value of MRI after recent diagnostic or surgical intervention in children with suspected osteomyelitis. *AJR Am J Roentgenol* 2008;191(5):1595-1600.

   MRI interpretation was not hindered by invasive interventions. MRI should be done before procedures, to improve the efficacy of patient management and avoid unnecessary procedures. Level of evidence: IV.

3. Connolly SA, Connolly LP, Drubach LA, Zurakowski D, Jaramillo D: MRI for detection of abscess in acute osteomyelitis of the pelvis in children. *AJR Am J Roentgenol* 2007;189(4):867-872.

   MRI is the diagnostic study of choice for children who may have pelvic acute hematogenous osteomyelitis. Level of evidence: III.

4. Klein JD, Leach KA: Pediatric pelvic osteomyelitis. *Clin Pediatr (Phila)* 2007;46(9):787-790.

   Children with pelvic osteomyelitis had a prolonged duration of illness and delayed diagnosis. MRI, bone scintigraphy, or CT was necessary for identifying the infection. Level of evidence: IV.

5. Gafur OA, Copley LA, Hollmig ST, Browne RH, Thornton LA, Crawford SE: The impact of the current epidemiology of pediatric musculoskeletal infection on evaluation and treatment guidelines. *J Pediatr Orthop* 2008;28(7):777-785.

   The annualized per capita incidence of osteomyelitis increased 2.8 times during a 20-year period in one community. MRSA was responsible for 30% of musculoskeletal infections. Level of evidence: III.

6. Castaldo ET, Yang EY: Severe sepsis attributable to community-associated methicillin-resistant Staphylococcus aureus: An emerging fatal problem. *Am Surg* 2007;73(7):684-688.

   The high mortality rate among children with MRSA sepsis requires a vigilant approach to management and a thorough search for sites of infection to prevent embolic spread. Level of evidence: IV.

7. Martínez-Aguilar G, Avalos-Mishaan A, Hulten K, Hammerman W, Mason EO Jr, Kaplan SL: Community-acquired, methicillin-resistant and methicillin-susceptible Staphylococcus aureus musculoskeletal infections in children. *Pediatr Infect Dis J* 2004;23(8):701-706.

   The rate of complications among children with a *PVL*-positive MRSA infection was 30.3%, compared with 0% in children with a *PVL*-negative MRSA infection. The *PVL* gene was identified in the MRSA of all five children with DVT. Level of evidence: II.

8. Saavedra-Lozano J, Mejías A, Ahmad N, et al: Changing trends in acute osteomyelitis in children: Impact of methicillin-resistant Staphylococcus aureus infections. *J Pediatr Orthop* 2008;28(5):569-575.

   MRSA infection was associated with increased length of hospitalization, duration of antibiotic treatment, and complication rate, compared with non-MRSA infection. Level of evidence: II.

9. Hawkshead JJ III, Patel NB, Steele RW, Heinrich SD: Comparative severity of pediatric osteomyelitis attributable to methicillin-resistant versus methicillin-sensitive Staphylococcus aureus. *J Pediatr Orthop* 2009;29(1):85-90.

   Disease severity was greater in children with MRSA osteomyelitis than in children with non-MRSA infection. More aggressive surgical and medical management was necessary. Level of evidence: II.

10. Afghani B, Kong V, Wu FL: What would pediatric infectious disease consultants recommend for management of culture-negative acute hematogenous osteomyelitis? *J Pediatr Orthop* 2007;27(7):805-809.

    Infectious disease specialists recommended empiric antibiotics based on the local prevalence of CA-MRSA. Level of evidence: V.

11. Weichert S, Sharland M, Clarke NM, Faust SN: Acute haematogenous osteomyelitis in children: Is there any evidence for how long we should treat? *Curr Opin Infect Dis* 2008;21(3):258-262.

    There is a lack of evidence-based data for the antibiotic dosage and route used in treating osteomyelitis in children. Only observational and retrospective studies are available. Four to 6 weeks of treatment is the standard therapy. Level of evidence: II.

12. Lazzarini L, Lipsky BA, Mader JT: Antibiotic treatment of osteomyelitis: What have we learned from 30 years of clinical trials? *Int J Infect Dis* 2005;9(3):127-138.

    Three decades of research have been inadequate to determine the best antibiotic selection, route, or duration for treating osteomyelitis, although most investigators recommend a course of approximately 6 weeks. Level of evidence: II.

13. Bachur R, Pagon Z: Success of short-course parenteral antibiotic therapy for acute osteomyelitis of childhood. *Clin Pediatr (Phila)* 2007;46(1):30-35.

    Uncomplicated osteomyelitis was successfully treated using a short parenteral antibiotic course (average, 4 days) followed by an oral antibiotic course (average, 28 days). Level of evidence: III.

14. Hollmig ST, Copley LA, Browne RH, Grande LM, Wilson PL: Deep venous thrombosis associated with osteomyelitis in children. *J Bone Joint Surg Am* 2007;89(7):1517-1523.

    The patient characteristics and clinical disease process of pediatric osteomyelitis and DVT are described. The children had advanced disease severity. Level of evidence: II.

15. Gonzalez BE, Teruya J, Mahoney DH Jr, et al: Venous thrombosis associated with staphylococcal osteomyelitis in children. *Pediatrics* 2006;117(5):1673-1679.

    Seven of nine children with DVT had isolated MRSA belonging to the USA300 clonal group, and seven of nine were positive for the *PVL* gene. Level of evidence: II.

16. Crary SE, Buchanan GR, Drake CE, Journeycake JM: Venous thrombosis and thromboembolism in children with osteomyelitis. *J Pediatr* 2006;149(4):537-541.

    Sixty percent of children with DVT had evidence of infection disseminated to the lung, brain, or heart. Prolonged hospitalization was required. Level of evidence: II.

17. Forlin E, Milani C: Sequelae of septic arthritis of the hip in children: A new classification and a review of 41 hips. *J Pediatr Orthop* 2008;28(5):524-528.

    A simplified classification of septic hip sequelae provides useful guidance. Level of evidence: II.

18. Saisu T, Kawashima A, Kamegaya M, Mikasa M, Moriishi J, Moriya H: Humeral shortening and inferior subluxation as sequelae of septic arthritis of the shoulder in neonates and infants. *J Bone Joint Surg Am* 2007;89(8):1784-1793.

Humeral shortening and inferior subluxation most commonly occurred in children who had a delay of at least 10 days from onset of infection until arthrotomy. Level of evidence: II.

19. Wada A, Fujii T, Takamura K, Yanagida H, Urano N, Surijamorn P: Operative reconstruction of the severe sequelae of infantile septic arthritis of the hip. *J Pediatr Orthop* 2007;27(8):910-914.

    Successful results were obtained by surgical correction in most children with a Choi type IIIA hip, but the results were less positive in those with a type IIIB, IVA, or IVB hip. Level of evidence: III.

20. Chometon S, Benito Y, Chaker M, et al: Specific real-time polymerase chain reaction places Kingella kingae as the most common cause of osteoarticular infections in young children. *Pediatr Infect Dis J* 2007;26(5):377-381.

    By using specific real-time polymerase chain reaction, *K kingae* was found to be the cause of 45% of bone and joint infections in a group of 131 children, and *S aureus* was the cause of 29%. Level of evidence: III.

21. Verdier I, Gayet-Ageron A, Ploton C, et al: Contribution of a broad range polymerase chain reaction to the diagnosis of osteoarticular infections caused by Kingella kingae: Description of twenty-four recent pediatric diagnoses. *Pediatr Infect Dis J* 2005;24(8):692-696.

    The characteristics of children with a *K kingae* infection diagnosed using polymerase chain reaction did not differ from those of children with a positive culture. Level of evidence: III.

22. Jeon IH, Choi CH, Seo JS, Seo KJ, Ko SH, Park JY: Arthroscopic management of septic arthritis of the shoulder joint. *J Bone Joint Surg Am* 2006;88(8):1802-1806.

    Arthroscopic treatment of the shoulder joint is safe and effective. Level of evidence: IV.

23. Forward DP, Hunter JB: Arthroscopic washout of the shoulder for septic arthritis in infants: A new technique. *J Bone Joint Surg Br* 2002;84(8):1173-1175.

24. Kim SJ, Choi NH, Ko SH, Linton JA, Park HW: Arthroscopic treatment of septic arthritis of the hip. *Clin Orthop Relat Res* 2003;407:211-214.

25. Vispo Seara JL, Barthel T, Schmitz H, Eulert J: Arthroscopic treatment of septic joints: Prognostic factors. *Arch Orthop Trauma Surg* 2002;122(4):204-211.

26. Ballock RT, Newton PO, Evans SJ, Estabrook M, Farnsworth CL, Bradley JS: A comparison of early versus late conversion from intravenous to oral therapy in the treatment of septic arthritis. *J Pediatr Orthop* 2009;29(6):636-642.

    Pediatric patients had similar outcomes regardless of whether conversion from intravenous to oral antibiotics was early or late during therapy for septic arthritis.

27. Kocher MS, Mandiga R, Murphy JM, et al: A clinical practice guideline for treatment of septic arthritis in children: Efficacy in improving process of care and effect on outcome of septic arthritis of the hip. *J Bone Joint Surg Am* 2003;85-A(6):994-999.

28. Ovadia D, Ezra E, Ben-Sira L, et al: Primary pyomyositis in children: A retrospective analysis of 11 cases. *J Pediatr Orthop B* 2007;16(2):153-159.

    Abscess formation is common in pyomyositis. Percutaneous or open surgical drainage followed by antibiotics led to complete resolution in almost all children. Level of evidence: IV.

29. Weinberg J, Friedman S, Sood S, Crider RJ: Tropical myositis (pyomyositis) in children in temperate climates: A report of 3 cases on Long Island, New York, and a review of the literature. *Am J Orthop (Belle Mead NJ)* 2007;36(5):E71-E75.

    Supplemental MRI or CT was helpful in diagnosing pyomyositis. CT or ultrasonography was useful in guiding percutaneous procedures. Level of evidence: IV.

30. Weber-Chrysochoou CW, Corti N, Goetschel P, Altermatt S, Huisman TA, Berger C: Pelvic osteomyelitis: A diagnostic challenge in children. *J Pediatr Surg* 2007;42(3):553-557.

    A diagnostic delay can be avoided by early use of MRI or bone scintigraphy whenever a child has pain referred to the hip, thigh, or abdomen. Level of evidence: II.

31. Park SD, Shatsky JB, Pawel BR, Wells L: Atraumatic compartment syndrome: A manifestation of toxic shock and infectious pyomyositis in a child. A case report. *J Bone Joint Surg Am* 2007;89(6):1337-1342.

    Streptococcal invasive infection is known to be associated with life- and limb-threatening invasive soft-tissue infections. Level of evidence: IV.

32. Yuksel H, Yilmaz O, Orguc S, Yercan HS, Aydogan D: A pediatric case of pyomyositis presenting with septic pulmonary emboli. *Joint Bone Spine* 2007;74(5):491-494.

    Pyomyositis caused by *S aureus*, with septic pulmonary emboli, is reported. Level of evidence: IV.

33. McCaskill ML, Mason EO Jr, Kaplan SL, Hammerman W, Lamberth LB, Hultén KG: Increase of the USA300 clone among community-acquired methicillin-susceptible Staphylococcus aureus causing invasive infections. *Pediatr Infect Dis J* 2007;26(12):1122-1127.

    The *S aureus* USA300 clone accounted for a growing proportion of invasive infections (67% of osteomyelitis by study year 5). Level of evidence: II.

34. Dohin B, Gillet Y, Kohler R, et al: Pediatric bone and joint infections caused by Panton-Valentine leukocidin-positive Staphylococcus aureus. *Pediatr Infect Dis J* 2007;26(11):1042-1048.

    Surgical drainage was required for 71% of PVL-positive *S aureus* musculoskeletal infections, and intravenous antibiotic treatment was required for 48 days. In contrast,

1: General Topics

surgical drainage was required for 17% of *PVL*-negative *S aureus* musculoskeletal infections, and intravenous antibiotic treatment was required for 11.3 days. Level of evidence: III.

35. Mitchell PD, Hunt DM, Lyall H, Nolan M, Tudor-Williams G: Panton-Valentine leukocidin-secreting Staphylococcus aureus causing severe musculoskeletal sepsis in children: A new threat. *J Bone Joint Surg Br* 2007;89(9):1239-1242.

   The *PVL* status of *S aureus* infections may be useful in identifying children with greater severity of disease as candidates for prolonged intravenous therapy or for early and aggressive surgical intervention. Level of evidence: IV.

36. Mishaan AM, Mason EO Jr, Martinez-Aguilar G, et al: Emergence of a predominant clone of community-acquired Staphylococcus aureus among children in Houston, Texas. *Pediatr Infect Dis J* 2005;24(3):201-206.

   TCH clone A was responsible for more than 90% of *S aureus* infections in the greater Houston area. Almost all of the severe infections were caused by *PVL*-positive strains. Level of evidence: II.

37. Asensi V, Alvarez V, Valle E, et al: IL-1 alpha (-889) promoter polymorphism is a risk factor for osteomyelitis. *Am J Med Genet A* 2003;119A(2):132-136.

38. Asensi V, Montes AH, Valle E, et al: The NOS3 (27-bp repeat, intron 4) polymorphism is associated with susceptibility to osteomyelitis. *Nitric Oxide* 2007;16(1):44-53.

   Genetic susceptibility to osteomyelitis is associated with *NOS3* polymorphism. Level of evidence: III.

39. Chapman SJ, Khor CC, Vannberg FO, et al: PTPN22 and invasive bacterial disease. *Nat Genet* 2006;38(5):499-500.

   PTPN22 polymorphism was identified in individuals with invasive bacterial disease. Level of evidence: III.

40. Montes AH, Asensi V, Alvarez V, et al: The Toll-like receptor 4 (Asp299Gly) polymorphism is a risk factor for Gram-negative and haematogenous osteomyelitis. *Clin Exp Immunol* 2006;143(3):404-413.

   Toll-like receptor 4 polymorphism is associated with hematogenous osteomyelitis. Level of evidence: III.

41. Ocaña MG, Valle-Garay E, Montes AH, et al: Bax gene G(-248)A promoter polymorphism is associated with increased lifespan of the neutrophils of patients with osteomyelitis. *Genet Med* 2007;9(4):249-255.

   Prolonged neutrophil life was identified in patients with *BAX* gene polymorphism and osteomyelitis. Level of evidence: IV.

Chapter 2

Bone and Soft-Tissue Neoplasms

Jennifer Lisle, MD   Scott C. Borinstein, MD, PhD   Douglas S. Hawkins, MD

1: General Topics

Introduction

Primary bone sarcomas are rare in children. The incidence of malignant pediatric bone tumors is approximately 0.2%, and less than one such tumor is diagnosed per 100,000 population per year.[1] Benign pediatric bone tumors are comparatively common, although their true incidence is unknown. Bone neoplasms are classified according to the type of cell or tissue involved, which may be osseous, cartilaginous, fibrous, round cell, giant cell, vascular, or undefined (Table 1). Soft-tissue sarcomas account for approximately 10% of all pediatric malignancies.[1] The major histologic soft-tissue categories include adipocytic, fibroblastic, fibrohistiocytic, smooth muscle, perivascular, skeletal muscle, vascular, chondro-osseous, and uncertain.

The etiology of bone and soft-tissue neoplasms is largely unknown. Environmental exposures, radiation, viral infection, and genetic associations have all been implicated. During the past two decades, considerable progress has been made in understanding the cytogenetics and molecular biology of these tumors.

Molecular Biology

The histologic diagnosis of a bone or soft-tissue tumor may involve immunohistochemistry, cytogenetics, reverse transcriptase polymerase chain reaction (RT-PCR), and fluorescence in situ hybridization (FISH), in addition to the evaluation of mitotic activity, cellular and nuclear atypia, and tissue architecture. Immunohistochemistry uses antibodies that are known tumor antigens, based on the specific subtype of the tumor, for narrowing the diagnosis (Table 2).

Cytogenetic and molecular genetic analysis of both benign and malignant bone and soft-tissue tumors has tremendously advanced the field of musculoskeletal oncology, leading to more accurate diagnostic techniques

as well as an improved understanding of the underlying tumor biology. New information about tumor biology has led to new and more effective treatments to complement conventional radiotherapeutic and cytotoxic treatments, and it may lead to additional novel therapeutic approaches.

Mutations leading to neoplasia may involve proto-oncogenes, antioncogenes, and chromosomal translocations. Proto-oncogenes normally stimulate cell proliferation but can mutate into oncogenes. This process has been well described in the breast cancer susceptibility (*BRCA-1* and *BRCA-2*), follicular B-cell lymphoma (*Bcl-2*), and C–Finkel osteogenic sarcoma (*c-Fos*) genes. Antioncogenes normally prevent cell proliferation. When a mutation occurs in these genes, uncontrolled proliferation can lead to neoplasia. The retinoblastoma (*Rb*) and protein 53 (*p53*) antioncogenes are associated with osteosarcoma.[2]

Sarcomas are a heterogenous group of tumors, and diagnosis based on morphologic features can be difficult. The identification of chromosomal translocations has been extremely helpful in establishing an accurate diagnosis in specific types of both benign and malignant musculoskeletal tumors. A chromosomal translocation is a break in two chromosomes and an exchange of the sequences, resulting in a translocation fusion gene that contributes to the specific malignant phenotype of the tumor[3] (Table 3).

The standard cytogenetic analysis is karyotyping, which can be used to identify chromosomal translocations. The large amount of fresh material required for karyotyping often is not available for retrospective diagnosis of sarcoma, as needle biopsies provide little tissue. The cell division required for cytogenetic analysis and the preparation and analysis of chromosomes can be technically difficult and time consuming, often taking several weeks.[4]

RT-PCR and FISH are more convenient and more widely used than karyotyping. These techniques can be used with a small amount of fresh or formalin-fixed, paraffin-embedded tissue. The results are available within 1 day. RT-PCR amplifies a defined piece of RNA and identifies demonic breakpoints by detecting fusion RNA transcripts. The diagnostic success of RT-PCR depends on appropriate primer design, RNA quality, and an uncontaminated reagent. FISH detects specific DNA target sequences in the nuclei of nondividing cells. The drawback of FISH is that it requires knowledge of the

Neither of the following authors nor any immediate family member has received anything of value from or owns stock in a commercial company or institution related directly or indirectly to the subject of this chapter: Dr. Lisle, Dr. Borinstein. Dr. Hawkins or an immediate family member has received research or institutional support from Pfizer.

Table 1

Classification of Bone Neoplasms by Cell or Tissue Type

Type	Classification			
	Latent	Active	Aggressive	Malignant
Osseous	Osteoid osteoma Osteoma	Osteoblastoma	Osteoblastoma	Osteosarcoma
Cartilaginous	Enchondroma Osteochondroma	Enchondroma Chondroblastoma	Chondroblastoma	Chondrosarcoma
Fibrous	Nonossifying fibroma Fibrous dysplasia Avulsive cortical irregularity	Nonossifying fibroma Fibrous dysplasia		
Miscellaneous	Eosinophilic granuloma Unicameral bone cyst	Eosinophilic granuloma Unicameral bone cyst Aneurysmal bone cyst	Eosinophilic granuloma Giant cell tumor Aneurysmal bone cyst	

Radiographic Features	Narrow zone of
	  transition
	Geographic
		Wide zone of
		  transition
			Permeative borders
			Cortical destruction
				Permeative borders
				Cortical destruction

Treatment	Observation	Extended curettage	Extended curettage Wide resection	Wide resection Limb salvage or amputation

suspected abnormality. The available FISH probes are the fusion proteins SYT, EWS, ETV6, FKHR, CHOP, and ALK.[3-6]

Clinical Evaluation

History and Examination

Bone Tumors

A well-conducted history and physical examination are important to formulating a differential diagnosis if a bone lesion is suspected. It is important to remember that infection (osteomyelitis) is by far the most common bone lesion in children. Most primary bone malignancies do not occur with fever, decreased appetite, or weight loss. A malignancy can, however, mimic infection with atraumatic onset of pain, swelling, limp or inability to bear weight, and increasing lethargy. An appropriate laboratory and radiographic workup is required to differentiate the two conditions.

The presence or absence of pain is important for the diagnosis. With most malignant lesions, there is a history of painful symptoms, whereas benign lesions are asymptomatic. Most benign bone lesions are detected as a painless incidental finding on a radiograph, but they may appear as a pathologic fracture. Nonossifying fibromas, avulsive cortical irregularities, osteochondromas, and latent simple bone cysts are examples of painless bone lesions commonly identified incidentally on radiographs after a traumatic event.

It is important to characterize the onset, progression, and severity of pain. Activity-related pain most com-

Table 2

Immunohistochemical Markers in Tumor Diagnosis

Marker	Tumor
CD1a	Langerhans cell histiocytosis
S100	Neural or nerve sheath tumor
Leukocyte common antigen	Lymphoma
CD99	Ewing sarcoma
Cytokeratin	Osteofibrous dysplasia Adamantinoma Some vascular tumors Some chondroblastomas
CD31 CD34	Vascular tumors
Vimentin	Mesenchymal cell tumors

monly is associated with a benign condition and must be differentiated from more worrisome night pain or rest pain. However, some benign bone lesions, most notably osteoid osteoma, produce night pain. Malignant lesions are more likely to produce insidiously progressive night and rest pain over weeks to months.

It may be difficult to determine how long the mass has been present. A slow-growing osteochondroma may not be noticed until just before the consultation, and the family therefore has the false impression that

Table 3

Chromosomal Translocations in Tumor Diagnosis

Chromosomal Translocation	Fusion Gene	Tumor
t(x;17)(q22;q13)	TFE3, ASPL	Alveolar soft-parts sarcoma
t(2:12)(q35;q14)	PAX3-FKHR	Rhabdomyosarcoma (alveolar)
t(x;18)(p11;q11)	SYT-SSX1 or SSX2	Synovial sarcoma
t(11;22)(q24;q12)	EWS-FLI1	Ewing sarcoma
t(17;22)(q22;q13)	COL1A1-PDGFB1	Dermatofibrosarcoma protuberans
t(12;22)(q13;q12)	ATF1-EWS	Clear cell sarcoma
t(11;22)	EWS-WT1	Desmoplastic small round cell sarcoma
t(12;16)	CHOP-TLS	Myxoid liposarcoma

the tumor has grown quickly. Because of the abundant soft-tissue camouflage, a mass in the proximal femur, humerus, or pelvis may be present for several months before being detected.

The age of the patient is relevant for the diagnosis. A bone lesion in a child younger than 5 years most commonly is an eosinophilic granuloma or simple bone cyst. Osteoblastoma, osteoid osteoma, and chondroblastoma more often occur in older children and adolescents.

Finally, the location of the tumor is extremely important. A bone lesion in the posterior element of the spine is most commonly an osteoid osteoma, osteoblastoma, or aneurysmal bone cyst. Eosinophilic granuloma most commonly is in the anterior elements of the spine. In the appendicular skeleton of children, the most common epiphyseal neoplasms are chondroblastoma and aneurysmal bone cyst; the most common diaphyseal lesions are fibrous dysplasia and eosinophilic granuloma. Nonossifying fibromas and simple cysts are extremely common metaphyseal bone neoplasms (Table 4).

Some bone neoplasms, including fibrous dysplasias, enchondromas, nonossifying fibromas, and osteochondromas, are associated with multifocal disease (Table 5). The clinician must fully inspect the skin and all extremities during the physical examination. Axillary freckling and café-au-lait spots of the coast-of-California type may be found in a child with Jaffe-Campanacci syndrome;[7] cutaneous hemangiomas, in a child with Maffucci disease; and café-au-lait spots of the coast-of-Maine type, in a child with McCune-Albright syndrome. The skin should be inspected for any overlying change, such as erythema or vascular engorgement from hyperemia, which may be associated with a primary bone sarcoma and is often seen in osteosarcoma. These changes may reflect a rapidly enlarging malignant tumor with vascular dilation causing increased heat and skin turgor.

If the patient has a single bony exostosis, the family history should be reviewed for multiple bony bumps that suggest hereditary multiple exostoses, an autosomal dominant condition. The patient's wrists and an-

Table 4

Common Tumors in the Epiphysis, Diaphysis, and Cortex of Bone

Epiphysis
Chondroblastoma
Aneurysmal bone cyst
Giant cell tumor
Infection

Diaphysis
Fibrous dysplasia
Osteofibrous dysplasia/adamantinoma
Round cell lesions
   Eosinophilic granuloma (Langerhans cell histiocytosis)
   Lymphoma
   Ewing sarcoma

Cortex
Osteoid osteoma
Nonossifying fibroma
Chondromyxoid fibroma
Osteofibrous dysplasia/adamantinoma
Fibrous cortical defect

kles should be carefully examined to detect angular deformity (ulnar deviation or valgus, respectively) caused by tethering of the exostosis. The tethering of the exostosis also can result in limb-length discrepancy and short stature.

Soft-Tissue Tumors
Soft-tissue masses in children are common and frequently are benign. However, it is extremely important and sometimes difficult to differentiate between benign and malignant soft-tissue lesions. Most pediatric soft-tissue sarcomas are painless until the mass becomes large enough to impinge on neurovascular structures. In contrast, some benign soft-tissue masses may present with pain. Intramuscular hemangiomas and synovial cysts can cause a dull ache or pain that waxes and wanes as the blood flow and size change during activity

Table 5

Neoplasms Characterized by Polyostotic Bone Lesions

Fibrous dysplasia
    Polyostotic fibrous dysplasia
    McCune-Albright syndrome
    Mazabraud syndrome

Langerhans cell histiocytosis
    Hans-Schüller-Christian syndrome
    Letterer-Siwe disease

Hereditary multiple exostoses

Ollier disease

Maffucci disease

Neurofibromatosis

Hemangioendothelioma

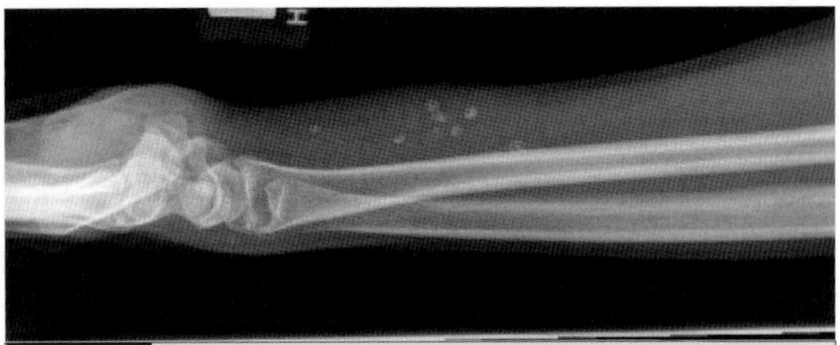

Figure 1 Lateral radiograph of the forearm showing phleboliths in a soft-tissue hemangioma.

and rest. Benign fibrous tumors such as nodular fasciitis, myositis ossificans, and glomus tumors can be very painful. Other soft-tissue processes can mimic a soft-tissue neoplasia. Epitrochlear lymph nodes secondary to a *Bartonella henselae* infection (cat scratch disease), foreign-body granulomas, and intramuscular inflammatory reactions to immunizations are infamous for their confusing clinical and radiologic appearance.

Most soft-tissue sarcomas metastasize primarily to the lungs. However, rhabdomyosarcoma, alveolar soft-parts sarcoma, clear cell sarcoma, epithelial sarcoma, and synovial sarcoma also can locally metastasize to regional lymph nodes. Palpation of regional lymph nodes for increased size, therefore, is an important part of the examination of patients with a suspicious mass.

The size, location, consistency, and mobility of the mass must be evaluated. A benign soft-tissue mass is soft and mobile; mobility of the tumor indicates that the tumor has not invaded the fascia and points to a benign character. Occasionally there is a palpable thrill or an audible bruit in a hemangioma. A mass that is larger than 5 cm, firm, fixed, and deep to the fascia should be considered sarcomatous until proven otherwise.[8] A large, firm, deep mass requires further workup and usually biopsy. A mass that has increased in size over time also should be considered for biopsy. A mass that has been present for a long period of time most likely is benign. Synovial and clear cell sarcomas are an exception, however, as they grow very slowly. Nodular fasciitis and desmoid tumors also are an exception; they are rapidly growing, locally invasive benign tumors.

Tenderness and pain of a mass around a joint can present a diagnostic dilemma. The joint should be assessed for effusion, range of motion, and muscle atrophy. Standard imaging, such as ultrasonography or MRI, is used to differentiate between lesional pain and intra-articular derangement. If necessary, an intra-articular injection of bupivacaine can be used to identify the source of pain.

Imaging

Plain radiographs are an essential starting point for diagnosing any bone or soft-tissue tumor. At least two orthogonal views centered over the lesion should be obtained. Plain radiographs combined with clinical examination are sufficient for diagnosing a benign bone tumor. Four characteristics of the lesion are used to evaluate bone and soft-tissue tumors on plain radiographs: its location, effect on the bone or soft tissue, and mineralization; and the reaction of normal tissue.[9] The geography of the lesion provides a clue to tumor aggressiveness. A well-defined lesion with a sclerotic border and narrow zone of transition implies an inactive benign tumor; a permeative lesion with extensive bony destruction and periosteal reaction implies an aggressive benign tumor or a malignant tumor. The presence of mature, well-corticated phleboliths implies a hemangioma (Figure 1). Liposarcoma and synovial sarcoma may have immature, ill-defined mineralization.

If the diagnosis cannot be established based on clinical and plain radiographic examination, more advanced imaging is required. Ultrasonography is painless and noninvasive, but it has limited utility for evaluating bone and soft-tissue tumors. Ultrasonography can be used to characterize an equivocal soft-tissue mass in a very young child so as to avoid the sedation required for MRI and the radiation generated by CT. A skilled technician and radiologist should be able to differentiate between a cystic and solid mass. Areas of high-velocity blood flow corresponding to feeding vessels can identify the presence of a vascular malformation or hemangioma.

CT is particularly useful for differentiating a benign lesion from a low-grade malignant cartilage lesion. Features of a benign lesion on CT include dense, widespread, uniformly distributed calcifications that form rings or spicules. Features of an aggressive, malignant lesion include faint amorphous calcification with cortical expansion and endosteal scalloping as well as large noncalcified areas.[10] Thin-cut (1-mm) chest CT slices are essential for staging a known primary bone or soft-tissue malignancy.

MRI is extremely useful for evaluating both bone and soft-tissue neoplasms. However, MRI is expensive, and sedation often is required for children younger than 8 years because of the length of time required (an

1: General Topics

average of 45 minutes, depending on the part of the body being examined). In a patient with a bone lesion, MRI can be used to detect an associated soft-tissue mass, the proximity of neurovascular structures, the extent of bone marrow involvement, and the presence of skip lesions.[11] In a patient with a soft-tissue lesion, MRI is useful for determining the site of tumor origin, the extent of disease, and the relationship of the lesion to adjacent anatomic structures.[12] In most patients, the contrast agent gadolinium should be added intravenously to further characterize the lesion. Gadolinium enhancement was found to be a sensitive screening tool for diagnosing benign lipoma and well-differentiated liposarcoma.[13] MRI characteristics are sufficient for diagnosing several types of soft-tissue masses, including lipoma, hemangioma, ganglion cyst, Baker cyst, myositis ossificans, neurolemmoma, and pigmented villonodular synovitis.[14] Tissue must be obtained to establish an accurate diagnosis if the lesion is larger than 5 cm on MRI; is deep to the fascia; is heterogenous with a high fluid content on T2-weighted studies; has a peripheral inflammatory zone or a poorly defined peripheral margin; or is hypointense with T1 weighting and hyperintense with T2 weighting, compared with muscle (suggesting a soft-tissue sarcoma)[14] (Figure 2).

Positron emission tomography (PET) allows tissue metabolism and physiology to be objectively evaluated in both soft-tissue and bone neoplasms. PET uses a radiolabeled molecule, most often [18]fluorodeoxyglucose (FDG), which is injected into the venous system and taken up within cells, where it becomes trapped. The accumulation of trapped FDG can be evaluated though PET.[15] Aggressive tumors usually have a higher rate of glycolysis than less aggressive lesions or normal tissue, and therefore metabolic evaluation with FDG-PET can be used to distinguish benign and malignant lesions.[16] An objective measure called a standard uptake value can be calculated from FDG-PET; this value is useful for predicting overall survival, risk of recurrence, and response to therapy in many types of bone and soft-tissue sarcomas.[17] In many sarcoma centers, combined PET-CT has replaced technetium bone scanning for pretherapy staging, assessment of the response to therapy, and posttherapy surveillance.[16]

Laboratory Studies

The need for a complete blood count with differential, erythrocyte sedimentation rate, and C-reactive protein level always should be considered when evaluating a bone tumor, especially an epiphyseal or metaphyseal lesion. Most laboratory studies are nonspecific for patients with a sarcoma, although pretherapy serum alkaline phosphatase and lactate dehydrogenase testing have prognostic value for patients with osteosarcoma.[18] A patient with Ewing sarcoma may have anemia, leukocytosis, or an increased erythrocyte sedimentation rate.[19] It is important to remember that osteomyelitis is far more common than bone neoplasm in children.

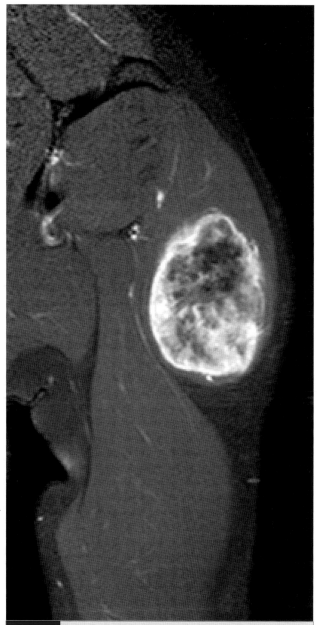

Figure 2   Coronal T2-weighted MRI of the shoulder showing a large, heterogenous soft-tissue mass that may represent a sarcoma.

Biopsy

Biopsy is necessary if the tissue diagnosis cannot be determined from the patient history, physical examination, and radiography. Biopsy should be performed only after considerable thought and planning. The hazards of inappropriate biopsy have been extensively described.[20] In general, the biopsy should be performed at the institution where the definitive treatment will occur. CT-guided or ultrasonography-guided percutaneous, open excisional, or incisional biopsy is chosen depending on the location and size of the tumor. The biopsy should provide an adequate amount of diagnostic tissue

1: General Topics

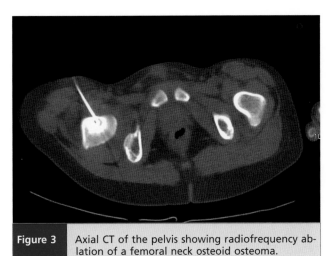

Figure 3 Axial CT of the pelvis showing radiofrequency ablation of a femoral neck osteoid osteoma.

without compromising subsequent reconstructive procedures. Culture at the time of biopsy is recommended.

Radiofrequency Ablation

Radiofrequency ablation (RFA) has gained importance as a minimally invasive treatment for certain benign bone tumors in children. RFA originally was developed for surgical coagulation and was a precursor of Bovie cautery.[21] RFA typically is performed as an outpatient procedure in the radiology suite using general anesthesia or monitored local anesthesia. A large peripheral lesion, as in the tibia or femur, can be located using fluoroscopy. A central lesion, as in the pelvis, spine, or femoral neck, is more easily located using CT. An MRI-compatible RFA probe has been developed in a porcine model but has not yet been used in clinical practice.[22] The size of the RFA probe is chosen based on the size and depth of the lesion. Multitined electrodes are available for larger lesions. The probe is activated, and a temperature of approximately 85° to 90°C is reached and sustained for 4 to 6 minutes (Figure 3). The recommended clearance between the electrode and vital structures such as nerves or vessels is 1 cm.[23] Complications are rare; the most commonly reported is skin burning.[24,25] Other reported complications include infection, necrosis of adjacent structures, and fracture.[24]

The first use of RFA in bone tumors was for percutaneous ablation of osteoid osteoma.[26] However, RFA is now also used in treating carefully selected patients with osteoblastoma, chondroblastoma, enchondroma, eosinophilic granuloma, or giant cell tumor.[27,28] Pain relief without tumor recurrence can be expected. Many of the reported treatment failures were caused by technical shortcomings, such as in needle positioning, or by suboptimal duration of treatment because of the proximity of vital structures.[29] It is imperative to confirm the diagnosis if RFA fails to relieve the symptoms or there is a recurrence. Conventional surgical treatment

with intralesional curettage and bone grafting can then be used.

RFA has been safely and effectively used to treat chondroblastoma in selected patients.[30] Three patients with chondroblastoma remained symptom free more than 2 years after percutaneous RFA.[31] In a study of four patients treated with RFA for chondroblastoma, two patients with a proximal tibial lesion had articular surface collapse.[32] In a third study, this complication was avoided by treating two patients with femoral head chondroblastoma using both percutaneous RFA and percutaneous bone graft augmentation.[33] As the use of RFA has expanded to include bone lesions other than osteoid osteoma, it has become increasingly important to establish a correct histologic diagnosis before treatment.

Benign Bone and Cartilage Neoplasms

Osteoid Osteoma
Osteoid osteoma appears during the first three decades of life. The lesions are believed to sometimes spontaneously burn out, although this occurrence is not well documented. The classic location of an osteoid osteoma is in the femur or tibia, in an intramedullary or subperiosteal position. Increased levels of prostaglandins and increased innervation have been associated with the development of the nidus. MRI is not helpful in diagnosing or staging the lesion. CT and bone scanning remain the preferred imaging modalities.

The current treatment of osteoid osteoma is with CT-guided RFA of the nidus. A lesion location near the spinal cord or nerve roots is a relative contraindication to RFA. The more traditional treatment of osteoid osteoma and the current treatment of a recurrent or inaccessible lesion is intralesional curettage. Identifying the lesion location often requires preoperative CT using a guidewire. Osteoid osteoma–induced scoliosis often spontaneously corrects itself after successful treatment of the lesion. Nonsteroidal anti-inflammatory drugs or salicylates alone can be successfully used for relieving pain, but symptom resolution often takes as long as 30 months.

Osteoblastoma
Like osteoid osteoma, osteoblastoma appears during the first three decades of life. This lesion is most common in the posterior elements of the spine and the metaphysis of the long bones of the lower extremity. The histologic features include disorganized seams of abundant osteoid production in the form of woven bone similar to that of the central nidus in osteoid osteoma but without the tendency toward organized mature trabeculae at the periphery. Vascular spaces and giant cells are often seen. Unlike osteoid osteoma, osteoblastoma progresses if not treated, and it has a higher incidence of local recurrence requiring repeat excision. Rarely, sarcomatous degeneration can occur. Complete intrale-

sional resection should be performed, with consideration of adjuvant treatment such as liquid nitrogen or phenol to reduce the risk of recurrence. Wide resection can be considered for an aggressive lesion in an expendable bone such as a rib or fibula.

Osteochondroma

Solitary osteochondroma is the most common bone tumor. A painless bony mass appears during the first two decades of life and may be associated with mechanical symptoms from adjacent bursitis. Inactivation of both copies of the exotosis-1 (EXT1) tumor suppressor gene causes a small herniation of physeal tissue in the metaphysis of a growing bone. Therefore, osteochondroma grows when the adjacent physis grows, and it should stop growing with skeletal maturity. A small number of exostoses occur after damage to the physis, most often from total body irradiation. Such an exostosis has a radiographic appearance different from that of developmental exostosis. Sarcomatous degeneration from the cartilaginous cap secondary to chondrosarcoma is rare. Intracanal lesions have occurred in association with multiple hereditary exostoses, with spontaneous paraparesis in several patients.[34]

Chondroblastoma

Chondroblastoma is most common in patients younger than 20 years. These tumors have a predilection for the epiphysis of long bones and less commonly are found in the tarsal bones and patella. They are considered benign tumors but in rare instances metastasize to the lungs. Approximately half of such metastases were found in patients with a recurrence or with a primary lesion in a flat bone.[35] The standard treatment is extended intralesional curettage, which can be augmented with liquid nitrogen or phenol.

Cystic Lesions
Simple Bone Cyst
A simple bone cyst (unicameral bone cyst) most often occurs in patients age 4 to 10 years; 85% occur within the first two decades of life. The reported recurrence rate is as high as 20%.[36] A randomized clinical study found significantly better radiographic healing when the cyst was treated with injection of methylprednisolone rather than bone marrow aspirate.[36] The rate of morbidity from pathologic fracture is highest in femoral neck and intertrochanteric lesions, and the threshold for curettage, bone grafting, and internal fixation therefore is lower for these lesions. Nonsurgical management should be used initially for a pathologic fracture of a simple bone cyst in the lower extremity; 15% to 20% of upper extremity lesions heal after pathologic fracture.[37]

Aneurysmal Bone Cyst
An aneurysmal bone cyst appears when a patient is age 1 to 20 years; the average age is 11 years. Primary aneurysmal bone cysts are most likely neoplastic, reflect-

ing a clonal chromosome band 17p13 translocation that places the ubiquitin-specific protease–6 (USP6) oncogene under the regulatory influence of the cadherin-11 (CDH11) promoter.[38] These chromosomal rearrangements are not seen in secondary aneurysmal bone cysts. It is of utmost importance to differentiate aneurysmal bone cysts from telangiectatic osteosarcoma. Because aneurysmal bone cysts are active and aggressive, intralesional curettage and bone grafting are recommended. Embolization and injection with bone marrow, with or without demineralized bone grafting, also have been described.

Fibrous Bone Lesions
Nonossifying Fibroma
Nonossifying fibroma is one of the most common benign lesions of bone. A metaphyseal fibrous cortical defect is a small (less than 0.5 cm), cortically based nonossifying fibroma that arises from a developmental defect in the periosteal cortical bone. An avulsive cortical irregularity has the same histology but is found only in the distal posteromedial femoral metaphysis. Avulsive cortical irregularity occurs as the result of repetitive avulsive microfracture from the distal adductor magnus insertion or the medial head of the gastrocnemius, and often it is bilateral.

Nonossifying fibromas spontaneously regress at skeletal maturity, sometimes with residual radiographic ossification and sclerosis. The treatment is based on the risk of fracture. Observation is recommended. Surgical curettage and bone grafting traditionally were recommended if the lesion occupied more than 50% of the volume of the bone on plain radiographs. CT-based evaluation of lesion size has been found to best predict fracture risk.[39,40]

Fibrous Dysplasia
Fibrous dysplasia is a benign fibro-osseous bone lesion that accounts for approximately 5% to 7% of benign bone tumors.[41] It is a developmental anomaly of bone formation caused by missense mutation in exon 8 of the GNAS gene (chromosome 20q13.2-13.3).[42] The traditional treatment includes observation of an asymptomatic or incidentally identified lesion. Curettage, bone grafting, and internal fixation are indicated if the patient has mono-ostotic disease, a symptomatic lesion, or a lesion with impending pathologic fracture.

Bisphosphonate therapy has been used for patients with a symptomatic large lesion or polyostotic disease.[43,44] Pamidronate, a second-generation bisphosphonate, has been most successful for relieving pain and improving radiographic findings in patients with symptomatic polyostotic fibrous dysplasia. Pamidronate is administered intravenously, usually over 3 days every 6 months in a dosage of 180 mg. Zoledronic acid can be administered intravenously over a shorter period of time. The recommended duration of this treatment is at least 2 years.[45] Patients should receive a daily dose of calcium and vitamin D to avoid secondary hyperthyroidism.[42] Clinical and radiologic symptoms improved in patients treated for several years with oral bisphosphonates such as alendronate, and there was an absence of new pathologic fractures.[46]

Although the results of bisphosphonate treatment are encouraging, potentially serious adverse effects have been reported. The US Food and Drug Administration in December 2004 warned that osteonecrosis of the jaw had been reported after intravenous zoledronic acid was used, mainly in patients with cancer. A dental examination and appropriate preventive dental treatment are recommended before treatment with bisphosphonates if the patient has a risk factor such as cancer, poor oral hygiene, or chemotherapeutic or corticosteroid treatment. In addition, a skeletally immature patient receiving a bisphosphonate should be monitored with serial radiographs for increased physeal plate thickening, indicating a transient mineralization defect.[41]

Malignant Bone and Soft-Tissue Neoplasms

Osteosarcoma

Osteosarcoma is the most common malignant pediatric bone tumor, most often occurring in adolescents and young adults. The US incidence is approximately 400 per year in individuals younger than 20 years and 600 per year in those age 15 to 25 years.[1] Osteosarcoma almost always is idiopathic. However, exposure to ionizing radiation significantly increases the risk of developing osteosarcoma. Patients with Li-Fraumeni syndrome (who have a germline mutation in the *p53* tumor suppressor gene) or retinoblastoma (who have loss of the tumor suppressor gene *Rb*) also are at increased risk for osteosarcoma. Patients with Rothmund-Thomson syndrome, an inherited condition characterized by poikiloderma, small stature, and skeletal dysplasia, have mutations in the DNA helicase gene *RECQL4* and a dramatically increased incidence of familial osteosarcoma.[47]

Patients with osteosarcoma usually have a hard mass as well as activity-associated intermittent pain. Less frequently, the patient has a pathologic fracture through the tumor. Although osteosarcoma can occur anywhere in the body, usually the tumor is in a long bone of an extremity; 80% occur around the knee (distal femur, proximal tibia, or proximal fibula), and 10% occur in the proximal humerus.[48] Patients rarely have overt metastatic disease. When metastasis does occur, the lungs and bones are the most common sites.

The diagnostic workup includes radiography and MRI of the primary lesion, CT of the chest to evaluate for pulmonary disease, and bone scintigraphy to evaluate for bony metastasis. FDG-PET is increasingly popular for use in osteosarcoma, as it is effective in identifying metastatic disease and assessing the response to chemotherapy.[17,49] Most tumors are intramedullary, arising within the marrow cavity. However, some tumors are on the surface of the bone; these parosteal or

periosteal tumors usually are low grade and can be treated with surgical resection alone. To confirm the diagnosis of osteosarcoma, a biopsy should be performed by an orthopaedic oncologist. Histologic examination reveals atypical cells surrounded by malignant osteoid. Although there are several histologic subtypes of osteosarcoma (osteoblastic, chondroblastic, fibroblastic, and telangiectatic), the subtype has no prognostic implication.

Osteosarcoma is treated with surgery and chemotherapy. Patients usually receive neoadjuvant chemotherapy to facilitate surgical resection. Most neoadjuvant chemotherapy protocols include cisplatin, doxorubicin, and methotrexate, sometimes with alkylating agents such as ifosfamide. Although one randomized study found no outcome benefit to neoadjuvant chemotherapy, compared with immediate surgery followed by adjuvant chemotherapy, the resulting delay often allows the surgeon time to prepare for an optimal limb salvage procedure.[50] Resection of metastatic disease is essential for long-term survival. Osteosarcoma is inherently radiation resistant, and radiation therapy is used only if surgical resection is not feasible.

Advances in imaging, surgery, and chemotherapy have led to modest improvement in survival rates. Patients with localized disease at diagnosis have an approximately 70% 5-year event-free survival rate when the most current chemotherapy protocols are used. However, patients with metastatic disease at diagnosis have a poor prognosis (an approximately 20% 5-year event-free survival rate).[48,50-52] An ongoing phase III clinical study by US and European cancer centers is designed to determine whether survival rates for patients with a poor histologic response to chemotherapy can be improved by the addition of ifosfamide and etoposide.[53] The importance of this study question is reinforced by the failure of earlier clinical studies to find a correlation between histologic response to different chemotherapy regimens and survival.[54,55] The current study also intends to determine whether the use of interferon α-2b, an agent that has demonstrated preclinical efficacy against osteosarcoma cell lines, improves overall survival in patients with localized osteosarcoma.[56] Additional research is under way to investigate the use of novel agents such as zoledronic acid and muramyl tripeptide for treating metastatic osteosarcoma.[57-59]

Ewing Sarcoma

Ewing sarcoma is the second most common malignant bone tumor in children. The annual US incidence is approximately 250, and the median patient age is 15 years. Individuals of European descent are six times more likely to develop Ewing sarcoma than those of African descent.[1] Unlike osteosarcoma, Ewing sarcoma almost always is idiopathic; there are no known genetic predispositions, and familial Ewing sarcoma is extremely rare.

Patients with Ewing sarcoma initially have pain, a mass, or pathologic fracture. Unlike osteosarcoma, in which most lesions occur near the knee, Ewing sarcoma can occur in bone or the surrounding soft tissue anywhere in the body. The most common site is the pelvis, which accounts for one fourth of all incidences. Metastatic disease is present at diagnosis in 15% to 30% of patients. The common sites of metastatic disease are the lungs, bone, and bone marrow. The diagnostic workup includes MRI or CT of the primary lesion as well as bone scan, FDG-PET, and chest CT. Bone marrow biopsy is recommended to rule out marrow involvement. Biopsy of the primary tumor should be sent for pathologic analysis in addition to FISH or RT-PCR. Histologic examination reveals small, round undifferentiated blue cells with immunohistochemical staining for CD99, which is a hematopoietic marker normally present on leukocytes. Ewing sarcoma tumors do not stain for neural-specific or muscle-specific markers. Cytogenetic or molecular characterization is critical in the diagnosis of Ewing sarcoma. More than 95% of patients with Ewing sarcoma have an identifiable chromosomal translocation between members of the Ewing sarcoma region 1 (EWSR1) and E–twenty-six (ETS) gene families. In more than 85% of patients, the translocation is between chromosomes 11 and 22. This translocation results in the generation of an abnormal fusion protein combining the EWSR1 and Friend leukemia virus integration 1 (Fli1) genes. This fusion protein is essential for the pathogenesis of the tumor. Most often, exon 7 of EWSR1 is fused with exon 6 of Fli1, generating a type I EWSR1-Fli1 fusion gene. Although some studies suggested that patients with the type I EWSR1-Fli1 translocation have a better prognosis than those with a non–type I EWSR1-Fli1 translocation, more recent studies found that the type of EWSR1-Fli1 fusion has no impact on survival.[60-63]

The treatment of Ewing sarcoma includes chemotherapy in conjunction with surgery and/or radiation therapy. Neoadjuvant chemotherapy usually is administered to shrink the primary tumor before surgical resection. Patients with an unresectable tumor or residual disease after resection usually require radiation therapy. The combination of cytotoxic agents used in chemotherapy regimens includes vincristine, doxorubicin, cyclophosphamide, ifosfamide, and etoposide. Recent studies found that interval-compressed chemotherapy regimens (administered at 2-week rather than 3-week intervals) and regimens that include intensive alkylator therapy are both safe and efficacious.[64,65] The 3-year event-free survival of patients with localized disease at diagnosis is approximately 75% when an interval-compressed chemotherapy regimen is used.[65] The prognosis for patients with metastatic disease at diagnosis remains poor,[66] and the outcome for patients with relapsed Ewing sarcoma is dismal, especially if recurrent or progressive disease occurs within 2 years of the initial diagnosis.[67]

Ongoing clinical investigations are attempting to determine the role of high-dose chemotherapy combined with hematopoietic stem cell rescue for treating Ewing sarcoma. Myeloablative chemotherapy followed by autologous stem cell transplantation may improve survival rates, although none of the available data are from prospective, randomized studies.[68-70] Conventional chemotherapy is being compared with two consolidation treatment regimens that include myeloablative chemotherapy followed by stem cell rescue, in an ongoing randomized prospective clinical study of patients with Ewing sarcoma who have isolated pulmonary metastatic disease. The study results should elucidate the role of stem cell transplantation in treating Ewing sarcoma.[70]

Rhabdomyosarcoma

Rhabdomyosarcoma is the most common soft-tissue sarcoma of childhood. The US incidence is approximately 350 per year. Unlike osteosarcoma or Ewing sarcoma, rhabdomyosarcoma has a peak incidence in children younger than 6 years.[1] Rhabdomyosarcoma usually is idiopathic, although individuals with neurofibromatosis or Li-Fraumeni syndrome have an increased incidence.

Rhabdomyosarcoma can occur in any part of the body. The clinical presentation depends on the location of the primary tumor. Head and neck rhabdomyosarcoma (including a parameningeal tumor) is most common in younger children, and it accounts for approximately 35% of all incidences of rhabdomyosarcoma. The patient has pain, often with a palpable mass, but vision changes or cranial nerve palsies occasionally are the presenting symptom. The genitourinary tract is the second most common primary site; the disease usually appears with a botryoid variant of embryonal sarcoma that arises in the bladder or vagina. Rhabdomyosarcoma also can arise from the skeletal musculature of the extremities, trunk, abdomen, or pelvis; and its appearance varies with the location and extent of disease. Most patients have localized disease, although one fourth of patients have metastasis at diagnosis. The common locations of metastasis include the lung, bone marrow, bone, and lymph nodes.

The workup for rhabdomyosarcoma includes CT or MRI of the primary lesion, bone scanning and/or FDG-PET, chest CT, and bone marrow evaluation. Patients with parameningeal rhabdomyosarcoma also should have a lumbar puncture for cytologic evaluation of the cerebral spinal fluid. Morphologic analysis reveals small, round, blue cells with immunoreactivity to muscle-specific markers such as myogenin, desmin, and MyoD.

Rhabdomyosarcoma has two main subtypes. Embryonal rhabdomyosarcoma (including the spindle cell and botryoid variants), which accounts for two thirds of all tumors, is stroma rich, less cellular, and in a spindle cell pattern. The remaining one third of patients have alveolar rhabdomyosarcoma, in which the more cellular, densely packed tumors resemble pulmonary alveoli. These tumors often are accompanied by metastatic disease and have a much worse prognosis than embryonal rhabdomyosarcoma. In 80% of alveolar rhabdomyosarcoma tumors, a characteristic chromosomal translocation between chromosomes 1 or 2 and 13 (t[1;13] or t[2;13]) results in the generation of an abnormal fusion protein between the paired box *(PAX)* 7 and forkhead box 1 *(FOXO1)* genes or the *PAX3* and *FOXO1* genes. The remaining 20% of alveolar rhabdomyosarcoma tumors do not harbor a *PAX-FOXO1* translocation and are defined as translocation-negative alveolar rhabdomyosarcoma. These tumors have gene expression profiles similar to that of embryonal rhabdomyosarcoma. Recent studies suggest that the clinical outcome of translocation-negative alveolar rhabdomyosarcoma is more similar to that of embryonal rhabdomyosarcoma than to that of other alveolar tumors.[71-74] In addition to histologic analysis, FISH or RT-PCR sometimes is required to confirm the diagnosis of alveolar rhabdomyosarcoma.

The staging of rhabdomyosarcoma is based on the location and extent of surgical resection at the time of diagnosis. Surgery is recommended first, if it can be completed without significant morbidity. Radiation therapy also is important in treating rhabdomyosarcoma. Patients with microscopic or gross residual disease after surgical resection usually require radiation therapy to achieve optimal local control. All patients with alveolar rhabdomyosarcoma require radiation therapy, regardless of surgical margins, because they have a high risk of local recurrence. Studies have suggested that patients have a better prognosis if radiation therapy is administered relatively early in treatment, and ongoing research is further investigating the optimal timing of radiation therapy.[75]

Tumor location and histology have important prognostic implications; tumors in a favorable site have a better outcome, as do embryonal tumors. Most institutions classify rhabdomyosarcoma as low, intermediate, or high risk so that the duration and intensity of treatment can be tailored to the extent of the disease.[76] Patients with low-risk rhabdomyosarcoma have an excellent prognosis, with a 5-year event-free survival rate approaching 90%. Patients with high-risk rhabdomyosarcoma have a 5-year event-free survival rate of less than 20%.[76]

Chemotherapy is effective in the treatment of rhabdomyosarcoma. Most regimens incorporate the cytotoxic agents vincristine, dactinomycin, cyclophosphamide, and ifosfamide. Ongoing investigations incorporate irinotecan, a topoisomerase I inhibitor shown in phase II studies to be effective for treating rhabdomyosarcoma when administered with vincristine.[77,78] Interval-compressed chemotherapy regimens were found to be safe and effective for patients with high-risk metastatic rhabdomyosarcoma.[79,80] No correlation has been found between the radiographically assessed response to chemotherapy and survival.[81,82] Current protocols are investigating the role of FDG-PET and treatment response.[81,82]

Novel Therapies and Long-Term Complications of Pediatric Sarcoma

Novel agents for treating pediatric sarcomas are being intensively investigated. One of the more exciting new therapies is the use of agents that block the insulinlike growth factor–1 (IGF-1) signaling pathway. Several anti–IGF-1 receptor antibodies have shown preclinical activity against osteosarcoma, Ewing sarcoma, and rhabdomyosarcoma,[83-85] and clinical activity has been found, especially in patients with Ewing sarcoma.[86-88] Studies are under way to determine the optimal use of these agents in combination chemotherapeutic regimens.

Improvements in the treatment of pediatric sarcomas have led to survival for many patients. However, these patients often have complications secondary to treatment. Many patients receive anthracycline-based chemotherapy, which is known to lead to long-term cardiac complications. Pediatric sarcoma survivors were found to have a fourfold increased risk of congestive heart failure, a threefold increased risk of myocardial infarction, a fivefold increased risk of pericardial disease, and a twofold increased risk of valvular abnormalities compared with the general population.[89] Patients with osteosarcoma often receive cisplatin, a well-established ototoxic agent. Although the reported incidence of hearing loss in survivors of osteosarcoma varies widely, patients treated with current protocols have a 30% incidence of hearing loss and a 4% incidence of severe impairment.[90,91] Exposure to an alkylating agent such as cyclophosphamide or ifosfamide and exposure to pelvic radiation contribute significantly to infertility; 71% of men were found to be infertile, and 49% of women had premature menopause.[92] Exposure to radiation and chemotherapy can lead to secondary malignancy. Survivors of Ewing sarcoma, osteosarcoma, and rhabdomyosarcoma have more than four times the risk of secondary neoplasm as the general population. The most common secondary malignancies are nonmelanoma skin cancer and breast cancer.[93]

Annotated References

1. Horner MJ, Ries LAG, Krapcho M, et al, eds: *SEER Cancer Statistics Review, 1975–2006.* Bethesda, MD, National Cancer Institute, 2009.

    This review of cancer statistics includes the incidence of bone malignancies.

2. Hanahan D, Weinberg RA: The hallmarks of cancer. *Cell* 2000;100(1):57-70.

3. Lazar A, Abruzzo LV, Pollock RE, Lee S, Czerniak B: Molecular diagnosis of sarcomas: Chromosomal translocations in sarcomas. *Arch Pathol Lab Med* 2006;130(8):1199-1207.

1: General Topics

Sarcomas are rare, heterogenous tumors that are difficult to classify. In a significant subset of sarcomas, specific chromosomal translocations are known to produce fusion genes with a role in the biology of the sarcoma. This information is helpful in differential diagnosis.

4. Slater O, Shipley J: Clinical relevance of molecular genetics to paediatric sarcomas. *J Clin Pathol* 2007; 60(11):1187-1194.

Specific fusion genes in pediatric bone and soft-tissue sarcomas are reviewed, with discussion of chromosomal translocations and the resultant gene fusion products. The technical application of FISH and RT-PCR is described. The future of clinical application markers and targets for novel therapeutic approaches are reviewed.

5. Bovée JV, Hogendoorn PC: Molecular pathology of sarcomas: Concepts and clinical implications. *Virchows Arch* 2010;456(2):193-199.

Recent advances in molecular genetic studies have had a major impact on identification, classification, and prognosis prediction in many types of sarcomas. Recent discoveries of reciprocal translocations, somatic mutations, and specific amplifications of sarcomas are reviewed. Histochemical staining, immunohistochemistry, and molecular diagnostics of small, round, blue-cell tumors and spindle cell tumors are reviewed and summarized.

6. Slominski A, Wortsman J, Carlson A, Mihm M, Nickoloff B, McClatchey K: Molecular pathology of soft tissue and bone tumors: A review. *Arch Pathol Lab Med* 1999;123(12):1246-1259.

7. Mankin HJ, Trahan CA, Fondren G, Mankin CJ: Nonossifying fibroma, fibrous cortical defect and Jaffe-Campanacci syndrome: A biologic and clinical review. *Chir Organi Mov* 2009;93(1):1-7.

Clinical, radiographic, and pathologic findings are reviewed for nonossifying fibroma, a common pediatric lesion of metaphyseal bone that is solitary, eccentric, and lytic. The lesion may be asymptomatic or present with pathologic fracture. The rarely encountered Jaffe-Campanacci syndrome can be seen in children as with multiple bony sites of nonossifying fibromas.

8. Damron TA, Beauchamp CP, Rougraff BT, Ward WG Sr: Soft-tissue lumps and bumps. *Instr Course Lect* 2004;53:625-637.

9. Enneking WF: The clinical presentation and initial management, in *Musculoskeletal Tumor Surgery*. Edinburgh, Scotland, Churchill Livingstone, 1983.

10. Rosenthal DI, Schiller AL, Mankin HJ: Chondrosarcoma: Correlation of radiological and histological grade. *Radiology* 1984;150(1):21-26.

11. Laffan EE, Ngan BY, Navarro OM: Pediatric soft-tissue tumors and pseudotumors: MR imaging features with pathologic correlation. Part 2: Tumors of fibroblastic/myofibroblastic, so-called fibrohistiocytic, muscular, lymphomatous, neurogenic, hair matrix, and uncertain origin. *Radiographics* 2009;29(4):e36.

The MRI findings of common soft-tissue tumors and pseudotumors in children are reviewed. MRI and pathologic findings are correlated in these tumors. MRI is useful in determining the site of origin, extent of disease, and treatment.

12. Wu JS, Hochman MG: Soft-tissue tumors and tumorlike lesions: A systematic imaging approach. *Radiology* 2009;253(2):297-316.

The radiographic findings of common soft-tissue lesions are characterized. A systematic approach to clinical history, lesion location, radiographic mineralization, and MRI signal intensity is used in the differential diagnosis. If the lesion cannot be characterized as benign, biopsy is required.

13. Panzarella MJ, Naqvi AH, Cohen HE, Damron TA: Predictive value of gadolinium enhancement in differentiating ALT/WD liposarcomas from benign fatty tumors. *Skeletal Radiol* 2005;34(5):272-278.

The predictive value of gadolinium enhancement for differentiating atypical lipomatous tumor from well-differentiated liposarcoma was reviewed in 32 patients. In contrast to biopsy, preoperative gadolinium-enhanced MRI of a homogenous fatty soft-tissue tumor was found to be a sensitive screening tool for determining a possible diagnosis of atypical lipomatous tumor or well-differentiated liposarcoma.

14. Papp DF, Khanna AJ, McCarthy EF, Carrino JA, Farber AJ, Frassica FJ: Magnetic resonance imaging of soft-tissue tumors: Determinate and indeterminate lesions. *J Bone Joint Surg Am* 2007;89(suppl 3):103-115.

Determinate and indeterminate soft-tissue masses are reviewed. Before MRI became available, patient history and physical examination, conventional radiographs, and CT were used in decision making, but biopsy often was required for definitive diagnosis. The characteristic MRI findings are described for a subset of soft-tissue tumors, including hemorrhagic, cysts, vascular malformations, and fatty tumors. MRI findings for these tumors may obviate biopsy or further delineate the surgical approach to biopsy.

15. Aoki J, Endo K, Watanabe H, et al: FDG-PET for evaluating musculoskeletal tumors: A review. *J Orthop Sci* 2003;8(3):435-441.

16. Bischoff M, Bischoff G, Buck A, et al: Integrated FDG-PET-CT: Its role in the assessment of bone and soft tissue tumors. *Arch Orthop Trauma Surg* 2010;130(7):819-827.

A prospective study evaluated the ability of FDG-PET with or without CT to differentiate benign and malignant lesions in 80 patients with a newly diagnosed musculoskeletal tumor. FDG-PET–CT reliably differentiated soft-tissue and bone tumors from benign lesions.

17. Hawkins DS, Conrad EU III, Butrynski JE, Schuetze SM, Eary JF: [F-18]-fluorodeoxy-D-glucose-positron emission tomography response is associated with outcome for extremity osteosarcoma in children and young adults. *Cancer* 2009;115(15):3519-3525.

This retrospective study found that FDG-PET findings are partially correlated with histologic response in extremity osteosarcoma.

18. Bacci G, Fabbri N, Balladelli A, Forni C, Palmerini E, Picci P: Treatment and prognosis for synchronous multifocal osteosarcoma in 42 patients. *J Bone Joint Surg Br* 2006;88(8):1071-1075.

In a retrospective review, 42 patients with synchronous multifocal osteosarcoma underwent two neoadjuvant chemotherapy protocols, followed by excision of primary and secondary tumors when feasible. The prognosis for synchronous multifocal osteosarcoma remains poor despite combined chemotherapy and surgery.

19. Maheshwari AV, Cheng EY: Ewing sarcoma family of tumors. *J Am Acad Orthop Surg* 2010;18(2):94-107.

This review of the Ewing sarcoma family of tumors summarizes presentation, staging, prognosis, and treatment. Improved understanding of the biology of the Ewing sarcoma family of tumors may lead to biologically targeted therapies.

20. Potter BK, Adams SC, Pitcher JD Jr, Temple HT: Local recurrence of disease after unplanned excisions of high-grade soft tissue sarcomas. *Clin Orthop Relat Res* 2008; 466(12):3093-3100.

A retrospective review of 203 consecutive patients with high-grade soft-tissue sarcoma, 64 of whom had undergone unplanned excision of the lesion, found that local recurrence occurred in 6% after planned excision and 34% after unplanned excision. More patients who underwent unplanned excision required flap coverage and/or skin grafting for limb salvage. Unplanned excision of a high-grade soft-tissue sarcoma was found to increase the risk of local recurrence but not disease-specific survival.

21. Wagshal AB, Pires LA, Huang SK: Management of cardiac arrhythmias with radiofrequency catheter ablation. *Arch Intern Med* 1995;155(2):137-147.

22. Cantwell CP, Flavin R, Deane R, et al: Radiofrequency ablation of bone with cooled probes and impedance control energy delivery in a pig model: MR imaging features. *J Vasc Interv Radiol* 2007;18(8):1011-1020.

Twelve pigs underwent multiple RFAs at the mid diaphysis of the long bones to determine coronal marrow ablation length and detect post-RFA cortical thinning. The change in the marrow signal intensity with impedance-controlled RFA was found to be larger than that reported for temperature-controlled protocols. RFA was found to lead to bone weakening.

23. Cantwell CP, Obyrne J, Eustace S: Current trends in treatment of osteoid osteoma with an emphasis on radiofrequency ablation. *Eur Radiol* 2004;14(4):607-617.

24. Pinto CH, Taminiau AH, Vanderschueren GM, Hogendoorn PC, Bloem JL, Obermann WR: Technical considerations in CT-guided radiofrequency thermal ablation of osteoid osteoma: Tricks of the trade. *AJR Am J Roentgenol* 2002;179(6):1633-1642.

25. Venbrux AC, Montague BJ, Murphy KP, et al: Image-guided percutaneous radiofrequency ablation for osteoid osteomas. *J Vasc Interv Radiol* 2003;14(3):375-380.

26. Rosenthal DI, Alexander A, Rosenberg AE, Springfield D: Ablation of osteoid osteomas with a percutaneously placed electrode: A new procedure. *Radiology* 1992; 183(1):29-33.

27. Corby RR, Stacy GS, Peabody TD, Dixon LB: Radiofrequency ablation of solitary eosinophilic granuloma of bone. *AJR Am J Roentgenol* 2008;190(6):1492-1494.

In the first report of RFA treatment for solitary eosinophilic granuloma of bone, the two patients were found to have a prompt clinical response without treatment-related complications.

28. Ruiz Santiago F, Del Mar Castellano García M, Guzmán Álvarez L, Martínez Montes JL, Ruiz García M, Tristán Fernández JM: Percutaneous treatment of bone tumors by radiofrequency thermal ablation. *Eur J Radiol* 2011;77(1):156-163.

The authors reviewed 22 benign and 4 malignant bone tumors after CT-guided RFA. Some patients underwent concurrent treatment with percutaneous cementation. Findings included successful resolution of pain within 1 month and no recurrence in 19 of the 21 benign tumors.

29. Cribb GL, Goude WH, Cool P, Tins B, Cassar-Pullicino VN, Mangham DC: Percutaneous radiofrequency thermocoagulation of osteoid osteomas: Factors affecting therapeutic outcome. *Skeletal Radiol* 2005;34(11):702-706.

Forty-five patients with osteoid osteoma were prospectively evaluated for relief of symptoms and recurrence after treatment with RFA. At a minimum 12-month follow-up after RFA, there were seven local recurrences, all of which were in a nondiaphyseal region.

30. Rybak LD, Rosenthal DI, Wittig JC: Chondroblastoma: Radiofrequency ablation: Alternative to surgical resection in selected cases. *Radiology* 2009;251(2):599-604.

When RFA was used to treat biopsy-proved chondroblastoma, all 17 patients reported relief of symptoms on the first postprocedure day. The patient with the largest lesion required surgical intervention, but all other patients had complete symptom relief, no further need for medication, and a full return to all activities.

31. Erickson JK, Rosenthal DI, Zaleske DJ, Gebhardt MC, Cates JM: Primary treatment of chondroblastoma with percutaneous radio-frequency heat ablation: Report of three cases. *Radiology* 2001;221(2):463-468.

32. Tins B, Cassar-Pullicino V, McCall I, Cool P, Williams D, Mangham D: Radiofrequency ablation of chondroblastoma using a multi-tined expandable electrode system: Initial results. *Eur Radiol* 2006;16(4):804-810.

This preliminary report of chondroblastoma treatment using a multitined expandable radiofrequency electrode system concludes that there is a risk of cartilage damage and mechanical weakening of the bone when RFA is used in weight-bearing joints and lesions near articular cartilage. However, RFA is promising for use in areas not adjacent to cartilage or a weight-bearing joint.

33. Petsas T, Megas P, Papathanassiou Z: Radiofrequency ablation of two femoral head chondroblastomas. *Eur J Radiol* 2007;63(1):63-67.

   The use of RFA for subarticular femoral head chondroblastoma led to healing without periarticular morbidity in two patients.

34. Roach JW, Klatt JW, Faulkner ND: Involvement of the spine in patients with multiple hereditary exostoses. *J Bone Joint Surg Am* 2009;91(8):1942-1948.

   Forty-four patients with multiple hereditary exostoses were evaluated with MRI or CT for spinal column exostosis involvement. Sixty-eight percent were found to have an exostosis arising from the spinal column, and 27% had a lesion encroaching into the spinal canal. The authors concluded that the risk of a patient with multiple hereditary exostoses having a lesion in the spinal canal was much greater than previously reported and suggested screening with advanced imaging at least once during the growing years.

35. Kirchhoff C, Buhmann S, Mussack T, et al: Aggressive scapular chondroblastoma with secondary metastasis: A case report and review of literature. *Eur J Med Res* 2006;11(3):128-134.

   A late-presenting scapular chondroblastoma with metastasis is described, with the differential diagnosis. The current literature on malignant transformation of chondroblastoma is reviewed.

36. Wright JG, Yandow S, Donaldson S, Marley L; Simple Bone Cyst Trial Group: A randomized clinical trial comparing intralesional bone marrow and steroid injections for simple bone cysts. *J Bone Joint Surg Am* 2008;90(4):722-730.

   Ninety patients with a unicameral bone cyst were randomly assigned to treatment with bone marrow or methylprednisolone acetate injection. At 2-year follow-up, the rate of healing was found to be better after methylprednisolone acetate injection but was low in both patient groups (methylprednisolone acetate, 42%; bone marrow, 23%). There was no significant difference between the two patient groups with respect to function, pain, number of injections, additional fractures, or complications

37. Hou HY, Wu K, Wang CT, Chang SM, Lin WH, Yang RS: Treatment of unicameral bone cyst: A comparative study of selected techniques. *J Bone Joint Surg Am* 2010;92(4):855-862.

   Forty patients with a unicameral bone cyst were treated with one of four surgical techniques and were followed clinically and radiographically for at least 18 months. Minimally invasive curettage, ethanol cauterization, disruption of the cyst boundary, insertion of synthetic calcium sulfate bone-graft substitute, and placement of a cannulated screw had the highest radiographically determined healing rate and the shortest time to union.

38. Oliveira AM, Perez-Atayde AR, Inwards CY, et al: USP6 and CDH11 oncogenes identify the neoplastic cell in primary aneurysmal bone cysts and are absent in so-called secondary aneurysmal bone cysts. *Am J Pathol* 2004;165(5):1773-1780.

39. Leong NL, Anderson ME, Gebhardt MC, Snyder BD: Computed tomography-based structural analysis for predicting fracture risk in children with benign skeletal neoplasms: Comparison of specificity with that of plain radiographs. *J Bone Joint Surg Am* 2010;92(9):1827-1833.

   Forty-one patients who had not received surgical treatment of a skeletal lesion were prospectively assessed for risk of fracture using an established CT rigidity analysis. There were no fractures among the patients without a predicted risk of fracture. The authors concluded that quantitative CT-based rigidity analysis is more specific than plain radiographic criteria for predicting risk of pathologic fracture.

40. Snyder BD, Hauser-Kara DA, Hipp JA, Zurakowski D, Hecht AC, Gebhardt MC: Predicting fracture through benign skeletal lesions with quantitative computed tomography. *J Bone Joint Surg Am* 2006;88(1):55-70.

   Using CT-based structural analysis, 18 patients who had a fracture through a benign skeletal lesion were compared with 18 patients who had a benign skeletal lesion that had not fractured over a 2-year period despite radiographic indications of increased fracture risk. The combined ratios of bending and torsional rigidities, as determined by CT, provided a sensitive and specific method of predicting fracture risk in children with a benign neoplasm of the skeleton.

41. DiCaprio MR, Enneking WF: Fibrous dysplasia: Pathophysiology, evaluation, and treatment. *J Bone Joint Surg Am* 2005;87(8):1848-1864.

   This is a comprehensive review of the pathophysiology, clinical presentation, diagnosis, natural history, and treatment of fibrous dysplasia. Treatment options are presented, with a literature review of bisphosphonate therapy specific to fibrous dysplasia.

42. Parekh SG, Donthineni-Rao R, Ricchetti E, Lackman RD: Fibrous dysplasia. *J Am Acad Orthop Surg* 2004;12(5):305-313.

43. Chapurlat RD, Orcel P: Fibrous dysplasia of bone and McCune-Albright syndrome. *Best Pract Res Clin Rheumatol* 2008;22(1):55-69.

   This review of the current treatment of patients with fibrous dysplasia focuses on nonsurgical management, specifically bisphosphonate therapy. Most studies of oral and intravenous agents found favorable results in pain relief, reduction of disability, and improvement of lytic lesions in both children and adults. Adverse effects were minimal, but all of these agents were still under clinical evaluation.

44. Liens D, Delmas PD, Meunier PJ: Long-term effects of intravenous pamidronate in fibrous dysplasia of bone. *Lancet* 1994;343(8903):953-954.

1: General Topics

45. Zacharin M, O'Sullivan M: Intravenous pamidronate treatment of polyostotic fibrous dysplasia associated with the McCune Albright syndrome. *J Pediatr* 2000; 137(3):403-409.

46. Lane JM, Khan SN, O'Connor WJ, et al: Bisphosphonate therapy in fibrous dysplasia. *Clin Orthop Relat Res* 2001;382:6-12.

47. Wang LL, Levy ML, Lewis RA, et al: Clinical manifestations in a cohort of 41 Rothmund-Thomson syndrome patients. *Am J Med Genet* 2001;102(1):11-17.

48. Bielack SS, Kempf-Bielack B, Delling G, et al: Prognostic factors in high-grade osteosarcoma of the extremities or trunk: An analysis of 1,702 patients treated on neoadjuvant cooperative osteosarcoma study group protocols. *J Clin Oncol* 2002;20(3):776-790.

49. Völker T, Denecke T, Steffen I, et al: Positron emission tomography for staging of pediatric sarcoma patients: Results of a prospective multicenter trial. *J Clin Oncol* 2007;25(34):5435-5441.

    A prospective multicenter study compared the use of FDG-PET to that of conventional imaging modalities in patients with Ewing sarcoma, osteosarcoma, or rhabdomyosarcoma. PET was equivalent to conventional imaging modalities for detecting primary tumors but superior for detecting bone and lymph node involvement.

50. Goorin AM, Schwartzentruber DJ, Devidas M, et al: Presurgical chemotherapy compared with immediate surgery and adjuvant chemotherapy for nonmetastatic osteosarcoma: Pediatric Oncology Group Study POG-8651. *J Clin Oncol* 2003;21(8):1574-1580.

51. Fuchs N, Bielack SS, Epler D, et al: Long-term results of the co-operative German-Austrian-Swiss osteosarcoma study group's protocol COSS-86 of intensive multidrug chemotherapy and surgery for osteosarcoma of the limbs. *Ann Oncol* 1998;9(8):893-899.

52. Kager L, Zoubek A, Pötschger U, et al: Primary metastatic osteosarcoma: Presentation and outcome of patients treated on neoadjuvant Cooperative Osteosarcoma Study Group protocols. *J Clin Oncol* 2003; 21(10):2011-2018.

53. Marina N, Bielack S, Whelan J, et al: International collaboration is feasible in trials for rare conditions: The EURAMOS experience. *Cancer Treat Res* 2009;152: 339-353.

    EURAMOS-1 is a fast-accruing clinical study of osteosarcoma designed to determine the effect on outcome of altering postoperative therapy based on histologic response.

54. Le Deley MC, Guinebretière JM, Gentet JC, et al: SFOP OS94: A randomised trial comparing preoperative high-dose methotrexate plus doxorubicin to high-dose methotrexate plus etoposide and ifosfamide in osteosarcoma patients. *Eur J Cancer* 2007;43(4):752-761.

    A randomized multicenter study found that etoposide and ifosfamide were effective in the treatment of extremity osteosarcoma. This study also investigated the role of histologic response at the time of surgery for risk stratification of patients.

55. Lewis IJ, Nooij MA, Whelan J, et al: Improvement in histologic response but not survival in osteosarcoma patients treated with intensified chemotherapy: A randomized phase III trial of the European Osteosarcoma Intergroup. *J Natl Cancer Inst* 2007;99(2):112-128.

    A randomized clinical study compared presurgery chemotherapy regimens of cisplatin and doxorubicin administered every 3 weeks to intensive therapy administered every 2 weeks. Good histologic response was more common in patients who received intensive therapy, but these patients did not have better survival.

56. Whelan J, Patterson D, Perisoglou M, et al: The role of interferons in the treatment of osteosarcoma. *Pediatr Blood Cancer* 2010;54(3):350-354.

    The evidence and rationale for using interferon α-2b in the treatment of osteosarcoma are reviewed.

57. Chou AJ, Kleinerman ES, Krailo MD, et al: Addition of muramyl tripeptide to chemotherapy for patients with newly diagnosed metastatic osteosarcoma: A report from the Children's Oncology Group. *Cancer* 2009; 115(22):5339-5348.

    A randomized phase III study compared three-drug chemotherapy (cisplatin, doxorubicin, and methotrexate) with four-drug chemotherapy (cisplatin, doxorubicin, methotrexate, and ifosfamide) in patients with localized osteosarcoma. No difference in event-free survival was found. The use of muramyl tripeptide phosphatidylethanolamine was evaluated in patients with metastatic osteosarcoma. There was a trend toward improved outcome in these patients, but it was not statistically significant.

58. Meyers PA, Schwartz CL, Krailo MD, et al: Osteosarcoma: The addition of muramyl tripeptide to chemotherapy improves overall survival: A report from the Children's Oncology Group. *J Clin Oncol* 2008;26(4):633-638.

    Patients with localized osteosarcoma who received muramyl tripeptide in conjunction with conventional chemotherapy had a statistically significant improvement in overall survival and a trend toward event-free survival.

59. Ory B, Heymann MF, Kamijo A, Gouin F, Heymann D, Redini F: Zoledronic acid suppresses lung metastases and prolongs overall survival of osteosarcoma-bearing mice. *Cancer* 2005;104(11):2522-2529.

    Preclinical data supports the use of zoledronic acid in the treatment of osteosarcoma.

60. de Alava E, Kawai A, Healey JH, et al: EWS-FLI1 fusion transcript structure is an independent determinant of prognosis in Ewing's sarcoma. *J Clin Oncol* 1998; 16(4):1248-1255.

61. Le Deley MC, Delattre O, Schaefer KL, et al: Impact of EWS-ETS fusion type on disease progression in Ewing's

sarcoma/peripheral primitive neuroectodermal tumor: Prospective results from the cooperative Euro-E.W.I.N.G. 99 trial. *J Clin Oncol* 2010;28(12):1982-1988.

Event-free survival and overall survival were compared in patients with type 1, type 2, and non–type 1 or 2 *EWS-Fli1* and *EWS-ERG* fusions. No difference in event-free or overall survival was found.

62. van Doorninck JA, Ji L, Schaub B, et al: Current treatment protocols have eliminated the prognostic advantage of type 1 fusions in Ewing sarcoma: A report from the Children's Oncology Group. *J Clin Oncol* 2010; 28(12):1989-1994.

The prognostic effect of *EWS-Fli1* fusion type was investigated in patients treated with Children's Oncology Group protocols after 1994. No survival advantage was observed in patients with non–type 1 *EWS-Fli1* fusions, contrary to the findings of earlier studies.

63. Zoubek A, Dockhorn-Dworniczak B, Delattre O, et al: Does expression of different EWS chimeric transcripts define clinically distinct risk groups of Ewing tumor patients? *J Clin Oncol* 1996;14(4):1245-1251.

64. Gupta AA, Pappo A, Saunders N, et al: Clinical outcome of children and adults with localized Ewing sarcoma: Impact of chemotherapy dose and timing of local therapy. *Cancer* 2010;116(13):3189-3194.

Outcomes were compared in adult and pediatric patients with localized Ewing sarcoma. Adults had inferior outcomes that could be related to lower doses of alkylating agents and the timing of local control.

65. Womer RB, West DC, Krailo MD, et al: Randomized comparison of every-two-week v. every-three-week chemotherapy in Ewing sarcoma family tumors (ESFT). *J Clin Oncol (Meeting Abstracts)* 2008:26(15, suppl): 10504.

This abstract describes early results from a Children's Oncology Group study. Patients with localized Ewing sarcoma can tolerate interval-compressed (every-2-week) chemotherapy and have a statistically significant improved event-free survival rate, compared with patients receiving conventional chemotherapy every 3 weeks.

66. Grier HE, Krailo MD, Tarbell NJ, et al: Addition of ifosfamide and etoposide to standard chemotherapy for Ewing's sarcoma and primitive neuroectodermal tumor of bone. *N Engl J Med* 2003;348(8):694-701.

67. Leavey PJ, Mascarenhas L, Marina N, et al: Prognostic factors for patients with Ewing sarcoma (EWS) at first recurrence following multi-modality therapy: A report from the Children's Oncology Group. *Pediatr Blood Cancer* 2008;51(3):334-338.

Patients with recurrent Ewing sarcoma treated in a multi-institutional study had a very poor 5-year event-free survival rate. Negative prognostic factors included time to relapse, combined local and distant recurrence, and an elevated lactate dehydrogenase level at diagnosis.

68. Burdach S, Thiel U, Schöniger M, et al: Total body MRI-governed involved compartment irradiation combined with high-dose chemotherapy and stem cell rescue improves long-term survival in Ewing tumor patients with multiple primary bone metastases. *Bone Marrow Transplant* 2010;45(3):483-489.

Total body MRI-governed involved-compartment irradiation and high-dose chemotherapy are feasible and may result in improved event-free survival in patients with high-risk Ewing sarcoma.

69. Fraser CJ, Weigel BJ, Perentesis JP, et al: Autologous stem cell transplantation for high-risk Ewing's sarcoma and other pediatric solid tumors. *Bone Marrow Transplant* 2006;37(2):175-181.

A retrospective review of 36 patients with a relapsed solid tumor treated with myeloablative chemotherapy followed by autologous stem cell transplantation found that those with Ewing sarcoma had a better overall survival rate than those with other solid tumors. Continued investigation is justified for autologous stem cell transplantation in the treatment of relapsed or metastatic Ewing sarcoma.

70. Ladenstein R, Pötschger U, Le Deley MC, et al: Primary disseminated multifocal Ewing sarcoma: Results of the Euro-EWING 99 trial. *J Clin Oncol* 2010;28(20):3284-3291.

Patients with high-risk metastatic Ewing sarcoma were treated with high-dose chemotherapy followed by autologous stem cell transplant. The risk factors for poor response included large tumor size, bone marrow metastasis, and multiple bone or lung metastases.

71. Davicioni E, Anderson JR, Buckley JD, Meyer WH, Triche TJ: Gene expression profiling for survival prediction in pediatric rhabdomyosarcomas: A report from the children's oncology group. *J Clin Oncol* 2010;28(7): 1240-1246.

A 34-metagene set was found to be predictive of outcome in patients with rhabdomyosarcoma.

72. Davicioni E, Anderson MJ, Finckenstein FG, et al: Molecular classification of rhabdomyosarcoma: Genotypic and phenotypic determinants of diagnosis. A report from the Children's Oncology Group. *Am J Pathol* 2009;174(2):550-564.

This study compared gene expression and loss-of-heterozygosity analyses from 160 patients with rhabdomyosarcoma. Patients with translocation-negative alveolar rhabdomyosarcoma had gene expression profiles indistinguishable from those of patients with embryonal rhabdomyosarcoma.

73. Davicioni E, Finckenstein FG, Shahbazian V, Buckley JD, Triche TJ, Anderson MJ: Identification of a PAX-FKHR gene expression signature that defines molecular classes and determines the prognosis of alveolar rhabdomyosarcomas. *Cancer Res* 2006;66(14):6936-6946.

A specific gene expression signature was identified in patients with *PAX-FKHR*–positive alveolar rhabdomyosarcoma.

74. Williamson D, Missiaglia E, de Reyniès A, et al: Fusion gene-negative alveolar rhabdomyosarcoma is clinically and molecularly indistinguishable from embryonal rhabdomyosarcoma. *J Clin Oncol* 2010;28(13):2151-2158.

Translocation-negative alveolar rhabdomyosarcoma was confirmed to have gene expression patterns similar to those of embryonal rhabdomyosarcoma. Patient outcomes are more similar to those of embryonal rhabdomyosarcoma than alveolar rhabdomyosarcoma.

75. Michalski JM, Meza J, Breneman JC, et al: Influence of radiation therapy parameters on outcome in children treated with radiation therapy for localized parameningeal rhabdomyosarcoma in Intergroup Rhabdomyosarcoma Study Group trials II through IV. *Int J Radiat Oncol Biol Phys* 2004;59(4):1027-1038.

76. Oberlin O, Rey A, Lyden E, et al: Prognostic factors in metastatic rhabdomyosarcomas: Results of a pooled analysis from United States and European cooperative groups. *J Clin Oncol* 2008;26(14):2384-2389.

Patients with metastatic rhabdomyosarcoma have poor event-free and overall survival. Adverse prognostic variables include older age, alveolar histology, location of primary tumor, presence of three or more sites of metastatic disease, and bone marrow involvement.

77. Pappo AS, Lyden E, Breitfeld P, et al: Two consecutive phase II window trials of irinotecan alone or in combination with vincristine for the treatment of metastatic rhabdomyosarcoma: The Children's Oncology Group. *J Clin Oncol* 2007;25(4):362-369.

Patients with rhabdomyosarcoma who received vincristine and irinotecan had a complete or partial response rate of 70%, showing high activity.

78. Vassal G, Couanet D, Stockdale E, et al: Phase II trial of irinotecan in children with relapsed or refractory rhabdomyosarcoma: A joint study of the French Society of Pediatric Oncology and the United Kingdom Children's Cancer Study Group. *J Clin Oncol* 2007;25(4):356-361.

Irinotecan, administered as a single agent in heavily pretreated patients with relapsed rhabdomyosarcoma, was well tolerated and resulted in an objective response in 11% of patients.

79. Arndt CA, Hawkins DS, Meyer WH, Sencer SF, Neglia JP, Anderson JR: Comparison of results of a pilot study of alternating vincristine/doxorubicin/cyclophosphamide and etoposide/ifosfamide with IRS-IV in intermediate risk rhabdomyosarcoma: A report from the Children's Oncology Group. *Pediatr Blood Cancer* 2008;50(1):33-36.

Vincristine, doxorubicin, and cyclophosphamide were alternated with ifosfamide and etoposide for patients with intermediate-risk rhabdomyosarcoma. Patients treated with this regimen had an event-free survival rate similar to that of patients treated with the comparison regimen.

80. Weigel B, Lyden E, Anderson JR, et al: Early results from Children's Oncology Group (COG) ARST0431: Intensive multidrug therapy for patients with metastatic rhabdomyosarcoma (RMS). *ASCO Meeting Abstracts* 2010:28(15, suppl):9503.

The early results of a Children's Oncology Group study of patients with high-risk rhabdomyosarcoma showed an 18-month event-free survival (20% higher than that of earlier studies). Longer term follow-up is required.

81. Burke M, Anderson JR, Kao SC, et al: Assessment of response to induction therapy and its influence on 5-year failure-free survival in group III rhabdomyosarcoma: The Intergroup Rhabdomyosarcoma Study-IV experience: A report from the Soft Tissue Sarcoma Committee of the Children's Oncology Group. *J Clin Oncol* 2007;25(31):4909-4913.

The response rate to induction chemotherapy in patients with group III rhabdomyosarcoma, as measured by radiographic methods, was independent of histology and had no influence on survival.

82. Rodeberg DA, Stoner JA, Hayes-Jordan A, et al: Prognostic significance of tumor response at the end of therapy in group III rhabdomyosarcoma: A report from the Children's Oncology Group. *J Clin Oncol* 2009;27(22):3705-3711.

Patients with rhabdomyosarcoma who had a complete radiographic response did not have a lower risk of recurrence. Second-look surgery to resect residual tumor was not correlated with improved survival.

83. Manara MC, Landuzzi L, Nanni P, et al: Preclinical in vivo study of new insulin-like growth factor-I receptor: Specific inhibitor in Ewing's sarcoma. *Clin Cancer Res* 2007;13(4):1322-1330.

This study describes the preclinical activity of the IGF-1R inhibitor NVP-AEW541 against Ewing sarcoma cell lines.

84. Houghton PJ, Morton CL, Gorlick R, et al: Initial testing of a monoclonal antibody (IMC-A12) against IGF-1R by the Pediatric Preclinical Testing Program. *Pediatr Blood Cancer* 2010;54(7):921-926.

Preclinical studies investigated the role of the anti–IGF-1R antibody IMC-A12 against pediatric tumor cell lines and xenographs. IMC-A12 was active against most pediatric solid tumors and was most active against rhabdomyosarcoma xenographs.

85. Wang Y, Lipari P, Wang X, et al: A fully human insulin-like growth factor-I receptor antibody SCH 717454 (Robatumumab) has antitumor activity as a single agent and in combination with cytotoxics in pediatric tumor xenografts. *Mol Cancer Ther* 2010;9(2):410-418.

SCH 717454, an anti–IGF-1R antibody, was active against neuroblastoma, osteosarcoma, and rhabdomyosarcoma tumor xenographs.

86. Kurzrock R, Patnaik A, Aisner J, et al: A phase I study of weekly R1507, a human monoclonal antibody insulin-like growth factor-I receptor antagonist, in patients with advanced solid tumors. *Clin Cancer Res* 2010;16(8):2458-2465.

A phase I clinical study investigated the toxicity of R1507, an anti–IGF-1R antibody that showed no dose-limiting toxicities and had antitumor activity in patients with Ewing sarcoma.

87. Pappo AS, Patel S, Crowley J, et al: Activity of R1507, a monoclonal antibody to the insulin-like growth factor-1 receptor (IGF1R), in patients (pts) with recurrent or refractory Ewing's sarcoma family of tumors (ESFT): Results of a phase II SARC study. *J Clin Oncol (Meeting Abstracts)* 2010:28(15, suppl):10000.

The role of the anti–IGF-1R antibody R1507 was studied in patients with refractory or recurrent Ewing sarcoma. R1507 was found to be active in approximately 15% of patients with Ewing sarcoma and had a very tolerable adverse effect profile.

88. Tolcher AW, Sarantopoulos J, Patnaik A, et al: Phase I, pharmacokinetic, and pharmacodynamic study of AMG 479, a fully human monoclonal antibody to insulin-like growth factor receptor 1. *J Clin Oncol* 2009;27(34): 5800-5807.

A phase I study was designed to determine the maximum tolerated dose of AMG 479, a monoclonal antibody to IGF-1R. This antibody was well tolerated, with no severe toxicities. Tumor responses were documented in two patients with Ewing sarcoma.

89. Mulrooney DA, Yeazel MW, Kawashima T, et al: Cardiac outcomes in a cohort of adult survivors of childhood and adolescent cancer: Retrospective analysis of the Childhood Cancer Survivor Study cohort. *BMJ* 2009;339:b4606.

Long-term cardiac adverse effects were investigated in patients treated with anthracyclines as part of a childhood cancer chemotherapy regimen. Survivors of childhood and adolescent cancer are at increased risk for cardiovascular disease and require follow-up medical care as adults.

90. Lewis MJ, DuBois SG, Fligor B, Li X, Goorin A, Grier HE: Ototoxicity in children treated for osteosarcoma. *Pediatr Blood Cancer* 2009;52(3):387-391.

This report describes the effect of cisplatin on hearing in patients treated for osteosarcoma.

91. Janeway KA, Grier HE: Sequelae of osteosarcoma medical therapy: A review of rare acute toxicities and late effects. *Lancet Oncol* 2010;11(7):670-678.

This excellent review describes common long-term adverse effects of osteosarcoma therapy, including effects on cardiac, renal, and gonadal function.

92. Mansky P, Arai A, Stratton P, et al: Treatment late effects in long-term survivors of pediatric sarcoma. *Pediatr Blood Cancer* 2007;48(2):192-199.

The long-term adverse effects of cancer therapy in survivors of pediatric sarcoma are described.

93. Friedman DL, Whitton J, Leisenring W, et al: Subsequent neoplasms in 5-year survivors of childhood cancer: The Childhood Cancer Survivor Study. *J Natl Cancer Inst* 2010;102(14):1083-1095.

Patients treated for childhood cancer have a long-term risk of developing a secondary neoplasm.

1: General Topics

Chapter 3
Pediatric Anesthesia

Sean H. Flack, MB ChB, DA, FCA

Introduction

Anesthesiologists and surgeons work together every day to provide safe, high-quality perioperative care to children undergoing an orthopaedic procedure. Complex cardiovascular and respiratory comorbidities are common, and maintenance of a normal airway can be difficult. Profound blood loss, protracted operating times, aspiration risk after trauma, fat embolism, concomitant chemotherapy, positioning challenges because of contractures or deformities, compartment syndrome, altered thermoregulation, and exposure to radiation may be encountered when caring for a child who is undergoing orthopaedic surgery.[1]

The long-held assumption that anesthetic agents do not carry a risk of long-term harm for the child recently has been challenged. Both animal laboratory and human epidemiologic studies have found possible neurotoxic effects on the developing brain. The use of regional anesthesia in children is increasingly common and has been facilitated by the development of portable ultrasonography devices capable of providing high-quality images of nerves and adjacent anatomy.

Children with an orthopaedic condition, including those undergoing scoliosis surgery, range from healthy adolescents to children with severely compromised health, including neuromuscular disease, respiratory failure, and cardiac complications. Consequently, it may be difficult to identify the best anesthetic technique and postoperative analgesic strategy.

Anesthetic Neurotoxicity and the Developing Brain

Inhaled or intravenous general anesthesia is required for most orthopaedic surgical procedures performed in children. Since the first public demonstration of ether anesthesia in 1846, millions of children have safely received anesthesia for procedures ranging from simple supracondylar fracture manipulation to anteroposterior spine reconstruction. Many children with an orthopae-

dic condition receive additional anesthetic exposure during diagnostic and interventional radiologic procedures. An exact understanding of the mechanisms by which various anesthetics act remains surprisingly elusive. It is known that complex interactions with the γ-aminobutyrate, glutamate, glycine, nicotinic, and serotonin neuronal receptors are involved.[2] Calcium, potassium, sodium, and numerous other ion channels also are anesthetic targets.[3]

It has been assumed that the effects of general anesthesia are entirely reversible and devoid of long-term consequences. Upon reversal of the anesthetic, the neurophysiology of the brain and spinal cord is believed to be indistinguishable from its preanesthetic state. There is, however, evidence that anesthesia has negative long-term effects. The adverse effects of halothane were reported 30 years ago.[4] Impaired synaptogenesis, reduced dendritic branching, suppressed axonal growth, and reduced myelination occurred after long-term prenatal and neonatal exposure to halothane in rodents.[4] This study did not cause great concern, however, because it was based on prolonged exposure to the anesthetic.

More recent research has reawakened concern as to the long-term effects of anesthesia. Seven-day-old rats were exposed to nitrous oxide, isoflurane, and midazolam, which are commonly used in pediatric anesthesia.[5] When the histopathologic, electrophysiologic, and behavioral effects were observed, the researchers found widespread apoptotic neurodegeneration in the developing brain, deficits in hippocampal synaptic function, and persistent memory and learning impairments. A study of 10-day-old mice found significant triggering of apoptosis with administration of ketamine and propofol, ketamine and thiopental, or a high dose of propofol alone.[6] Disruption of spontaneous activity and learning subsequently was observed. Diazepam was found to have less effective anxiolytic action if adult mice had neonatal exposure to propofol. Blood gas analyses were normal, and therefore these results could not be attributed to physiologic parameter disturbances such as hypotension, hypoxia, or hypercarbia.

These adverse effects are not species specific. Ketamine was administered as a 24-hour infusion to rhesus monkeys at three points of development (gestational day 122, postnatal day 5, and postnatal day 35).[7] Other rhesus monkeys were exposed to 3 hours of ketamine anesthesia at postnatal day 5. Significant evidence of neuronal cell death was found in the cortices

Neither Dr. Flack nor any immediate family member has received anything of value from or owns stock in a commercial company or institution related directly or indirectly to the subject of this chapter.

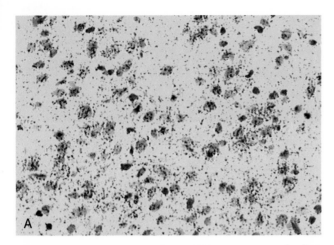

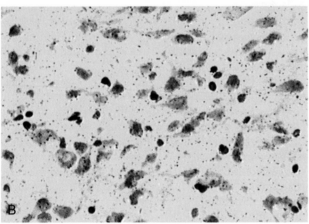

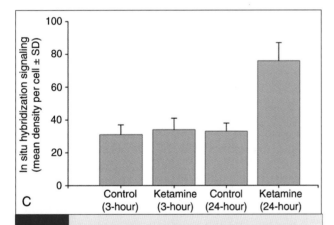

Figure 1 Evidence of increased neuronal death appears as greater autoradiograph grain density in rhesus monkeys exposed to 24-hour ketamine infusion (**A**) compared with control monkeys (**B**). **C**, Quantitative analysis reveals evidence of increased neuronal cell death in monkeys exposed to 24-hour ketamine infusion ($P < 0.05$); monkeys with 3-hour exposure and control monkeys had no significant difference in cell death. (Adapted with permission from Slikker WJ Jr, Zou X, Hotchkiss CE, et al: Ketamine-induced neuronal cell death in the perinatal rhesus monkey. *Toxicol Sci* 2007;98[1]:145-158.)

of the animals exposed to the 24-hour ketamine infusion at gestational day 122 or postnatal day 5. This effect was not found in the animals exposed to the 24-hour ketamine infusion at postnatal day 35 or exposed to 3 hours of ketamine anesthesia at postnatal day 5[7] (Figure 1). A recent review concluded that available data indicate "that anesthetic agents are toxic to the brain and that this injury results in a long-term impairment of cognitive function. Such neurotoxicity has now been demonstrated not only for isoflurane but also for ketamine, midazolam, diazepam, pentobarbital, thiopental, nitrous oxide, and propofol."[8]

These study results have caused consternation among pediatric anesthesiologists and within the US Food and Drug Administration. However, no prospective studies have causally linked surgery under anesthesia in children with clinically relevant impairment in neurodevelopment. It is unknown whether the animal studies can be extrapolated to humans, although two recent studies attempted to answer this question. A birth cohort study of children in Olmsted County, MN, examined whether there was an association between exposure to anesthesia before age 4 years and the development of a learning disability.[9] After exclusions, data related to 5,357 children were included in the final report. Children with a single exposure to anesthesia were not at increased risk, but those exposed two or more times were almost twice as likely to develop a learning disability as those who had never received anesthesia. The increased risk was found even after children with an American Society of Anesthesiologists physical status classification of III or higher were excluded from the analysis.[9] A retrospective birth cohort review of approximately 229,000 children found that children who underwent inguinal hernia repair when they were younger than 2 years were almost twice as likely to be diagnosed with a developmental or behavioral disorder than children in a random sample of 5,000 who had never undergone surgery.[10]

Because of the lack of rigorously conducted prospective, randomized trials, no clinical practice recommendations can be made.[11] The epidemiologic studies emphasize the urgent need for large-scale human studies to examine the effects of anesthesia on the cognitive development of children. The US Food and Drug Administration recently established the Safety of Key Inhaled and Intravenous Drugs in Pediatrics (SAFEKIDS) initiative to provide initial funding for several clinical projects. It is hoped that subsequent clinical investigations will provide data on the safety of anesthesia in children sufficient to guide clinicians' and parents' decision making.

Regional Anesthesia

Regional anesthesia was used in children more than 4,000 years ago to relieve the pain of circumcision. The first study of pediatric regional anesthesia was pub-

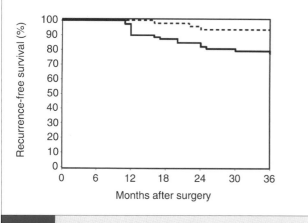

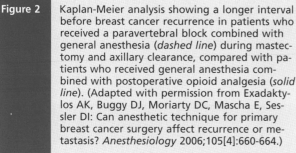

Figure 2 Kaplan-Meier analysis showing a longer interval before breast cancer recurrence in patients who received a paravertebral block combined with general anesthesia (*dashed line*) during mastectomy and axillary clearance, compared with patients who received general anesthesia combined with postoperative opioid analgesia (*solid line*). (Adapted with permission from Exadaktylos AK, Buggy DJ, Moriarty DC, Mascha E, Sessler DI: Can anesthetial technique for primary breast cancer surgery affect recurrence or metastasis? *Anesthesiology* 2006;105[4]:660-664.)

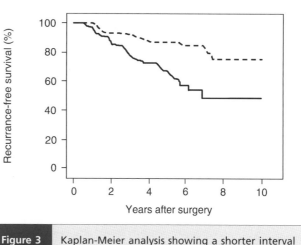

Figure 3 Kaplan-Meier analysis showing a shorter interval before prostate cancer recurrence in patients who received general anesthesia and epidural analgesia (*dashed line*) during radical prostatectomy, compared with patients who received general anesthesia combined with postoperative opioid analgesia (*solid line*). (Adapted with permission from Biki B, Mascha E, Moriarty DC, Fitzpatrick JM, Sessler DI, Buggy DJ: Anesthetic technique for radical prostatectomy surgery affects cancer recurrence: A retrospective analysis. *Anesthesiology* 2008;109[2]:180-187.)

lished by August Bier in 1899, and the urologic use of caudal blocks was reported in the early 1930s. More recent studies debunked the belief that neonates and children do not feel pain. This finding has led to important advances in pediatric pain management, especially in the use of regional anesthesia.[12]

Benefits and Safety

The advantages of regional anesthesia over traditional narcotic-based analgesia regimens include superior pain control and a reduction in the neuroendocrine stress response. In adults, reductions in morbidity and mortality were reported when regional anesthesia was used rather than general anesthesia. Regional anesthesia was found to reduce or eliminate the adverse effects of opioids, including nausea, vomiting, pruritus, sedation, respiratory depression, and urinary retention.[13]

Recent small, level III studies suggested that adults who undergo surgical resection of a malignant tumor have a lower recurrence rate if both general and regional anesthesia are used rather than general anesthesia alone.[14,15] These studies have led to questions concerning the means by which regional anesthesia might alter the host immune response. One proposed mechanism is related to the immune function depression caused by general anesthesia, which is avoided if regional anesthesia is used.[14,15] Similarly, opioids have been reported to inhibit both cellular and humoral immune function;[16,17] strategies that reduce the need for opioids, therefore, may improve immune function. Larger prospective studies are needed (**Figures 2 and 3**).

Regional anesthesia currently is used in as many as 25% of pediatric surgical procedures.[18] The safety of regional anesthesia techniques in children has been confirmed in several single-center and multicenter studies. Most notably, a prospective study in France collected data from 85,412 procedures, of which only general anesthesia was used in 61,003 and anesthesia including a regional block was used in 24,409.[19] A central block, usually a caudal block, was used in 15,013 procedures (more than 60% of the regional anesthetic procedures), and peripheral nerve blocks and local anesthesia techniques represented 38% of the regional blocks. The types of surgical procedures were not recorded. Complications were both rare (0.9 per 1,000 procedures) and minor. There were no complications when peripheral nerve blocks were used; this finding has encouraged pediatric anesthesiologists to substitute peripheral nerve blocks, when appropriate, for neuraxial techniques such as caudal and epidural blocks. The caudal block, formerly the most popular technique, now is used much less frequently than the peripheral nerve block.

The use of continuous postoperative analgesia also has increased. Formerly an epidural block was typically used to deliver continuous postoperative analgesia, but a peripheral nerve catheter now is used much more frequently (**Figure 4**). Families and patients may encounter difficulties during in-home use of a peripheral nerve catheter, including inadequate analgesia, insertion site leakage, local anesthetic toxicity, infection, difficult catheter removal, and injury resulting from a fall or

1: General Topics

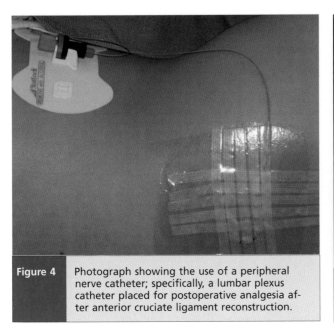

Figure 4   Photograph showing the use of a peripheral nerve catheter; specifically, a lumbar plexus catheter placed for postoperative analgesia after anterior cruciate ligament reconstruction.

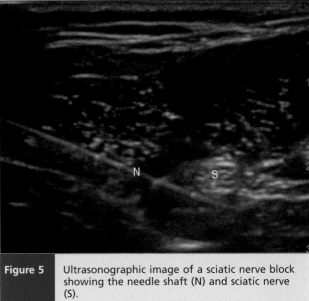

Figure 5   Ultrasonographic image of a sciatic nerve block showing the needle shaft (N) and sciatic nerve (S).

trauma to an insensate limb. A study of 217 children discharged home with a peripheral nerve catheter found a 6.6% rate of neurologic complications.[20] All of these complications resolved spontaneously without residual effects. An appropriate follow-up program must be available to support the patient and to recognize and manage any difficulties. There is increasing interest in the use of peripheral nerve catheters for children undergoing orthopaedic extremity procedures. Recent studies suggested that implementing an at-home program is feasible, despite the significant risk of complications.[21-26] However, appropriate expertise for insertion, patient-family education, and comprehensive follow-up are crucial for the prompt detection and treatment of adverse events.

Regional anesthesia for the lower limb can be achieved using a femoral, sciatic, and/or saphenous nerve block, depending on the required analgesia distribution. Because of the relative frequency of lower limb orthopaedic procedures in children, these are the most commonly used blocks. For an upper limb procedure, supraclavicular, infraclavicular, or axillary approaches to the brachial plexus can be used. The precise indications for and application of these techniques are institution specific.

Ultrasonographic guidance is increasingly popular in pediatric regional anesthesia for the purpose of shortening block performance and onset times and reducing the number of needle punctures (Figures 5 and 6). The use of ultrasonography has been found to hasten the onset of an upper extremity block, prolong analgesia after upper or lower extremity blockade, and lower the anesthetic requirement.[27]

Compartment Syndrome

The most controversial aspect of regional anesthesia in children and adults may be the use of nerve blocks in

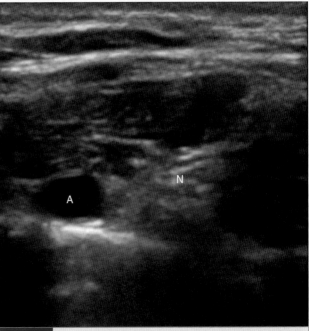

Figure 6   Ultrasonographic image of a supraclavicular block showing the brachial plexus (N) lateral to the subclavian artery (A).

patients who are at risk for compartment syndrome. Both nerve blocks and other analgesic modalities, such as intravenous morphine, have been implicated in delaying the diagnosis of compartment syndrome.[28] Clinical assessment generally is considered the cornerstone for diagnosing compartment syndrome. Pain disproportionate to the injury is the most important early symptom, with increasing pain from passive stretching or palpation of the involved muscles.[29] Diagnosis can be difficult in a child who is crying, nonverbal, or obtunded. An increasing requirement for analgesia may be useful as a diagnostic tool. It is recommended that prophylactic fasciotomies be performed whenever a child undergoes an orthopaedic procedure that carries a significant risk of compartment syndrome. Pressure monitoring remains the most objective and accurate diagnostic test for compartment syndrome, and it has an important role in patients with nerve blocks or other forms of regional or epidural anesthesia.

The concentration of local anesthetic required to block ischemic pain and mask a compartment syndrome is unknown, although a dilute concentration (0.1% to 0.2% ropivacaine) is unlikely to do so. A concentrated local anesthetic should not be used in any procedure for which there is a recognized postsurgical risk of developing a compartment syndrome. An increasing need for rescue analgesia in the presence of a functioning nerve block or epidural block should alert the nursing and clinical staff to the possibility of an evolving compartment syndrome.

Anesthesia and Analgesia for Spine Surgery

An anesthesiologist who is taking care of a child undergoing scoliosis surgery must determine the ideal anesthetic to allow neuromonitoring during surgery as well as the best means of meeting the child's postoperative analgesic requirements. Surgery to correct scoliosis may be complicated by a spinal cord injury and the resulting neurologic deficits. Identifying spinal cord injury under anesthesia is vital; the techniques include intraoperative neurophysiologic monitoring (IOM) using somatosensory and/or motor-evoked potentials, intraoperative wake-up testing, and ankle clonus testing.[30] In most centers, IOM is an integral component of scoliosis surgery. Because the reliability of IOM techniques can be adversely affected by inhalational anesthetic agents or nitrous oxide, a completely intravenous anesthetic technique including propofol is commonly used if IOM is required. Although propofol is efficacious, it can have dosage-related adverse effects including delayed wakening, lipemia, and alteration of platelet function. The intraoperative risk of propofol infusion syndrome is an even greater concern. High doses of propofol, as are commonly required for scoliosis surgery, may impair mitochondrial respiratory chain function, leading to propofol infusion syndrome. The clinical manifestation of propofol infusion syndrome is acute refractory bradycardia leading to asystole, in the presence of metabolic acidosis (base deficit greater than 10 mmol/L), rhabdomyolysis, hyperlipidemia, and/or an enlarged or fatty liver.[31] Consequently, strategies to lower the dose of propofol required are frequently used. The adjunctive agents for this purpose include the short-acting opioid remifentanil; desflurane or another low-dosage volatile anesthetic; and the α-2 adrenergic agonist dexmedetomidine, which provides both sedation and analgesia.[32]

The length of the surgical incision and the extent of tissue trauma required for pediatric scoliosis surgery can be related to severe postoperative pain.[33] A patient-controlled or nurse-controlled intravenous analgesia pump usually is used to administer opioids, supplemented by acetaminophen and nonsteroidal anti-inflammatory drugs as appropriate. Benzodiazepines often are prescribed to treat muscle spasms.

A single dose of neuraxial morphine is effective for postoperative analgesia in some patients. A randomized prospective study found that intrathecal morphine provided better analgesia than patient-controlled analgesia with intravenous morphine alone.[34] When intrathecal morphine was used, pain scores were significantly better at rest but not during coughing. Epidural infusion of either opioids or local anesthetics was found to be highly effective in controlling postoperative pain after spine or abdominal surgery, but there is no consensus on the best use of epidural catheters after scoliosis surgery because of variations in surgical and analgesic technique.[35]

The variables in analgesic technique relate to the types of drugs (opioids and/or local anesthetics), their dosages, and the number of epidural catheters. A continuous infusion of local anesthetics through a single epidural catheter, with or without morphine, was found to provide better analgesia than intravenously administered opioids.[36] The surgeon typically places the catheter in the epidural space under direct visualization through a laminotomy site (a newly created site or an existing site adjacent to a sublaminar hook or wire). The use of a single epidural catheter has had questionable results; improved pain control and early return of bowel function have been accompanied by a high incidence of adverse effects including pruritus, nausea, and vomiting.[33] These adverse effects probably are caused by the addition of opioids to the epidural infusate. A single epidural catheter apparently is insufficient for the entire length of the surgical incision; many patients had significant pain at the upper and lower edges of the incision.[33] These results suggest that the concentration of local anesthetics in the infusate was too low and the concentration of opioids was too high for optimal analgesia.

In a small study of 14 patients, two epidural catheters were placed before surgical wound closure to provide analgesia extending the entire length of the wound.[37] One catheter was inserted at the T6-8 level with the tip directed cephalad to T1-4, and the other was inserted at T12 with the tip positioned at the L1-4 level. A 1-mg/kg dose of hydromorphone was followed by a continuous infusion of 0.1% ropivacaine and 10 mg/mL hydromorphone in each catheter. A satisfactory level of postoperative pain control was achieved; the average median and maximum pain scores during the first 5 days were lower than 2 and lower than 4, respectively (maximum score = 10). However, some patients had episodes of severe pain (scored as high as 6 to 7).

The efficacy of a double epidural catheter was investigated in 23 adolescent patients.[38] The cephalad catheter was positioned at T4-6, and the lower catheter was positioned at T10-L1. After a normal postoperative neurologic examination, an initial 5- or 8-mL bolus of 0.0625% bupivacaine was administered. (The dosage was based on whether the patient weighed more or less than 50 kg.) The bolus was followed by a continuous infusion of 0.0625% bupivacaine with fentanyl (2 mg/mL) and clonidine (3 mg/mL) at 10 mL/h. All patients had complete analgesia at rest. The analgesia remained adequate in 83% of the patients during mobilization and respiratory physiotherapy. Postoperative nausea and vomiting were observed in 17%, but no excessive sedation, pruritus, or respiratory depression was recorded. In a prospective study of 30 patients undergoing posterior correction of scoliosis, the double epidural catheter technique using plain ropivacaine was compared with continuous intravenous administration of morphine for postoperative analgesia.[39] When neurologic status returned to normal on the first postoperative day, patients received either a continuous epidural infusion of 0.3% ropivacaine or a continuous intravenous infusion of morphine at 0.05 mg/kg/h. The results were compelling. In patients who received epidural analgesia, the pain scores at rest were significantly lower at almost all time points during the first 72 hours after surgery; these patients also recovered bowel function more quickly. In patients who received morphine, the pain scores with motion were significantly higher at 24, 48, and 72 hours, and there was a greater incidence of postoperative nausea and vomiting as well as pruritus. The same researchers conducted a similar study of 30 patients undergoing anterior correction of thoracic scoliosis.[40] In one group of patients, two epidural catheters were placed transforaminally at the end of scoliosis correction. Compared with the patients receiving continuous intravenous morphine, those receiving epidural 0.3% ropivacaine had significantly less pain at rest and with motion, required less rescue morphine, had better bowel activity, and were more satisfied with their pain control.

These studies confirm that the use of double epidural catheters can improve pain control. It is preferable to use local anesthetics without opioids to facilitate bowel recovery and decrease the incidence and severity of adverse effects. Further investigation is needed to determine the value of using clonidine or patient-controlled epidural analgesia.

Summary

Pediatric anesthesiologists and orthopaedic surgeons must make quality improvement a cornerstone of their professional work. Delivering safe anesthesia is pivotal to the quality of care, but concerns about neurotoxicity have not been resolved. It is reasonable to delay surgery until the child reaches 6 months of age if the delay does not place the child at additional risk.[41] Anesthesia and analgesia should be provided in accordance with the in-

stitution's best practice guidelines. Regional anesthesia can be used as an alternative to parenteral analgesia. The use of regional anesthesia can facilitate early hospital discharge, particularly with an in-home program using a peripheral nerve catheter. The neurotoxicity of regional anesthesia remains to be determined. Scoliosis surgery continues to challenge anesthesiologists because of the complexities of individual patient physiology, surgical procedures, neuromonitoring requirements, and postoperative analgesic delivery.

Annotated References

1. Wilton N, Anderson B: Orthopedic and spine surgery, in Coté CJ, Lerman J, Todres ID, eds: *A Practice of Anesthesia for Infants and Children.* Philadelphia, PA, Saunders Elsevier, 2009, pp. 633-644.

   Anesthesia for spine and other orthopaedic surgery in children is comprehensively reviewed.

2. Istaphanous GK, Loepke AW: General anesthetics and the developing brain. *Curr Opin Anaesthesiol* 2009; 22(3):368-373.

   This is an excellent review of the current evidence regarding anesthetic neurotoxicity and the developing brain.

3. Campagna JA, Miller KW, Forman SA: Mechanisms of actions of inhaled anesthetics. *N Engl J Med* 2003; 348(21):2110-2124.

4. Uemura E, Bowman RE: Effects of halothane on cerebral synaptic density. *Exp Neurol* 1980;69(1):135-142.

5. Jevtovic-Todorovic V, Hartman RE, Izumi Y, et al: Early exposure to common anesthetic agents causes widespread neurodegeneration in the developing rat brain and persistent learning deficits. *J Neurosci* 2003; 23(3):876-882.

6. Fredriksson A, Pontén E, Gordh T, Eriksson P: Neonatal exposure to a combination of N-methyl-D-aspartate and gamma-aminobutyric acid type A receptor anesthetic agents potentiates apoptotic neurodegeneration and persistent behavioral deficits. *Anesthesiology* 2007; 107(3):427-436.

   Neonatal mice exposed to a variety of commonly used anesthetics had brain cell death as well as functional deficits in adulthood.

7. Slikker WJ Jr, Zou X, Hotchkiss CE, et al: Ketamine-induced neuronal cell death in the perinatal rhesus monkey. *Toxicol Sci* 2007;98(1):145-158.

   Long-term (but not short-term) exposure to ketamine in perinatal monkeys was found to induce neuronal cell death.

8. Patel P, Sun L: Update on neonatal anesthetic neurotoxicity: Insight into molecular mechanisms and relevance to humans. *Anesthesiology* 2009;110(4):703-708.

The molecular mechanisms for anesthetic neurotoxicity in rodents are discussed, with the potential relevance for humans.

9. Wilder RT, Flick RP, Sprung J, et al: Early exposure to anesthesia and learning disabilities in a population-based birth cohort. *Anesthesiology* 2009;110(4):796-804.

    A population-based, retrospective birth cohort study found that anesthetic exposure was a significant risk factor for the later development of a learning disability in children receiving multiple, but not single, anesthetic exposure.

10. Kalkman CJ, Peelen L, Moons KG, et al: Behavior and development in children and age at the time of first anesthetic exposure. *Anesthesiology* 2009;110(4):805-812.

    A retrospective pilot study found an increase in behavioral disturbances in children younger than 2 years who were undergoing urologic surgery, in comparison with children undergoing surgery after age 2 years.

11. Sun LS, Li G, Dimaggio C, et al; Coinvestigators of the Pediatric Anesthesia Neurodevelopment Assessment (PANDA) Research Network: Anesthesia and neurodevelopment in children: Time for an answer? *Anesthesiology* 2008;109(5):757-761.

    An editorial discusses the design of clinical studies of the effect of anesthesia on the developing brain.

12. Suresh S, Ivani G: Regional anesthesia in pediatric patients, in Hadzic A, ed: *Textbook of Regional Anesthesia and Acute Pain Management*. New York, NY, McGraw Hill, 2007, p. 721.

    This chapter was written by international experts in pediatric regional anesthesia.

13. Rodgers A, Walker N, Schug S, et al: Reduction of postoperative mortality and morbidity with epidural or spinal anaesthesia: Results from overview of randomised trials. *BMJ* 2000;321(7275):1493-1496.

14. Exadaktylos AK, Buggy DJ, Moriarty DC, Mascha E, Sessler DI: Can anesthetic technique for primary breast cancer surgery affect recurrence or metastasis? *Anesthesiology* 2006;105(4):660-664.

    This retrospective analysis suggests that paravertebral anesthesia and analgesia for breast cancer surgery reduces the risk of recurrence or metastasis during the first years of follow-up.

15. Biki B, Mascha E, Moriarty DC, Fitzpatrick JM, Sessler DI, Buggy DJ: Anesthetic technique for radical prostatectomy surgery affects cancer recurrence: A retrospective analysis. *Anesthesiology* 2008;109(2):180-187.

    A retrospective review found that substituting epidural analgesia for postoperative opioids was associated with substantially less risk of biochemical cancer recurrence.

16. Sacerdote P, Bianchi M, Gaspani L, et al: The effects of tramadol and morphine on immune responses and pain after surgery in cancer patients. *Anesth Analg* 2000; 90(6):1411-1414.

17. Yeager MP, Colacchio TA, Yu CT, et al: Morphine inhibits spontaneous and cytokine-enhanced natural killer cell cytotoxicity in volunteers. *Anesthesiology* 1995; 83(3):500-508.

18. Rochette A, Dadure C, Raux O, Capdevila X: Changing trends in paediatric regional anaesthetic practice in recent years. *Curr Opin Anaesthesiol* 2009;22(3):374-377.

    Emerging epidemiologic data on regional anesthesia techniques in children are reviewed.

19. Giaufré E, Dalens B, Gombert A: Epidemiology and morbidity of regional anesthesia in children: A one-year prospective survey of the French-Language Society of Pediatric Anesthesiologists. *Anesth Analg* 1996;83(5):904-912.

20. Ganesh A, Rose JB, Wells L, et al: Continuous peripheral nerve blockade for inpatient and outpatient postoperative analgesia in children. *Anesth Analg* 2007;105(5):1234-1242.

    A continuous peripheral nerve blockade program was implemented at a single institution to provide postoperative analgesia after orthopaedic procedures in children.

21. Ludot H, Berger J, Pichenot V, Belouadah M, Madi K, Malinovsky JM: Continuous peripheral nerve block for postoperative pain control at home: A prospective feasibility study in children. *Reg Anesth Pain Med* 2008; 33(1):52-56.

    An observational study demonstrated the feasibility of shortening hospital stays by using at-home continuous peripheral nerve blockade.

22. Khoury CE, Dagher C, Ghanem I, Naccache N, Jawish D, Yazbeck P: Combined regional and general anesthesia for ambulatory peripheral orthopedic surgery in children. *J Pediatr Orthop B* 2009;18(1):37-45.

    A prospective study found low pain scores and good postoperative comfort after ambulatory peripheral pediatric orthopaedic surgery under general anesthesia combined with regional anesthesia.

23. Dadure C, Pirat P, Raux O, et al: Perioperative continuous peripheral nerve blocks with disposable infusion pumps in children: A prospective descriptive study. *Anesth Analg* 2003;97(3):687-690.

24. Dadure C, Motais F, Ricard C, Raux O, Troncin R, Capdevila X: Continuous peripheral nerve blocks at home for treatment of recurrent complex regional pain syndrome I in children. *Anesthesiology* 2005;102(2):387-391.

    Ambulatory continuous peripheral nerve block combined with an initial Bier block provided complete pain relief, early mobilization, and rapid return home in 13 children with recurrent pediatric complex regional pain syndrome I.

25. Dadure C, Bringuier S, Raux O, et al: Continuous peripheral nerve blocks for postoperative analgesia in children: Feasibility and side effects in a cohort study of 339 catheters. *Can J Anaesth* 2009;56(11):843-850.

In a 5-year single-institution review of 339 nerve catheters in 292 children, prolonged analgesia without major adverse effects was achieved in most patients.

26. Capdevila X, Macaire P, Aknin P, Dadure C, Bernard N, Lopez S: Patient-controlled perineural analgesia after ambulatory orthopedic surgery: A comparison of electronic versus elastomeric pumps. *Anesth Analg* 2003; 96(2):414-417.

27. Tsui BC, Pillay JJ: Evidence-based medicine: Assessment of ultrasound imaging for regional anesthesia in infants, children, and adolescents. *Reg Anesth Pain Med* 2010; 35(suppl 2):S47-S54.

    A meta-analysis found some evidence to support the use of ultrasonographic imaging for different outcomes in pediatric regional anesthesia.

28. Lejus C: What does analgesia mask? *Paediatr Anaesth* 2004;14(8):622-624.

29. Bae DS, Kadiyala RK, Waters PM: Acute compartment syndrome in children: Contemporary diagnosis, treatment, and outcome. *J Pediatr Orthop* 2001;21(5):680-688.

30. Tobias JD, Goble TJ, Bates G, Anderson JT, Hoernschemeyer DG: Effects of dexmedetomidine on intraoperative motor and somatosensory evoked potential monitoring during spinal surgery in adolescents. *Paediatr Anaesth* 2008;18(11):1082-1088.

    A retrospective review of prospectively collected data found that dexmedetomidine can be used as a component of total intravenous anesthesia during posterior spinal fusion without affecting neurophysiologic monitoring.

31. Kam PC, Cardone D: Propofol infusion syndrome. *Anaesthesia* 2007;62(7):690-701.

    This review article summarizes the history, mechanisms, pathophysiologic features, and management of propofol infusion syndrome.

32. Ngwenyama NE, Anderson J, Hoernschemeyer DG, Tobias JD: Effects of dexmedetomidine on propofol and remifentanil infusion rates during total intravenous anesthesia for spine surgery in adolescents. *Paediatr Anaesth* 2008;18(12):1190-1195.

    A surgical database review found that concomitant use of dexmedetomidine in patients undergoing spinal fusion reduces propofol infusion requirements, in comparison with patients receiving only propofol and remifentanil.

33. Borgeat A, Blumenthal S: Postoperative pain management following scoliosis surgery. *Curr Opin Anaesthesiol* 2008;21(3):313-316.

    In a review of pain management strategies for scoliosis surgery, double epidural catheters and 0.2% or 0.3% ropivacaine infusions provided very good analgesia, with few adverse effects and no motor block.

34. Gall O, Aubineau JV, Bernière J, Desjeux L, Murat I: Analgesic effect of low-dose intrathecal morphine after spinal fusion in children. *Anesthesiology* 2001;94(3): 447-452.

35. Shaw BA, Watson TC, Merzel DI, Gerardi JA, Birek A: The safety of continuous epidural infusion for postoperative analgesia in pediatric spine surgery. *J Pediatr Orthop* 1996;16(3):374-377.

36. Sucato DJ, Duey-Holtz A, Elerson E, Safavi F: Postoperative analgesia following surgical correction for adolescent idiopathic scoliosis: A comparison of continuous epidural analgesia and patient-controlled analgesia. *Spine (Phila Pa 1976)* 2005;30(2):211-217.

    An 11-year retrospective review found that continuous epidural analgesia provided better postoperative pain control than patient-controlled analgesia.

37. Tobias JD, Gaines RW, Lowry KJ, Kittle D, Bildner C: A dual epidural catheter technique to provide analgesia following posterior spinal fusion for scoliosis in children and adolescents. *Paediatr Anaesth* 2001;11(2):199-203.

38. Ekatodramis G, Min K, Cathrein P, Borgeat A: Use of a double epidural catheter provides effective postoperative analgesia after spine deformity surgery. *Can J Anaesth* 2002;49(2):173-177.

39. Blumenthal S, Min K, Nadig M, Borgeat A: Double epidural catheter with ropivacaine versus intravenous morphine: A comparison for postoperative analgesia after scoliosis correction surgery. *Anesthesiology* 2005; 102(1):175-180.

    A prospective, unblinded study found that double epidural catheters provide better postoperative analgesia, earlier recovery of bowel function, fewer adverse effects, and greater patient satisfaction after scoliosis correction, compared with continuous intravenous morphine.

40. Blumenthal S, Borgeat A, Nadig M, Min K: Postoperative analgesia after anterior correction of thoracic scoliosis: A prospective randomized study comparing continuous double epidural catheter technique with intravenous morphine. *Spine (Phila Pa 1976)* 2006; 31(15):1646-1651.

    A prospective, randomized comparative study found significant advantages to the use of continuous epidural analgesia through two epidural catheters compared with intravenous morphine after anterior correction of thoracic scoliosis.

41. Sanders RD, Davidson A: Anesthetic-induced neurotoxicity of the neonate: Time for clinical guidelines? *Paediatr Anaesth* 2009;19(12):1141-1146.

    Editorials discuss a US Food and Drug Administration suggestion and encourage postponing elective surgery until a child reaches age 6 months.

Section 2

Basic Science

SECTION EDITOR:
HARRY K.W. KIM, MD, MS, FRCSC

Chapter 4

Genetics

Carol A. Wise, PhD   Swarkar Sharma, PhD

Genetics Principles and Laboratory Methods

Genes are DNA sequences that encode RNA and proteins, which are the functional cellular molecules (**Table 1**). The term gene mapping refers to the process of locating or pinpointing the chromosomal or genomic regions harboring specific DNA sequences. Disease gene mapping is the process of identifying the deleterious changes in DNA sequence that cause a specific disease. Three components are required for disease gene mapping: known starting loci (markers) in the human genome, laboratory methods of detecting these markers, and statistical methods for relating the resulting data to disease status in an affected individual. During the past 5 years, there have been dramatic breakthroughs in these three components.

Formerly, the primary means of mapping disease genes was to analyze a sparse set of markers, as found in a large multigenerational family with multiple cases of a particular mendelian disease. Markers for each family member were statistically assessed to identify the markers that were inherited along with the disease more often than expected by chance. Positional cloning methods were then used to isolate and study linked regions until causative genetic mutations were found. The positional cloning method is quite powerful if large multiply affected families are available for study, with only one possible causative mutation per family. More than 2,500 human disease genes have been identified, mostly through positional cloning.[1] However, this approach has little power when applied to a disease caused by many simultaneous mutations in a family (or individual) or when applied to a disease for which no families with multiple affected members are available. This difficulty is present for most common diseases of interest, such as rheumatoid arthritis or hypertension. These so-called complex genetic diseases are thought to be caused by variable combinations of genetic and environmental susceptibility factors. Gene mapping for these diseases requires powerful methods that are effective regardless of family structure.

One approach to genetic mapping of complex diseases relies on the so-called common disease–common variant hypothesis, which states that a common disease may be caused by frequently occurring DNA sequence variations rather than by rare or unique mutations.[2] Naturally occurring DNA sequence changes (variants or polymorphisms) that contribute to the development of disease may be retained in the genome because there is no means of selection against them. That is, either the symptoms of the disease appear after an affected person has procreated, or the ability to produce offspring is not limited by the disease. For example, HLA B27 is a common variant known to be associated with ankylosing spondylitis. Genetic risk factors thus should be identifiable by identifying sequence variants in the genome that occur with different frequencies in affected and unaffected individuals; the genetic changes can thereby be associated with the disease.

The most common DNA variant in the human genome is a change of a single nucleotide, known as a single nucleotide polymorphism (SNP). SNPs were identified and their chromosomal locations were mapped as a part of the Human Genome Sequencing Project.[3] The International Haplotype Mapping (HapMap) Project continued this work by cataloging genetic variation in multiple anonymous individuals of African, Asian, or European ancestry.[4] The HapMap Project also identified haplotypes, which are combinations of variants that are typically inherited together in a genetic segment (a chromosomal region). By 2007, more than 3 million SNPs had been cataloged. Because many SNPs are correlated with one another, only a fraction of these markers must be tested to effectively interrogate most genetic variation in the genome. Genotyping of SNPs has become popular because of the great frequency of SNPs in the genome and the ease of screening for them with high-throughput methods.

Detailed examination of the human genome has revealed another type of DNA polymorphism, called copy number variation (CNV). CNVs are contiguous losses or gains of DNA sequence, ranging from one base pair to entire chromosomes. Extreme CNVs have long been known in the context of disease; examples include trisomy 21 (diagnostic for Down syndrome) and chromosome 15 deletions (diagnostic for Angelman

Dr. Wise or an immediate family member serves as a board member, owner, officer, or committee member of Wise Orthodontics, Stonebridge Orthodontics, and OrthoDent 3D Imaging; and has received research or institutional support from Medtronic Sofamor Danek. Dr. Sharma or an immediate family member has received research or institutional support from Medtronic Sofamor Danek.

Table 1

Common Genetics Terms

Term	Definition and Characteristics
Caspase	A family of intracellular enzymes that specifically cleave peptides at a cysteine amino acid that follows an aspartic acid residue.
Chromosome	A structure consisting of or containing DNA, which carries the genetic information essential to the cell.
Complex genetic disease	A genetic disease caused by multiple genetic variations in a single individual.
Copy number variation (CNV)	Contiguous losses or gains of DNA between individuals at certain places in the genome.
Deoxyribonucleic acid (DNA)	A molecule composed of repeating units of phosphate, sugar, and the nitrogen bases guanine, adenine, thymine, and cytosine. Strands of DNA form a double helical structure. Sequences may form a code transcribed into RNA.
DNA variant	Difference in DNA between individuals at certain places in the genome; common variants are called polymorphisms.
Gene	A heritable physical and functional unit within a genome.
Genetic association	DNA sequence variants that occur with different frequencies in groups of patients with a specific disease, compared with control subjects.
Genetic linkage	Regions of the genome that co-segregate with a particular trait in families.
Genome	The entire DNA of a complete set of chromosomes.
Genotype	The genetic constitution of an individual at a locus.
Haplotype	Combinations of variants that are typically inherited together in a genetic segment. Example: In a given population, two neighboring SNPs with sequence A or G could be more common as a G-G sequence than as a G-A sequence.
Mendelian genetic disease	A genetic disorder caused by a single genetic variation in a single individual.
Positional cloning	Method of identifying the DNA sequences responsible for a trait or disease by mapping in the genome relative to known markers
Ribonucleic acid (RNA)	A molecule made by copying regions of DNA but differing slightly from DNA in chemical structure. Certain RNAs function as templates for decoding into functional proteins. Different RNAs and proteins are produced in different cell types.
Single nucleotide polymorphism (SNP)	Variant consisting of a change of one nucleotide between individuals. SNPs are the most common DNA polymorphism in the human genome.

and Prader-Willi syndromes). It is now clear that more moderate CNVs are common in healthy individuals and may be genetic risk factors for certain diseases.[5,6]

The use of SNP- and CNV-based detection systems is possible because of new laboratory and analysis methods. By 2006, several microchip-based platforms could determine the genotype of as many as 1 million SNPs per sample per microchip, with more than 99% accuracy and efficiency. The cost of determining one genotype has dropped well below $0.01. Cost per genotype is critically important because very large cohorts must be studied to detect true genetic disease associations, for at least two reasons. Several genetic risk factors may contribute to the development of a disease, and large numbers therefore are required to detect a collective signal with statistical significance. In addition, large-scale analysis requires multiple tests that can produce many false-positive results; in a genomewide analysis, very large sample sizes (on the order of 1,000 or more) are typically required to definitively identify true-positive results.

Numerous studies have used SNP- and CNV-based methods. The genetic variations associated with many common diseases have been discovered, including diabetes mellitus types I and II, psoriasis, and Crohn disease.[7] Most such studies must now attempt to discover the actual DNA sequence changes causing the disease and to understand their biologic consequences.

Discovering genetic risk factors ultimately will be a matter of generating and analyzing a complete DNA sequence in an individual human. Although the cost and technologic challenges until recently were insurmountable, they are being addressed by emerging next-generation methods of DNA sequencing. So-called massively parallel sequencing can determine the entire DNA sequence of an individual human within several days.[8]

Most DNA sequencing research is limited by cost considerations, but efforts are under way to achieve whole-genome sequencing for less than $1,000 per sample.[9] Direct DNA sequencing is expected to become the norm within the next 5 to 10 years. Developing appropriate analytic tools for finding disease-causing DNA changes remains challenging, but the process has begun for rare diseases. Proof-of-concept identification of disease-causing mutations in Freeman-Sheldon syndrome recently was achieved by sequencing all protein-coding regions of the genome in only four unrelated affected individuals.[10]

Complex Orthopaedic Diseases

Genetic insights are becoming available for some complex orthopaedic disorders, including the idiopathic forms of talipes equinovarus and scoliosis. Like other complex diseases, these diseases are believed to result from a combination of genetic and environmental changes.

Idiopathic talipes equinovarus (ITEV), known as clubfoot, is a common congenital deformity that occurs in one child per 1,000 live births, generally via complex inheritance. For unknown reasons, the incidence of ITEV is twice as high in boys as in girls. Multiple epidemiologic studies have found that maternal smoking is an environmental risk factor.[11] A study of one multigenerational family in which several members had ITEV found some evidence for the existence of disease genes on chromosomes 3 and 13, but follow-up analyses have not yet confirmed the presence of ITEV-related genes on these chromosomes.[12,13] Several large deleted chromosomal regions have been identified in patients with ITEV; this finding suggests that the absence of genes normally found in the deleted regions may be important in ITEV pathogenesis. In patients with ITEV who do not have the chromosomal deletion, studies of SNPs suggested a role for CASP8, CASP10, and CFLAR, which encode caspases 8, 10, and CASP8 and FADD-like apoptosis regulator, respectively. The encoded proteins of these genes all participate in apoptosis (cell death). It has been hypothesized that variation in the genes involved in apoptosis may contribute to ITEV; some evidence of association was found for SNPs in other apoptosis-related genes.[14] An examination of the relationship between ITEV susceptibility and the genes involved in smoking biometabolism found some suggestion of association with variants in the NAT2 gene.[11] The NAT2 gene encodes an N-acetyltransferase involved in acetylation and, therefore, in the metabolism of arylamines. Further study is needed to determine the importance of this pathway in the development of ITEV.

A disease-causing mutation in the PITX1 gene was identified in a five-generation family having members with a variety of lower limb malformations including clubfoot, bilateral foot preaxial polydactyly, right-sided tibial hemimelia in the proband and clubfoot, pes planus, bilateral hypoplastic patella, and developmental hip dysplasia.[15] No upper extremity anomalies were noted, and clubfoot was the only orthopaedic finding in most of the affected family members. In mice, the PITX1 gene was found to be expressed predominantly in the developing hindlimb, and loss-of-function PITX1 mutations caused predominantly right-sided malformations including reduction in hip structures, femur shortening, and abnormal numbers of digits.[16,17] The findings for both humans and mice illustrate the well-established concept that multigenerational families can provide great power for disease gene identification, and they provide a testable hypothesis that PITX1 may be an important contributor to ITEV in the absence of a family history.

Adolescent-onset idiopathic scoliosis (AIS) is the most common pediatric spine deformity, affecting approximately 3% of children worldwide. Twin studies and observations of familial aggregation reveal that the genetic contribution to AIS is significant. The role of possible environmental factors in disease susceptibility is assumed but still undefined. Autosomal-dominant and X-linked inheritance models were previously believed to account for some occurrences of AIS, but the currently prevailing belief is that a genetically complex model is necessary to explain AIS.[18] Although traditional methods of analysis usually lack sufficient power for studying complex genetic diseases, in AIS they have detected chromosomal regions worthy of further investigation. The results of genomewide scans of 202 families varied depending on the stratification of the data, but the researchers were able to conclude that regions of chromosomes 6, 9, 16, and 17 are of primary interest.[19] A study of targeted regions in members of 53 families led to significant findings related to a large region of chromosome 8q12. Follow-up analysis revealed significant evidence of association with SNPs in the gene encoding the chromodomain-helicase-DNA-binding protein 7 (CHD7).[20] CHD7 currently is the only candidate gene identified for AIS susceptibility. The identified SNPs were associated with a range of disease severity; this factor suggests that in AIS the genetic factors controlling susceptibility and severity are distinct or not entirely overlapping. The CHD7 protein binds to DNA, and its cellular function is beginning to be understood. One study found that the CHD7 protein is likely to control the transcription of other genes in a developmental manner (by controlling the timing or tissue specificity of gene expression).[21]

The question of disease severity (curve progression) is central to treating AIS. The known clinical markers, including bone age and curve magnitude at first appearance of symptoms, are somewhat predictive of progression. The relevance of underlying biologic-genetic factors is assumed.[22,23] A commercially available genetic test claims to predict the likelihood of curve nonprogression (ScoliScore; Axial Biotech, Salt Lake City, UT). Further study is needed to determine the value of this test and its applicability to patients with AIS. Well-characterized patient cohorts and appropriate statistical methods are now available for studying AIS, and new

2: Basic Science

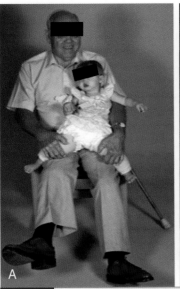
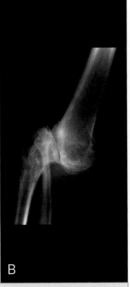

Figure 1 **A,** Photograph of two family members affected by autosomal-dominant Larsen syndrome. Both the man and the child (his grandniece) have the characteristic flattened nasal bridge and prominent forehead. Multiple joint dislocations are a hallmark of the disease; the child is being treated with casts for dislocated hips. **B,** Lateral radiograph showing knee dislocation in the man.

Figure 2 Photograph of a man with MOPD and an unrelated, unaffected woman of approximately the same age.

genetic modifiers of the disease course are likely to be discovered within the next few years.

Genetic discoveries related to complex orthopaedic diseases will have a future clinical impact. The testing of hypotheses suggested by the nature of associated variants and genes is expected to guide new treatment protocols. Whether this information will be useful in predicting disease risk is less certain. An individual's risk of developing a specific complex genetic disease will continue to be difficult to assess until there is a better understanding of the interactions of genes with one another and the environment.

Very Rare Orthopaedic Diseases

The mapping of mendelian single-gene disease mutations by traditional positional cloning is reasonably straightforward. Most of these mutations correspond to a rare disease that has a dominant, recessive, X-linked, or other clear inheritance pattern. It is generally accepted that most such diseases have been discovered, and identifying additional diseases is particularly difficult because of the rarity of live-born patients. However, recently there have been some interesting findings.

The International Skeletal Dysplasia Registry has existed for decades and has accumulated more than 12,000 cases of 50 different diseases.[24] During the past 5 years, data in the registry have led to multiple rare gene discoveries, including the linking of five registry

diseases through the same causative gene. The *FLNB* gene, encoding the filamin B protein, is a large cytoskeletal protein with a distinct actin-binding homology domain followed by 24 repeating domains. Filamin B apparently is expressed in all tissues, including chondrocytes within vertebral growth plates. Rare diseases caused by *FLNB* mutations include Larsen syndrome (**Figure 1**), perinatal lethal atelosteogenesis types I and III, spondylocarpotarsal syndrome, and perinatal lethal boomerang dysplasia. *FLNB* mutational analysis does not explain differences in clinical appearance or phenotype. At least once, the same mutation separately caused atelosteogenesis types I and III. It is anticipated that further study of filamin B and its biochemical pathways will increase the basic understanding of bone-chondrocyte biology.[25,26]

New discoveries recently were reported for certain forms of primordial dwarfism. Patients with primordial dwarfism have a pattern of extremely short stature with proportional bones and organs, beginning before birth. This skeletal condition may be characterized by microcephaly, bony dysplasia, and limb shortening. The body size of affected children is approximately 8 standard deviations below normal. Patients with Seckel syndrome or one of the three types of Majewski osteodysplastic primordial dwarfism (MOPD) have especially small stature[27] (**Figure 2**). Primordial dwarfism is rare; for example, recessively inherited MOPD type II is estimated to affect 40 to 50 individuals in the United States. Two separate studies mapped both Seckel syn-

2: Basic Science

drome and MOPD type II to the *PCNT2* gene, which is located on chromosome 21 and encodes a protein called pericentrin.[28,29] Like filamin B, pericentrin appears to be expressed in all tissues, but clearly it has profound effects on skeletal growth. Within individual cells, pericentrin localizes to complexes known as centrosomes, which organize and coordinate DNA replication and cell division during mitosis. The cells of people with Seckel syndrome or MOPD type II lack pericentrin, and mitotic deficiencies can be seen in vitro. These observations have led to the hypothesis that mitotically deficient cells are lost in these patients during fetal development and childhood; the results are an overall reduced cellularity and small body size.

The discovery of mutations related to very rare mendelian diseases underscores the recurring observation that one mutation can lead to different phenotypes. Very little is understood about the biologic relationship between mutation (genotype) and phenotype. The clinical implications of these studies include the ability to provide molecular diagnosis and genetic counseling. Genetic counseling is important to inform patients of the spectrum of possible clinical features in the presence of a given mutation, particularly as related to sporadically occurring disease or a disease that can be subtle or severe (for example, Larsen syndrome). Carrier testing may also be warranted for disorders that have recessive inheritance or otherwise reduced penetrance. Genetic mutations related to disease severity are less well understood, and further work is needed in this area. The discovery of mutations related to very rare diseases may improve understanding of the disease process and lead to treatments based on the molecular pathways affected by the mutation. It remains to be determined whether clinical diagnosis eventually will be superseded by molecular diagnosis.

Summary

The genetic causes of human diseases are rapidly being discovered as the result of remarkable advances in technology and statistical methodologies, leading to a fundamental understanding of the human genome. Most notable are the advances in understanding complex diseases such as AIS and ITEV, which probably are caused by several genetic and environmental factors. Several biologic pathways important in these diseases are likely to be discovered within the next 5 years, and this knowledge will inform new treatments. Breakthroughs also are occurring in studies of very rare skeletal diseases such as MOPD type II, in part because new technologies allow researchers to discover rare causative mutations by analysis involving relatively few patients. The discovery of rare disease mutations is important for genetic counseling in families and insight into disease mechanisms.

Annotated References

1. Altshuler D, Daly MJ, Lander ES: Genetic mapping in human disease. *Science* 2008;322(5903):881-888.

   The scientific principles underlying disease gene mapping are outlined, with historical perspective, current progress, and online sources of continually updated information.

2. Collins FS, Guyer MS, Charkravarti A: Variations on a theme: Cataloging human DNA sequence variation. *Science* 1997;278(5343):1580-1581.

3. Collins FS, Patrinos A, Jordan E, Chakravarti A, Gesteland R, Walters L: New goals for the U.S. Human Genome Project: 1998-2003. *Science* 1998;282(5389): 682-689.

4. Frazer KA, Ballinger DG, Cox DR, et al: A second generation human haplotype map of over 3.1 million SNPs. *Nature* 2007;449(7164):851-861.

   The second phase of the HapMap project characterized more than 3 million SNPs in 270 individuals of four major ethnic groups. The correlation between SNPs is included, as well as the effectiveness of commercially available genotyping systems for coverage of the entire human genome.

5. Kidd JM, Cooper GM, Donahue WF, et al: Mapping and sequencing of structural variation from eight human genomes. *Nature* 2008;453(7191):56-64.

   This study analyzed DNA duplications, deletions, and inversions of intermediate size (thousands to millions of base pairs) in the chromosomes of eight normal individuals of diverse ethnicity (four Yoruban Africans and four non-Africans). Approximately half of the structural variations were common to at least two individuals. Numerous structural variations found across all chromosomes of all humans form the basis of studies to relate them to traits such as disease.

6. Lupski JR: Schizophrenia: Incriminating genomic evidence. *Nature* 2008;455(7210):178-179.

   Two genetic studies of schizophrenia were significant because they found that CNVs in the human genome contribute to a relatively common and previously intractable disease.

7. Hindorff LA, Mehta JP, Manolio TA: A catalog of published genome-wide association studies. http//: www.genome.gov/gwastudies. Accessed Sept 18, 2009.

   This list of published genomewide association studies includes the studied disease, study population, implicated genes and SNPs, and most significant findings.

8. Mardis ER: Next-generation DNA sequencing methods. *Annu Rev Genomics Hum Genet* 2008;9:387-402.

   The intellectual basis and molecular mechanisms of three so-called next-generation sequencing methods are described, with their benefits and limitations. These methods can be applied to previously intractable research difficulties.

2: Basic Science

9. 1000 Genomes Project: 1000 genomes: A deep catalog of human genetic variation. http://www.1000genomes.org. Accessed Nov 17, 2009.

The 1000 Genomes Project Website provides a browser tool and data downloads that allow researchers to directly compare their sequencing and genotyping data to similar data. The project is expected to enhance disease mutation discovery.

10. Ng SB, Turner EH, Robertson PD, et al: Targeted capture and massively parallel sequencing of 12 human exomes. *Nature* 2009;461(7261):272-276.

Methods were developed for rapid, highly efficient DNA sequencing of all protein-coding regions of the human genome. Using bioinformatics, DNA from four unrelated individuals with Freeman-Sheldon syndrome was sequenced and compared. The discovery of a single mutation in the four people established that certain mutations can be discovered by comprehensive analysis of unrelated patients, without the need to include other family members.

11. Hecht JT, Ester A, Scott A, et al: NAT2 variation and idiopathic talipes equinovarus (clubfoot). *Am J Med Genet A* 2007;143A(19):2285-2291.

Maternal smoking is a risk factor for idiopathic clubfoot. The hypothesis that genes involved in tobacco metabolism are altered in individuals with ITEV was tested by analyzing DNA polymorphisms that create amino acid changes in two proteins involved in tobacco biometabolism. The results provided some evidence for an association with ITEV.

12. Dietz FR, Cole WG, Tosi LL, et al: A search for the gene(s) predisposing to idiopathic clubfoot. *Clin Genet* 2005;67(4):361-362.

A four-generation family with ITEV was studied by linkage analysis with testing of 77 polymorphic DNA markers. Two regions on chromosomes 3 and 13 were found to be most likely to harbor an ITEV gene, although neither identification had statistical significance.

13. Shyy W, Dietz F, Dobbs MB, Sheffield VC, Morcuende JA: Evaluation of CAND2 and WNT7a as candidate genes for congenital idiopathic clubfoot. *Clin Orthop Relat Res* 2009;467(5):1201-1205.

No disease-causing mutations were found in two candidate genes for ITEV implicated by an earlier study.[12] These genes were excluded as likely candidates for ITEV in the studied families.

14. Ester AR, Tyerman G, Wise CA, Blanton SH, Hecht JT: Apoptotic gene analysis in idiopathic talipes equinovarus (clubfoot). *Clin Orthop Relat Res* 2007;462:32-37.

The investigators earlier observed a chromosome 2q31-33 deletion in a patient with ITEV as well as evidence of linkage with association to *CASP10*, a gene in the region in other patients. In this study, seven other genes involved in apoptotic (cell death) functions also were investigated. Some evidence of association with ITEV was found, suggesting that apoptotic pathways may be involved in the development of ITEV.

15. Gurnett CA, Alaee F, Kruse LM, et al: Asymmetric lower-limb malformations in individuals with homeobox PITX1 gene mutation. *Am J Hum Genet* 2008;83(5):616-622.

Predominant right-sided clubfoot, accompanied by other lower limb malformations, was mapped to a mutation in the *PITX1* gene in a five-generation family. *PITX1* alters limb development in animal models. Results suggest that *PITX1* may be important in the development of ITEV.

16. Szeto DP, Rodriguez-Esteban C, Ryan AK, et al: Role of the Bicoid-related homeodomain factor Pitx1 in specifying hindlimb morphogenesis and pituitary development. *Genes Dev* 1999;13(4):484-494.

17. Lanctôt C, Moreau A, Chamberland M, Tremblay ML, Drouin J: Hindlimb patterning and mandible development require the Ptx1 gene. *Development* 1999;126(9):1805-1810.

18. Wise CA, Gao X, Shoemaker S, Gordon D, Herring JA: Understanding genetic factors in idiopathic scoliosis, a complex disease of childhood. *Curr Genomics* 2008;9(1):51-59.

The current understanding of the genetics of idiopathic scoliosis is summarized. Genetic contributions are quantified relative to other complex diseases such as rheumatoid arthritis, and methods for discovering idiopathic scoliosis disease genes are outlined.

19. Miller NH, Justice CM, Marosy B, et al: Identification of candidate regions for familial idiopathic scoliosis. *Spine (Phila Pa 1976)* 2005;30(10):1181-1187.

Linkages were tested for 202 families affected by idiopathic scoliosis. The results were compared with linkage results after stratification by scoliosis curve severity. Several identified regions of the genome may harbor genetic variants contributing to idiopathic scoliosis.

20. Gao X, Gordon D, Zhang D, et al: CHD7 gene polymorphisms are associated with susceptibility to idiopathic scoliosis. *Am J Hum Genet* 2007;80(5):957-965.

Linkage analysis in a three-generation family with multiple cases of idiopathic scoliosis identified three candidate chromosomal regions. Follow-up linkage studies of the chromosome 8 region produced positive results in an additional 52 families. The *CHD7* gene encoded in this region was significantly associated with idiopathic scoliosis in these families, suggesting a pathogenic role in the disease.

21. Schnetz MP, Bartels CF, Shastri K, et al: Genomic distribution of CHD7 on chromatin tracks H3K4 methylation patterns. *Genome Res* 2009;19(4):590-601.

The *CHD7* gene encodes a protein that was predicted to bind to chromosomes and thereby alter the behavior of nearby genes. This study is the first to conclusively show that *CHD7* binds chromosomes and delineates specific regions of binding in different cell types.

22. Lonstein JE, Carlson JM: The prediction of curve progression in untreated idiopathic scoliosis during growth. *J Bone Joint Surg Am* 1984;66(7):1061-1071.

23. Peterson LE, Nachemson AL: Prediction of progression of the curve in girls who have adolescent idiopathic scoliosis of moderate severity: Logistic regression analysis based on data from The Brace Study of the Scoliosis Research Society. *J Bone Joint Surg Am* 1995;77(6): 823-827.

24. Biesecker LG: Phenotype matters. *Nat Genet* 2004; 36(4): 323-324.

25. Zhang D, Herring JA, Swaney SS, et al: Mutations responsible for Larsen syndrome cluster in the FLNB protein. *J Med Genet* 2006;43(5):e24.

    FLNB mutations were discovered in patients and families with a diagnosis of Larsen syndrome or ITEV. This finding highlighted the need for molecular diagnosis by *FLNB* mutation screening to diagnosis Larsen syndrome and provide appropriate genetic counseling.

26. Winer N, Kyndt F, Paumier A, et al: Prenatal diagnosis of Larsen syndrome caused by a mutation in the filamin B gene. *Prenat Diagn* 2009;29(2):172-174.

    Larsen syndrome was suspected after abnormalities were detected on fetal ultrasonic screening at weeks 22 through 31 of gestation. Physical examination at birth confirmed the findings. *FLNB* screening revealed a de novo mutation previously associated with Larsen syndrome. Mutation screening is crucial for confirming the diagnosis of Larsen syndrome and for appropriate genetic counseling.

27. Hall JG, Flora C, Scott CI Jr, Pauli RM, Tanaka KI: Majewski osteodysplastic primordial dwarfism type II (MOPD II): Natural history and clinical findings. *Am J Med Genet A* 2004;130A(1):55-72.

28. Griffith E, Walker S, Martin CA, et al: Mutations in pericentrin cause Seckel syndrome with defective ATR-dependent DNA damage signaling. *Nat Genet* 2008; 40(2):232-236.

    Linkage analysis of two consanguineous families revealed a locus for Seckel syndrome on human chromosome 21. The *PCNT2* gene in this region was known to encode a centrosomal protein, and other such proteins are involved in related conditions of primary microcephaly. *PCNT2* mutations were discovered in these families and other individuals with Seckel syndrome. Cells from these patients also were found to be defective in responding to DNA damage.

29. Rauch A, Thiel CT, Schindler D, et al: Mutations in the pericentrin (PCNT) gene cause primordial dwarfism. *Science* 2008;319(5864):816-819.

    Linkage analysis of three consanguineous families revealed a locus for MOPD type II on human chromosome 21. Mutations were identified in the *PCNT2* gene encoded in this region. Abnormal mitotic morphology was observed in cells from patients with MOPD type II, consistent with defects in *PCNT*-mediated cell division. The authors hypothesize that ancient *Homo floresiensis* hominids from the island of Flores, Indonesia, may have had MOPD type II.

2: Basic Science

Chapter 5

Stem Cells in Pediatric Orthopaedics

Benjamin A. Alman, MD

Introduction

Stem cells are undifferentiated cells that are capable of self-renewal and differentiation. These cells have the potential to aid in the regeneration of musculoskeletal tissues and in the treatment of a number of conditions managed by orthopaedic surgeons. Much remains to be learned about the optimal and safe use of stem cells in patients, however. Widespread clinical use of stem cells should be reserved until their efficacy and safety are well supported by additional clinical evidence.

Stem Cells

A stem cell is an undifferentiated cell that is capable of dividing into an undifferentiated and a differentiated daughter cell. The undifferentiated daughter cell is capable of dividing to produce a differentiated cell of another type. This capacity to produce a daughter cell whose own daughter cells can differentiate to different pathways while retaining the ability to self-renew is a cardinal feature of stem cells. A pluripotent stem cell can differentiate into any of the body's cell types, but a multipotent stem cell can become only certain types of cells (**Figure 1**). Some other types of cells also can differentiate into other cell types, but these precursor cells lack the ability to self-renew.[1-3]

Embryonic Stem Cells

Embryonic stem cells are pluripotent. They have the ability to differentiate into all derivatives of the three primary germ layers (the ectoderm, endoderm, and mesoderm). Embryonic stem cells are derived from the inner cell mass of the blastocyst, which is an early-stage embryo; human embryos reach the blastocyst stage 4 to 5 days after fertilization, when they consist of 50 to 150 cells. The ability of embryonic stem cells to self-renew means that they can be maintained as stem cells in long-term cell cultures. Their ability to differentiate into all cell types means that they can be used to repair or replace tissue damaged by injury or disease. The use of stem cells for these purposes is called regenerative

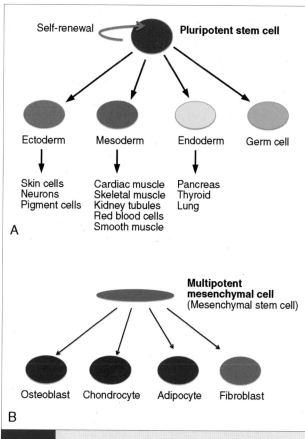

Figure 1 **A**, Pluripotent stem cells can divide by differentiation down one of the three main cell lineages (mesoderm, ectoderm, endoderm), differentiation into germ cells, and self-renewal (in which one daughter cell remains a stem cell). **B**, Mesenchymal stem cells are multipotent; they can become multiple cell types but cannot become cells from all three main cell lineages. An ability to self-renew has not been established.

Dr. Alman or an immediate family member serves as a board member, owner, officer, or committee member of the American Orthopaedic Association, the Scoliosis Research Society, and the Shriners Hospitals for Children; and has received research or institutional support from Amgen, AO, Biomet, and the Canadian Institutes of Health Research.

2: Basic Science

medicine, and it has been shown to have great potential. Studies in mice have suggested several potential uses for stem cells, including motor function improvement after spinal cord injury.[4] However, the use of human embryonic stem cells has been controversial in some countries because of their derivation from human blastocysts.[4-6]

Induced Pluripotent Stem Cells

The recent finding that mature cells can be induced to behave like embryonic stem cells caused a paradigm shift in the understanding of cell differentiation.[7-9] Previously it was believed that a differentiated cell could never become pluripotent. Induced pluripotent stem cells typically are derived by inserting stem cell–associated genes into nonpluripotent cells using a virus vector. This transfection technique was initially described in adult fibroblasts, using viral vectors expressing the stem cell–associated genes *Oct-3/4*, *SOX2*, *c-Myc*, and *Klf4*. Since the initial process was described, researchers have derived induced pluripotent stem cells from a variety of mature cell types, using several transfection protocols. These induced pluripotent cells behave much like embryonic stem cells, with the ability to differentiate into all cell types. Induced pluripotent cells from mice have even been used to generate an entirely new mouse, in a manner similar to the use of embryonic stem cells.[7-9] The discovery of induced pluripotent stem cells raises the possibility that all cells have the capacity to dedifferentiate. Dedifferentiation may be important in repairing wounds and fractures, and it may have a role in the initiation of neoplasia.[7-9]

Mesenchymal Stem Cells

Muscle, bone, cartilage, fat, and fibrous tissue are derived from the mesoderm. A long-standing hypothesis suggests that cells of these types are maintained by a population of mesenchymal stem cells. Mesenchymal stem cells are multipotent; they are tissue specific and able to produce only a limited number of cell types. Multipotent cells exist in mature organisms, in contrast to embryonic stem cells. Also in contrast to embryonic stem cells, multipotent cells have not been definitively found to self-renew. As a result, there is controversy as to whether multipotent cells are true stem cells.

The existence of mesenchymal stem cells has been hypothetical, and identification of a true mesenchymal stem cell, as opposed to a precursor cell, has proved elusive. Only recently, a cell type identified in vitro was found to behave like a mesenchymal stem cell derived from pericytes on blood vessels; its daughter cells retain the ability to form multiple lineages and are self-renewing. Mesenchymal stem cells have yet to be found in vivo. The possible reasons include the different behavior of cells in vivo and in vitro as well as the absence of markers for mesenchymal stem cells. In contrast, other tissue-specific stem cells, such as those in the colon, have been identified based on cell-surface markers.[10]

The Stem Cell Niche

Self-renewal and differentiation are regulated both by the stem cells themselves and by their environment. The environmental effect may be specific to a stem cell's location and immediately surrounding area, which are called its niche. The effect of the niche is well known in the hematopoietic system, where the niche is maintained by cancellous bone and osteoblasts, and hematopoiesis can be regulated by modulating bone density.[11]

The Therapeutic Potential of Stem Cells

Stem cells are believed to be responsible for maintaining mature tissues. The cellular cascade involved in this process has been well characterized for the hematopoietic system, endothelium, and some specialized tissues, such as the hair follicle, but not for the musculoskeletal tissues. Stem cells maintain these tissues by providing daughter cells to replace the differentiated cells that have died from injury or senescence. This process is most easily seen in the hematopoietic system, where stem cells produce new blood cells; without this process, fatal anemia and thrombocytopenia would rapidly develop.

Replacing Damaged Cells

The ability of stem cells to maintain mature organs means that it may become possible to harness stem cells to repair or replace damaged organs. This concept has been researched in the central nervous system, the endocrine system, the heart, the muscles, and the bones and joints. The strategies include harvesting stem cells from the patient and placing them at the site of injury, using stem cells from another person to repair a patient's damaged organ, or removing stem cells from the patient or another person and placing them in an artificial extracellular environment to engineer a new organ. The last approach is a type of tissue engineering.[12,13]

Improving Innate Repair Processes

Orthopaedic surgeons activate innate stem cells during every surgical procedure, as stem cells are responsible for healing most of the tissues affected by the surgery. The repair process can be improved by increasing the number of participating cells or increasing the speed of repair. Improving the stem cell niche could achieve this goal; for example, the hematopoietic stem cell niche can be improved by increasing the patient's bone density, leading to better hematopoiesis activation. Pharmacologic agents can be used to activate stem cell differentiation; for example, erythropoietin can be used to increase the number of red blood cells. The mechanisms by which bone morphogenetic protein repairs a fracture may include activation of mesenchymal stem cells using pharmacologic agents.

The discovery of induced pluripotent stem cells raises the possibility that mature cells are induced to act like stem cells by locally released factors during normal repair processes. This theory may provide important insight into the normal repair process, and it has important implications for stem cell generation for therapeutic use. By learning more about the process by which mature cells behave like precursor cells, researchers probably will be able to develop improvements to the normal healing process.[14]

Stem cells may produce factors that improve the healing of other innate cells. Mesenchymal stem cells transplanted into a damaged heart were found to help activate the innate repair cells and thereby improve cardiac function, without any of the stem cells becoming cardiomyocytes.[15,16]

Modulating Immune Functions

Mesenchymal stem cells have an intriguing ability to modulate normal immune functions, although the underlying cellular mechanism is not understood. This property is one reason that mesenchymal stem cells can be transplanted from one person into another without immunosuppression, and it has led to the use of mesenchymal stem cells in treating autoimmune diseases. The earliest clinical studies of stem cell use were undertaken for treating such disorders.[17,18]

The Pitfalls of Stem Cell Use

Stem cells have strong potential for use in regenerative medicine, but their ability to differentiate into many cell types also creates pitfalls. The molecular and cellular pathways controlling the differentiation of stem cells have not been completely elucidated. Stem cell differentiation into cells of an undesired type usually leads to treatment failure;[19] for example, if stem cells differentiate into fibroblasts instead of osteoblasts in bone repair, the outcome will be poor. Stem cells have the potential to differentiate into neoplastic cells,[20] with a detrimental effect. Several studies found that some mesenchymal stem cells maintained in long-term culture undergo sarcomatous transformation. The risk appears to be greater if the stem cells were derived from donor cells expanded in culture ex vivo.[21,22] The risks and benefits of stem cell therapy must be balanced. The use of so-called off-the-shelf donor-derived cells probably should be reserved for life-threatening conditions or research investigations. Informed consent is essential before the clinical use of stem cell therapy.

Cancer Stem Cells

Tumors, like mature tissues, may be maintained by a subpopulation of stem cells. This theory first was confirmed in malignancies of the hematopoietic system and later in breast cancer, brain tumors, and sarcomas.[23,24] Cancer stem cells were first identified by their ability to initiate tumor formation in immunodeficient mice.[23,24] Like other stem cells, cancer stem cells are defined by their capacity to self-renew and produce a heterogeneous lineage. Only a few cancer stem cells are required to maintain, expand, and disseminate the tumor. This property may explain why tumors often persist or recur after treatment; only a few remaining cancer stem cells can cause disease recurrence. Like most other types of cells, differentiated cancer cells have a limited life span. However, cancer stem cells have an unlimited life span. Targeting cancer stem cells is a novel, exciting concept. This approach to eliminating tumors and preventing recurrence is an area of intense research, and the initial results are extremely promising.[23,24]

Sources of Mesenchymal Stem Cells

In pediatric patients, mesenchymal stem cells frequently are used for bone grafting or bone marrow injection. Mesenchymal stem cells can be derived from several endogenous sources, although not all of these sources have the same multipotent properties. The bone marrow, in which mesenchymal stem cells exist as stromal cells, is commonly used as an enriched source of therapeutic cells. Each 2 mL of bone marrow aspirate contains approximately 2,000 mesenchymal stem cells.[25] There are fewer mesenchymal stem cells in bone marrow aspirates from older people, however, and their stem cells do not differentiate as efficiently.[26] The pericyte cells that line the blood vessels are another source of mesenchymal stem cells. These cells can be derived from adipose tissue in adults or from umbilical cords,[27-30] and umbilical cord tissue is being developed as a commercial source of stem cells.[31] Because mesenchymal stem cells do not incite an immune response, they are readily transplantable to patients.

Therapeutic Uses in Pediatric Orthopaedics

Endogenous stem cells are thought to be frequently used in orthopaedic therapies, including distraction osteogenesis, fracture repair, or bone marrow injection of bone cysts. The use of a patient's own mesenchymal stem cells has been promoted for bone healing after fracture or spine fusion, but it is not clear that this approach is preferable to traditional autologous bone grafting. There is no clinical evidence that mesenchymal stem cells can differentiate into cartilage cells.

In vitro expanded mesenchymal stem cells are commercially available. The use of commercial cells should be considered experimental until well-designed clinical studies have determined their safety and efficacy. These cells should be used only when no other treatments are available. Understanding the possible long-term complications of using these cells is even more important for a pediatric patient than for an adult patient.[32]

The first routine use of allograft stem cell transplantation probably will be for improving neurologic recovery after nerve injury or paralysis or for inhibiting the immune response in autoimmune disorders.[33,34] The future uses of allograft stem cell transplantation in pediatric orthopaedics are likely to include difficult bone repairs and pathologic bone treatment. Mesenchymal stem cell transplantation has been used to treat osteogenesis imperfecta,[35] and it has been proposed for pathologic conditions such as fibrous dysplasia.[36] Animal studies suggest that mesenchymal stem cells can improve wound healing after radiation therapy.[37] These cells could be used for repairing damaged articular cartilage or growth plates[38-40] or for managing osteonecrosis.[41]

Summary

Stem cells hold tremendous promise for the development of therapies that could revolutionize orthopaedic care. Before stem cells can be brought into widespread clinical use, basic science studies must provide an understanding of ways in which the differentiation and proliferation of these cells can be regulated. Careful comparative clinical studies to determine the effectiveness of stem cell treatments also are required.

Annotated References

1. Stent GS: The role of cell lineage in development. *Philos Trans R Soc Lond B Biol Sci* 1985;312(1153):3-19.

2. Allegrucci C, Young LE: Differences between human embryonic stem cell lines. *Hum Reprod Update* 2007; 13(2):103-120.

3. Alison MR, Islam S: Attributes of adult stem cells. *J Pathol* 2009;217(2):144-160.

4. Yu J, Thomson JA: Pluripotent stem cell lines. *Genes Dev* 2008;22(15):1987-1997.

5. Jung KW: Perspectives on human stem cell research. *J Cell Physiol* 2009;220(3):535-537.

6. Lo B, Parham L: Ethical issues in stem cell research. *Endocr Rev* 2009;30(3):204-213.

7. Verfaillie C: Pluripotent stem cells. *Transfus Clin Biol* 2009;16(2):65-69.

8. Hochedlinger K, Plath K: Epigenetic reprogramming and induced pluripotency. *Development* 2009;136(4): 509-523.

9. Yamanaka S: Induction of pluripotent stem cells from mouse fibroblasts by four transcription factors. *Cell Prolif* 2008;41(suppl 1):51-56.

This is an excellent review article by the researcher who first discovered that mature differentiated cells can be induced to act as stem cells. The process is useful in regenerative medicine strategies and may explain how normal repair processes occur.

10. Caplan AI: Why are MSCs therapeutic? New data: New insight. *J Pathol* 2009;217(2):318-324.

11. Garrett RW, Emerson SG: Bone and blood vessels: The hard and the soft of hematopoietic stem cell niches. *Cell Stem Cell* 2009;4(6):503-506.

12. Andersson ER, Lendahl U: Regenerative medicine: A 2009 overview. *J Intern Med* 2009;266(4):303-310.

13. Prockop DJ: Repair of tissues by adult stem/progenitor cells (MSCs): Controversies, myths, and changing paradigms. *Mol Ther* 2009;17(6):939-946.

This is a comprehensive review of the potential clinical uses of mesenchymal stem cells.

14. Branski LK, Gauglitz GG, Herndon DN, Jeschke MG: A review of gene and stem cell therapy in cutaneous wound healing. *Burns* 2009;35(2):171-180.

15. Fazel S, Chen L, Weisel RD, et al: Cell transplantation preserves cardiac function after infarction by infarct stabilization: Augmentation by stem cell factor. *J Thorac Cardiovasc Surg* 2005;130(5):1310.

16. Fazel S, Cimini M, Chen L, et al: Cardioprotective c-kit+ cells are from the bone marrow and regulate the myocardial balance of angiogenic cytokines. *J Clin Invest* 2006;116(7):1865-1877.

17. Bartholomew A, Polchert D, Szilagyi E, Douglas GW, Kenyon N: Mesenchymal stem cells in the induction of transplantation tolerance. *Transplantation* 2009;87(9, suppl):S55-S57.

18. Kuo TK, Ho JH, Lee OK: Mesenchymal stem cell therapy for nonmusculoskeletal diseases: Emerging applications. *Cell Transplant* 2009;18(9):1013-1028.

19. Cuomo AV, Virk M, Petrigliano F, Morgan EF, Lieberman JR: Mesenchymal stem cell concentration and bone repair: Potential pitfalls from bench to bedside. *J Bone Joint Surg Am* 2009;91(5):1073-1083.

20. Tasso R, Augello A, Caridà M, et al: Development of sarcomas in mice implanted with mesenchymal stem cells seeded onto bioscaffolds. *Carcinogenesis* 2009; 30(1):150-157.

This is one of a number of studies raising the possibility that a small number of mesenchymal stem cells can become neoplastic. Although the chance of this occurrence probably is relatively small, it must be seriously considered, especially for young patients.

21. Baker M: Tumours spark stem-cell review. *Nature* 2009; 457(7232):941.

22. Mishra PJ, Mishra PJ, Glod JW, Banerjee D: Mesenchymal stem cells: Flip side of the coin. *Cancer Res* 2009; 69(4):1255-1258.

23. Wu C, Wei Q, Utomo V, et al: Side population cells isolated from mesenchymal neoplasms have tumor initiating potential. *Cancer Res* 2007;67(17):8216-8222.

    This is the first study to find that a variety of musculoskeletal tumors contain a subpopulation of cells with stem cell–like properties. This finding is important because therapeutic targeting of these cells could decrease the metastatic potential of sarcomas, thus substantially improving patient outcomes.

24. Marotta LL, Polyak K: Cancer stem cells: A model in the making. *Curr Opin Genet Dev* 2009;19(1):44-50.

25. Muschler GF, Boehm C, Easley K: Aspiration to obtain osteoblast progenitor cells from human bone marrow: The influence of aspiration volume. *J Bone Joint Surg Am* 1997;79(11):1699-1709.

26. Stolzing A, Jones E, McGonagle D, Scutt A: Age-related changes in human bone marrow-derived mesenchymal stem cells: Consequences for cell therapies. *Mech Ageing Dev* 2008;129(3):163-173.

27. Franco Lambert AP, Fraga Zandonai A, Bonatto D, Cantarelli Machado D, Pêgas Henriques JA: Differentiation of human adipose-derived adult stem cells into neuronal tissue: Does it work? *Differentiation* 2009; 77(3):221-228.

28. Brooke G, Rossetti T, Pelekanos R, et al: Manufacturing of human placenta-derived mesenchymal stem cells for clinical trials. *Br J Haematol* 2009;144(4):571-579.

29. Ruhil S, Kumar V, Rathee P: Umbilical cord stem cell: An overview. *Curr Pharm Biotechnol* 2009;10(3):327-334.

30. Tsai PC, Fu TW, Chen YM, et al: The therapeutic potential of human umbilical mesenchymal stem cells from Wharton's jelly in the treatment of rat liver fibrosis. *Liver Transpl* 2009;15(5):484-495.

31. Zweigerdt R: Large scale production of stem cells and their derivatives. *Adv Biochem Eng Biotechnol* 2009; 114:201-235.

32. Lepperdinger G, Brunauer R, Jamnig A, Laschober G, Kassem M: Controversial issue: is it safe to employ mesenchymal stem cells in cell-based therapies? *Exp Gerontol* 2008;43(11):1018-1023.

33. Kim SU, de Vellis J: Stem cell-based cell therapy in neurological diseases: a review. *J Neurosci Res* 2009; 87(10):2183-2200.

34. Kastrinaki MC, Papadaki HA: Mesenchymal stromal cells in rheumatoid arthritis: biological properties and clinical applications. *Curr Stem Cell Res Ther* 2009; 4(1):61-69.

35. Satija NK, Singh VK, Verma YK, et al: Mesenchymal stem cell-based therapy: A new paradigm in regenerative medicine. *J Cell Mol Med* 2009;13(11-12):4385-4402.

36. Waese EY, Kandel RA, Kandel RR, Stanford WL: Application of stem cells in bone repair. *Skeletal Radiol* 2008;37(7):601-608.

37. Greenberger JS, Epperly M: Bone marrow-derived stem cells and radiation response. *Semin Radiat Oncol* 2009; 19(2):133-139.

38. Richardson SM, Hoyland JA, Mobasheri R, Csaki C, Shakibaei M, Mobasheri A: Mesenchymal stem cells in regenerative medicine: Opportunities and challenges for articular cartilage and intervertebral disc tissue engineering. *J Cell Physiol* 2010;222(1):23-32.

39. Hwang NS, Elisseeff J: Application of stem cells for articular cartilage regeneration. *J Knee Surg* 2009;22(1): 60-71.

40. Chen WH, Lai MT, Wu AT, et al: In vitro stage-specific chondrogenesis of mesenchymal stem cells committed to chondrocytes. *Arthritis Rheum* 2009;60(2):450-459.

41. Lee K, Chan CK, Patil N, Goodman SB: Cell therapy for bone regeneration: Bench to bedside. *J Biomed Mater Res B Appl Biomater* 2009;89(1):252-263.

2: Basic Science

Chapter 6

The Biology of Bone Morphogenetic Proteins

David G. Little, PhD, FRACS (Orth)   Aaron Schindeler, PhD

Introduction

The discovery of bone morphogenetic proteins (BMPs) dates from the mid 1960s, when ectopic bone was found to be inducible using demineralized bone matrix.[1] This and later research led to an understanding that there are intrinsically osteoinductive factors within bone. Specific genes encoding for bone-inductive proteins were isolated during the 1980s and 1990s, accompanied by significant advancements as to the nature and mechanism of action of these proteins.[2,3] BMP research has been clinically applied in orthopaedics and bone tissue engineering. The clinical applications of BMPs continue to evolve, particularly as new delivery systems and adjunctive agents are developed.

BMP Structure and Function

BMPs are members of the transforming growth factor–β superfamily of proteins. A BMP is classified as osteogenic or nonosteogenic based on whether it has the ability to stimulate osteoblast differentiation and bone gene expression. Of the original 15 bone-derived BMPs, BMP-2, BMP-4, BMP-5, BMP-6, BMP-7, and BMP-9 are considered osteoinductive. BMP-2 and BMP-7 are approved for clinical applications. Some BMPs have been renamed; for example, BMP-14 is more commonly referred to as growth differentiation factor–5 (GDF-5), and BMP-7 originally was known as osteogenic protein–1 (OP-1).

BMPs are synthesized as precursor proteins that are proteolytically cleaved to yield disulfide-linked protein dimers.[4,5] BMP proteins are extremely stable and can retain their biologic osteogenic activity after being dis-

solved in organic solvents or impregnated in a variety of carriers. BMPs also are heat stable, retaining their activity even after prolonged exposure to temperatures as high as 70°C.[6]

BMPs bind to BMP receptors (BMPRs) and activate the BMP signal to induce changes in gene expression within the cell. BMPs cannot affect cells that do not express BMPRs. A variety of BMP antagonists have been found; they bind directly to BMPs or BMPRs and inhibit their activity.[7] These molecules have critical roles in bone and joint development.

The interactions between the BMPs and their receptors are complex, with a variety of BMPR subunits interacting in different combinations.[8] Once activated, BMPRs activate canonical signaling via the SMAD family of proteins. Noncanonical pathways, including Ras-MAPK, WNT, and others, also can be activated.[9-11] These signaling systems are able to effect changes in gene expression that regulate numerous cellular processes, including cell proliferation, cell differentiation, extracellular matrix production, and cell death.

The Physiologic Roles of BMPs

Early Embryonic Patterning and Skeletogenesis

BMP family members are expressed in a distinct but overlapping series of patterns during embryonic development.[12,13] BMPs and their receptors are critical for normal development, as revealed by gene disruption experiments. The *BMP-2* and *BMP-4* genes are critical for normal cardiac and mesodermal differentiation, respectively, and mouse embryos fail to develop if deficient in these genes.[14,15] *BMPR-1a* is important for early embryonic development (gastrulation), cartilage development, and bone mass regulation.[16-19] Studies using more advanced mouse conditional knockout models to examine the role of BMPs in bone healing found that BMP-2 is critical for fracture healing, but BMP-7 is not critical.[20,21] Several mutations in BMP genes or pathway members have been reported to cause skeletal manifestations in humans (**Table 1**).

Dr. Little or an immediate family member has received royalties from Novartis; is a member of a speakers' bureau or has made paid presentations on behalf of Amgen Co., Eli Lilly, Novartis, and Stryker; serves as an unpaid consultant to Amgen Co. and Novartis; and has received research or institutional support from Amgen Co., Novartis, and Stryker. Dr. Schindeler or an immediate family member has received research or institutional support from Amgen Co., Novartis, Celgene, and Acceleron.

2: Basic Science

Table 1

Diseases Associated With BMP Anomalies

Disease	Gene	Study
Polydactyly, syndactyly	*BMP-4*	Bakrania et al[22]
Acromesomelic chondrodysplasia	*CDMP-1/GDF-5*	Costa et al[23]
Acromesomelic chondrodysplasia	*BMPR-1b*	Demirhan et al[24]
Brachydactyly type A2	*BMP-2* regulatory element	Dathe et al[25]
Fibrodysplasia ossificans progressiva	*ALK-2* (type-I BMP receptor family member)	Kaplan et al[26]

Bone Cell Differentiation

BMPs are potent stimulators of osteoblastic differentiation from precursor cells. In vitro studies found that BMP-2, BMP-6, and BMP-9 have the greatest effect on preosteoblastic cells and that BMP-7 is osteogenic for more mature cells. In vivo studies found that BMP-2, BMP-6, BMP-7, and BMP-9 produce ectopic bone but that BMP-3 is inhibitory.[27] In addition to their role in promoting osteoblast differentiation, the osteoinductive BMPs are able to promote osteoclast formation.[28] Increases in osteoclast activity may be indirectly mediated by increased secretion of the receptor activator of nuclear factor κ-β ligand (RANKL) by osteoblasts or by the direct effects of BMPs on osteoclasts or their precursors.[29] A BMP-induced increase in osteoclast activity may be a mechanistic explanation of the increased bone resorption reported in some animal and clinical studies.

Fracture Repair

BMPs are expressed during normal fracture repair; early expression of BMP-2 has been observed with later expression of BMP-4, BMP-5, and BMP-6 and even later expression of BMP-7.[30] BMP antagonists are expressed in bone repair as part of a negative feedback control mechanism.[31] The expression of BMPs as well as their antagonists, receptors, and downstream signaling was recently described in murine fracture repair.[32] BMP inhibitors such as BMP-3 and noggin also are expressed with BMPs. Granulation tissues express BMPs but do not express their receptors or downstream SMAD signals (**Table 2**).

BMPs as Pharmaceutical Agents

Preclinical Models

Studies using a variety of animal models have investigated potential clinical uses of BMPs, focusing on the capacity of BMPs for healing segmental or critical-size bone defects that cannot heal without intervention. BMP-2 and BMP-7 have been studied in rodent, large mammal (sheep or goat), and nonhuman primate models. Most of these studies used collagen or polylactide-polyglycolide polymers as carrier or delivery systems.

BMPs are potent bone-inducing agents, and they were found in animal models to be effective in treating some of the most challenging orthopaedic insults. BMPs were capable of restoring function in the presence of large diaphyseal bone defects,[33,34] and they were effective in preventing nonunion after severe open fractures.[35] Even in orthopaedic treatments having a lower intrinsic failure rate, such as distraction osteogenesis and closed fracture repair, BMPs were found to accelerate the healing response.[36,37] BMPs were effective as an alternative to bone graft in animal models of spine fusion[38,39] and have been used in conjunction with allograft and autograft to produce enhanced results. BMPs were found to be effective in the osseointegration of prosthetic devices.[40] Because BMPs have been found effective for treating a variety of orthopaedic indications, emerging preclinical studies are focusing on generating new or improved delivery systems, applying BMP gene- and cell-based therapies, or combining recombinant human BMP (rhBMP) with other compounds that can stimulate bone or blood vessel formation.

Clinical Studies of rhBMP-2 and rhBMP-7

The orthopaedic use of rhBMP-2 and rhBMP-7 has been investigated in randomized, controlled studies. The surgical use of 3.5 mg of rhBMP-7 was compared with the use of autogenous bone graft in 122 patients with a tibia nonunion.[41] No significant difference was found; the treatment was successful in 81% of the patients treated with rhBMP-7 and 85% of the patients treated with bone graft. A more recent study of 40 patients suggests that rhBMP-7 also is effective in treating externally fixed tibia fractures.[42]

Perhaps the most convincing evidence for the orthopaedic efficacy of BMP is in a large, prospective study of BMP-2 used in open tibia fractures. In 450 patients treated with intramedullary fixation (the standard of care) or intramedullary fixation with the addition of 6 mg or 12 mg of rhBMP-2 in a collagen sponge, the patients treated with 12 mg of rhBMP-2 had a 44% reduction in the risk of failure, in comparison with control subjects.[43] Treatment with 12 mg of rhBMP-2 also was associated with lower rates of infection and hardware failures and with accelerated wound healing.

Both rhBMP-2 and rhBMP-7 have been tested for spine applications. In a prospective but nonblinded study, 90 adults were treated with rhBMP-2 during an-

2: Basic Science

Table 2

Immunoreactivity of BMPs and BMP Antagonists, Receptors, and Effectors During Nonstabilized Fracture Healing*

BMP or Related Factor	Periosteal Cells		Granulation Tissue		Chondrocytes				Osteoblasts or Osteocytes in New Bone			
	Day 3	Day 5	Day 3	Day 5	Day 5	Day 7	Day 10	Day 14	Day 7	Day 10	Day 14	Day 21
BMP-2	+	–	+	++	++	+++	+++	+	++	+	+	–
BMP-3	+	–	–	–	+	++	++	+	+	++	–	–
BMP-4	+	–	–	+	–	+	+++	–	+	++	–	–
BMP-5	+	+	+	++	–	+++	+++	+	+++	+	–	–
BMP-6	–	–	+	++	++	+++	+++	+	+++	+	+	–
BMP-7	–	–	+	+	++	+++	+++	+	+++	+	–	–
BMP-8	++	–	–	+	+	+++	+++	+	+++	+++	–	–
Noggin	+	–	+	++	++	++	+++	–	+	+	–	–
BMPR-1a	+	+	–	–	++	+++	++	++	+++	+	+	–
BMPR-1b	–	–	–	–	++	+++	+++	+	+++	+	+	–
BMPR-2	+	+	–	–	++	+++	+++	++	+++	+++	+	–
pSMAD 1/5/8	++	+	–	–	++	+++	++	+	++	+++	+	–

* – = negative staining, + = weak staining, ++ = moderate staining, +++ = strong staining.
(Adapted with permission from Yu YY, Lieu S, Lu C, Miclau T, Marcucio RS, Colnot C: Immunolocalization of BMPs, BMP antagonists, receptors, and effectors during fracture repair. *Bone* 2010;46:841-851.)

terior fusion (47 patients) or posterior fusion (43 patients); the fusion rate was 91% or 97%, respectively.[44] In several small clinical studies, rhBMP-7 used in OP-1 putty (Stryker Biotech; Hopkinton, MA) was found to be similarly effective in adult degenerative lumbar spine fusion.[45,46] BMPs are particularly advantageous for spine fusion, in comparison with traditional bone grafting, because they allow the complications associated with donor site morbidity to be avoided.

Complications Associated With rhBMPs
The pharmaceutical use of rhBMPs has a good safety record. Continued monitoring is warranted, however, as both on-label and off-label uses continue to expand. The number of reported failures and complications has recently increased. In the long bones, periarticular use can lead to heterotopic ossification if the BMP is not contained; a heterotopic ossification incidence of more than 50% and a reoperation rate of 24% were reported after BMP-2 was used to augment tibial plateau fractures.[47]

Redness and inflammation may be confused with infection in long bone open fractures, before or after surgical treatment. Inflammation with greater-than-expected swelling has been particularly noticeable in the cervical spine. A retrospective study using the Nationwide Inpatient Sample database found a 1.22% rate of wound-related complications when BMP was used in spine fusion surgery, compared with a 0.65% rate when BMP was not used (adjusted odds ratio, 1.67; 95% confidence interval, 1.10–2.53); and a 4.35% rate of dysphagia or hoarseness when BMP was used, compared with a 2.45% rate when BMP was not used (adjusted odds ratio, 1.63; 95% confidence interval, 1.30–2.05).[48] Airway complications have been reported after BMP was used in the anterior cervical spine.[49-51]

Synergy With Antiresorptive Agents
BMPs can stimulate bone resorption; the osteogenic BMPs are able to directly and/or indirectly enhance osteoclast formation, activation, and activities. However, BMP-associated resorption before formation has been reported in several patients, leading to loss of position and a need for further surgery.[52-54] Thus, it has been speculated that the effects of BMPs can be maximized by concurrent prevention of premature or excessive resorption.[55] Several preclinical studies suggested that the results of BMP therapy can be improved by combining it with the use of an antiresorptive agent such as a bisphosphonate.[34,56,57] In a rat critical-size femoral defect model, the addition of zoledronic acid to rhBMP-7 increased the ultimate size and strength of the callus.[34] No prospective, randomized studies are available, however.

2: Basic Science

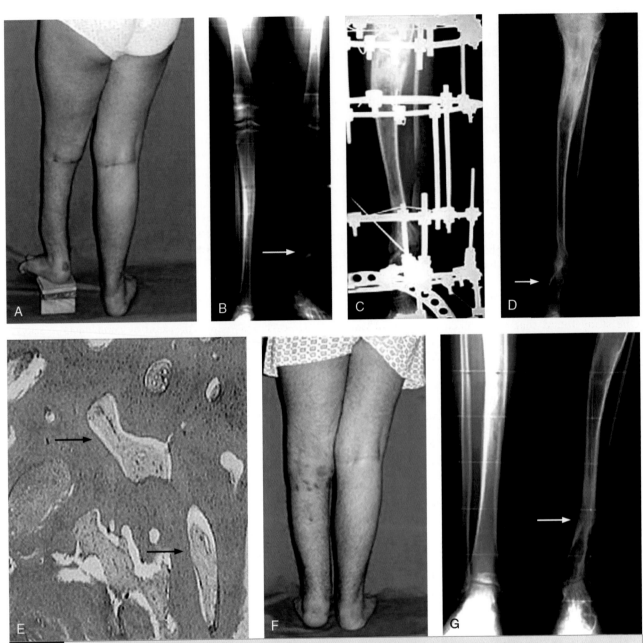

Figure 1 After undergoing 12 earlier surgical procedures, a patient with congenital pseudarthrosis of the tibia was treated using OP-1 (BMP-7), a proximal tibial corticotomy, and an Ilizarov device. Presurgical photograph (**A**) and radiograph (**B**) showing differences in leg length, valgus of the ankle joint, and pseudarthrosis of the tibia (*arrow*). Radiographs showing postsurgical fixation using an Ilizarov device (**C**) and bridging of the bone ends (*arrow*) when the Ilizarov frame was removed 8 months after surgery (**D**). **E**, Histologic slide showing Von Kossa staining (25× magnification) of bone taken during frame removal; fibrous tissue (*arrows*) has infiltrated into cortical and trabecular bone. **F**, Photograph showing equal limb length 12 months after surgery. **G**, Radiograph showing continued improvement (*arrow*) 45 months after surgery. (Adapted with permission from Anticevic D, Jelic M, Vukicevic S: Treatment of a congenital pseudarthrosis of the tibia by osteogenic protein-1 [bone morphogenetic protein-7]: A case report. *J Pediatr Orthop B* 2006;15:220-221.)

Antagonism of BMP Effects

Heterotopic ossification can arise for a genetic reason, as in fibrodysplasia ossificans progressiva; spontaneously after trauma, as in myositis ossificans; or after surgical trauma, as in a hip replacement. BMP release and/or aberrant BMP signaling probably contributes to the formation of heterotopic bone in these conditions. Heterotopic ossification can be challenging to manage, but emerging anti-BMP agents hold promise for its prevention and treatment.[58] A retinoic acid receptor agonist was found to inhibit heterotopic ossification in a BMP-2 induced model.[59]

The Pediatric Use of BMPs

There are no approved indications for the therapeutic use of BMPs in children, and robust evidence of efficacy is lacking. Neither BMP-2 nor BMP-7 has been approved by the US Food and Drug Administration for use in children. The main areas of interest for the pediatric use of BMPs in children mirror the adult uses, but very little information is available. The potential use of BMPs in children with congenital pseudarthrosis of the tibia associated with neurofibromatosis type I (NF1) represents a unique situation, however. Preclinical studies found that, although NF1 is somewhat resistant to BMP application, BMPs are still capable of stimulating osteoblasts affected by NF1. The ectopic bone formed in response to rhBMP-2 in NF1-deficient animals was approximately half of that in wild-type animals.[60]

A few reports have described the use of BMP-7 in patients with congenital pseudarthrosis of the tibia. One study found that union occurred only in one of five patients when BMP-7 was used alone.[61] The use of BMP-7 alone or BMP-7 plus autogenous bone graft was reported as successful in several individual patients[62-64] (Figure 1). Five of seven pediatric patients with congenital pseudarthrosis had union after index treatment with intramedullary rod fixation, autogenous bone grafting, and the application of BMP-2 in a collagen sponge; one additional patient had union after a subsequent application.[65] Given the poor outcomes usually associated with congenital pseudarthrosis of the tibia, clinical studies to establish the efficacy and safety of the use of BMPs in treating this disorder should be a priority.

Only a few pediatric case reports have described the use of BMPs in the spine. In a child with Down syndrome who had undergone multiple failed occipitocervical fusions, fusion was achieved by application of BMP-2.[66] The routine use of BMP in pediatric spine fusion is unlikely to become necessary or affordable, however.

A recently published review of BMP-2 use at a tertiary institution found that in 81 patients younger than 18 years, a total of 16 complications might be attributable to the use of rhBMP-2.[67] Nine of the patients had a complication at the surgical site, three had a deep infection, one had a postsurgical compartment syndrome, and two had neurologic sequelae (progressive myelopathy or weakness and dural fibrosis); one patient with neurofibromatosis and previously diagnosed intracranial gliomas had subsequent enlargement of these gliomas. A review of these complications led to the conclusion that only the dural fibrosis with subsequent weakness had a possible direct relationship to the use of BMP-2.

There is concern about the potential for oncogenesis when potent growth factors are used in children. Such uses have been off-label and sporadic; although malignancy has not been reported, it remains a possibility.

Several reports have suggested that BMP-7, as a differentiation factor, may suppress tumor formation.[68,69] Antibodies to BMPs and collagen delivery materials have been detected;[41,70] although allergic reactions have not been reported, repeated BMP application may not be successful if neutralizing antibodies are present.

Summary

BMPs are an advanced therapeutic modality with the potential to improve the outcome of bone repair. However, the indications for use must be further refined, and clinical studies in children are required before BMPs can be recommended as standard treatment for pediatric patients with an orthopaedic condition.

Annotated References

1. Urist MR: Bone: Formation by autoinduction. *Science* 1965;150(698):893-899.

2. Rosen V, Wozney JM, Wang EA, et al: Purification and molecular cloning of a novel group of BMPs and localization of BMP mRNA in developing bone. *Connect Tissue Res* 1989;20(1-4):313-319.

3. Ozkaynak E, Rueger DC, Drier EA, et al: OP-1 cDNA encodes an osteogenic protein in the TGF-beta family. *EMBO J* 1990;9(7):2085-2093.

4. Sampath TK, Coughlin JE, Whetstone RM, et al: Bovine osteogenic protein is composed of dimers of OP-1 and BMP-2A, two members of the transforming growth factor-beta superfamily. *J Biol Chem* 1990;265(22):13198-13205.

5. Jones WK, Richmond EA, White K, et al: Osteogenic protein-1 (OP-1) expression and processing in Chinese hamster ovary cells: Isolation of a soluble complex containing the mature and pro-domains of OP-1. *Growth Factors* 1994;11(3):215-225.

6. Ohta H, Wakitani S, Tensho K, et al: The effects of heat on the biological activity of recombinant human bone morphogenetic protein-2. *J Bone Miner Metab* 2005;23(6):420-425.

   In an experimental preclinical study, heat-treated rhBMP-2 in collagen discs was implanted into mice to assay the amount of bone formed.

7. Rosen V: BMP and BMP inhibitors in bone. *Ann N Y Acad Sci* 2006;1068:19-25.

   The actions of BMP antagonists such as noggin, sclerostin, chordin, connective tissue growth factor, follistatin, and gremlin are discussed in detail.

8. Feng XH, Derynck R: Specificity and versatility in tgf-beta signaling through Smads. *Annu Rev Cell Dev Biol* 2005;21:659-693.

2: Basic Science

The structural and functional relationships of transforming growth factor–β receptors and their downstream signaling targets are discussed.

9. Schindeler A, Little DG: Ras-MAPK signaling in osteogenic differentiation: Friend or foe? *J Bone Miner Res* 2006;21(9):1331-1338.

   A range of in vitro and in vivo data supports an agonistic or antagonistic role for Ras-MAPK signaling in bone cell differentiation.

10. Löwik CW, van Bezooijen RL: Wnt signaling is involved in the inhibitory action of sclerostin on BMP-stimulated bone formation. *J Musculoskelet Neuronal Interact* 2006;6(4):357.

    This brief review notes that, although sclerostin initially was postulated to affect BMP-SMAD signaling, emerging evidence suggests its action is mediated by WNT signaling.

11. Guo X, Wang XF: Signaling cross-talk between TGF-beta/BMP and other pathways. *Cell Res* 2009;19(1):71-88.

    This is a detailed summary of the downstream signaling pathways involved in transducing BMP action.

12. Lyons KM, Hogan BL, Robertson EJ: Colocalization of BMP 7 and BMP 2 RNAs suggests that these factors cooperatively mediate tissue interactions during murine development. *Mech Dev* 1995;50(1):71-83.

13. Dudley AT, Robertson EJ: Overlapping expression domains of bone morphogenetic protein family members potentially account for limited tissue defects in BMP7 deficient embryos. *Dev Dyn* 1997;208(3):349-362.

14. Zhang H, Bradley A: Mice deficient for BMP2 are non-viable and have defects in amnion/chorion and cardiac development. *Development* 1996;122(10):2977-2986.

15. Winnier G, Blessing M, Labosky PA, Hogan BL: Bone morphogenetic protein-4 is required for mesoderm formation and patterning in the mouse. *Genes Dev* 1995;9(17):2105-2116.

16. Mishina Y, Suzuki A, Ueno N, Behringer RR: Bmpr encodes a type I bone morphogenetic protein receptor that is essential for gastrulation during mouse embryogenesis. *Genes Dev* 1995;9(24):3027-3037.

17. Yoon BS, Ovchinnikov DA, Yoshii I, Mishina Y, Behringer RR, Lyons KM: Bmpr1a and Bmpr1b have overlapping functions and are essential for chondrogenesis in vivo. *Proc Natl Acad Sci U S A* 2005;102(14):5062-5067.

    In *BMPR-1a* conditional knockout and *BMPR-1b* knockout mouse models, these receptors were found to have functional redundancy, although loss of both genes prevents normal cartilage formation.

18. Mishina Y, Starbuck MW, Gentile MA, et al: Bone morphogenetic protein type IA receptor signaling regulates postnatal osteoblast function and bone remodeling. *J Biol Chem* 2004;279(26):27560-27566.

19. Kamiya N, Ye L, Kobayashi T, et al: Disruption of BMP signaling in osteoblasts through type IA receptor (BMPRIA) increases bone mass. *J Bone Miner Res* 2008;23(12):2007-2017.

    In a detailed phenotypic analysis of conditional knockout mice, *BMPR-1a* was removed from osteoblasts.

20. Tsuji K, Bandyopadhyay A, Harfe BD, et al: BMP2 activity, although dispensable for bone formation, is required for the initiation of fracture healing. *Nat Genet* 2006;38(12):1424-1429.

    This seminal study used conditional knockout mice in which *BMP-2* was removed from mature bone cells. The mice were born skeletally normal, but spontaneous fractures developed that showed deficient bone healing.

21. Tsuji K, Cox K, Gamer L, Graf D, Economides A, Rosen V: Conditional deletion of BMP7 from the limb skeleton does not affect bone formation or fracture repair. *J Orthop Res* 2010;28(3):384-389.

    Unlike *BMP-2* conditional knockout mice, *BMP-7* conditional knockout mice did not have spontaneous fractures or abnormal bone repair.

22. Bakrania P, Efthymiou M, Klein JC, et al: Mutations in BMP4 cause eye, brain, and digit developmental anomalies: Overlap between the BMP4 and hedgehog signaling pathways. *Am J Hum Genet* 2008;82(2):304-319.

    BMP-4 mutations were found in a screening of 215 patients with ocular malformation defects.

23. Costa T, Ramsby G, Cassia F, et al: Grebe syndrome: Clinical and radiographic findings in affected individuals and heterozygous carriers. *Am J Med Genet* 1998;75(5):523-529.

24. Demirhan O, Türkmen S, Schwabe GC, et al: A homozygous BMPR1B mutation causes a new subtype of acromesomelic chondrodysplasia with genital anomalies. *J Med Genet* 2005;42(4):314-317.

    A novel mutation was discovered in a 16-year-old girl from a consanguineous family who had skeletal abnormalities.

25. Dathe K, Kjaer KW, Brehm A, et al: Duplications involving a conserved regulatory element downstream of BMP2 are associated with brachydactyly type A2. *Am J Hum Genet* 2009;84(4):483-492.

    A genetic screening study of two separate families found that BMP-2 regulatory elements are associated with brachydactyly type A2.

26. Kaplan FS, Le Merrer M, Glaser DL, et al: Fibrodysplasia ossificans progressiva. *Best Pract Res Clin Rheumatol* 2008;22(1):191-205.

    A topical review discusses the clinical treatment of fibrodysplasia ossificans progressiva, with a focus on emerging therapies.

27. Kang Q, Sun MH, Cheng H, et al: Characterization of the distinct orthotopic bone-forming activity of 14 BMPs using recombinant adenovirus-mediated gene delivery. *Gene Ther* 2004;11(17):1312-1320.

28. Paul S, Lee JC, Yeh LC: A comparative study on BMP-induced osteoclastogenesis and osteoblastogenesis in primary cultures of adult rat bone marrow cells. *Growth Factors* 2009;27(2):121-131.

    An in vitro study used a primary cell culture system to illustrate that the osteogenic BMPs (BMP-2, -4, -5, -6, and -7) are able to induce osteoblastic and osteoclast markers.

29. Kaneko H, Arakawa T, Mano H, et al: Direct stimulation of osteoclastic bone resorption by bone morphogenetic protein (BMP)-2 and expression of BMP receptors in mature osteoclasts. *Bone* 2000;27(4):479-486.

30. Gerstenfeld LC, Cullinane DM, Barnes GL, Graves DT, Einhorn TA: Fracture healing as a post-natal developmental process: Molecular, spatial, and temporal aspects of its regulation. *J Cell Biochem* 2003;88(5):873-884.

31. Fajardo M, Liu CJ, Egol K: Levels of expression for BMP-7 and several BMP antagonists may play an integral role in a fracture nonunion: A pilot study. *Clin Orthop Relat Res* 2009;467(12):3071-3078.

    Preliminary data suggest that fracture union or nonunion is related to BMP-7 concentration.

32. Yu YY, Lieu S, Lu C, Miclau T, Marcucio RS, Colnot C: Immunolocalization of BMPs, BMP antagonists, receptors, and effectors during fracture repair. *Bone* 2010;46(3):841-851.

    A detailed experimental study examined the expression levels and tissue distribution of a range of BMPs and related factors during mouse fracture healing.

33. Lane JM, Yasko AW, Tomin E, et al: Bone marrow and recombinant human bone morphogenetic protein-2 in osseous repair. *Clin Orthop Relat Res* 1999;361:216-227.

34. Little DG, McDonald M, Bransford R, Godfrey CB, Amanat N: Manipulation of the anabolic and catabolic responses with OP-1 and zoledronic acid in a rat critical defect model. *J Bone Miner Res* 2005;20(11):2044-2052.

    Combining BMPs with an anticatabolic agent was found to increase the amount of bone formation.

35. Hak DJ, Makino T, Niikura T, Hazelwood SJ, Curtiss S, Reddi AH: Recombinant human BMP-7 effectively prevents non-union in both young and old rats. *J Orthop Res* 2006;24(1):11-20.

    In a severe nonunion model produced using electrocautery, BMP-7 application alone was sufficient for recruiting and differentiating bone cells at the site to permit repair; control rats had nonunion.

36. Mandu-Hrit M, Haque T, Lauzier D, et al: Early injection of OP-1 during distraction osteogenesis accelerates new bone formation in rabbits. *Growth Factors* 2006; 24(3):172-183.

    In a preclinical study in rabbits, purified OP-1 was directly injected in the early stages of distraction osteogenesis.

37. Einhorn TA, Majeska RJ, Mohaideen A, et al: A single percutaneous injection of recombinant human bone morphogenetic protein-2 accelerates fracture repair. *J Bone Joint Surg Am* 2003;85-A(8):1425-1435.

38. Hidaka C, Goshi K, Rawlins B, Boachie-Adjei O, Crystal RG: Enhancement of spine fusion using combined gene therapy and tissue engineering BMP-7-expressing bone marrow cells and allograft bone. *Spine (Phila Pa 1976)* 2003;28(18):2049-2057.

39. Zhu W, Rawlins BA, Boachie-Adjei O, et al: Combined bone morphogenetic protein-2 and -7 gene transfer enhances osteoblastic differentiation and spine fusion in a rodent model. *J Bone Miner Res* 2004;19(12):2021-2032.

40. Matin K, Senpuku H, Hanada N, Ozawa H, Ejiri S: Bone regeneration by recombinant human bone morphogenetic protein-2 around immediate implants: A pilot study in rats. *Int J Oral Maxillofac Implants* 2003; 18(2):211-217.

41. Friedlaender GE, Perry CR, Cole JD, et al: Osteogenic protein-1 (bone morphogenetic protein-7) in the treatment of tibial nonunions. *J Bone Joint Surg Am* 2001; 83-A(suppl 1, pt 2):S151-S158.

    In the healing of nonunions, OP-1 (BMP-7) alone in a collagen carrier is equivalent to autograft in most respects. There was some difference in radiology scores after OP-1 and autograft treatment.

42. Ristiniemi J, Flinkkilä T, Hyvönen P, Lakovaara M, Pakarinen H, Jalovaara P: RhBMP-7 accelerates the healing in distal tibial fractures treated by external fixation. *J Bone Joint Surg Br* 2007;89(2):265-272.

    A small study of 20 patients found that fractures repaired more rapidly when rhBMP-7 was used.

43. Govender S, Csimma C, Genant HK, et al: Recombinant human bone morphogenetic protein-2 for treatment of open tibial fractures: A prospective, controlled, randomized study of four hundred and fifty patients. *J Bone Joint Surg Am* 2002;84-A(12):2123-2134.

44. Mulconrey DS, Bridwell KH, Flynn J, Cronen GA, Rose PS: Bone morphogenetic protein (RhBMP-2) as a substitute for iliac crest bone graft in multilevel adult spinal deformity surgery: Minimum two-year evaluation of fusion. *Spine (Phila Pa 1976)* 2008;33(20):2153-2159.

    In a prospective comparison study of three different treatment approaches to spine fusion, rhBMP-2 was used with or without local bone grafting.

45. Johnsson R, Strömqvist B, Aspenberg P: Randomized radiostereometric study comparing osteogenic protein-1 (BMP-7) and autograft bone in human noninstrumented

posterolateral lumbar fusion: 2002 Volvo Award in clinical studies. *Spine (Phila Pa 1976)* 2002;27(23):2654-2661.

46. Vaccaro AR, Patel T, Fischgrund J, et al: A pilot safety and efficacy study of OP-1 putty (rhBMP-7) as an adjunct to iliac crest autograft in posterolateral lumbar fusions. *Eur Spine J* 2003;12(5):495-500.

47. Boraiah S, Paul O, Hawkes D, Wickham M, Lorich DG: Complications of recombinant human BMP-2 for treating complex tibial plateau fractures: A preliminary report. *Clin Orthop Relat Res* 2009;467(12):3257-3262.

    Treatment with BMP-2 increased the incidence of heterotopic ossification in tibial plateau fractures.

48. Cahill KS, Chi JH, Day A, Claus EB: Prevalence, complications, and hospital charges associated with use of bone-morphogenetic proteins in spinal fusion procedures. *JAMA* 2009;302(1):58-66.

    BMPs were used in approximately 25% of all spine fusions in 2006 in the United States; use was associated with a greater frequency of complications after anterior cervical fusion and higher costs after all types of fusions.

49. Shields LB, Raque GH, Glassman SD, et al: Adverse effects associated with high-dose recombinant human bone morphogenetic protein-2 use in anterior cervical spine fusion. *Spine (Phila Pa 1976)* 2006;31(5):542-547.

    BMP use in anterior cervical spine fusion is associated with swelling that can obstruct the airway.

50. Perri B, Cooper M, Lauryssen C, Anand N: Adverse swelling associated with use of rh-BMP-2 in anterior cervical discectomy and fusion: A case study. *Spine J* 2007;7(2):235-239.

    A 54-year-old patient had severe neck swelling after cervical spine fusion involving rhBMP-2 application.

51. Smucker JD, Rhee JM, Singh K, Yoon ST, Heller JG: Increased swelling complications associated with off-label usage of rhBMP-2 in the anterior cervical spine. *Spine (Phila Pa 1976)* 2006;31(24):2813-2819.

    A retrospective evaluation of swelling in 234 patients who underwent cervical spine fusion found that clinically significant swelling occurred after 27.5% of procedures involving rhBMP-2, compared with 3.6% of control procedures.

52. Pradhan BB, Bae HW, Dawson EG, Patel VV, Delamarter RB: Graft resorption with the use of bone morphogenetic protein: Lessons from anterior lumbar interbody fusion using femoral ring allografts and recombinant human bone morphogenetic protein-2. *Spine (Phila Pa 1976)* 2006;31(10):E277-E284.

    When BMPs were used with structural allograft, BMP-associated resorption interfered with fixation and outcome.

53. Vaidya R, Weir R, Sethi A, Meisterling S, Hakeos W, Wybo CD: Interbody fusion with allograft and rhBMP-2 leads to consistent fusion but early subsidence. *J Bone Joint Surg Br* 2007;89(3):342-345.

    A nonrandomized sequential study examined spine fusion with allograft or autograft and rhBMP-2. Early subsidence was noted in the patients treated with rhBMP-2.

54. Laursen M, Høy K, Hansen ES, Gelineck J, Christensen FB, Bünger CE: Recombinant bone morphogenetic protein-7 as an intracorporal bone growth stimulator in unstable thoracolumbar burst fractures in humans: Preliminary results. *Eur Spine J* 1999;8(6):485-490.

55. Little DG, Ramachandran M, Schindeler A: The anabolic and catabolic responses in bone repair. *J Bone Joint Surg Br* 2007;89(4):425-433.

    This key review discusses the application of an anabolic-catabolic concept of bone to orthopaedic medicine and adjunctive drug therapies.

56. Chen WJ, Jingushi S, Hirata G, Matsumoto Y, Iwamoto Y: Intramuscular bone induction by the simultaneous administration of recombinant human bone morphogenetic protein 2 and bisphosphonate for autobone graft. *Tissue Eng* 2004;10(11-12):1652-1661.

57. Jeppsson C, Astrand J, Tägil M, Aspenberg P: A combination of bisphosphonate and BMP additives in impacted bone allografts. *Acta Orthop Scand* 2003;74(4):483-489.

58. Yu PB, Deng DY, Lai CS, et al: BMP type I receptor inhibition reduces heterotopic [corrected] ossification. *Nat Med* 2008;14(12):1363-1369.

    A BMP type I receptor inhibitor was effective in treating a mouse model of fibrodysplasia ossificans progressiva.

59. Shimono K, Morrison TN, Tung WE, et al: Inhibition of ectopic bone formation by a selective retinoic acid receptor alpha-agonist: A new therapy for heterotopic ossification? *J Orthop Res* 2010;28(2):271-277.

    Ectopic bone formed by rhBMP-2 could be inhibited using NRX195183, a potent and highly selective RAR-α agonist.

60. Schindeler A, Ramachandran M, Godfrey C, et al: Modeling bone morphogenetic protein and bisphosphonate combination therapy in wild-type and Nf1 haploinsufficient mice. *J Orthop Res* 2008;26(1):65-74.

    A preclinical animal study found that rhBMP-2 is less effective in an NF1-deficient mouse model but revealed a dramatic retention of BMP-induced bone by cotreatment with zoledronic acid.

61. Lee FY, Sinicropi SM, Lee FS, Vitale MG, Roye DP Jr, Choi IH: Treatment of congenital pseudarthrosis of the tibia with recombinant human bone morphogenetic protein-7 (rhBMP-7): A report of five cases. *J Bone Joint Surg Am* 2006;88(3):627-633.

    In a small case study, treatment with rhBMP-7 had limited success in patients with congenital pseudarthrosis of the tibia.

62. Kujala S, Vähäsarja V, Serlo W, Jalovaara P: Treatment of congenital pseudarthrosis of the tibia with native bovine BMP: A case report. *Acta Orthop Belg* 2008;74(1):132-136.

In an anecdotal report, a 7-year-old boy with congenital pseudarthrosis of the tibia was treated using native bovine BMP extract.

63. Anticevic D, Jelic M, Vukicevic S: Treatment of a congenital pseudarthrosis of the tibia by osteogenic protein-1 (bone morphogenetic protein-7): A case report. *J Pediatr Orthop B* 2006;15(3):220-221.

Persistent congenital pseudarthrosis of the tibia in an 11-year-old boy was successfully treated using rhBMP-7 and an external frame.

64. Fabeck L, Ghafil D, Gerroudj M, Baillon R, Delincé P: Bone morphogenetic protein 7 in the treatment of congenital pseudarthrosis of the tibia. *J Bone Joint Surg Br* 2006;88(1):116-118.

Persistent congenital pseudarthrosis of the tibia in a 9-year-old boy was successfully treated using rhBMP-7 and autologous bone graft.

65. Richards BS, Oetgen ME, Johnston CE: The use of rhBMP-2 for the treatment of congenital pseudarthrosis of the tibia: A case series. *J Bone Joint Surg Am* 2010;92(1):177-185.

Five of seven patients with congenital pseudarthrosis treated with intramedullary rod fixation, autogenous bone grafting, and the application of BMP-2 in a collagen sponge had union at the index procedure, and one had union in a subsequent application.

66. Lu DC, Sun PP: Bone morphogenetic protein for salvage fusion in an infant with Down syndrome and craniovertebral instability: Case report. *J Neurosurg* 2007;106(suppl 6):480-483.

A 4-month-old boy with Down syndrome was treated with BMP-induced fusion of the craniovertebral junction after two unsuccessful operations resulting in a nonunion.

67. Oetgen ME, Richards BS: Complications associated with the use of bone morphogenetic protein in pediatric patients. *J Pediatr Orthop* 2010;30(2):192-198.

The use of BMP-2 in children and adolescents was associated with typical complications, only one of which was attributed to BMP use.

68. Bleuming SA, He XC, Kodach LL, et al: Bone morphogenetic protein signaling suppresses tumorigenesis at gastric epithelial transition zones in mice. *Cancer Res* 2007;67(17):8149-8155.

Conditional knockout of *BMPR-1a* in the stomachs of mice led to neoplastic lesions, suggesting BMPR-1A signaling is important for suppressing tumorigenesis.

69. Buijs JT, Rentsch CA, van der Horst G, et al: BMP7, a putative regulator of epithelial homeostasis in the human prostate, is a potent inhibitor of prostate cancer bone metastasis in vivo. *Am J Pathol* 2007;171(3):1047-1057.

BMP-7 was found to be upregulated in primary human prostate cancer samples. In a nude mouse model, BMP-7 administration inhibited the growth of cancer cells in bone.

70. Jones AL, Bucholz RW, Bosse MJ, et al: Recombinant human BMP-2 and allograft compared with autogenous bone graft for reconstruction of diaphyseal tibial fractures with cortical defects: A randomized, controlled trial. *J Bone Joint Surg Am* 2006;88(7):1431-1441.

Antibodies to bovine collagen were detected in a randomized controlled trial for BMP-2.

Chapter 7

Bisphosphonate Treatment in Children and Adolescents

Frank Rauch, MD

Introduction

The drugs classified as bisphosphonates are primarily used to treat adult skeletal disorders such as postmenopausal osteoporosis, Paget disease, and skeletal metastasis. Bisphosphonates also have been used off-label during the past 20 years to treat a range of disorders in children and adolescents, particularly osteogenesis imperfecta (OI).

Bisphosphonates

Chemical Structure and Types

Bisphosphonates are potent antiresorptive agents that inhibit osteoclast function.[1] The chemical structure of all bisphosphonates is based on a phosphorus-calcium-phosphorus base molecule that resembles the phosphorus-oxygen-phosphorus structure of pyrophosphate. Pyrophosphate is a naturally occurring molecule involved in the mineralization process (**Figure 1**). The chemical structure of bisphosphonates explains their affinity for mineralized surfaces.

The members of the bisphosphonate family differ in the structure of the two side chains (R_1 and R_2) attached to the base molecule.[1] More than a dozen types of bisphosphonates have been used clinically; some of the currently popular bisphosphonates are listed in **Table 1**. For clinical purposes, a bisphosphonate can be classified as oral or intravenous. This distinction reflects the marketing decisions of the pharmaceutical companies that produce bisphosphonates rather than fundamental differences among the physicochemical characteristics of the compounds.

Pharmacokinetics

Orally administered bisphosphonates are poorly absorbed by the digestive system. Studies of adults found that the bioavailability of oral bisphosphonates is ap-

proximately 1%.[1] The findings were similar in children with OI; the mean oral bioavailability of alendronate tablets was found to be approximately 0.6%. Individual bioavailability varied widely in children, however, ranging from 0.2% to 2.0%.[2] Therefore, the amount of systemically active bisphosphonate after oral administration can differ between patients by a factor of 10. To circumvent this variability in the amount of drug reaching systemic circulation, bisphosphonates can be administered by intravenous infusion.[3]

Bisphosphonates are rapidly cleared from the circulation, whether they are administered orally or intravenously.[1] They are resistant to enzymatic and chemical breakdown and therefore are not metabolized in the body. Approximately half of the systemically administered dose is taken up by the skeleton, and the other half is excreted unmetabolized through the kidneys. The distribution of bisphosphonates in the skeleton depends on the metabolic activity of bone and the regional blood flow. Consequently, there is greater deposition of the drug in the growth plate region.

Mechanism of Action

Bisphosphonates primarily act on the bone-resorbing osteoclasts, which are the only type of cells that take up large quantities of bone mineral. The drug becomes attached to mineralized surfaces and subsequently is taken up by osteoclasts.[1] Once inside the osteoclasts, bisphosphonates interfere with biochemical processes.

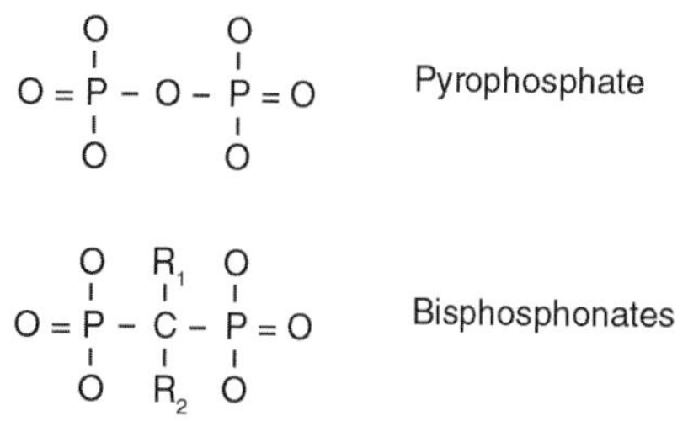

Figure 1 The chemical structures of pyrophosphate and bisphosphonates.

Dr. Rauch or an immediate family member has received research or institutional support from Novartis and Procter & Gamble.

Table 1

Commonly Used Bisphosphonates

Drug	Trade Name (Manufacturer)	Method of Administration
Alendronate	Fosamax (Merck, Whitehouse Station, NJ)	Oral
Ibandronate	Boniva (Roche, Nutley, NJ)	Oral
Pamidronate	Aredia (Novartis, East Hanover, NJ)	Intravenous
Risedronate	Actonel (Proctor & Gamble, Cincinnati, OH)	Oral
Zoledronic acid	Reclast (Novartis, East Hanover, NJ)	Intravenous

Bisphosphonates that contain nitrogen in the R_2 side chain act by interfering with farnesyl pyrophosphate synthase, an intercellular enzyme that has a key role in the functioning of important intracellular proteins. Most of the newer bisphosphonates, including those listed in **Table 1**, belong to the nitrogen-containing group. Non–nitrogen-containing bisphosphonates act by incorporation into adenosine triphosphate. Loss of osteoclast activity ensues after either type of bisphosphonate is administered.

The bisphosphonates differ in how strongly they inhibit farnesyl pyrophosphate synthase or bind to hydroxyapatite.[1] This factor may explain the variations in retention and persistence of effect among the bisphosphonates. For example, zoledronic acid binds to bone mineral more strongly than do other bisphosphonates and, consequently, is the most potent available bisphosphonate.

The bisphosphonate molecules that are not immediately taken up by osteoclasts can remain buried in bone mineral for many years.[1] When the bone mineral eventually is resorbed, the drug is released and can inhibit osteoclast activity. This turnover may explain the long duration of action of these drugs. Bisphosphonates are released from bone very slowly; pamidronate was detected in urine samples of young patients as late as 8 years after the cessation of treatment.[4]

The effect of bisphosphonates on individual osteoclasts presumably is similar in children and adults, although the effect on bone mass and density is much more dramatic in children.[5] The explanation is that bisphosphonates act on bone modeling and endochondral ossification, both of which primarily occur in growing children. Modeling is the shaping mechanism through which, for example, the shaft of a long bone is increased in diameter. The actions of osteoblasts and osteoclasts are not directly coupled in modeling. Therefore, bisphosphonates can be used to inhibit the action of osteoclasts without interfering with the action of osteoblasts. In growing children treated with bisphosphonates, the result is a marked increase in cortical thickness. In contrast, bone metabolic activity in adults is largely limited to remodeling, in which osteoblast activity is coupled to earlier osteoclast action. Using bisphosphonates to inhibit the action of osteoclasts leads to a decrease in bone formation, and the gains in bone mass are modest.

In growing children, bisphosphonate treatment not only affects the cortical bone but also increases the number of trabeculae in the metaphysis.[5] Bone resorption normally is very active immediately adjacent to the growth plate, where most of the primary trabeculae formed by endochondral ossification are completely remodeled into mature trabeculae. During bisphosphonate treatment, a larger percentage of primary trabeculae survive because the remodeling process is inhibited. The persistence of primary trabeculae and calcified cartilage produces radiodense metaphyseal lines below the growth plate in children receiving periodic bisphosphonate therapy. This effect is specific to children because it requires the presence of an active growth plate.

Pediatric Indications for Bisphosphonate Treatment

Bisphosphonates have been used in growing children for treating three types of conditions, with three distinct goals: in acute hypercalcemia, to decrease serum calcium levels; in conditions that lead to general low bone mass and bone fragility, to increase bone mass; and in localized bone disorders, usually to prevent bone removal or to decrease bone turnover.

Hypercalcemia

Intravenous bisphosphonates have been successfully used to treat hypercalcemia secondary to a wide variety of conditions, as reported in many pediatric case studies.[6] For a child with acute hypercalcemia, bisphosphonates are used to diminish the influx of calcium into the circulatory system and thereby to quickly decrease bone resorption. A decrease in serum calcium levels was observed within a few hours to a few days after the infusion, depending on the type of bisphosphonate and the dosage.[6]

Bone Fragility

General bone fragility can be a primary disorder, most often caused by a genetic defect, or it can occur as a result of a wide variety of chronic conditions.

Osteogenesis Imperfecta

As the prototype of primary general bone fragility disorder, OI is the condition for which pediatric bisphosphonate use has been most studied. Usually, OI is caused by a mutation affecting collagen type I production in osteoblasts. The hypothesis underlying the use of an antiosteoclast medication in osteoblast disorders such as OI is that a decrease in the activity of the bone-resorbing system can compensate for the weakness of the bone-forming cells. Physical therapy and surgical intervention remain the mainstay treatments for OI, but bisphosphonate treatment has been established as a beneficial supportive therapy.[5] Consequently, the use of bisphosphonates has become a de facto standard of care for severe forms of OI.

Pamidronate is the most widely used bisphosphonate in children with OI. Several intravenous regimens are used. The most-studied regimen consists of a 3-day cycle of infusions administered every 2 to 4 months, depending on the age of the patient.[5] Most reports agree that intravenous pamidronate infusions lead to a marked and rapid decrease in chronic bone pain, a rapid rise in vertebral bone mineral mass, and an increased sense of well-being. Collapsed vertebral bodies regain a relatively normal size and shape. At present there is insufficient evidence to judge the effect of bisphosphonate treatment on the incidence of long bone fractures. Some studies reported that mobility improved in more than half of the patients treated with intravenous pamidronate.[7,8] It is unknown whether pamidronate treatment delays the progression of scoliosis.

Intravenous bisphosphonates other than pamidronate recently have been investigated. In a randomized study, the use of neridronate, which is similar to pamidronate but is available in only a few countries, was found to lead to higher bone mineral density and a decrease in the overall number of fractures in children with OI.[9]

Zoledronic acid, a newer intravenously administered bisphosphonate, is marketed for the treatment of postmenopausal osteoporosis. The available evidence suggests that the effects of zoledronic acid are similar to those of pamidronate. The primary advantages of using zoledronic acid are that each cycle consists of a single infusion requiring less than 1 hour (rather than the usual pamidronate cycle of three infusions on 3 successive days) and that the interval between cycles is 6 to 12 months (rather than 2 to 4 months).

Oral bisphosphonates also have been studied in children with OI. Small observational studies found that orally administered alendronate increases bone mineral density in the lumbar spine and decreases the number of fractures in children with OI. Oral olpadronate, a bisphosphonate that is not widely available, was tested in a randomized, placebo-controlled study of 34 children and adolescents with OI.[10] After 2 years, the patients who received active treatment had a higher bone mineral density in the lumbar spine and a lower incidence of long bone fractures. No difference was detected in functional outcomes such as mobility and muscle force. A recent placebo-controlled study of pediatric patients with mild OI found that treatment with oral risedronate led to significantly increased lumbar spine bone density but had no effect on the fracture rate.[11]

Secondary Osteoporosis

Low bone mass and bone fragility can result from many chronic diseases of childhood and adolescence. Many clinicians use bisphosphonates to treat secondary forms of osteoporosis, despite the relative lack of scientific evidence. Several observational studies and a few small randomized studies assessed the effect of different bisphosphonates on bone fragility secondary to cerebral palsy, Duchenne muscular dystrophy, extensive burns, rheumatologic disease, chronic graft-versus-host disease after hematopoietic cell transplantation, or steroid-induced osteoporosis.[3] Almost invariably, bisphosphonate treatment was found to lead to higher bone mineral density. However, none of the studies had sufficient power to determine more clinically relevant outcomes such as fracture rate, pain, or mobility. A systematic review concluded that the data are insufficient to support the standard use of bisphosphonate therapy for children with secondary osteoporosis; nonetheless, the short-term safety and efficacy data (extending as long as 3 years) were believed to be sufficient to justify the use of bisphosphonates as a compassionate measure in patients with severe bone fragility.[12]

Local Conditions

The immediate goal of bisphosphonate treatment for OI or secondary osteoporosis is to systemically improve bone mass. These drugs also have been used to treat more local conditions.

Fibrous Dysplasia

Observational studies found that treatment with intravenous pamidronate is promising for adults with fibrous dysplasia; the patients had decreased intensity of bone pain and a radiographically apparent refilling of osteolytic sites.[13] It is unclear whether bisphosphonates work as well in children with fibrous dysplasia. Refilling of dysplastic lesions appears to occur rarely, if ever, in growing children; most lesions increase in size despite bisphosphonate therapy. However, bisphosphonates usually are effective in decreasing the bone pain associated with fibrous dysplasia, and this beneficial effect may provide a sufficient rationale for offering bisphosphonate therapy.[14]

Chronic Recurrent Multifocal Osteomyelitis

Chronic recurrent multifocal osteomyelitis is an idiopathic, aseptic, inflammatory bone condition that can cause significant bone pain, a reduction in bone mass, and vertebral compression fracturing. Recent observational studies suggest that intravenous pamidronate may be useful in treating patients with significant vertebral involvement.[15]

Distraction Osteogenesis

In animal studies of distraction osteogenesis, the use of an intravenous bisphosphonate was found to improve the mechanical properties of newly formed bone.[16] Distraction osteogenesis stimulates both bone formation and bone resorption; this factor probably accounts for the beneficial effect of bisphosphonates. Clinical experience with bisphosphonate treatment for distraction osteogenesis is limited. However, intravenous administration of pamidronate or zoledronic acid was associated with regenerate healing in some patients with protracted regenerate insufficiency.[17]

Osteonecrosis

In patients with femoral head osteonecrosis, osteoclastic resorption of necrotic subchondral bone can lead to mechanical weakening and collapse of the femoral head. Several animal studies found that inhibition of osteoclast activity by bisphosphonates can attenuate or prevent the collapse and improve functional outcomes.[18,19] Observational studies in children and adolescents with traumatic osteonecrosis of the femoral head found that intravenous pamidronate or zoledronic acid therapy was associated with preservation of femoral head sphericity in some patients.[20] However, it is difficult to judge the contribution of the bisphosphonate to these outcomes in the absence of data from randomized studies. The blood supply is impaired in femoral head osteonecrosis, and intravenous application of bisphosphonates therefore may be less effective than administration of bisphosphonates directly into the lesion.[21] Although animal studies using this approach yielded encouraging results, clinical data are lacking.

Adverse Effects of Pediatric Bisphosphonate Treatment

A bisphosphonate infusion causes an immediate decrease in serum calcium levels, often to values slightly below the reference range. However, clinical manifestations of this effect are rare in patients with an adequate vitamin D level and good calcium intake. Many children experience flulike fever, rash, and vomiting after the first pamidronate infusion, typically 12 to 36 hours after the infusion began.[5] Usually these symptoms can be controlled with standard antipyretic therapy and do not recur with later treatments. This reaction may be of concern in an infant or young child with respiratory difficulty or a compromised general condition.

The growth-suppressive effect of high-dosage bisphosphonates in animals is well known, and there was initial concern about the long-term safety of bisphosphonate treatment in humans. Fortunately, no negative effect of bisphosphonate treatment on growth has been detected in children.[22]

Antiresorptive drugs such as bisphosphonates inevitably decrease bone-remodeling activity. A sustained decrease in remodeling activity during growth may be harmful over the long term. The remnants of mineralized growth plate cartilage accumulate in trabecular bone. Because calcified cartilage is less resistant to fracturing than is normal bone, theoretically the bone could become more brittle after prolonged bisphosphonate use.

Bisphosphonate treatment in growing children is associated with several radiologic and histologic adverse effects, including metaphyseal lines corresponding to each bisphosphonate infusion, modeling defects at the metaphyses, and the presence of unusually large osteoclasts in bone tissue. The clinical significance of these findings is unclear.

Because bisphosphonates remain in the skeleton for many years, their effect on female reproductive health is of concern. It is unknown whether bisphosphonate released from the maternal skeleton affects a fetus. A recent review of the available studies found 51 patients who had been exposed to bisphosphonates before or during pregnancy. No signs of skeletal abnormality or other congenital malformation were detected in the infants, but the limited number of patients did not allow full assessment of the reproductive risk of bisphosphonate treatment.[23] Adolescent girls should use an effective means of birth control while receiving bisphosphonates, and each bisphosphonate infusion should be preceded by a pregnancy test.

Osteonecrosis of the jaw has been reported in adults who received bisphosphonates, particularly in patients being treated for cancer. Osteonecrosis of the jaw has not been reported in children or adolescents who received bisphosphonate treatment. Bisphosphonate therapy during early childhood may delay the eruption of secondary teeth, but the clinical significance of the delay is unknown.[24]

The standard pamidronate treatment was found not to delay the healing of spontaneous fractures but possibly to delay osteotomy healing in children with OI.[25] It may be prudent to avoid bisphosphonate treatment after an osteotomy until the osteotomy site is well consolidated. The effect of bisphosphonate treatment on consolidation after spinal fusion has not been systematically assessed. However, some centers have adopted a policy of refraining from administering bisphosphonates during the first 4 months after spinal fusion to avoid interference with bone healing.

Selecting an Intravenous or Oral Bisphosphonate

The choice of an intravenous or oral bisphosphonate to some extent depends on the clinical context. An intravenous bisphosphonate is the obvious choice if rapid action is important, as it is in treating hypercalcemia or regenerate failure in distraction osteogenesis. Both oral and intravenous bisphosphonates are acceptable for the long-term treatment of a chronic condition. Little published evidence is available to guide the selection of a bisphosphonate regimen. The studies that directly compared the efficacy and safety of different therapeutic approaches were too small to detect any differences between oral and intravenous therapy.[26] Many clinicians believe that intravenous pamidronate has a more marked effect on bone pain than oral bisphosphonate therapy and that bone mineral density increases more quickly when intravenous treatment is used.

Oral treatment has practical advantages over intravenous infusion if the patient is able to swallow pills and observe requirements such as drinking a large glass of water with the pill and maintaining an upright position for at least 30 minutes thereafter. The drawbacks of oral therapy include uncertain compliance, low and variable drug bioavailability, and the possibility of gastrointestinal adverse effects. Oral treatment exposes the skeleton to small, frequent doses of medication, whereas intravenous treatment provides larger doses with less frequency. In growing children, this difference results in specific radiographic features: intravenous treatment leads to discrete metaphyseal lines that correspond to horizontal trabecula, and oral treatment can lead to a blurry zone of dense-appearing bone adjacent to the growth plate (**Figure 2**). It is unknown whether there are other differences in the skeletal effects of oral and intravenous bisphosphonate therapy in children.

Duration of Treatment

The duration of bisphosphonate therapy depends on the condition for which the drug is used. A single dose of an intravenous bisphosphonate often is sufficient to treat hypercalcemia or regenerate failure after distraction osteogenesis. If the purpose of bisphosphonate therapy is to increase bone mass after high-dose steroid therapy or a transient condition, it is reasonable to discontinue the treatment when the transient condition improves.

The decision to stop bisphosphonate treatment is more difficult if the underlying condition, such as OI, is unlikely to improve. In a growing child, the bone produced after treatment is not exposed to the drug and therefore is of lower density than the bone that was present during therapy. The result can be localized bone weaknesses, especially in the metaphyses of long bones. Several children were reported to have metaphyseal fractures after bisphosphonate treatment ended.[27] Growing patients with OI who received bisphosphonates for several years frequently report lack of stamina and a recurrence of bone pain after cessation of treatment. These symptoms appear to diminish in importance after growth plate activity ceases.

The negative effects of treatment cessation must be weighed against the risks associated with prolonged bisphosphonate therapy. The policy in some institutions is to decrease the bisphosphonate dosage after 2 to 4 years of treatment and to continue a maintenance regimen as long as growth continues. It is unknown

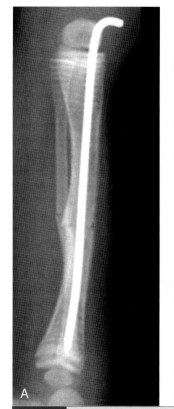
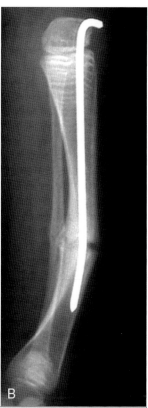

| Figure 2 | Intramedullary rodding of the tibia was done in a 3-year-old boy with OI type IV, and the child received pamidronate treatment. **A,** One year after the surgical intervention, the osteotomy site is still visible. **B,** Two years after the intervention, the osteotomy site has opened further and deformity has occurred. The metaphyseal lines resulting from each pamidronate infusion cycle are visible. |

whether this approach is effective in preventing either fractures or adverse effects.

Summary

Bisphosphonates have been used in growing children for the treatment of acute hypercalcemia, conditions that lead to generalized low bone mass, and some localized bone disorders causing high bone turnover. Most of the published research pertains to the treatment of OI, in which bisphosphonate treatment appears to decrease fracture incidence. The clinical research for most other pediatric indications is limited to small case studies. Although few adverse treatment effects have been reported in children, bisphosphonate use may delay the healing of osteotomy sites. It may be prudent to delay bisphosphonate treatment after an osteotomy until the site is well consolidated. In considering the use of bisphosphonates, the risk of unknown long-term adverse effects must be weighed against the severity of the condition.

2: Basic Science

Annotated References

1. Russell RG: Bisphosphonates: Mode of action and pharmacology. *Pediatrics* 2007;119(suppl 2):S150-S162.

   The pharmacology of bisphosphonates is described, with a focus on pediatric treatment.

2. Ward LM, Denker AE, Porras A, et al: Single-dose pharmacokinetics and tolerability of alendronate 35- and 70-milligram tablets in children and adolescents with osteogenesis imperfecta type I. *J Clin Endocrinol Metab* 2005;90(7):4051-4056.

   This is the only study of bisphosphonate pharmacokinetics in children. Approximately 1% of orally administered alendronate was found to enter the systemic circulation.

3. Bachrach LK, Ward LM: Clinical review 1: Bisphosphonate use in childhood osteoporosis. *J Clin Endocrinol Metab* 2009;94(2):400-409.

   This is an overview of bisphosphonate treatment in children who have osteoporosis secondary to a chronic disorder.

4. Papapoulos SE, Cremers SC: Prolonged bisphosphonate release after treatment in children. *N Engl J Med* 2007;356(10):1075-1076.

5. Rauch F, Glorieux FH: Osteogenesis imperfecta. *Lancet* 2004;363(9418):1377-1385.

6. Shaw NJ, Bishop NJ: Bisphosphonate treatment of bone disease. *Arch Dis Child* 2005;90(5):494-499.

   Approximately 124 clinical practice and research articles on the pediatric use of bisphosphonates were published before this article, almost 100 of them since 1997.

7. Glorieux FH, Bishop NJ, Plotkin H, Chabot G, Lanoue G, Travers R: Cyclic administration of pamidronate in children with severe osteogenesis imperfecta. *N Engl J Med* 1998;339(14):947-952.

8. Land C, Rauch F, Montpetit K, Ruck-Gibis J, Glorieux FH: Effect of intravenous pamidronate therapy on functional abilities and level of ambulation in children with osteogenesis imperfecta. *J Pediatr* 2006;148(4):456-460.

   A 3-year study of 59 children with moderate or severe OI found that cyclic treatment with pamidronate improved mobility, ambulation, and muscle force.

9. Gatti D, Antoniazzi F, Prizzi R, et al: Intravenous neridronate in children with osteogenesis imperfecta: A randomized controlled study. *J Bone Miner Res* 2005;20(5):758-763.

   A 3-year randomized controlled study of 64 children with OI found that quarterly infusions of neridronate led to increased bone mineral density and decreased risk of fracture.

10. Sakkers R, Kok D, Engelbert R, et al: Skeletal effects and functional outcome with olpadronate in children with osteogenesis imperfecta: A 2-year randomised placebo-controlled study. *Lancet* 2004;363(9419):1427-1431.

11. Rauch F, Munns CF, Land C, Cheung M, Glorieux FH: Risedronate in the treatment of mild pediatric osteogenesis imperfecta: A randomized placebo-controlled study. *J Bone Miner Res* 2009;24(7):1282-1289.

    Risedronate was found to increase bone mineral density but not to lower the risk of fracture in children with mild OI.

12. Ward L, Tricco AC, Phuong P, et al: Bisphosphonate therapy for children and adolescents with secondary osteoporosis. *Cochrane Database Syst Rev* 2007;4:CD005324.

    Nine studies were examined and found not to support the use of bisphosphonates as standard therapy in children with secondary osteoporosis. Short-term use (3 years or less) was well tolerated.

13. Chapurlat RD, Hugueny P, Delmas PD, Meunier PJ: Treatment of fibrous dysplasia of bone with intravenous pamidronate: Long-term effectiveness and evaluation of predictors of response to treatment. *Bone* 2004;35(1):235-242.

14. Plotkin H, Rauch F, Zeitlin L, Munns C, Travers R, Glorieux FH: Effect of pamidronate treatment in children with polyostotic fibrous dysplasia of bone. *J Clin Endocrinol Metab* 2003;88(10):4569-4575.

15. Gleeson H, Wiltshire E, Briody J, et al: Childhood chronic recurrent multifocal osteomyelitis: Pamidronate therapy decreases pain and improves vertebral shape. *J Rheumatol* 2008;35(4):707-712.

    Seven children with chronic recurrent multifocal osteomyelitis benefited from intravenous pamidronate treatment.

16. Little DG, Smith NC, Williams PR, et al: Zoledronic acid prevents osteopenia and increases bone strength in a rabbit model of distraction osteogenesis. *J Bone Miner Res* 2003;18(7):1300-1307.

17. Kiely P, Ward K, Bellemore CM, Briody J, Cowell CT, Little DG: Bisphosphonate rescue in distraction osteogenesis: A case series. *J Pediatr Orthop* 2007;27(4):467-471.

    In six of seven patients with protracted regenerate insufficiency after distraction osteogenesis, the regenerate healed rapidly after bisphosphonate infusion.

18. Kim HK, Randall TS, Bian H, Jenkins J, Garces A, Bauss F: Ibandronate for prevention of femoral head deformity after ischemic necrosis of the capital femoral epiphysis in immature pigs. *J Bone Joint Surg Am* 2005;87(3):550-557.

    In a piglet model, radiographic and histomorphometric assessment revealed that ibandronate treatment prevented femoral head deformity and preserved the trabecular structure of the osseous epiphysis early in the repair of ischemic necrosis.

19. Little DG, McDonald M, Sharpe IT, Peat R, Williams P, McEvoy T: Zoledronic acid improves femoral head sphericity in a rat model of perthes disease. *J Orthop Res* 2005;23(4):862-868.

Treatment with zoledronic acid favorably altered femoral head shape in an established rat model of Perthes disease. In children with Perthes disease, the need for surgical intervention might be reduced by using zoledronic acid.

20. Ramachandran M, Ward K, Brown RR, Munns CF, Cowell CT, Little DG: Intravenous bisphosphonate therapy for traumatic osteonecrosis of the femoral head in adolescents. *J Bone Joint Surg Am* 2007;89(8):1727-1734.

In this observational study, adolescents with traumatic osteonecrosis of the femoral head were found to have a positive outcome after treatment with intravenous bisphosphonate.

21. Kim HK, Sanders M, Athavale S, Bian H, Bauss F: Local bioavailability and distribution of systemically (parenterally) administered ibandronate in the infarcted femoral head. *Bone* 2006;39(1):205-212.

In a piglet model, induced ischemic osteonecrosis of the femoral head was followed by ibandronate administration at 1, 3, and 6 weeks. Revascularization and repair were found to produce significant alterations in ibandronate local bioavailability and distribution.

22. Zeitlin L, Rauch F, Plotkin H, Glorieux FH: Height and weight development during four years of therapy with cyclical intravenous pamidronate in children and adolescents with osteogenesis imperfecta types I, III, and IV. *Pediatrics* 2003;111(5, pt 1):1030-1036.

23. Djokanovic N, Klieger-Grossmann C, Koren G: Does treatment with bisphosphonates endanger the human pregnancy? *J Obstet Gynaecol Can* 2008;30(12):1146-1148.

A search of the Medline and Embase databases identified 51 incidences of maternal exposure to bisphosphonates before or during pregnancy. No skeletal or other abnormalities were identified in the infants.

24. Kamoun-Goldrat A, Ginisty D, Le Merrer M: Effects of bisphosphonates on tooth eruption in children with osteogenesis imperfecta. *Eur J Oral Sci* 2008;116(3):195-198.

Tooth emergence was analyzed in 33 children with OI who were treated with bisphosphonates, compared with strictly matched control subjects. The children treated with bisphosphonates had a mean 1.67-year delay in tooth eruption.

25. Munns CF, Rauch F, Zeitlin L, Fassier F, Glorieux FH: Delayed osteotomy but not fracture healing in pediatric osteogenesis imperfecta patients receiving pamidronate. *J Bone Miner Res* 2004;19(11):1779-1786.

26. DiMeglio LA, Peacock M: Two-year clinical trial of oral alendronate versus intravenous pamidronate in children with osteogenesis imperfecta. *J Bone Miner Res* 2006;21(1):132-140.

Oral and intravenous bisphosphonates were found to have equivalent effectiveness in children with OI. Children with mild OI had a greater response to therapy than those with severe OI.

27. Rauch F, Cornibert S, Cheung M, Glorieux FH: Long-bone changes after pamidronate discontinuation in children and adolescents with osteogenesis imperfecta. *Bone* 2007;40(4):821-827.

Bone density in the metaphysis of the radius was found to decrease rapidly after pamidronate treatment was discontinued in growing children, and some patients had a subsequent metaphyseal fracture.

2: Basic Science

Chapter 8
Skeletal Dysplasias

Wagner A.R. Baratela, MD   William G. Mackenzie, MD

Introduction

The skeletal dysplasias are a large, heterogeneous group of bone disorders with a proven or probable genetic basis. The most recent "Nosology and Classification of Genetic Skeletal Disorders"[1] included 372 different skeletal dysplasias classified into 37 groups defined by clinical, radiographic, histopathologic, biochemical, and molecular criteria. An abnormality of skeletal development can be categorized as dysostosis (malformation of a single bone caused by signaling factor expression during embryogenesis), disruption (caused by a toxic substance or infectious agent), or dysplasia (caused by postnatal expression of a defect in a prenatally expressing gene).[2] Although individual skeletal dysplasias are rare, as a group they are significant in number, with a prevalence of approximately 2 to 3 per 10,000 newborns.[3] The inheritance pattern is variable and may be autosomal dominant, autosomal recessive, or X linked. Some teratogenic exposures, such as maternal lupus erythematosus and uniparental disomy, can mimic skeletal dysplasia as a phenocopy.[4]

Clinical Evaluation

Growth deficiency or short stature is a major concern to parents, and the possibility of a disorder in skeletal development or the endocrine system must be considered. The evaluation should include the patient and family history, a physical examination, and full skeletal radiographs, if indicated. It is important to determine whether the growth deficiency is of prenatal or postnatal onset. Some skeletal dysplasias, such as achondroplasia and diastrophic dysplasia, are evident at birth, but others, such as hypochondroplasia, usually are diagnosed later in childhood. All findings from the pa-

tient's history and physical examination should be evaluated in relation to other family members.

The evaluation should include the patient's anthropometric measurements: occipitofrontal circumference, weight, standing and sitting heights, arm span, ratio of upper and lower body segments, and ratio of arm span to height. These measurements are helpful in determining whether the growth deficiency is proportionate or disproportionate; skeletal dysplasias frequently are of the latter type. It also is important to classify the limb-shortening pattern based on whether the most affected region of the limb is proximal (rhizomelic), middle (mesomelic), or distal (acromelic).

For a child with proportionate short stature, several possible diagnoses should be considered: intrauterine growth restriction, a dysmorphic syndrome, a chromosomal disorder, malnutrition, a chronic disease, the use of various growth-inhibiting drugs, psychosocial dwarfism (a well-recognized form of growth arrest involving endocrine hormone control and related to child abuse, neglect, or stress), and other endocrine disorders.

The presence of disproportionate short stature should prompt radiographic and bone metabolic assessments. A full skeletal radiographic survey is recommended for purposes of differential diagnosis. The survey should include lateral skull, AP and lateral thorax, complete lateral spine, and AP pelvis, long bones, hands, and feet radiographs. The form, shape, and size of the individual bones should be assessed. Few radiographic findings are specific, however. The skeletal survey is useful in classifying a patient with a skeletal dysplasia as having spondylo-, epiphyseal, metaphyseal, and/or diaphyseal involvement. The skeletal survey also is useful in determining spine involvement (Table 1). Useful diagnostic clues can be derived from other specific radiologic findings including bone age; punctuate calcifications, as in chondrodysplasia punctata; cone-shaped epiphyses of the hand bones, as in type II trichorhinophalangeal syndrome; and abnormal nail size and proportions of the phalanges, as in chondroectodermal dysplasia (Ellis–van Creveld syndrome).

Because skeletal dysplasias involve the growth and development of bones, radiographic findings may be dynamic and age related. Radiographs obtained after the bones have matured often are less useful than those obtained during the growth period. In some patients, the phenotypic expression of a genetic disorder continues to change throughout life. A skeletal survey should

Neither Dr. Baratela nor any immediate family member has received anything of value from or owns stock in a commercial company or institution related directly or indirectly to the subject of this chapter. Dr. Mackenzie or an immediate family member is a member of a speakers' bureau or has made paid presentations on behalf of Smith & Nephew and Biomet; serves as an unpaid consultant to Biomet and Smith & Nephew; and has received research or institutional support from Biomet and DePuy, a Johnson & Johnson company.

2: Basic Science

Table 1

Spine Involvement in the Skeletal Dysplasias

Skeletal Dysplasia	Foramen Magnum Stenosis	Atlantoaxial Instability or Odontoid Hypoplasia	Kyphosis	Kyphoscoliosis	Lordosis	Spinal Stenosis
Achondroplasia	XX		X		X	XX
Hypochondroplasia	X				X	X
Spondyloepiphyseal dysplasia congenita		XX		XX	X	
Stickler syndrome				X		
Diastrophic dysplasia			X	XX	X	X
Pseudoachondroplasia		XX		X		
Osteogenesis Imperfecta				XX		
Mucopolysaccharidosis type IV		XX	X	XX	X	XX

X = may be present, XX = common.

be performed at different ages during infancy and childhood. However, the survey should not be repeated within 12 months of the initial examination.[2]

Bone mineral density must be assessed in some patients. An increased bone density appears in many heterogeneous disorders, such as pycnodysostosis and the various forms of osteopetrosis. Osteopenia characterizes several other disorders, such as the various forms of osteogenesis imperfecta and hypophosphatasia.

Metabolic bone studies should be performed to rule out nutritional rickets (vitamin D deficiency), hypophosphatemic rickets, and hypophosphatasia (alkaline phosphatase deficiency), which may have clinical and radiographic features resembling those of the skeletal dysplasias, including growth failure, brachycephaly, hypotonia, lax ligaments, scoliosis, costochondral enlargement (so-called rachitic rosary), flared metaphyses resulting in thickening of joints, and bowing of long bones.

A biochemical investigation is imperative for obtaining an accurate diagnosis of some skeletal dysplasias, including mucopolysaccharidosis type IV (Morquio-Brailsford syndrome), other mucopolysaccharidoses, mucolipidosis, chondrodysplasia punctata of the Conradi-Hünermann-Happle type (*CDPX2*), and others. Blood and urine are qualitatively screened for oligosaccharides and mucopolysaccharides, but the diagnosis is obtained with quantitative enzyme assays, usually of leukocytes or fibroblasts.[5]

Before the advent of molecular biology, histologic examination of the growth plate cartilage and the extracellular matrix was used to distinguish the phenotypes of conditions with similar clinical and radiologic findings. Molecular biology has revolutionized the nosology and classification of hereditary bone disorders. Genetic testing for the skeletal dysplasias provides not

only accurate diagnostic input but also a better understanding of the pathogenetic mechanisms. Almost 400 different bone conditions are now recognized, of which more than half are associated with 140 different genes.[1] Genetic testing allows better patient management. When fetal abnormalities are found on ultrasonography, genetic testing can be used to confirm or rule out the presence of certain skeletal dysplasias. If the fetus is found to have a lethal form of skeletal dysplasia during the early stages of gestation, the family is able to make a decision regarding pregnancy termination. In addition, the risk of the condition affecting a subsequent pregnancy can be determined.

Specific Skeletal Dysplasias

Achondroplasia

Achondroplasia is the most common skeletal dysplasia, occurring in 1 of every 30,000 live births.[6] The condition is inherited in an autosomal dominant fashion with complete penetrance, and it is associated with advanced paternal age.[7] In the past, the diagnosis of achondroplasia was mistakenly applied to many types of short-limbed dwarfism. The underlying cause has now been well described as a "gain of function" mutation resulting from substitution of an arginine for a glycine residue (the G380R mutation) in the transmembrane domain of fibroblast growth factor receptor-3 (*FGFR3*), located at 4p16.3.[8] Genetic studies using knockout mice revealed that *FGFR3* is a negative regulator of chondrocyte proliferation and differentiation. The mutation activates the receptor function, producing the mutation as well as further inhibition of chondrocyte proliferation and differentiation.[9] The consequent phenotype is a disproportionately short stature

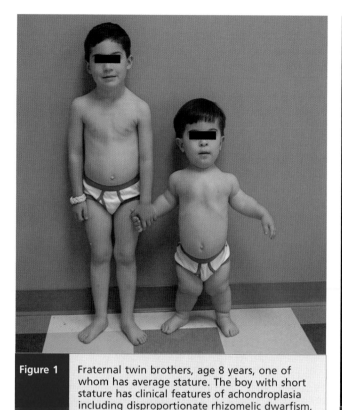

Figure 1 Fraternal twin brothers, age 8 years, one of whom has average stature. The boy with short stature has clinical features of achondroplasia including disproportionate rhizomelic dwarfism, a larger-than-normal cranium, frontal bossing, midface hypoplasia, and excessive skin folding.

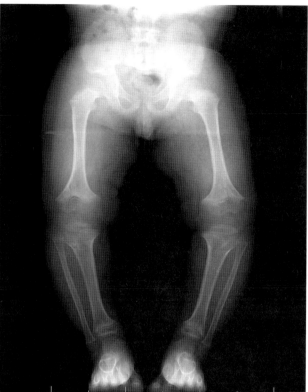

Figure 2 Standing AP radiograph of the lower extremities of a 5-year-old girl with achondroplasia, showing the typical genu vara, short tubular bones with a chevron sign in the distal femora, long fibulae, and squared pelvis with small sacrosciatic notches.

with shortened long bones, especially in the proximal portions, leading to rhizomelia (**Figure 1**). Frontal bossing, macrocephaly, hypoplasia of the midface, a short nasal dorsum, a trident shape of the hands, and thoracolumbar kyphosis are among the other clinical features. The child usually achieves developmental milestones later than is normal, with independent walking at an average age of 17 months. A skeletal survey generally reveals shortening of the tubular bones, chevron-shaped physes of the distal femurs with normal epiphyses, flared metaphyses, narrowing of the spine interpediculate distance from L1 to L5, a notchlike sacroiliac groove, and squared iliac wings (**Figure 2**).

One of the most serious manifestations of achondroplasia during early infancy is foramen magnum stenosis caused by the small skull base (**Table 1**). The transverse and sagittal dimensions of the foramen magnum can be 3 to 5 standard deviations below average in children with achondroplasia.[10] Unexpected infant death was found to occur in 2% to 5% of affected children when an aggressive evaluation was not performed.[11] The foramen magnum stenosis can cause chronic brainstem compression symptoms such as apnea, dysfunction of the lower cranial nerve, difficulty in swallowing, hyperreflexia, hypotonia, weakness or paresis, and clonus.[12,13] A baseline CT or MRI of the brain and cervical spine is recommended for young children.[14] Polysomnography also is indicated. To avoid the need for sedation, polysomnography may be preferred as the initial

study; CT or MRI can be performed if the sleep study is positive.[13] In a retrospective study of 43 patients with achondroplasia who underwent foramen magnum decompression and upper cervical laminectomy, with or without duraplasty, 20 (46.5%) had an obstructive (more commonly) or central respiratory difficulty, ranging from excessive snoring to sleep apnea.[12] Ventriculomegaly is common, generally with no clinical evidence of increased intracranial pressure; this condition also is known as compensated hydrocephalus.

Thoracolumbar kyphosis is common in patients with achondroplasia, with a prevalence of 87% at age 1 to 2 years, 39% at age 2 to 5 years, and 11% at age 5 to 10 years[15] (**Figure 3**). It has been proposed that the combination of a disproportionately large head, a flat chest, truncal hypotonia, and a protuberant abdomen promotes thoracolumbar kyphosis. Anterior vertebral wedging is common, probably secondary to anterior compressive forces. One study recommended that unsupported sitting should be prohibited during the first year of life and that the C-sitting position should be avoided by using a 60° sitting angle and a hard-back seat with lumbar support.[16] The study recommends bracing if the fixed component of the kyphosis is greater than 30°, the anterior vertebral wedging progresses, or there is substantial posterior displacement of

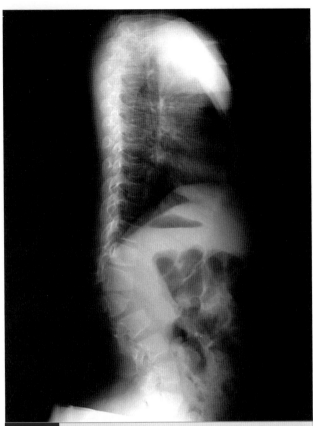

Figure 3 Standing lateral spine radiograph of an 8-year-old boy with achondroplasia showing fixed thoracolumbar kyphosis and lumbar vertebrae wedging, especially at L1.

the vertebrae at the kyphotic apex. In addition, bracing is recommended until the child can walk independently, the anterior corners of the vertebral bodies are reconstituted, and the residual fixed component of the curve is no longer decreasing. Surgical treatment traditionally is indicated if the child has kyphosis with neurologic compromise, or is older than 4 years and has a curve greater than 50°, because of the risk of a progression to a rigid kyphosis with neurologic compromise.[13] The surgical methods include anterior instrumentation and fusion; posterior decompression, instrumentation, and fusion; and combined anterior and posterior instrumentation and fusion. Lumbosacral hyperlordosis affects approximately 80% of children with achondroplasia and usually is associated with hip flexion contractures. Treatment is rarely required.

Spinal stenosis generally appears during the third or fourth decade of life but may develop earlier. The prevalence ranges from 37% to 89%, and approximately 25% of patients may require surgical intervention.[17,18] A decreased interpedicular distance from L1 to L5, short and thickened pedicles, and hyperplastic intervertebral disks and ligamentum flavum result in a 40% reduction in the sagittal and coronal diameters of the spinal canal.[19] It is common for a child with achondroplasia to squat in an attempt to decrease the hyperlor-

dosis and obtain relief from symptoms of neurogenic claudication, especially after exercise or a long walk. The indications for surgical intervention include progressive symptoms of neurogenic claudication, urinary retention, and neurologic symptoms at rest.[13] In the past, myelography was used to assess the level of stenosis and the extent of spinal cord compromise. However, myelography in patients with achondroplasia is a technically difficult and painful procedure with complications including neurologic compromise, herniation of the cauda equina roots through the puncture defect, and failure of the contrast medium to progress to severely stenotic regions because of poor cerebrospinal fluid flow.[20] Multilevel laminectomies combined with arthrodesis appear to be the best surgical option for a skeletally immature patient; the arthrodesis prevents postlaminectomy thoracolumbar kyphosis.[21,22] Pedicle screw fixation should be used instead of laminar hooks and wires because of the narrowing of the spinal canal.[13]

Genu varum is very common in patients with achondroplasia and can be associated with pain, knee instability, limitation of joint function, and a waddling gait. The cause may be multifactorial and includes asymmetric physeal growth, obesity, lateral collateral ligament laxity, and fibular overgrowth.[23] Surgical correction is indicated to treat a symptomatic or progressive deformity or a valgus thrust at the knee. The level of deformity defines the level of tibial osteotomy, and the concurrent tibial torsion must be managed (**Figure 4**).

The height discrepancy between patients with achondroplasia and unaffected individuals ranges from −1.5 standard deviation at birth to −5.0 standard deviations at age 2 years. Specifically designed height, weight, and head circumference growth charts must be used to predict adult height in these patients.[24,25] Growth hormone therapy and limb lengthening have been used to increase adult stature and ameliorate the impairments resulting from short limbs.[26,27] Although limb lengthening is technically difficult and controversial, it can be successful in increasing height. In 140 patients, an average length increase of 20.5 cm (± 4.7 cm) was reported for the lower limb (femur or tibia), with an average treatment duration of 31 months; an increase of 10.2 cm (± 1.25 cm) was reported for the upper limb (humerus), with an average treatment duration of 9 months.[26] Complications including fracture, malalignment, early consolidation, failed union, joint stiffness, and infection were observed in 43% of the patients.[26]

Maintaining an ideal body weight often is a challenge for patients with achondroplasia, and participation in low-impact physical activities and sports is strongly recommended.[11]

Hypochondroplasia

Hypochondroplasia is another nonlethal *FGFR3*-related disorder. This condition was considered a milder form of achondroplasia until evidence of allelism with achondroplasia was described. The inheri-

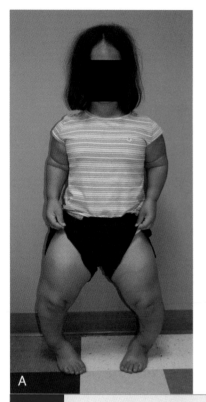
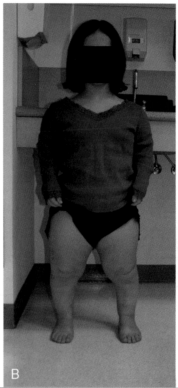
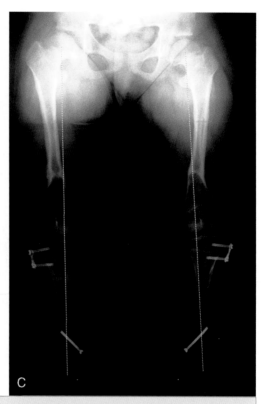

Figure 4 **A,** Preoperative photograph of a 12-year-old girl with achondroplasia, showing typical bilateral bowing of the lower limbs. **B,** Photograph of the same girl showing straighter lower limbs after bilateral distal femoral osteotomies with external fixation, bilateral lateral proximal tibial hemiepiphysiodesis, and bilateral distal tibial and fibular realignment osteotomies with external fixation. **C,** Standing AP radiograph of the girl's lower extremities 6 months after the procedure, showing union of the osteotomy sites and an improved mechanical axis passing just medial to the center of the knee.

tance of hypochondroplasia is autosomal dominant. In approximately 65% of patients, a lysine is substituted for asparagine in codon 540 in *FGFR3*.[28,29] However, hypochondroplasia is genetically heterogenous and sometimes is caused by mutation in a gene other than *FGFR3*. The clinical and radiologic features of hypochondroplasia are not as striking as those of achondroplasia; they include short stature, rhizomelic shortening of the limbs, lordosis, and a large head circumference with a normal face.[30] The pelvis is normal, and the only significant radiologic finding in the spine is a lumbar narrowing of the interpedicular distance. The medical issues and treatment are similar to those for patients with achondroplasia but may require modification because hypochondroplasia is less severe.

Spondyloepiphyseal Dysplasia Congenita

Spondyloepiphyseal dysplasia congenita is a representative type of disproportionate short-trunk dwarfism with vertebral and epiphyseal abnormalities. The genetic defect is in the type 2 collagen αI chain (*COL2A1*) gene located on chromosome 12.q13.1-q13.2, and it results in defective procollagen type 2 subunits.[31] Collagen type 2 is found in the vitreous, as well as the cartilage, and as a result patients have ocular abnormalities. Myopia with membranous vitreous anomaly occurs in

as many as 50% of patients.[32] Retinal detachment, hearing loss, and cleft palate also are common.[33] The short trunk is a result of platyspondyly, and the limb shortening results from epiphyseal and physeal involvement (**Figure 5**).

Atlantoaxial instability is common because of odontoid hypoplasia and ligamentous laxity. Myelopathy with atlantoaxial subluxation has been reported to occur in as many as 42% of patients.[34-36] Posterior decompression and fusion is the surgical procedure of choice.[35] Several other features are common in patients with spondyloepiphyseal dysplasia congenita: coxa vara and hip flexion contractures with hip pain and dysfunction, which can be treated with hip osteotomies; premature osteoarthritis, which is treated with joint arthroplasty; and genu valgum, treated using guided growth or osteotomy. Although total hip arthroplasty is technically demanding in these patients, generally it has a positive outcome, with significant improvement in pain and function.[37]

Stickler Syndrome

Stickler syndrome, or hereditary arthro-ophthalmopathy of Stickler, is characterized by a marfanoid build, enlargement of the joints, epiphyseal abnormalities with premature degenerative changes in various joints, liga-

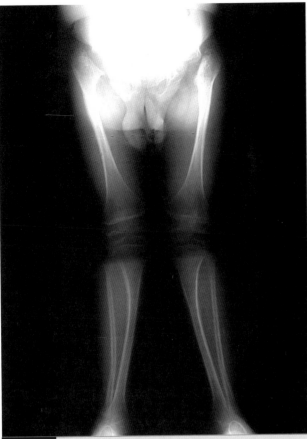

Figure 5   Standing AP radiograph of the lower extremities of a 17-year-old boy with spondyloepiphyseal dysplasia congenita, showing the typical small pelvis with horizontal acetabular roofs, poorly ossified capital femoral epiphysis, coxa vara, and flattened epiphysis in the distal femora and proximal tibiae.

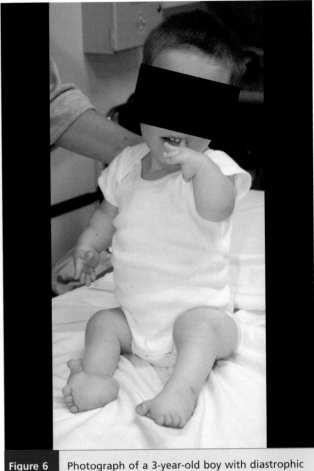

Figure 6   Photograph of a 3-year-old boy with diastrophic dysplasia, showing the typical rhizomelic micromelia, brachydactyly with hitchhiker thumb, and bilateral hallux adductus.

mentous laxity, cleft palate, hearing impairment, and ocular involvement including congenital vitreous gel abnormalities and retinal detachment.[38-40] The three described types, based on ocular abnormalities and genetic findings, involve *COL2A1, COL11A1,* and *COL11A2* gene mutations.[38] Mild spondyloepiphyseal dysplasia is common in these patients. One third of patients were found to have scoliosis, which tends to be self-limiting.[41] Hyperkyphosis was found in 43% of patients, often progressing through childhood. In adult patients, kyphotic deformities are assumed to be caused by vertebral body malformation during spine growth. Spondylolisthesis occurred in a small number of patients.[41] When hip pain was assessed in a large group of patients, 79% were found to have chronic hip pain as adults.[42] Varus or valgus deformity of the femoral neck and protrusio acetabuli also occurred. Slipped capital femoral epiphysis and Legg-Calvé-Perthes disease were found to be more common in patients with Sticker syndrome than in the general population, and total hip replacement was frequently required.[42]

Diastrophic Dysplasia

The Greek term diastrophic means "crooked and bent." Diastrophic dysplasia is a short-limb rhizomelic dwarfism characterized by multiple joint contractures, progressive scoliosis and kyphosis, brachydactyly, so-called hitchhiker thumbs, abducted halluces, talipes equinovarus, cleft palate, swelling of the ear pinnae (so-called cauliflower ears), and abnormalities of the tracheal-laryngeal-bronchial tract (**Figure 6**). The genetic defect is in the sulfate transporter gene *SCL26A2,* and inheritance is autosomal recessive, usually with compound heterozygosity. Cervical kyphosis is relatively common but usually resolves spontaneously. The reported prevalence of scoliosis in patients with diastrophic dysplasia ranges from 33% to 88%, with varying degrees of severity and progression.[43] The treatment of a progressive curve includes spine instrumentation and fusion. Bracing is not successful for treating spine deformities in diastrophic dysplasia.[44] Growth-oriented fusionless treatment using a growing rod system can achieve as much spine length as possible and prevent the pulmonary function impairment associated with spine fusion in young children.[45] Posterior instru-

Table 2

The Clinical Features of Achondroplasia and Pseudoachondroplasia

Condition	Craniofacial Dysmorphism	Spine Deformity	Rhizomelia	Angular Deformity
Achondroplasia	Frontal bossing Macrocrania Midface hypoplasia Orthodontic issues	Close-to-normal trunk height	Pronounced since birth	Genu varum
Pseudoachondroplasia	None	Platyspondyly Atlantoaxial instability Anterior vertebral body protrusion	Apparent at age 2 to 3 years	Windswept deformity Genu valgum Genu varum

mentation and fusion are effective in adolescents and adults.

The foot deformity is complex and distinct from idiopathic clubfoot. The most common foot deformity is tarsal valgus and metatarsus adductovarus, which in one study was found in 44 of 102 patients (43%).[46] The characteristic radiographic finding is a lateral displacement of the navicular on the talus. Surgical treatments have limited success. The recurrence rate was 87% in 40 patients who underwent procedures such as Achilles tendon lengthening, posteromedial release, talectomy, supramalleolar osteotomy, and triple arthrodesis.[47] Joint contractures in the lower extremities are among the most common orthopaedic complications. In 50 patients with diastrophic dysplasia, 93% had a hip flexion contracture; the mean contracture was 23°, and all contractures progressed with patient growth.[48] These contractures are related to the abnormal femoral head shape (flattened with a double-hump deformity) as well as contractures of flexors and periarticular soft tissues.[48,49] The knee joints are severely affected, generally with flexion contractures, excessive valgus deformity, and lateral patellar subluxation. In 46 patients, anteroposterior tibiofemoral instability was found in 85% of the knees, with 28 (60%) of the patients having spontaneous subluxation.[50] Progressive osteoarthritis, disabling pain, and impaired walking are common among these patients, and joint arthroplasties often are required. Technical difficulties involving the femoral components of the prosthesis are to be expected.[34,48-50]

Multiple Epiphyseal Dysplasia

All autosomal dominant types of multiple epiphyseal dysplasia (MED) and pseudoachondroplasia recently were classified into the same group because of their clinical and genetic similarities. These disorders share a defect in the cartilage oligomeric matrix protein (COMP) gene. In addition, mutations in the collagen type 9 (COL9A1, COL9A2, COL9A3) and matrilin-3 (MATN3) genes have been found in patients with an autosomal dominant type of MED. The autosomal recessive type of MED is classified as a sulphation disorder

because the genetic defect is in the sulfate transporter gene SLC26A2. Children with MED have short stature, brachydactyly, genu valgum, and joint laxity. The radiographic findings include widening of the joint spaces, delayed epiphyseal ossification, and small epiphyses, particularly in the lateral part of the distal tibia ossification center. A small epiphysis in this location leads to valgus deformity of the distal tibia in adults. The most significant bone abnormalities are in the epiphyses, leading to early-onset degenerative osteoarthritis.[51] MED has both a milder and a more severe form (the Ribbing and Fairbank types, respectively).

Patients with MED may require joint arthroplasty early in life. Some technical difficulties should be expected, such as a diaphyseal-metaphyseal mismatch; the use of a conic narrow stem may be required to achieve an ideal diaphyseal anchorage, rotational stability, and osseous integration.[52] Hemiepiphysiodesis has long been used to correct angular deformity in the knee. A correction of 20° or more can be achieved if the patient has sufficient remaining growth.[53]

Pseudoachondroplasia

Pseudoachondroplasia is an autosomal dominant osteochondrodysplasia characterized by disproportionate short stature, with rhizomelic shortening of the limbs resembling that of achondroplasia (Table 2). The COMP gene is defective. The clinical features include joint laxity, increased thoracic kyphosis, accentuated lumbar lordosis, and atlantoaxial instability.[54] These features are not evident until the child reaches age 1 to 3 years. The radiologic findings include small, irregular capital femoral epiphyses; shortening of the tubular bones with irregular metaphyses; small, deformed epiphyses; and platyspondyly, with a tonguelike anterior protrusion of the central portion of the vertebral bodies. Spine instability at C1-C2 is found in 10% to 20% of patients. If neurologic compromise or myelopathy is present, the conventional treatment is arthrodesis and decompression.[55] The prevalence of lower limb deformities such as genu varum, genu valgum, or windswept deformity is as high as 84%. A natural history study found that 69% of patients with limb deformity

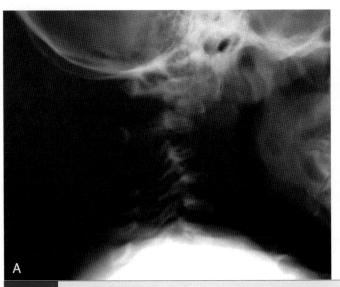
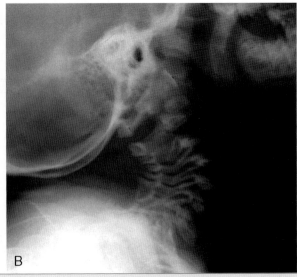

Figure 7   Lateral cervical spine radiographs of a 3-year-old girl with Morquio-Brailsford syndrome, showing mild atlantoaxial instability and platyspondyly. **A**, Hyperflexion view. **B**, Hyperextension view.

needed surgery, and 33% of those older than 19 years had a total hip arthroplasty.[56]

Osteogenesis Imperfecta

Osteogenesis imperfecta is an inherited disease of the connective tissue; 90% of patients have a genetic defect in a type I collagen gene (*COL1A1* or *COL1A*). Osteogenesis imperfecta is characterized by bone fragility and low-impact–related fractures. The range of severity is wide, from a lethal perinatal form to a near-normal form with infrequent fractures. Family variability is commonly found. The most recent classification system describes seven types, based on age at onset of symptoms, severity and progression, short stature, and associated clinical findings such as blue sclerae, hearing loss, and dentinogenesis imperfecta.[57] The differential diagnosis should include metabolic bone disorders such as vitamin D–resistant rickets and perinatal hypophosphatasia, Bruck syndrome (characterized by bone fragility and multiple contractures), and child abuse–related fracture. A careful physical examination and a radiographic survey are necessary to make a diagnosis. Establishing the family history can be difficult because a family member may have mild, undiagnosed osteogenesis imperfecta. Radiographs reveal generalized demineralization; slender, tubular bones with thin cortex; poor trabecular spongiosa; wormian bones; and bone fragility with secondary deformities. Bisphosphonates have been used with relative success to reduce the risk of fracture and improve pain control, mobility, and participation in daily activities. The goals of surgical treatment, especially in a child with severe osteogenesis imperfecta who has the potential ability to stand, are to prevent recurrent fractures and correct severe bowing deformities. The basic surgical realignment procedures for the bone deformities are multiple osteotomies with intramedullary fixation. A new telescoping rod offers some advantages over earlier instrumentation and has been recommended.[58,59]

Mucopolysaccharidosis Type IV

Mucopolysaccharidosis type IV, also known as Morquio-Brailsford syndrome, is an autosomal recessive lysosomal storage disease with intracellular accumulation of glycosaminoglycans. The characteristic clinical features are a short trunk, disproportionate short stature, progressive osseous dystrophy, corneal clouding, and aortic valve disease, in a child with generally normal intelligence.[60] Mucopolysaccharidosis type IV has three subtypes. In types A and B, a deficiency is present in the N-acetylgalactosamine-6-sulfatase (GALNS) and β-galactosidase (GLB1) enzymes, respectively. More than 150 different mutations have been associated with these enzyme deficiencies. There is excessive urinary excretion of keratan sulfate in both types A and B. In type C, keratan sulfate is not excreted. The radiologic findings resemble those of the spondyloepiphyseal dysplasias, including platyspondyly in the thoracic and lumbar spine, anterior tonguelike protrusions of the vertebral bodies, odontoid hypoplasia, coxa valga, progressive hip dysplasia, and genu valgum (**Figure 7**).

The skeletal abnormalities are progressive and appear within the first 2 to 3 years of life. Cervical spine instability caused by odontoid hypoplasia and ligamentous laxity is common and requires surgical intervention. A combination of cervical spine instability and glycosaminoglycan deposition in the extradural soft tissues leads to upper cervical spine stenosis and consequent myelopathy. Decompression and fusion may be preferred in an asymptomatic patients if the space available for the spinal cord is less than 14 mm, the

C1-C2 instability is more than 8 mm, or lateral cervical flexion-extension radiographs and MRI show spinal cord impingement. Early osteoarthrosis in the lower extremities is to be expected, necessitating joint arthroplasty in adulthood. A retrospective study with CT assessment of the hip in seven patients found a global acetabular deficiency, predominantly in the anterosuperior region. This finding suggests that the treatment should focus on increasing the acetabular depth and containing the femoral head.[61] The success of enzyme replacement in animal models of mucopolysaccharidosis type IV raises the prospect of new medical therapies for this condition.

Social and Psychological Considerations

Every professional involved in the care of patients with a skeletal dysplasia should be aware of the social and psychological implications of short stature. "Living in a world of giants" is a useful phrase for understanding many of the daily barriers and difficulties these patients experience. The wide spectrum of height among individuals with skeletal dysplasia requires different types of adaptation. The primary goal is to create the most accessible possible environment by targeting all aspects, situations, and physical settings of the child's life, including the home, the school, and recreational facilities. Respect for obvious physical limitations can increase the professional's ability to assist a child in attaining independence and a productive, socially integrated life. The many available opportunities for functional improvement should be discussed with the parents. A multidisciplinary approach including occupational and psychological therapy is necessary.

Although attitudes in modern societies have evolved, some old values persist. Success still may be equated with height and physical strength, and the effect on a growing child's personality can be devastating. A child's awareness of having short stature usually begins at age 4 to 6 years. Psychological support, primarily directed toward the parents and focused on understanding and accepting the condition, is beneficial. Parents should be encouraged to investigate patient- and parent-support groups (for example, Little People of America). The opportunity to meet other people with short stature and their families and to exchange information and personal experiences can be educational for the family and offer the child an early opportunity to associate with others who have a similar condition. Even the most understanding parents may need professional psychological assistance during turbulent times such as adolescence.

Annotated References

1. Superti-Furga A, Unger S: Nosology and classification of genetic skeletal disorders: 2006 revision. *Am J Med Genet A* 2007;143(1):1-18.

This is a thorough overview of the classification of dysplasias.

2. Offiah AC, Hall CM: Radiological diagnosis of the constitutional disorders of bone: As easy as A, B, C? *Pediatr Radiol* 2003;33(3):153-161.

3. Orioli IM, Castilla EE, Barbosa-Neto JG: The birth prevalence rates for the skeletal dysplasias. *J Med Genet* 1986;23(4):328-332.

4. Krakow D, Lachman RS, Rimoin DL: Guidelines for the prenatal diagnosis of fetal skeletal dysplasias. *Genet Med* 2009;11(2):127-133.

These guidelines provide an approach to the fetal diagnosis of a skeletal dysplasia, which can allow a management plan to be developed and the recurrence risk to be accurately determined.

5. Unger S, Superti-Furga A, Rimoin D: A diagnostic approach to skeletal dysplasias, in Glorieux FH, Pettifor JM, Jüppner H, eds: *Pediatric Bone: Biology and Disease*. New York, NY, Academic Press, 2003, pp 375-400.

6. Oberklaid F, Danks DM, Jensen F, Stace L, Rosshandler S: Achondroplasia and hypochondroplasia: Comments on frequency, mutation rate, and radiological features in skull and spine. *J Med Genet* 1979;16(2):140-146.

7. Risch N, Reich EW, Wishnick MM, McCarthy JG: Spontaneous mutation and parental age in humans. *Am J Hum Genet* 1987;41(2):218-248.

8. Rousseau F, Bonaventure J, Legeai-Mallet L, et al: Mutations in the gene encoding fibroblast growth factor receptor-3 in achondroplasia. *Nature* 1994;371(6494):252-254.

9. Horton WA: Recent milestones in achondroplasia research. *Am J Med Genet A* 2006;140(2):166-169.

Research in achondroplasia is comprehensively reviewed.

10. Hecht JT, Nelson FW, Butler IJ, et al: Computerized tomography of the foramen magnum: Achondroplastic values compared to normal standards. *Am J Med Genet* 1985;20(2):355-360.

11. Trotter TL, Hall JG; American Academy of Pediatrics Committee on Genetics: Health supervision for children with achondroplasia. *Pediatrics* 2005;116(3):771-783.

This review article from the American Academy of Pediatrics Committee on Genetics provides information on anticipatory care in children with achondroplasia.

12. Bagley CA, Pindrik JA, Bookland MJ, Camara-Quintana JQ, Carson BS: Cervicomedullary decompression for foramen magnum stenosis in achondroplasia. *J Neurosurg* 2006;104(3, suppl)166-172.

Decompression of the cervical medullary junction in achondroplasia can be accomplished safely, with minimal morbidity. The clinical benefit is significant.

2: Basic Science

13. Shirley ED, Ain MC: Achondroplasia: Manifestations and treatment. *J Am Acad Orthop Surg* 2009;17(4): 231-241.

    The orthopaedic issues in achondroplasia and their management are reviewed.

14. Pauli RM, Horton VK, Glinski LP, Reiser CA: Prospective assessment of risks for cervicomedullary-junction compression in infants with achondroplasia. *Am J Hum Genet* 1995;56(3):732-744.

15. Kopits SE: Thoracolumbar kyphosis and lumbosacral hyperlordosis in achondroplastic children. *Basic Life Sci* 1988;48:241-255.

16. Pauli RM, Breed A, Horton VK, Glinski LP, Reiser CA: Prevention of fixed, angular kyphosis in achondroplasia. *J Pediatr Orthop* 1997;17(6):726-733.

17. Bethem D, Winter RB, Lutter L, et al: Spinal disorders of dwarfism: Review of the literature and report of eighty cases. *J Bone Joint Surg Am* 1981;63(9):1412-1425.

18. Hunter AG, Bankier A, Rogers JG, Sillence D, Scott CI Jr: Medical complications of achondroplasia: A multicentre patient review. *J Med Genet* 1998;35(9):705-712.

19. Lutter LD, Longstein JE, Winter RB, Langer LO: Anatomy of the achondroplastic lumbar canal. *Clin Orthop Relat Res* 1977;126:139-142.

20. Suss RA, Udvarhelyi GB, Wang H, Kumar AJ, Zinreich SJ, Rosenbaum AE: Myelography in achondroplasia: Value of a lateral C1-2 puncture and non-ionic, water-soluble contrast medium. *Radiology* 1983;149(1):159-163.

21. Ain MC, Shirley ED, Pirouzmanesh A, Hariri A, Carson BS: Postlaminectomy kyphosis in the skeletally immature achondroplast. *Spine (Phila Pa 1976)* 2006;31(2): 197-201.

    Skeletally immature children with achondroplasia are at high risk of developing thoracolumbar kyphosis after thoracolumbar laminectomy for spinal stenosis. Concurrent spinal fusion and instrumentation is indicated.

22. Pyeritz RE, Sack GH Jr, Udvarhelyi GB: Thoracolumbosacral laminectomy in achondroplasia: Long-term results in 22 patients. *Am J Med Genet* 1987;28(2):433-444.

23. Kopits SE: Orthopedic aspects of achondroplasia in children. *Basic Life Sci* 1988;48:189-197.

24. Horton WA, Rotter JI, Rimoin DL, Scott CI, Hall JG: Standard growth curves for achondroplasia. *J Pediatr* 1978;93(3):435-438.

25. Paley D, Matz AL, Kurland DB, Lamm BM, Herzenberg JE: Multiplier method for prediction of adult height in patients with achondroplasia. *J Pediatr Orthop* 2005; 25(4):539-542.

    A method is described for quickly predicting the future height of a child with achondroplasia, at any age.

26. Aldegheri R, Dall'Oca C: Limb lengthening in short stature patients. *J Pediatr Orthop B* 2001;10(3):238-247.

27. Kanazawa H, Tanaka H, Inoue M, Yamanaka Y, Namba N, Seino Y: Efficacy of growth hormone therapy for patients with skeletal dysplasia. *J Bone Miner Metab* 2003;21(5):307-310.

28. Bellus GA, McIntosh I, Smith EA, et al: A recurrent mutation in the tyrosine kinase domain of fibroblast growth factor receptor 3 causes hypochondroplasia. *Nat Genet* 1995;10(3):357-359.

29. Le Merrer M, Rousseau F, Legeai-Mallet L, et al: A gene for achondroplasia-hypochondroplasia maps to chromosome 4p. *Nat Genet* 1994;6(3):318-321.

30. Cohen MM Jr: Some chondrodysplasias with short limbs: Molecular perspectives. *Am J Med Genet* 2002; 112(3):304-313.

31. Tiller GE, Rimoin DL, Murray LW, Cohn DH: Tandem duplication within a type II collagen gene (COL2A1) exon in an individual with spondyloepiphyseal dysplasia. *Proc Natl Acad Sci U S A* 1990;87(10):3889-3893.

32. Hamidi-Toosi S, Maumenee IH: Vitreoretinal degeneration in spondyloepiphyseal dysplasia congenita. *Arch Ophthalmol* 1982;100(7):1104-1107.

33. Meredith SP, Richards AJ, Bearcroft P, Pouson AV, Snead MP: Significant ocular findings are a feature of heritable bone dysplasias resulting from defects in type II collagen. *Br J Ophthalmol* 2007;91(9):1148-1151.

    Bone dysplasias caused by a defect of type II collagen carry a high risk of retinal detachment, with retinal tears occurring at a young age.

34. Kopits SE: Orthopedic complications of dwarfism. *Clin Orthop Relat Res* 1976;114:153-179.

35. Miyoshi K, Nakamura K, Haga N, Mikami Y: Surgical treatment for atlantoaxial subluxation with myelopathy in spondyloepiphyseal dysplasia congenita. *Spine (Phila Pa 1976)* 2004;29(21):E488-E491.

36. Spranger JW, Langer LO Jr: Spondyloepiphyseal dysplasia congenita. *Radiology* 1970;94(2):313-322.

37. Ain MC, Andres BM, Somel DS, Fishkin Z, Frassica FJ: Total hip arthroplasty in skeletal dysplasias: Patient selection, preoperative planning, and operative techniques. *J Arthroplasty* 2004;19(1):1-7.

38. Rose PS, Levy HP, Liberfarb RM, et al: Stickler syndrome: Clinical characteristics and diagnostic criteria. *Am J Med Genet A* 2005;138A(3):199-207.

39. Stickler GB, Belau PG, Farrell FJ, et al: Hereditary progressive arthro-ophthalmopathy. *Mayo Clin Proc* 1965; 40:433-455.

40. Stickler GB, Hughes W, Houchin P: Clinical features of hereditary progressive arthro-ophthalmopathy (Stickler syndrome): A survey. *Genet Med* 2001;3(3):192-196.

41. Rose PS, Ahn NU, Levy HP, et al: Thoracolumbar spinal abnormalities in Stickler syndrome. *Spine (Phila Pa 1976)* 2001;26(4):403-409.

42. Rose PS, Ahn NU, Levy HP, et al: The hip in Stickler syndrome. *J Pediatr Orthop* 2001;21(5):657-663.

43. Remes V, Poussa M, Peltonen J: Scoliosis in patients with diastrophic dysplasia: A new classification. *Spine (Phila Pa 1976)* 2001;26(15):1689-1697.

44. Jalanko T, Remes V, Peltonen J, Poussa M, Helenius I: Treatment of spinal deformities in patients with diastrophic dysplasia: A long-term, population based, retrospective outcome study. *Spine (Phila Pa 1976)* 2009; 34(20):2151-2157.

Thoracic spine deformities are rigid in diastrophic dysplasia, and brace treatment does not alter the natural history. Anterior and posterior surgery may be necessary for severe deformity. The risk of major complications is high in patients with kyphosis.

45. Yazici M, Emans J: Fusionless instrumentation systems for congenital scoliosis: Expandable spinal rods and vertical expandable prosthetic titanium rib in the management of congenital spine deformities in the growing child. *Spine (Phila Pa 1976)* 2009;34(17):1800-1807.

Expandable growing rods or vertical expandable prosthetic rib devices have both advantages and limitations for the fusionless management of spine deformity. If the patient has significant thoracic compromise as well as significant remaining growth, the vertical expandable prosthetic rib device is the best choice.

46. Ryöppy S, Poussa M, Merikanto J, Marttinen E, Kaitila I: Foot deformities in diastrophic dysplasia: An analysis of 102 patients. *J Bone Joint Surg Br* 1992;74(3):441-444.

47. Weiner DS, Jonah D, Kopits S: The 3-dimensional configuration of the typical foot and ankle in diastrophic dysplasia. *J Pediatr Orthop* 2008;28(1):60-67.

The typical foot-and-ankle deformity in diastrophic dysplasia is unlike that of idiopathic clubfoot. The hindfoot is in equinovalgus, the navicular is displaced laterally on the talus, and the forefoot is in varus.

48. Vaara P, Peltonen J, Poussa M, et al: Development of the hip in diastrophic dysplasia. *J Bone Joint Surg Br* 1998;80(2):315-320.

49. Helenius I, Remes V, Tallroth K, Peltonen J, Poussa M, Paavilainen T: Total hip arthroplasty in diastrophic dysplasia. *J Bone Joint Surg Am* 2003;85(3):441-447.

50. Peltonen J, Vaara P, Marttinen E, Ryöppy S, Poussa M: The knee joint in diastrophic dysplasia: A clinical and radiological study. *J Bone Joint Surg Br* 1999;81(4): 625-631.

51. Deere M, Blanton SH, Scott CI, Langer LO, Pauli RM, Hecht JT: Genetic heterogeneity in multiple epiphyseal dysplasia. *Am J Hum Genet* 1995;56(3):698-704.

52. Pavone V, Costarella L, Privitera V, Sessa G: Bilateral total hip arthroplasty in subjects with multiple epiphyseal dysplasia. *J Arthroplasty* 2009;24(6):868-872.

Patients with multiple epiphyseal dysplasia develop secondary hip osteoarthritis during the third or fourth decade of life. Total hip arthroplasty is successful for these patients.

53. Cho TJ, Choi IH, Chung CY, Yoo WJ, Park MS, Lee DY: Hemiepiphyseal stapling for angular deformity correction around the knee joint in children with multiple epiphyseal dysplasia. *J Pediatr Orthop* 2009;29(1): 52-56.

Hemiepiphyseal stapling is effective for correcting genu valgum in a patient with multiple epiphyseal dysplasia. Overcorrection should be avoided, and close monitoring is mandatory until skeletal maturity.

54. Wynne-Davies R, Hall CM, Young ID: Pseudoachondroplasia: Clinical diagnosis at different ages and comparison of autosomal dominant and recessive types. A review of 32 patients (26 kindreds). *J Med Genet* 1986; 23(5):425-434.

55. Shetty GM, Song HR, Unnikrishnan R, Suh SW, Lee SH, Hur CY: Upper cervical spine instability in pseudoachondroplasia. *J Pediatr Orthop* 2007;27(7):782-787.

Os odontoideum is present in 60% of patients with pseudoachondroplasia. Upper cervical instability is more common with increased age.

56. McKeand J, Rotta J, Hecht JT: Natural history study of pseudoachondroplasia. *Am J Med Genet* 1996;63(2): 406-410.

57. Van Dijk FS, Pals G, Van Rijn RR, Nikkels PG, Cobben JM: Classification of osteogenesis imperfecta revisited. *Eur J Med Genet* 2010;53(1):1-5.

A revision of the existing classification of osteogenesis imperfecta was based on clinical, radiologic, and histologic criteria, with consideration of genetic factors.

58. Cho TJ, Choi IH, Chung CY, Yoo WJ, Lee KS, Lee DY: Interlocking telescopic rod for patients with osteogenesis imperfecta. *J Bone Joint Surg Am* 2007;89(5):1028-1035.

A new interlocking telescopic rod system was found to be comparable to conventional telescopic rod systems.

59. Esposito P, Plotkin H: Surgical treatment of osteogenesis imperfecta: Current concepts. *Curr Opin Pediatr* 2008;20(1):52-57.

2: Basic Science

This is an excellent review of the medical and surgical management of osteogenesis imperfecta.

60. Morquio L: Sur une forme de dystrophie osseuse familiale. *Bull Soc Pediat* 1929;27:142-152.

61. Borowski A, Thacker MM, Mackenzie WG, Littleton AG, Grissom L: The use of computed tomography to assess acetabular morphology in Morquio-Brailsford syndrome. *J Pediatr Orthop* 2007;27(8):893-897.

In patients with Morquio-Brailsford syndrome, CT of the hip reveals a severe dysplasia of the anterior acetabular wall and roof of the acetabulum. CT is helpful in preoperative decision making.

Chapter 9

The Modulation of Skeletal Growth

David D. Aronsson, MD   Ian A.F. Stokes, PhD

Introduction

The anatomic, biomechanical, and biochemical mechanisms regulating the growth of the skeleton include growth plate anatomy, blood supply, function, and endocrine regulation. Experimental studies are improving the understanding of the mechanical modulation of growth of the spine and extremities, and this understanding is being extended to clinical applications. Methods including permanent and reversible epiphysiodesis and hemiepiphysiodesis have been developed for modulating growth and treating angular deformities and growth arrest.

Skeletal Growth

The skeleton is composed of four organs: bone, cartilage, ligaments, and tendons. The skeleton thus is an example of an organ system in which two or more organs work together to provide a common function. Growth (the process by which organs enlarge) is better understood in bones than in other organs such as the heart.[1] The term bone growth is used to indicate an increase in the external dimensions of a bone before skeletal maturity; modeling describes the establishment of a refined architecture of bone tissue after its initial formation; and remodeling describes a change in the architecture of a bone in response to a functional, pathologic, or iatrogenic environmental stimulus, whether internal (systemic) or external. Although longitudinal bone growth ends at skeletal maturity, anabolic and catabolic processes continue constantly throughout life.

Dr. Aronsson or an immediate family member serves as a board member, owner, officer, or committee member of the International Federation of Pediatric Orthopaedic Societies and the International Society of Orthopaedic Surgery and Traumatology; has received research or institutional support from Spineology, Stryker, DePuy, a Johnson & Johnson company, and Synthes; and owns stock or stock options in Abbott, Bristol-Myers Squib, Eli Lilly, Johnson & Johnson, Medtronic, Merck, and Pfizer. Dr. Stokes or an immediate family member has received research or institutional support from unknown companies or suppliers.

Adaptive remodeling occurs as osteoclasts gradually remove bone tissue and osteoblasts gradually make bone tissue. The remodeling process is of tremendous interest. Recent research has focused on osteoporosis, in which osteoclastic resorption outpaces osteoblastic formation and leads to a net loss of the bone tissue critical for movement and calcium storage.

The two essential processes in new bone formation are endochondral (cartilaginous) and intramembranous ossification. Some bones are formed by intramembranous ossification in the embryonic stage, and others are formed by endochondral ossification of the cartilage anlage or the cartilage model. The cartilage anlage grows in all three dimensions (length, width, and height). Cartilage growth occurs in the epiphyseal plates, apophyseal plates, and articular cartilage. Endochondral ossification also occurs in fracture healing, when vascular invasion brings oxygen essential for the complex, coordinated process of calcifying the cartilage cells and producing bone tissue or callus.

In intramembranous ossification, the cartilage intermediate is absent, and mesenchymal stem cells differentiate directly into osteoblasts that form bone tissue. Intramembranous ossification is primarily responsible for producing the clavicles and flat bones of the skull. The periosteum of long bones appears at 8 weeks' gestation with the primary bone collar. The periosteum contains an outer fibrous layer and an inner cambium layer. The cambium layer contains progenitor cells that develop into osteoblasts responsible for increasing the width of long bones. These progenitor cells also participate in fracture healing, where they develop into both callus-forming chondroblasts and osteoblasts. Fracture callus forms from both endochondral and intramembranous ossification.

Growth Plate Anatomy

The growth plate (physis) develops as the remnant of the cartilage that remains between the primary and secondary ossification centers. During embryogenesis, condensation and chondrification of mesenchymal cells form a three-dimensional cartilaginous anlage. Subsequent vascular invasion into the center of the cartilaginous anlage results in calcification of the cartilage to

2: Basic Science

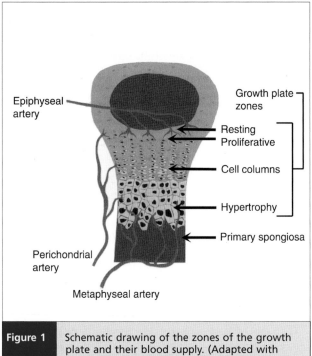

Epiphyseal artery

Growth plate zones

Resting
Proliferative

Cell columns

Hypertrophy

Primary spongiosa

Perichondrial artery

Metaphyseal artery

Figure 1	Schematic drawing of the zones of the growth plate and their blood supply. (Adapted with permission from Hefti F: Basic principles: Growth, in Hefti F, ed: *Pediatric Orthopaedics in Practice*. Berlin and Heidelberg, Germany, Springer Medizin Verlag, 2007, p 42.)

create the primary center of ossification. The primary center of ossification gradually replaces the surrounding cartilage, converting it first into bone and then into the medullary cavity. Cartilaginous growth cannot occur in width because of the primary bone collar. The bone grows longitudinally at the ends through endochondral growth; it grows in width by appositional growth, in which new layers of bone tissue are added onto those previously formed. Vascular invasion of the cartilage at the ends of long bones calcifies the cartilage to form secondary centers of ossification.

The growth plates are formed at the junction between the limits of the primary and secondary centers of ossification. The growth plates are responsible for endochondral cartilage growth, which accounts for most longitudinal growth of the upper and lower extremities. The four zones of the growth plate are the resting zone, the proliferative zone, the zone of cell columns, and the zone of hypertrophy. The zone of cell columns and zone of hypertrophy account for approximately one half of the total height of the growth plate. The metaphysis begins subjacent to the zone of hypertrophy, where the chondrocytes undergo apoptosis and subsequently are invaded by blood vessels from the metaphysis. The vascular invasion of the terminal hypertrophic chondrocytes in the zone of hypertrophy calcifies the cartilaginous matrix in the region, creating the primary spongiosa. Modeling of the primary spongiosa with further ossification gradually creates the secondary spongiosa and the metaphyseal bone (Figure 1).

These zones are clinically important because the proliferative zone has potential for cell proliferation, which is almost absent in the zone of hypertrophy.[2] On the epiphyseal side of the physis, matrix predominates over the cellular elements, whereas on the metaphyseal side the cellular elements predominate over the matrix.[3] As a result, a fracture or infection that involves the proliferative zone may affect growth, whereas a fracture or infection that involves the zone of hypertrophy is unlikely to affect growth. Because the growth plate is weakest at the level of the zone of hypertrophy, most fractures propagate through this zone, with a low frequency of growth disturbance. A pediatric bone infection (osteomyelitis) most often develops in the metaphysis because it is an area of relative vascular stasis. The zone of hypertrophy is a relative barrier to blood flow, so there is a low frequency of growth disturbance in association with osteomyelitis.

The growth plate is circumferentially supported by the perichondrial fibrocartilaginous complex.[4] The perichondrial fibrocartilaginous complex includes the ossification groove of Ranvier, which provides appositional growth expanding the bone circumference; and the perichondrial ring of LaCroix, which provides circumferential support for the growth plate. These structures are clinically important because a traumatic injury involving the ossification groove of Ranvier can affect growth on one side of the bone, thus creating an angulation deformity such as a varus deformity of the ankle (a Salter type VI fracture). At puberty the perichondrial ring of LaCroix provides less support to the growth plate, making it susceptible to a shear stress. Repetitive shear stresses during puberty can create a slipped capital femoral epiphysis.[4] Similarly, a large shear stress involving the spine can cause a slipped vertebral apophysis having signs and symptoms similar to those of an acute herniated disk.

Blood Supply to the Growth Plate

Blood is supplied to the growth plate by the epiphyseal, metaphyseal, and perichondrial arteries. The central part of the growth plate is supplied by the epiphyseal arteries on the epiphyseal side and the metaphyseal arteries on the metaphyseal side. The periphery of the growth plate is supplied by the perichondrial arteries (Figure 1). The metaphyseal and epiphyseal vascular systems communicate with each other through a rich network of vessels from the perichondrial system. In infants, there is also a vascular communication between the epiphysis and metaphysis through vessels that directly cross the growth plate. This communication decreases with growth, and the zone of hypertrophy is relatively avascular in older children.

The vascular supply is responsible for transporting the nutrients and molecules that regulate the activity of the growth plate through systemic endocrine mechanisms. In a classic study, the epiphyseal and metaphyseal arterial supply to the growth plate of the proximal tibia was disrupted in rabbits.[5] Disruption of the epi-

2: Basic Science

physeal arteries caused the death of bony trabeculae as early as the second day and was followed by chondrocyte death, a decrease in matrix staining, and the formation of osseous bridges between the epiphysis and metaphysis. Disruption of the metaphyseal arteries caused an increase in the height of the zone of hypertrophy that was apparent on the first day and was followed by a lack of calcification of the matrix in the primary spongiosa. There was no evidence of death of any of the osteocytes in the metaphysis. The authors concluded that the epiphyseal arteries supplied the essential nutritive and metabolic requirements of the growth plate.[5] More recent investigators have noted that the proximal femoral growth plate does not always develop a complete growth arrest in patients with Legg-Calvé-Perthes disease. The hypothesis that disruption of the epiphyseal vasculature does not inevitably lead to a complete growth arrest was tested in piglets, with the finding that complete disruption of the epiphyseal vasculature did not lead to diffuse growth plate damage in most femoral heads.[6] Most of the animals did not develop a growth arrest, but they had decreased growth in comparison with the normal side. The authors concluded that the epiphyseal vasculature is not the sole source of nutrition for the proximal femoral growth plate, as was traditionally believed.[6] Laboratory studies of the delivery of fluoresceinated dextrans to the murine growth plate confirmed these findings. A study of the epiphyseal, metaphyseal, and perichondrial vascular supply to the murine growth plate found that small molecules (as large as 10 kDa) pass freely to the growth plate from the metaphyseal and epiphyseal sides.[7] In contrast, larger dextrans (40 kDa or larger) did not enter the growth plate at all. These findings suggest that molecules of low molecular weight, such as basic nutrients and systemic hormones no larger than 10 kDa, have access to the growth plate from the epiphyseal and metaphyseal sides. Larger dextrans can enter the growth plate by diffusion through large physiologic pores for the transport of proteins or through the metaphyseal capillaries, which lack a basement membrane and are permeable even to high molecular weight molecules.

In an infant, the vessels crossing the growth plate may allow an osteomyelitis developing in the metaphysis to rapidly decompress into the epiphysis and adjacent joint, leading to osteonecrosis and septic arthritis. These vessels persist into childhood, although they become less patent; as a result, the growth plate, unlike the articular cartilage, does not form an absolute barrier to the spread of tumors. Vascular communication between the metaphysis and epiphysis gradually diminishes during childhood, and the perichondrial vascular system gradually begins to break down. Any injury to the perichondrial vascular system during this time can have disastrous consequences for the epiphysis, including osteonecrosis (as in patients with Legg-Calvé-Perthes disease), an unstable slipped capital femoral epiphysis, or femoral neck fracture.

Growth Plate Function

The endochondral growth of an epiphyseal growth plate is monopolar, with longitudinal growth directed away from the resting zone. In contrast, the endochondral growth of the apophyseal growth plate is bipolar, with the resting zone in the middle and growth in both directions. The approximate rate of epiphyseal endochondral growth can be calculated as the final chondrocyte height, in microns, multiplied by the chondrocyte proliferation rate over a given period of time.[8] Higher growth rates are associated with an increase in chondrocyte height, matrix synthesis, height of the zone of hypertrophy, and chondrocyte proliferation rate.[2]

Endocrine Regulation of Growth

The process of longitudinal bone growth is governed by a complex network of endocrine signals produced by growth hormone, insulin-like growth factor–I (IGF-I), glucocorticoid, thyroid hormone, estrogen, androgen, vitamin D, and leptin.[9] Some of the local hormonal effects are mediated by paracrine factors that control chondrocyte proliferation and differentiation. Nutritional factors, mechanical loading, and soft-tissue constraints also modulate longitudinal growth, but their effects are ultimately mediated by complex endocrine controls; for example, IGF-I levels decline in malnourished patients. Maturation of the growth plate and the eventual cessation of growth are associated with changing levels of systemic hormones, especially estrogen; it also appears that the growth plate chondrocytes can undergo only a finite number of cell divisions.[9]

Clinical studies of diseases characterized by deficient growth hormone and IGF-I, as well as animal studies, have established the importance of these hormones in regulating longitudinal bone growth.[9,10] Recombinant forms of growth hormone and IGF-I are available for clinical use in augmenting longitudinal bone growth, and they have a positive effect in reversing the deleterious effects of hormone deficiency. Both hormones act directly on the growth plate, although the exact biochemical pathways by which they affect bone growth remain to be elucidated. Growth hormone appears to act both directly, by causing an increase in the chondrocyte proliferation rate; and indirectly, by stimulating local production of IGF-I, which primarily stimulates chondrocyte differentiation and hypertrophy. The stimulatory effects of IGF-I on longitudinal bone growth also may be related to its antiapoptotic effects in the growth plate.[10] Increasing the height of the zone of hypertrophy may decrease the ability of the physis to resist shear forces, and these anatomic changes may contribute to the increased risk of scoliosis progression and slipped capital femoral epiphysis in patients taking growth hormone.[11]

The proliferation of chondrocytes in the growth plate is under the control of a local feedback loop that determines the rate at which cells leave the proliferative zone and enter the zone of cell columns.[12] This feed-

2: Basic Science

back loop primarily involves three signaling molecules synthesized by growth plate chondrocytes: parathyroid hormone–related peptide, Indian hedgehog, and transforming growth factor–β.

During puberty, increases in growth hormone and testosterone can negatively affect the strength of the growth plate. Growth hormone not only stimulates growth by increasing the activity of the growth plate but also lowers the loading capacity of the growth plate. Testosterone promotes growth and reduces the mechanical strength of the growth plate. Although estrogen promotes maturation, indirectly increasing the mechanical strength of the growth plate, the negative effects of growth hormone and testosterone may overpower the positive effects of estrogen.[1] The decrease in mechanical strength during puberty creates a predisposition to epiphyseal separation, particularly in growth plates that are subjected to high shear loads. Slipped capital femoral epiphysis occurs with relative frequency in overweight individuals.[4]

The Mechanical Modulation of Skeletal Growth

Growth alteration by mechanical forces was first identified in the early 19th century by Jacques Delpech, at the University of Montpellier, France. Delpech stated that the release of abnormal pressure from a physis causes growth stimulation. The concept was expanded into the Hueter-Volkmann law, which states that growth is inhibited by compression and stimulated by distraction;[13] and Wolff's law, which states that bone tissue remodels over time in response to prevailing mechanical demands.[14] Decreased physical activity rapidly leads to osteopenia; conversely, bone density increases in physically active individuals. The internal architecture of bones includes both cortical thickness and trabecular parameters such as density, connectivity, and trajectories. The strength of a bone is determined by a complex interplay of these architectural variables so that a simple measurement of bone mineral density is not an accurate predictor of bone strength. Although it appears that the remodeled bone architecture is optimal for providing maximal strength in relation to tissue mass, neither experimental studies nor analytical simulations have discovered any objective rules governing the adaptation of bone to mechanical demands.[14,15] Repetitive loading, rather than static loading, is necessary to maintain homeostasis and induce remodeling.[13]

Quantification of the Hueter-Volkmann Effect

Several studies have confirmed that sustained loading in distraction causes an increase in the growth rate, whereas loading in compression causes a decrease. Growth rates were compared using two different compression and distraction loads in two anatomic locations (tibia and vertebra) in rats, rabbits, and calves at two different ages.[16] The modulation of growth was found not to differ between species or by age. The

growth rate sensitivity to stress averaged 17% per 0.1 MPa, and the range was 9% to 24% per 0.1 MPa for different growth plates. The fast-growing proximal tibia appeared to be slightly more sensitive to stress than the slow-growing vertebra.

The mechanical modulation of growth by sustained compression or distraction is associated with alterations in the growth plate. The reduction or increase in growth rate with compression or distraction, respectively, is associated with a corresponding change in the number of proliferative chondrocytes, the mean chondrocytic height, and the height of the zone of hypertrophy.[17,18] Compression loading causes a decrease in the chondrocyte proliferation rate, chondrocyte cell height, and height of the zone of hypertrophy; distraction loading causes an increase in these parameters.[19]

Dynamic Loading and Growth Modulation

The effect of dynamic loading on growth is unclear. One study reported decreased growth, but another found no change in growth in animals subjected to three different levels of physical activity.[20,21] In a lamb model, 90% of proximal tibia growth occurred during periods of recumbency, when the growth plate was not subjected to dynamic loading.[3] Further study is needed to determine the overall effects of dynamic loading relative to the effects of continuous or sustained loading.

The Effect of Periosteal Resection on Growth

Longitudinal growth can be influenced by the integrity of the periosteum, possibly through a vascular effect or, in part, the growth-inhibiting effect of tension in the periosteum.[13,22] Periosteal stripping alone has a limited clinical effect. In a lamb model, the proximal tibial periosteum was resected, and subsequent growth velocity was measured using implanted microtransducers or fluorochrome labeling.[23] The average growth velocity was 273 microns per day after periosteal resection, compared with 201 microns per day in the contralateral limb of the same animals. This growth rate difference had only a small effect on overall bone length, however. The increased growth was secondary to increased chondrocyte height rather than to an increase in chondrocyte proliferation or matrix production.

Growth Modulation and Scoliosis

The Cobb angle measurement of scoliosis represents the sum of the angular wedging of each vertebra and disk between the end vertebrae.[24] The progression of the vertebral-wedging component of scoliosis during growth is often attributed to the operation of the Hueter-Volkmann law of mechanically modulated endochondral growth. As a result, the rapid progression of scoliosis during the adolescent growth spurt may occur because a scoliotic spine has greater loading on the concave side. This asymmetric loading causes asymmetric growth, which causes vertebral wedging and leads to a vicious cycle of scoliosis progression.[25] To test the vicious cycle hypothesis, an Ilizarov-type external fixator with an imposed 30° scoliosis and axial compression was applied to the tail vertebrae of 10 immature rats for 6 weeks.[26] The tail vertebrae gradually developed a vertebral wedge deformity averaging 15°, which was reported to be secondary to asymmetric growth. The reversibility of the growth disturbance was studied by reversing the loading in one group of rats and removing the loading in a second group.[27] The mean vertebral wedging was 0° when the loading was reversed, and the mean wedging was 7° when the loading was removed.

Part-Time Versus Full-Time Loading

A study of the effect of compression loading on the longitudinal growth of rat tibiae and vertebrae found that full-time loading (24 hours a day) had twice the effect of part-time loading (12 hours a day).[28] Part-time loading had the same effect regardless of whether it was applied during daytime or nighttime hours. The findings of this laboratory study cast doubt on the clinical value of part-time (night) bracing, compared with full-time bracing. If the appropriate loading can be applied, full-time bracing should lead to the most rapid possible correction of skeletal deformity.

Procedures to Modulate Skeletal Growth

Physeal Bar Resection

Physeal bar resection is recommended for children if a bony bridge across a growth plate is tethering growth and causing deformity. The procedure involves surgical resection of the bony bar that is tethering the growth plate, with placement of a spacer such as fat to allow normal growth to resume. If the bony bridge involves less than 50% of the growth plate and the child has considerable remaining growth, physical bar resection is reported to be 70% successful in restoring some longitudinal growth.[29] In a young child with a bony bar that has caused a severe deformity, physeal bar resection can be combined with an osteotomy to simultaneously correct the deformity and allow growth resumption.

Epiphysiodesis

In the traditional Phemister epiphysiodesis, a block of bone was removed from the medial and lateral sides of the bone, including a portion of the metaphysis, growth plate, and epiphysis. The entire growth plate was then ablated using curets, and the bone blocks were rotated 90° and reinserted into the bone. An epiphysiodesis treated a limb-length discrepancy by creating a growth arrest in one growth plate to allow a gradual correction as normal growth occurred on the opposite side. The Phemister technique was modified as a percutaneous technique that had similar results and caused less scarring.[30]

The results of a growth arrest procedure depend on an accurate assessment of the amount of remaining growth. Chronologic age is unreliable for estimating remaining growth; skeletal age, as depicted in the Greulich and Pyle atlas, is more accurate.[31] An evaluation of the growth centers of the elbow and hand, in association with skeletal age determined using the Greulich and Pyle atlas, was found to increase the accuracy of estimates of remaining growth.[32,33]

Reversible Epiphysiodesis

Epiphyseal stapling has been used to arrest growth, with resumption of growth allowed by removing the staples.[34] The initial tendency of the staples to break was remedied by reinforcing the corners where most breaks occurred. The currently used Blount staples (Zimmer; Warsaw, IN) are constructed of cobalt-chromium and are more durable than earlier staples.

Minimally invasive procedures for reversibly arresting bone growth include reinforced Blount stapling and percutaneous epiphysiodesis using transphyseal screws (PETS).[35] Growth is arrested while the implant is in place but is allowed to resume when the implant is removed. This innovation allows for a limb-length discrepancy to be corrected before a major deformity develops. It is no longer necessary to perform the surgery at the precise skeletal age at which there is just enough remaining growth in the contralateral extremity to correct the limb-length discrepancy. In the newer procedures, accurate placement of the staples is crucial (if staples are used). In 50% of patients, a mechanical axis deviation of 1 cm or more was found after staple epiphysiodesis, compared with preoperative measurements;[36] 89% of these mechanical axis deviations were varus in nature. Most of the axis deviations occurred in the proximal tibia, and particular caution therefore is required when placing staples in this location.

Hemiepiphysiodesis

Angular deformities of the lower extremity or spine can be treated using hemiepiphysiodesis. The lower extremity procedure is similar to epiphysiodesis, and it requires an accurate assessment of remaining growth to avoid undercorrection or overcorrection. Blount staples and PETS have been successfully used to induce a reversible hemiepiphysiodesis. The recently developed 8-plate (eight-Plate; Orthofix, McKinney, TX) can be used to create guided growth.[37] This implant is similar to a staple except that the screws toggle in the holes in the plate, using a tension band concept to move the fulcrum of asymmetric growth to the bone surface (**Figure 2**). The technique slows growth on one side of the bone while allowing normal growth on the opposite side to correct a deformity such as genu varum. A slight overcorrection is recommended because some rebound growth stimulation has been reported after the removal of a guided-growth implant.[37] If too much dissection is used to place the implant, growth arrest is a possible complication. Therefore, a careful approach is

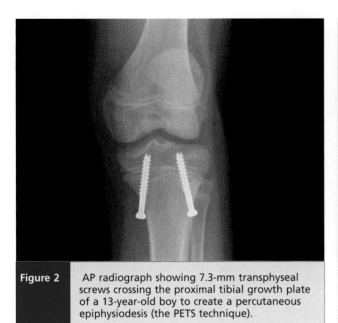

Figure 2 AP radiograph showing 7.3-mm transphyseal screws crossing the proximal tibial growth plate of a 13-year-old boy to create a percutaneous epiphysiodesis (the PETS technique).

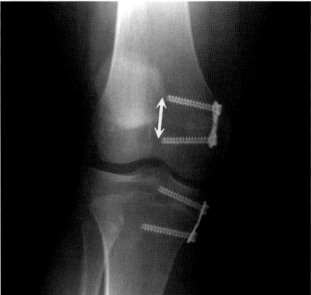

Figure 3 AP radiograph showing 8-plates in the distal medial femur and proximal medial tibia, as used to create a hemiepiphysiodesis for correcting genu valgum by guided growth in a 12-year-old girl. Although the screws are diverging with growth (arrow), no growth is allowed at the medial cortices.

recommended, with limited dissection during implant insertion.

The PETS Technique

The PETS technique involves placing 7.3-mm cannulated, threaded screws across the growth plate to tether growth. A screw may be placed on one side to function as a hemiepiphysiodesis for correcting an angular deformity, or screws may be placed on both sides to function as an epiphysiodesis for correcting a limb-length discrepancy (**Figure 3**).[35] The advantages of the minimally invasive PETS technique include percutaneous screw placement through small incisions; a minimal risk of screw dislodgement; reversible growth arrest; and the use of reverse-cutting threads, which permit easy screw removal, if necessary. Percutaneous hemiepiphysiodesis using the PETS technique was found to be simple, fast, and reproducible, with a low morbidity rate and rapid rehabilitation.[38] The screws can cause pain if they are left protruding, particularly in the proximal medial tibia, where the screw can irritate the pes anserinus tendons. The PETS technique is designed to arrest growth, and it will fail if there is insufficient remaining growth to achieve the desired effect. In one study, complete angular correction occurred early in 13 growth plates of 6 patients who had significant remaining growth; growth resumed in all growth plates when the screws were removed.[39]

The 8-Plate Technique

The 8-plate is a tension band plate construct designed to allow guided growth in deformity correction.[37] The cannulated screw-plate device was designed to decrease the frequency of staples backing out of the bone, particularly in young children. The 8-plate is positioned on the cortex of the bone, moving the fulcrum of correc-

tion to the side of the bone, to allow more rapid correction of angular deformities (**Figure 2**). The toggling of the screws allows most of the growth plate to grow normally while preventing growth directly under the 8-plate.

Breakage of the titanium screws was reported in large patients treated with the 8-plate, and the study authors concluded that staple hemiepiphysiodesis is as effective with respect to rates of correction and complications as the 8-plate for guided correction of angular deformity.[40]

Surgical planning for any type of guided growth procedure to correct skeletal deformity must simultaneously address the postoperative asymmetric growth and the amount of growth remaining. If the surgery is performed too early with respect to remaining growth, an overcorrection may develop; this can be rectified by removing the implant if the hemiepiphysiodesis or guided growth procedure is reversible. If the surgery is performed too late, an undercorrection or failure may develop; this cannot easily be reversed. Lateral hemiepiphysiodesis was reported to be unsuccessful in 66% of patients with adolescent tibia vara who were at least 10 years of age at the time of surgery; 94% of the patients had a body mass index above the 95th percentile.[41] The high failure rate was associated with patient age of 14 years or older, severe tibia vara, and patient obesity, which contributed to the Hueter-Volkmann effect of decreased growth on the compression side of the physis.

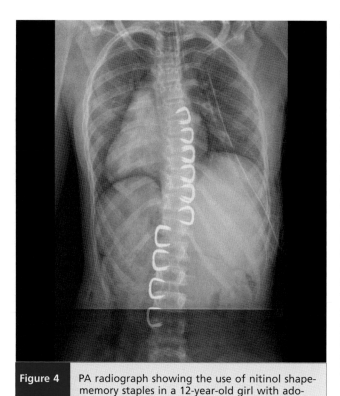

Figure 4 PA radiograph showing the use of nitinol shape-memory staples in a 12-year-old girl with adolescent idiopathic scoliosis. A convex vertebral hemiepiphysiodesis was created to correct the scoliosis by growth modulation. (Courtesy of John T. Braun, MD, Burlington, VT.)

Methods to Modulate Spine Growth

Hemiepiphysiodesis

A combined anterior and posterior hemiepiphysiodesis of the spine has been successful in treating children with congenital scoliosis caused by a hemivertebra or an unsegmented bar. This procedure allows for gradual correction of the scoliosis with growth. Fusionless instrumentation systems using a growing rod or vertical expandable prosthetic titanium rib (VEPTR) have been developed for treating congenital scoliosis.[42-44]

Vertebral Stapling

Vertebral stapling is designed to span the disk and growth plates of two adjacent vertebrae to tether growth on the convex side of a scoliosis deformity. This technique was used as a model of spine hemiepiphysiodesis in creating a thoracic scoliosis in pigs; the staple was supplemented by two screws to preclude staple dislodging.[45] The height of the zone of hypertrophy, the chondrocyte cell height, and the cell width were found to be decreased on the stapled side compared with either the contralateral side or control vertebrae.

In principle, the process of convex tethering of growth to allow gradual correction of a scoliosis secondary to growth on the concave side appears to be sound. Early experience with vertebral stapling was disappointing, however. There was limited correction be-cause the patients had severe scoliosis and little remaining growth. Staples dislodged because they spanned the disk spaces; investigators speculated that the forces generated by the staples might be absorbed by the flexible disks, thus minimizing the forces across the growth plates, as observed in a porcine model of spine stapling.[45]

A staple constructed of nitinol, which is a shape-memory alloy, was designed to prevent vertebral staple dislodgement. The prongs of the nitinol staple are a standard straight shape when cool, to allow easy insertion. At body temperature, the prongs clamp down into the bone in a C-shape to prevent staple dislodgement (**Figure 4**). In an uncontrolled case series, curve progression of more than 10° was reported in 18% of curves greater than 30° and 0% of curves smaller than 30° after nitinol vertebral stapling.[46] Thoracoscopic insertion is recommended for nitinol staples. The role of vertebral stapling has not been determined, and no intermediate- or long-term results are available. This procedure currently is recommended only for a low-grade scoliosis if the alternative is observation, bracing, or casting. The device has not been approved by the US Food and Drug Administration for this use.

Anterolateral Vertebral Tethering

A novel fusionless treatment method for scoliosis attempts to modulate growth by tethering the anterolateral aspect of the spine.[47] An anterolateral tether was created in 12 minipigs by placing four staple-screws connected by a polyethylene tether over the anterolateral aspect of four consecutive thoracic vertebrae. After 12 months, radiographs showed an average scoliosis of 30°, with associated vertebral wedging in all four vertebrae. This fusionless procedure can be performed thoracoscopically.

A recent case report described an intriguing preliminary outcome of treatment for a boy with juvenile idiopathic scoliosis, whose right thoracic curve from T6 to T12 had progressed from 25° to 40° in 3 years.[48] He was treated with a minithoracotomy, and vertebral body screws were placed at each level. A polypropylene tether 4.5 mm in diameter was secured into the screw heads to create an anterior tether without fusion. The postoperative curve was 25°; 4 years later, the curve was 6°.

Limitations of Growth-Tethering Techniques

A potential limitation of the use of growth modulation procedures involving vertebral staples, nitinol staples, or anterolateral flexible tethering is the limited remaining spine growth in a patient with progressive adolescent idiopathic scoliosis. The ideal time for a growth-tethering procedure is 1 to 2 years before peak growth velocity, the onset of menses, and closure of the triradiate cartilage. However, most patients have a small curve at this age, and the clinician cannot be certain whether the scoliosis will continue to be mild or will progress to a large curve.

Summary

There is tremendous potential for developing less invasive surgical techniques to modulate growth and correct skeletal deformities, following basic science principles. In the future, an understanding of the biochemical feedback mechanisms involved in growth will allow the development of nonsurgical techniques to modulate growth and correct skeletal deformities. Novel techniques will be extremely valuable for the fusionless treatment of spine deformities, but care must be taken to responsibly develop and apply these techniques.

Acknowledgment

The authors thank Keith M. Bagnall, PhD for his constructive critique of the contents of this chapter and Paul J. Zimakas, MD for his contribution to the hormonal regulation of longitudinal growth.

Annotated References

1. Hefti F: Basic principles: Growth, in Hefti F, ed: *Pediatric Orthopedics in Practice*. Berlin and Heidelberg, Germany, Springer Medizin Verlag, 2007, pp 41-48.

   This comprehensive and comprehensible textbook covers all aspects of pediatric orthopaedics. A strong interest in growth and development permeates the book, which includes many references from international journals.

2. Wilsman NJ, Farnum CE, Green EM, Lieferman EM, Clayton MK: Cell cycle analysis of proliferative zone chondrocytes in growth plates elongating at different rates. *J Orthop Res* 1996;14(4):562-572.

3. Noonan KJ, Farnum CE, Leiferman EM, Lampl M, Markel MD, Wilsman NJ: Growing pains: Are they due to increased growth during recumbency as documented in a lamb model? *J Pediatr Orthop* 2004;24(6):726-731.

4. Chung SM, Batterman SC, Brighton CT: Shear strength of the human femoral capital epiphyseal plate. *J Bone Joint Surg Am* 1976;58(1):94-103.

5. Trueta J, Amato VP: The vascular contribution to osteogenesis: III. Changes in the growth cartilage caused by experimentally induced ischaemia. *J Bone Joint Surg Br* 1960;42-B:571-587.

6. Kim HK, Stephenson N, Garces A, Aya-ay J, Bian H: Effects of disruption of epiphyseal vasculature on the proximal femoral growth plate. *J Bone Joint Surg Am* 2009;91(5):1149-1158.

   Disruption of the epiphyseal vasculature of the proximal femoral growth plate in a porcine model did not lead to diffuse growth plate damage. The proximal part of the femur continued to elongate, although more slowly than on the normal side. These findings suggest that the epiphyseal vasculature may not be the sole source of nutrition for the proximal femoral growth plate.

7. Farnum CE, Lenox M, Zipfel W, Horton W, Williams R: In vivo delivery of fluoresceinated dextrans to the murine growth plate: Imaging of three vascular routes by multiphoton microscopy. *Anat Rec A Discov Mol Cell Evol Biol* 2006;288(1):91-103.

   This is an analysis of the real-time dynamics of entrance of fluoresceinated tracers of different molecular weight into the growth plate from the systemic vasculature. Small molecules (as large as 10 kDa) entered the growth plate from both the epiphyseal and metaphyseal vessels, whereas dextrans molecules of 40 kDa or larger did not enter from either the epiphyseal or metaphyseal vessels.

8. Kember NF, Sissons HA: Quantitative histology of the human growth plate. *J Bone Joint Surg Br* 1976;58-B(4):426-435.

9. Nilsson O, Marino R, De Luca F, Phillip M, Baron J: Endocrine regulation of the growth plate. *Horm Res* 2005;64(4):157-165.

   Longitudinal bone growth is governed by a complex network of endocrine signals, including growth hormone, IGF-I, glucocorticoid, thyroid hormone, estrogen, androgen, vitamin D, and leptin. The mechanism by which each of these endocrine signals regulates longitudinal growth is reviewed.

10. Wu S, Fadoju D, Rezvani G, De Luca F: Stimulatory effects of insulin-like growth factor-I on growth plate chondrogenesis are mediated by nuclear factor-kappaB p65. *J Biol Chem* 2008;283(49):34037-34044.

    IGF-I is reported to increase longitudinal growth by two main cellular events: stimulation of the chondrocyte proliferation rate and stimulation of chondrocyte differentiation and hypertrophy. The longitudinal growth stimulatory effects also may be related to antiapoptotic effects, further increasing the chondrocyte height in the zone of hypertrophy.

11. Bowlby DA, Rapaport R: Safety and efficacy of growth hormone therapy in childhood. *Pediatr Endocrinol Rev* 2004;2(suppl 1):68-77.

12. Ballock RT, O'Keefe RJ: The biology of the growth plate. *J Bone Joint Surg Am* 2003;85-A(4):715-726.

13. Wilson-MacDonald J, Houghton GR, Bradley J, Morscher E: The relationship between periosteal division and compression or distraction of the growth plate: An experimental study in the rabbit. *J Bone Joint Surg Br* 1990;72(2):303-308.

14. Huiskes R: If bone is the answer, then what is the question? *J Anat* 2000;197(Pt 2):145-156.

15. Rubin CT, Lanyon LE: Osteoregulatory nature of mechanical stimuli. Function as a determinant for adaptive remodeling in bone. *J Orthop Res* 1987;5(2):300-310.

2: Basic Science

16. Stokes IA, Aronsson DD, Dimock AN, Cortright V, Beck S: Endochondral growth in growth plates of three species at two anatomical locations modulated by mechanical compression and tension. *J Orthop Res* 2006; 24(6):1327-1334.

    An apparently linear relationship between stress and growth rate was found. Vertebrae and the proximal tibiae had relatively small differences in growth rate sensitivity to stress despite large differences in growth rates. The results may apply to human growth plates.

17. Stokes IA, Mente PL, Iatridis JC, Farnum CE, Aronsson DD: Enlargement of growth plate chondrocytes modulated by sustained mechanical loading. *J Bone Joint Surg Am* 2002;84-A(10):1842-1848.

18. Stokes IA, Clark KC, Farnum CE, Aronsson DD: Alterations in the growth plate associated with growth modulation by sustained compression or distraction. *Bone* 2007;41(2):197-205.

    Growth plates that had been subjected to sustained loading were examined histologically. Reduced growth rate with compression and increased growth rate with distraction were associated with corresponding changes in the number of proliferative chondrocytes and the final (maximum) hypertrophic chondrocytic height. Chondrocytic enlargement was the most important contributor to altered growth rates.

19. Apte SS, Kenwright J: Physeal distraction and cell proliferation in the growth plate. *J Bone Joint Surg Br* 1994;76(5):837-843.

20. Akyuz E, Braun JT, Brown NA, Bachus KN: Static versus dynamic loading in the mechanical modulation of vertebral growth. *Spine (Phila Pa 1976)* 2006;31(25): E952-E958.

    Tail vertebrae of immature rats were subjected to a static or dynamic (1 Hz) asymmetric load. The resulting wedge angles were greater in the dynamically loaded vertebrae. This finding suggests that growth modulation devices applied to a spine with scoliosis should use dynamic loading.

21. Niehoff A, Kersting UG, Zaucke F, Morlock MM, Brüggemann GP: Adaptation of mechanical, morphological, and biochemical properties of the rat growth plate to dose-dependent voluntary exercise. *Bone* 2004; 35(4):899-908.

22. Foolen J, van Donkelaar CC, Murphy P, Huiskes R, Ito K: Residual periosteum tension is insufficient to directly modulate bone growth. *J Biomech* 2009;42(2):152-157.

    This study of growth plates of chick embryotic tibiotarsi refuted the generally accepted hypothesis that growth augmentation after division of the periosteum results from release of compressive force created by tensioned periosteum. The measured residual stress would not have produced substantial growth rate alteration based on present understanding of stress-induced growth modulation.

23. Sansone JM, Wilsman NJ, Leiferman EM, Noonan KJ: The effect of periosteal resection on tibial growth velocity measured by microtransducer technology in lambs. *J Pediatr Orthop* 2009;29(1):61-67.

    The authors circumferentially resected the proximal tibial metaphyseal periosteum in five lambs. Sustained growth acceleration developed secondary to axial elongation of the hypertrophic chondrocytes, but its limited magnitude suggests that this technique should be considered as an adjunct to other procedures.

24. Stokes IA, Aronsson DD: Disc and vertebral wedging in patients with progressive scoliosis. *J Spinal Disord* 2001;14(4):317-322.

25. Stokes IA: Analysis and simulation of progressive adolescent scoliosis by biomechanical growth modulation. *Eur Spine J* 2007;16(10):1621-1628.

    Different rates of growth were simulated in the convex and concave sides of vertebrae in a scoliosis, using published data on spine load asymmetry and growth sensitivity to altered stress. The rate of scoliosis progression was similar to that observed in adolescents, suggesting that biomechanical factors are responsible for progression during the growth spurt.

26. Mente PL, Stokes IA, Spence H, Aronsson DD: Progression of vertebral wedging in an asymmetrically loaded rat tail model. *Spine (Phila Pa 1976)* 1997;22(12):1292-1296.

27. Mente PL, Aronsson DD, Stokes IA, Iatridis JC: Mechanical modulation of growth for the correction of vertebral wedge deformities. *J Orthop Res* 1999;17(4):518-524.

28. Stokes IA, Gwadera J, Dimock A, Farnum CE, Aronsson DD: Modulation of vertebral and tibial growth by compression loading: Diurnal versus full-time loading. *J Orthop Res* 2005;23(1):188-195.

    The growth plates of growing rats were compression loaded for 8 days, during 12 daytime hours, 12 nighttime hours, or all 24 hours. Growth suppression (modulation) was in proportion to the duration of loading and was approximately half as much in the growth plates that received part-time loading.

29. Marsh JS, Polzhofer GK: Arthroscopically assisted central physeal bar resection. *J Pediatr Orthop* 2006;26(2): 255-259.

    After 37 central physeal bars were resected using an arthroscopically assisted technique, growth occurred in 70% of patients, with failure in 13%. Failures occurred when the bar was caused by infection or its size approached 50% of the physeal surface. This technique provides the best visualization of the bar.

30. Timperlake RW, Bowen JR, Guille JT, Choi IH: Prospective evaluation of fifty-three consecutive percutaneous epiphysiodeses of the distal femur and proximal tibia and fibula. *J Pediatr Orthop* 1991;11(3):350-357.

2: Basic Science

31. Greulich WW: *Radiographic Atlas of Skeletal Development of the Hand and Wrist*, ed 2. Stanford, CA, Stanford University Press, 1959.

32. Charles YP, Diméglio A, Canavese F, Daures JP: Skeletal age assessment from the olecranon for idiopathic scoliosis at Risser grade 0. *J Bone Joint Surg Am* 2007; 89(12):2737-2744.

    A simplified olecranon method was developed to assess skeletal age at 6-month intervals during puberty. The method was evaluated in 100 boys and 100 girls with idiopathic scoliosis and was found to be simple, reliable, and precise, complementing the Risser sign and triradiate cartilage evaluation. Level of evidence: II.

33. Sanders JO, Khoury JG, Kishan S, et al: Predicting scoliosis progression from skeletal maturity: A simplified classification during adolescence. *J Bone Joint Surg Am* 2008;90(3):540-553.

    A simplified skeletal maturity staging system using the Tanner-Whitehouse–III descriptors was found to correlate more strongly with the curve progression behavior of patients with idiopathic scoliosis than the Risser sign or Greulich and Pyle skeletal ages. Level of evidence: I.

34. Blount WP, Clarke GR: Control of bone growth by epiphyseal stapling; a preliminary report. *J Bone Joint Surg Am* 1949;31A(3):464-478.

35. Métaizeau JP, Wong-Chung J, Bertrand H, Pasquier P: Percutaneous epiphysiodesis using transphyseal screws (PETS). *J Pediatr Orthop* 1998;18(3):363-369.

36. Gorman TM, Vanderwerff R, Pond M, MacWilliams B, Santora SD: Mechanical axis following staple epiphysiodesis for limb-length inequality. *J Bone Joint Surg Am* 2009;91(10):2430-2439.

    The preoperative and final radiographs of 54 patients who underwent staple epiphysiodesis revealed a mechanical axis shift of 1 cm or more in 50%, most of which were into varus. Poor proximal lateral tibial staple placement accounted for some of the deformities. Level of evidence: IV.

37. Stevens PM, Klatt JB: Guided growth for pathological physes: Radiographic improvement during realignment. *J Pediatr Orthop* 2008;28(6):632-639.

    The authors performed a guided growth procedure in 14 children with rickets. Of the 53 deformities treated with staple fixation (in 10 children), 45% had staple migration. Of the 15 deformities treated with 8-plate fixation (in 4 children), none had migration. Guided growth to maintain alignment is recommended to avoid later surgery. Level of evidence: IV.

38. Mesa PA, Yamhure FH: Percutaneous hemiepiphysiodesis using transphyseal cannulated screws for genu valgum in adolescents. *J Child Orthop* 2009.

    The authors conducted a prospective evaluation of 52 patients (100 knees) using the PETS technique to create a distal femoral hemiepiphysiodesis. The tibiofemoral angle was satisfactorily corrected, and the authors concluded that PETS is a simple, fast, and reproducible technique with a low morbidity rate.

39. Khoury JG, Tavares JO, McConnell S, Zeiders G, Sanders JO: Results of screw epiphysiodesis for the treatment of limb length discrepancy and angular deformity. *J Pediatr Orthop* 2007;27(6):623-628.

    The PETS technique was used in 30 patients to treat a limb-length discrepancy and 30 patients to treat an angular deformity. Improvement occurred in all patients. In 13 growth plates of 6 patients, screws were removed after correction and growth resumed. PETS combines a minimally invasive percutaneous technique with reversibility.

40. Wiemann JM IV, Tryon C, Szalay EA: Physeal stapling versus 8-plate hemiepiphysiodesis for guided correction of angular deformity about the knee. *J Pediatr Orthop* 2009;29(5):481-485.

    The authors compared 39 limbs treated with staple hemiepiphysiodesis and 24 limbs treated with an 8-plate. There was no difference between the two groups in the rate of correction or the frequency of complications. The rate of complications was greater in patients with pathologic physes. Level of evidence: III.

41. McIntosh AL, Hanson CM, Rathjen KE: Treatment of adolescent tibia vara with hemiepiphysiodesis: Risk factors for failure. *J Bone Joint Surg Am* 2009;91(12): 2873-2879.

    Lateral hemiepiphysiodesis was unsuccessful in 66% of 49 patients with adolescent tibia vara who were at least 10 years of age and had an average body mass index of 40.7. Lateral hemiepiphysiodesis may be an option for thin patients with mild tibia vara, but it is likely to fail in older adolescents with a high body mass index and greater deformity. Level of evidence: II.

42. Thompson GH, Akbarnia BA, Campbell RM Jr: Growing rod techniques in early-onset scoliosis. *J Pediatr Orthop* 2007;27(3):354-361.

    Early onset scoliosis can be treated using a single growing rod, dual growing rods, or a VEPTR. Dual growing rods with lengthening every 6 months had better results than single growing rods. The VEPTR was particularly beneficial for treating congenital scoliosis and fused ribs or for children with severe thoracic insufficiency syndrome.

43. Campbell RM Jr, Smith MD, Mayes TC, et al: The effect of opening wedge thoracostomy on thoracic insufficiency syndrome associated with fused ribs and congenital scoliosis. *J Bone Joint Surg Am* 2004;86-A(8):1659-1674.

44. Yazici M, Emans J: Fusionless instrumentation systems for congenital scoliosis: Expandable spinal rods and vertical expandable prosthetic titanium rib in the management of congenital spine deformities in the growing child. *Spine (Phila Pa 1976)* 2009;34(17):1800-1807.

    A review of research articles and presentations was used to compare growing rods and VEPTR. The authors conclude that growing rods should be used if the primary deformity is in the spine. Expansion thoracostomy and VEPTR should be used if the primary deformities include rib fusions and thoracic insufficiency syndrome.

45. Bylski-Austrow DI, Wall EJ, Glos DL, Ballard ET, Montgomery A, Crawford AH: Spinal hemiepiphysiodesis decreases the size of vertebral growth plate hypertrophic zone and cells. *J Bone Joint Surg Am* 2009; 91(3):584-593.

     Staples were applied unilaterally to midthoracic vertebrae of skeletally immature pigs. After 8 weeks, the vertebral hypertrophic zone height was reduced in inverse proportion to the distance from the staples, indicating a graded growth modulation across the vertebra.

46. Betz RR, D'Andrea LP, Mulcahey MJ, Chafetz RS: Vertebral body stapling procedure for the treatment of scoliosis in the growing child. *Clin Orthop Relat Res* 2005; 434:55-60.

     After vertebral body stapling in 39 patients with adolescent idiopathic scoliosis, 87% had curve stability (progression of no more than 10°). A fusion was necessary in 2 patients. Stapling is recommended for immature patients with adolescent idiopathic scoliosis who have curves of 20° to 45°, with 5° of progression for curves of less than 25°. Level of evidence: IV.

47. Newton PO, Upasani VV, Farnsworth CL, et al: Spinal growth modulation with use of a tether in an immature porcine model. *J Bone Joint Surg Am* 2008;90(12): 2695-2706.

     A staple-screw construct connected by a polyethylene tether was applied over four consecutive thoracic vertebrae of 7-month-old minipigs. There was a progressive increase in Cobb angle to 30° at 12 months, along with an unexpected wedging of disks opposite to that of the vertebrae, with nucleus migration to the side of the tether.

48. Crawford CH III, Lenke LG: Growth modulation by means of anterior tethering resulting in progressive correction of juvenile idiopathic scoliosis: A case report. *J Bone Joint Surg Am* 2010;92(1):202-209.

     This case report describes the treatment of a boy with juvenile scoliosis using an anterior tethering procedure without fusion, which caused a gradual correction of the scoliosis from 40° preoperatively to 6° at 48-month follow-up. The authors were not aware of any similar earlier report.

2: Basic Science

Chapter 10
Cerebral Palsy

David E. Westberry, MD   Jon R. Davids, MD

Introduction

The term cerebral palsy (CP) describes a group of permanent disorders of movement and posture that are attributed to nonprogressive disturbances originating in the fetal or infant brain. The motor disorders often are accompanied by disturbances of sensation, perception, cognition, communication, and behavior. Seizure activity and secondary musculoskeletal problems also may be present.[1]

CP is the most common cause of physical disability in children, with an incidence of 1 to 3 per 1,000 live births.[2] Extremely premature birth increases the risk of CP approximately 100-fold, compared with near-term birth.[2] The prevalence of CP was stable in developed countries from the 1950s until the 1970s, when neonatal intensive care units became widely available. During the late 1970s and early 1980s, the incidence of CP rose secondary to increased survival rates for vulnerable infants who earlier would have died. During the past two decades in developed countries, the rates of CP have been stable or have decreased. The lower rates of birth-related injury resulting from improved obstetric care have been offset by higher rates of survival for preterm infants as a result of improved neonatal care.

Although the growing child's cerebral lesion is static, the associated musculoskeletal deformities and impairment can be progressive. The care of a child with CP requires a multidisciplinary approach that emphasizes early developmental therapies, tone management, orthotic devices, and musculoskeletal surgery. Orthopaedic surgeons, physical and occupational therapists, neurologists, neurosurgeons, pediatricians, and orthotists must contribute if a child with CP is to reach the highest possible level of function. Treatment during the child's early years focuses on tone management, prevention of contractures, assisted walking, and multilevel bony and soft-tissue surgeries to improve gait.

The literature on the treatment of adult patients with CP is limited. Many adults with CP continue to have spasticity and pain, which contribute to deterioration of the ability to ambulate. Often the patient loses the ability to walk independently or with support after reaching adulthood. The care of adults with CP is affected by a lack of dedicated health and rehabilitation services.[3]

Pathophysiology and Medical Comorbidities

CP can occur as a consequence of intrauterine factors, perinatal infection, premature birth, or anoxic birth injury. MRI evaluation of the brain of a child with CP who was born prematurely may reveal periventricular leukomalacia. However, the etiology of CP is unidentifiable in many patients, and this fact can be a source of great frustration for the child's parents. The severity and distribution of CP vary greatly, depending on the extent of the underlying central nervous system injury.

Bone mineral density in children with CP can be impaired by factors including short-term immobilization and lack of weight bearing after orthopaedic surgery. Poor nutrition, low calcium intake, and anticonvulsant drugs also can have a negative effect. An increased incidence of fractures was found in children with CP who were nonambulatory and taking antiseizure medication. Delays in diagnosing low bone mineral density were common.[4] Poor coordination of the tongue and pharyngeal muscles, gastroesophageal reflux, or an inability to hold utensils independently may limit the ability of a child with severe CP to receive nutrition adequate for normal growth and development. Nutritional supplementation, speech therapy training, or placement of a gastrostomy tube sometimes is necessary to allow adequate caloric intake.

Children with mild or moderate CP may be at risk for childhood obesity. A recent retrospective study found that the prevalence of obesity in ambulatory children with CP increased significantly during the past decade, as it did in the general pediatric population.[5] Children with relatively little neuromuscular involvement and a relatively high level of function were more likely to be obese.

Classification and Outcomes Assessment

The clinical spectrum of CP ranges from very minor impairment to significant cognitive deficits and motor function limitations. Patients with severe CP often have

2: Basic Science

comorbid conditions such as seizures, recurrent pneumonia, and feeding dysfunction (often requiring the use of a feeding tube). CP can be classified on the basis of physical examination findings, anatomic location of musculoskeletal involvement, ambulatory ability, or functional status. On the basis of physical examination, CP is classified as spastic, dystonic, dyskinetic, ataxic, or hypotonic. The spastic form of CP is the most common, and mixed forms are increasingly being diagnosed. The anatomic classification reflects the number of involved extremities and uses the terms quadriplegic (equal involvement of all four extremities), diplegic (greater involvement of the lower extremities than the upper extremities), and hemiplegic (unilateral upper and lower extremity involvement). Triplegic (three-extremity involvement), monoplegic (single-extremity involvement), and asymmetric forms also occur.

CP also can be classified based on the child's ability to walk and sit. The Gross Motor Function Classification System (GMFCS) is a five-level grading system based on an assessment of self-initiated movement[6] (**Figure 1**). The GMFCS is used to determine the child's level of function by assessing functional limitations, the need for walking aids or wheeled mobility equipment, and quality of movement as related to the child's age. The GMFCS originally was intended for use in children age 12 years or younger, but recently it was expanded and revised to apply to children as old as 18 years.[6] Children with CP may decline in gross motor function over time, especially during the adolescent growth spurt, with a corresponding change in the GMFCS level.

Although many methods are available for evaluating and measuring a child with CP, there is no comprehensive tool for assessment across multiple domains. The International Classification of Functioning, Disability, and Health is a framework for outcome assessment in which "cerebral palsy" is considered among domains that can be affected by environmental, personal, and other factors, including "body structure and function" and "activity participation versus limitation."[7] Body function traditionally has been assessed using radiographs and measures of range of motion, strength, and spasticity. These can be complemented by functional outcome assessment tools including the Gross Motor Function Measure and the Functional Mobility Scale. Parent- and child-report questionnaires are used to assess quality of life. These tools are not specific to CP, however, and their overall value in outcome assessment has not been established.

Treatment Modalities

Pharmacologic Therapy

Botulinum Toxin A
Botulinum toxin A (BoNT-A) is a protein-polypeptide chain extracted from *Clostridium botulinum* that irreversibly binds to the cholinergic terminals at the neuromuscular junction and effectively inhibits the release of acetylcholine from the synaptic vesicles. Botulinum toxin has seven known serotypes, of which types A and B are approved by the US Food and Drug Administration for the treatment of spasticity in humans and are commercially available. The toxin can be locally injected into spastic muscles, causing a rapid onset of weakness that may last 3 to 6 months. In children with CP, the muscles most commonly treated with BoNT-A injection are spastic ankle plantar flexors, posterior tibialis, hamstrings, hip adductors, and wrist flexors. The risks of repeated injections include a lessening of the positive effect of the toxin and possible antibody formation. Some children appear to develop a tolerance after repeated injections.

The therapeutic benefit of BoNT-A for patients with CP is unclear. A recent literature review concluded that clinical outcomes of BoNT-A use were better than those of placebo treatment.[8] Outcomes were better when BoNT-A was combined with casting or a structured physical therapy program. Few adverse events have been reported after BoNT-A use at the recommended dosages.

BoNT-A is commonly used to treat children with dynamic spastic equinus or equinus contracture. A recent randomized, controlled study found that outcomes were better when casting was delayed at least 4 weeks after BoNT-A injection; immobilization of the ankle by immediate casting was believed to reduce the effective uptake of BoNT-A and thereby lessen its clinical effectiveness.[9]

Baclofen
Oral baclofen is a gamma-aminobutyric acid analogue that binds to gamma-aminobutyric acid receptors in the spinal cord after crossing the blood-brain barrier. Baclofen acts at the spinal cord level to impede the release of excitatory neurotransmitters that cause spasticity. Because of the blood-brain barrier, a large dose of oral baclofen is required to reduce spasticity. The use of oral baclofen is limited by the adverse effects associated with large dosages, including somnolence, hypotonia, weakness, and nausea. Physiologic dependence can develop, and careful weaning is necessary to prevent rebound spasticity, hallucinations, or seizures.

Intrathecal administration allows an effective dose of baclofen to reach the target tissues with decreased systemic adverse effects. The dosage of intrathecal baclofen (ITB) is 30 times lower than the oral baclofen dosage. A synchronized infusion system is used, with an implantable infusion pump, a spinal catheter, and an external programmer. Complications occur in as many as 20% of patients and can be life threatening; they include cerebrospinal fluid leakage, infection, catheter fracture, catheter dislodgement, wound dehiscence, and baclofen overdose.[10] ITB pumps most often are implanted in patients with severe spasticity that interferes with function and positioning. In patients with dystonic CP, ITB can lead to dystonia reduction and postural improvement, thus facilitating care of the patient.[11] The

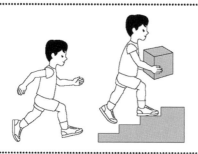

GMFCS Level I

Children walk at home, in school, outdoors, and in the community. They can climb stairs without the use of a railing. Children perform gross motor skills such as running and jumping, but speed, balance, and coordination are limited.

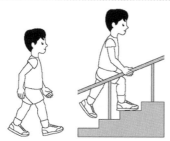

GMFCS Level II

Children walk in most settings and climb stairs holding onto a railing. They may experience difficulty walking long distances and balancing on uneven terrain, on inclines, in crowded areas, or in confined spaces. Children may walk with physical assistance or a handheld mobility device, or use wheeled mobility equipment over long distances. Children have only minimal ability to perform gross motor skills such as running and jumping.

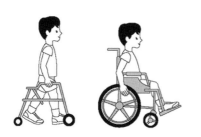

GMFCS Level III

Children walk using a handheld mobility device in most indoor settings. They may climb stairs holding onto a railing with supervision or assistance. Children use wheeled mobility equipment when traveling long distances and may self-propel for shorter distances.

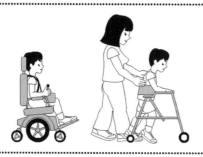

GMFCS Level IV

Children use methods of mobility that require physical assistance or powered mobility equipment in most settings. They may walk for short distances at home with physical assistance or use powered mobility equipment or a body-support walker when positioned. At school, outdoors, and in the community, children are transported in a manual wheelchair or use powered mobility equipment.

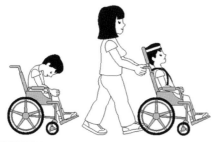

GMFCS Level V

Children are transported in a manual wheelchair in all settings. Children are limited in their ability to maintain antigravity head and trunk postures and to control leg and arm movements.

Figure 1   The Expanded and Revised Gross Motor Function Classification System (GMFCS) for children between their 6th and 12th birthdays. (Adapted with permission from Palisano R, Rosenbaum P, Walter S, Russell D, Wood E, Galuppi B: Development and reliability of a system to classify gross motor function in children with cerebral palsy. *Dev Med Child Neurol* 1997;39[4]:214-223. Drawings courtesy of Kerr Graham, Bill Reid, and Adrienne Harvey, Melbourne, Australia.)

2: Basic Science

effect of ITB on the ambulatory function of children with CP has not been reported.

The effect of ITB on spine alignment is controversial. Some studies reported an increased incidence of rapid scoliosis progression after pump placement, but other studies suggested that the natural progression of neuromuscular scoliosis is unaffected by ITB.[12] Close monitoring of spine deformity with serial radiographs of the spine is warranted after placement of a baclofen pump.

Treatment of Dystonia

Dystonic CP is the second most common form of CP, after the spastic form. Its characteristic feature is abnormal twisting or posturing caused by sustained involuntary muscle contractions. Dystonia is clinically classified based on the location of abnormal muscle activity. Focal dystonia may involve the upper extremity or the lower extremity. Approximately 90% of patients with dystonic CP have the generalized form, and most of these patients are nonambulatory. Hemidystonia is easily confused with spastic hemiparesis, but the characteristic flexion deformities at multiple joints typically are not present.

Dystonia is treated using oral medications, intramuscular injections, intrathecal medications, nerve transaction, and deep brain stimulation. Oral medications usually are ineffective for focal dystonia. The primary nonsurgical treatment is BoNT-A injection, which was reported to be effective for several years.[13] ITB is the recommended treatment for severe, generalized dystonic CP.[14] The effective dosage of ITB to treat dystonia typically is twice the dosage required to treat spasticity, and a higher frequency of complications therefore is to be expected.

Orthotic Devices

An ankle-foot orthosis (AFO) is commonly prescribed to improve gait and stability, prevent deformity, and protect surgical repairs during the postoperative period. Solid or hinged AFOs improve gait in children with spastic diplegic CP. Floor-reaction AFOs are effective in correcting a crouch gait secondary to weakness of the ankle plantar flexors. An AFO can be used in a young child to try to prevent the development of equinus contractures. In addition, an AFO can be used to prevent recurrence of deformity after BoNT-A injection and serial casting for dynamic or mild myostatic deformities of the ankle plantar flexors.

AFOs were found to be ineffective in improving static alignment of the foot and ankle, as measured by radiographs.[15] Only orthotic devices that extend to the knee and have a rigid ankle, leaf spring, or hinged design were found to prevent equinus deformity. Prevention of equinus deformity improves walking speed and stride length for most children with an appropriate orthotic device.[16]

A hinged AFO offers foot and ankle control throughout the gait cycle while allowing increased dorsiflexion of the ankle. The disadvantages of the hinged design include the cost and the difficulty of fitting shoes over the brace. A dynamic AFO offers foot and ankle control during the swing phase of gait while allowing a modest amount of motion during the stance phase. A dynamic AFO typically is lighter than a hinged-design AFO and provides improved contours around the hindfoot and ankle. Both AFO designs were found to be effective at improving ankle kinematics and kinetics in children with CP who were at GMFCS level I.[17]

Physical Therapy

Physical therapy is believed to be critical in the treatment of a child with motor dysfunction. Several routine physical therapy sessions every week allow the child to improve range of motion, strengthen the involved muscles, undergo gait training, and receive assistance with activities of daily living. Some aspects of physical therapy are controversial. The intensity (number of weekly sessions), modalities, and goals of therapy are a current focus of study. In a recent randomized controlled study, specific goal-directed therapy on an intensive level was compared with generalized therapy sessions in a group of 56 children with CP at GMFCS level III or better.[18] As assessed using the Gross Motor Function Measure and Gross Motor Performance Measure, there was no significant difference in the function and performance outcomes of the two groups of patients.[18] Increasing the duration and frequency of therapy sessions for children with CP offered no significant benefits in motor or general development.[19]

Children with CP have generalized weakness in comparison with normally developing children. Children with spasticity can benefit from strengthening programs involving progressive resistance exercises. Strengthening programs were found to lead to improved overall muscle strength and improved gait function.[20]

Neurosurgery

Some children with CP can benefit from selective dorsal rhizotomy, in which dorsal rootlets from L1 to S2 are selectively cut. As a result, the patient's heightened responses to afferent impulses from muscle spindles can be interrupted and spasticity can be lessened. There is controversy as to the precise indications, techniques, and surgical approach for selective dorsal rhizotomy, as well as the specific rootlets that should be cut. In most centers, selective dorsal rhizotomy is recommended for ambulatory children with significantly increased tone and spasticity, good motor control and strength, and the ability to participate in intensive physical therapy after surgery. Significant weakness of the lower extremities and poor selective motor control are relative contraindications to the procedure.

Randomized clinical studies found that patients with CP had functional improvement and reduced spasticity after selective dorsal rhizotomy and physical therapy, compared with patients who underwent physical therapy alone.[21] In the short term after selective dorsal rhizotomy, patients had reduction in spasticity, improvement in gait quality, reduction in energy cost, and improvement in overall ambulatory function.[22] Long-term studies found that tone reduction was maintained without recurrent spasticity, passive range of motion was improved, and functional skills and independence were improved.[23]

The complications associated with selective dorsal rhizotomy include transient or permanent bowel or bladder incontinence, dysesthesia, dural leakage, weakness, and musculoskeletal deformities including hip subluxation and spine deformity. Mild scoliosis occurs in 44% of patients, and spondylolisthesis occurs in 19%.[24] These deformities typically are mild and clinically insignificant, but the risk warrants routine radiographic evaluation during the remaining years of growth.

Orthopaedic Surgery

Presurgical Gait Analysis

Gait analysis is an evolving diagnostic and research tool for ambulatory patients in which computers, cameras, reflective markers, in-floor force plates, dynamic electromyographs, and pedobarographs are used to capture and analyze movement in multiple planes. A gait analysis includes a detailed physical examination; videotaped observation of gait; gathering of temporal, kinematic, and kinetic data; and pedobarographic measurement of foot pressure. A preoperative assessment provides information on multiple joints and can guide the treating physician in the selection of procedures such as muscle-tendon lengthening and rotational osteotomy. In level II and III studies, gait analysis was found to be useful in confirming clinical indications for surgery, defining indications for surgery that had not been clinically proposed, and excluding or delaying surgery that had been clinically proposed. Subsequent surgery was less frequently applied when gait analysis was done before the index procedure, and gait analysis therefore was considered to be cost-effective.[25]

Musculoskeletal Surgery

Single-event multilevel surgery (SEMLS) is the current paradigm for orthopaedic treatment of children with ambulatory CP. Normal gait patterns typically are established after age 5 years, and surgical intervention is delayed until children have achieved their neurologic potential and are able to comply with the preoperative evaluation and postoperative rehabilitation. The goal is to treat all primary gait deviations during one procedure, thereby minimizing the psychological trauma to the child, the disruption to the family, and the number of hospital admissions. Optimal results can be achieved with accurate preoperative planning and surgical technique, followed by a successful rehabilitation program. Parents were most satisfied with SEMLS if the child had mild, unilateral CP (hemiplegia at GMFCS level I).[26] SEMLS can be effective for treating recurrent deformity or gait dysfunction in an adolescent or young adult.

Treatment of Specific Musculoskeletal Deformities

Spine

Spine deformity is most common among patients with severe CP (at GMFCS level V). The typical pattern of neuromuscular scoliosis in CP is a long, C-shaped thoracolumbar curve that often is resistant to bracing and is relentlessly progressive. A spine deformity greater than 60° can disrupt sitting balance because of associated pelvic obliquity. Nonsurgical measures such as soft thoracolumbar bracing and modifications to the wheelchair seating system may provide temporary improvement in sitting balance but do not affect curve progression.

The deformity can be corrected by posterior spine fusion with fixation to the pelvis. Adequate correction of rigid, severe deformities (more than 90°) may require anterior releases. Alternatively, a severe deformity can be treated using temporary internal distraction, in which a posterior release of the rigid segment is followed by placement of temporary spine instrumentation under distraction. Definitive fixation is done several weeks later. This two-stage procedure may lead to better overall correction of the deformity. The standard method for spine fusion in neuromuscular scoliosis has been segmental spine fixation with sublaminar wires and pelvic fixation using the Galveston technique. Alternative methods of fixation to the pelvis, such as the use of iliac screws, leads to correction equivalent to that obtained with the Galveston method.

Because children with CP and severe scoliosis commonly have associated comorbidities, the decision to pursue surgical correction must be individualized. The patient's quality of life, sitting ability and balance, and level of pain must be considered. A thorough medical evaluation must be performed in order to optimize the patient's preoperative medical and nutritional status. Surgical complications are common, including perioperative morbidity related to blood loss, pulmonary compromise, wound infection, and gastrointestinal problems such as ileus and pancreatitis.[27] The late complications include hardware prominence, hardware breakage, and loss of correction.

Outcome studies found that spine fusion to correct scoliosis in children with CP corrects the spine deformity and consequently improves the patient's physical appearance and self-esteem.[28] Parents and other caregivers typically report positive outcomes related to ease of care, appearance, and overall quality of life.

Hip

Hip subluxation may appear in children with CP at age 2 to 4 years, secondary to spasticity of the hip adductors and hip flexors. AP radiographs of the pelvis should be obtained at 6-month intervals to monitor for subluxation. Radiographic findings indicating neuromuscular hip subluxation include acetabular dysplasia (usually superior or posterosuperior), increased femoral

2: Basic Science

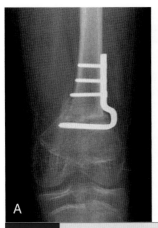
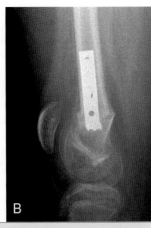

Figure 2 AP (**A**) and lateral (**B**) radiographs showing correction of a persistent knee flexion contracture after distal femoral extension osteotomy in a child with crouch gait.

anteversion, and increased femoral neck-shaft angle. In younger children with CP, hip displacement usually is asymptomatic. However, the incidence of pain secondary to hip displacement increases with longer follow-up of these patients.

The risk of hip displacement is directly related to the severity of neurologic involvement and is directly correlated with the level of gross motor function, as measured using the GMFCS. A recent study of 323 children with CP found no hip displacement among children who were at GMFCS level I but a 90% incidence among children at GMFCS level V.[29]

The natural history of hip subluxation involves a progression from mild subluxation to complete dislocation, possibly with severe arthritic changes and pain in the hip. Mild or moderate hip subluxation can be treated with soft-tissue releases of the adductor muscles, but the failure rate of this procedure approaches 30%.[30] Nonsurgical measures such as bracing or BoNT-A injections into the adductors are ineffective.[31] When performed with acetabular osteotomies, varus-producing osteotomies of the proximal femur improve the coverage and stability of the developing hip. Outcome studies found that quality of life and pain improved after successful hip reconstruction, with minimal changes in level of function or independence.[32]

Hip dislocation in a teenager or young adult is difficult to diagnose and treat. Not all dislocated hips are painful, and it may be difficult to determine the extent of pain from a dislocated hip in a child with severe CP. The treatment may be palliative and can include a salvage procedure to reduce the contact forces surrounding the hip joint. The modified Hass procedure redirects the femoral head laterally away from the acetabulum through a valgus-producing subtrochanteric osteotomy. This procedure leads to a reduction in pain and improves caregivers' ability to position the patient.[33] However, complications are frequent and include failure of fixation, infection, and heterotopic ossification. Femoral head resection is an alternative salvage procedure for painful hip dislocation, although complications including heterotopic ossification and proximal femoral migration can occur. Perioperative use of an external fixator across the hip does not offer any advantage over the use of a postoperative spica cast in reducing the likelihood of femoral migration.[34] The long-term benefits of these salvage procedures have not been determined. Hip fusion can be considered for a patient with unilateral hip dislocation but no spine deformity.

Knee

Spasticity of the hamstrings can lead to increased knee flexion during the stance phase of gait. Untreated knee flexion contractures and a worsening crouch gait increase the load across the patellofemoral joint, resulting in pain and late arthritis. A decrease in the dynamic range of the knee and a poor transition from the swing to stance phase of gait are common secondary to rectus femoris spasticity. The treatment is medial hamstring lengthening with a concomitant posterior transfer of the rectus tendon.[35] After hamstring lengthening, residual knee flexion contractures of less than 15° can be treated with postoperative serial stretch casting. Transient, and occasionally permanent, neurapraxic injury to the nerve structures of the popliteal fossa can occur after medial hamstring lengthening. Older children and children who cannot communicate, cannot walk, or require postoperative epidural pain management are at increased risk of postoperative nerve palsy.[36] Lateral hamstring release is reserved for an older patient with resistant knee flexion contractures or a patient who has undergone medial hamstring release. Lateral hamstring lengthening carries a risk of excessive weakness leading to knee hyperextension in the stance phase.

Severe crouch gait with fixed knee flexion deformity can be treated with distal femoral extension osteotomy (**Figure 2**). An anterior closing wedge osteotomy of the distal femur with crossed-wire or lateral blade plate fixation can correct a fixed knee contracture. Patients with open physes may have a recurrence. Concomitant shortening or advancement of the patellar tendon may reduce the risk of recurrence and improve knee extension during gait.[37]

Ankle and Foot

The equinus deformity, which adversely affects standing and gait, is the most common ankle and foot deformity in children with CP. The treatment is primarily based on the child's age. For a child who is younger than 3 years, developmental therapy and orthotic devices are used. For a child age 3 to 6 years, a combination of serial casting, BoNT-A injection, and orthotic devices is recommended. Definitive muscle tendon surgery for persistent equinus deformity is delayed until the child is at least 6 years old. The choice of surgical procedure depends on the extent of deformity and contracture. A selective gastrocnemius or gastrocnemius-soleus recession is most common. Nonselective Achilles tendon lengthening is reserved for a severe myostatic deformity (generally more than 15° of plantar flexion). Compared with gastrocnemius-soleus recession, Achilles tendon lengthening carries a greater risk of over-lengthening the ankle plantar flexors. The resulting disruption of the ankle plantar flexion–knee extension couple leads to a crouch gait pattern.

Planovalgus deformity is a common foot malalignment in patients with CP. Severe deformity may prevent a nonambulatory patient from wearing shoes or sitting comfortably in a wheelchair. The treatment of an ambulatory patient is directed at correcting skeletal lever arm deficiency to maximize ankle plantar flexion and facilitate the use of an orthotic device. A soft-tissue procedure such as posterior calf muscle lengthening may be done in addition to skeletal realignment of the foot. Lateral column lengthening through the neck of the calcaneus can provide multisegment correction of a planovalgus deformity. A severe or rigid deformity may require additional skeletal surgery, including arthrodesis of one or more joints.

Complete correction of a severe pes planus deformity may require selective arthrodesis of the foot. In conjunction with triple arthrodesis, lateral column lengthening through the calcaneocuboid joint is effective for correcting an extreme equinoplanovalgus deformity in an older child or teenager. Isolated talonavicular fusion is an effective alternative for correction of a severe pes planus deformity. A recent 40-month review of this procedure found that the correction had been maintained and that few complications had occurred.[38] Lateral column lengthening and subtalar arthrodesis were recently compared in children with CP undergoing treatment of hindfoot valgus deformity.[39] Extra-articular subtalar arthrodesis was effective in treating the hindfoot valgus but failed to correct forefoot supination or calcaneal equinus deformities. Lateral column lengthening was found to provide multisegment correction on radiography and to improve loading patterns, as measured by dynamic pedobarography.

Hallux valgus is an acquired deformity in children with CP that results from intrinsic muscle imbalance and abnormal extrinsic loading of the forefoot during the stance phase of gait. The definitive treatment is metatarsophalangeal arthrodesis. A recent review of short-term results after metatarsophalangeal arthrodesis found stable radiographic correction with improvements in pain, cosmesis, functional activity, footwear use, callosities, and hygiene.[40]

Equinovarus foot deformity most commonly is seen in children with hemiplegic CP. It can be challenging to determine whether the anterior or posterior tibialis is the primary deforming force. Dynamic fine wire electromyography of the posterior tibialis is helpful, as is the confusion test. In the confusion test, the seated patient is asked to flex the hip against gravity and against resistance applied from the examiner's hand. Cocon-traction of the hip and ankle dorsiflexors is a hard-wired motor synergy persistently present in most children with CP. Straight, normal ankle dorsiflexion during the test suggests that activity of the tibialis anterior is not contributing to the dynamic varus deformity seen during gait. In contrast, ankle dorsiflexion and inversion during the confusion test suggest that tibialis anterior activity is contributing to the dynamic varus deformity.

Dynamic pedobarography is an evolving tool for evaluating foot abnormalities. As the patient ambulates across a pressure-sensitive floor mat, quantitative data are gathered across the foot over time. The data provide a measure of the loading pattern of the foot that can be useful in preoperative planning and postoperative objective assessment.

The treatment for a mild or moderate equinovarus deformity is surgical lengthening of the gastrocnemius-soleus complex and fractional lengthening of the posterior tibialis. A pure dynamic deformity can be treated with split-tendon transfer of the anterior tibialis or the posterior tibial tendon. Correcting a fixed deformity to produce a plantigrade, braceable foot may require a combination of sequential soft-tissue releases and skeletal surgery.

Transverse Plane

In some children with ambulatory CP, the normal neonatal increase in femoral anteversion is not resolved with growth. The result is a lever deficiency at the level of the hip. Assessing the extent of pathologic femoral anteversion may require clinical examination, two-dimensional CT, and gait analysis. The patient compensates during the gait cycle by internal rotation of the hip and external rotation of the pelvis to restore the lever arm. Correction of these deviations can be achieved after correction of the increased anteversion by derotational osteotomy of the femur. This procedure is done proximally below the lesser trochanter or distally above the metaphyseal flare. Blade plate fixation at the subtrochanteric level provides stability adequate for early postoperative weight bearing. Ambulatory children undergoing proximal femoral osteotomies had an earlier return to standing and walking as well as reduced pain if they were allowed to bear weight immediately after surgery.[41]

An intoeing gait pattern may be secondary to incomplete resolution of internal tibial torsion in ambulatory children with CP. Tibial torsion is clinically assessed by evaluation of the thigh-foot axis and transmalleolar axis as well as the second-toe test. Two-dimensional CT and three-dimensional gait analysis are used for further assessment of the torsional profile of the lower extremities. The validity and reliability of these clinical measures were recently compared with CT evaluation. All methods were found to have substantial validity; assessment of the transmalleolar axis was the most reliable and valid measure.

Summary

A multidisciplinary approach is required to provide treatment and optimize outcomes for a child with CP. Medical management and surgical interventions are available to treat musculoskeletal dysfunction that may develop as the child grows. The quality of life of a child with CP can be improved through appropriate diagnosis and timing of interventions.

Annotated References

1. The definition and classification of cerebral palsy. *Dev Med Child Neurol* 2007;49(S109):1-44.

   This review of the currently accepted definition of CP includes the use and value of classification schemes for the diagnosis, prognosis, and treatment of children.

2. Washburn LK, Dillard RG, Goldstein DJ, Klinepeter KL, deRegnier RA, O'Shea TM: Survival and major neurodevelopmental impairment in extremely low gestational age newborns born 1990-2000: A retrospective cohort study. *BMC Pediatr* 2007;7:20.

   In a regionally based sample, survival rates for infants born at an extremely low gestational age were found to improve during the 1990s, with a minor decrease in the rate of neurodevelopmental impairment.

3. Young NL: The transition to adulthood for children with cerebral palsy: What do we know about their health care needs? *J Pediatr Orthop* 2007;27(4):476-479.

   This is an overview of current knowledge concerning the health care needs of adults with CP.

4. Presedo A, Dabney KW, Miller F: Fractures in patients with cerebral palsy. *J Pediatr Orthop* 2007;27(2):147-153.

   A retrospective review of the incidence of fractures in children with CP found that nonambulatory patients and those using anticonvulsive medications are at increased risk of fracture. Level of evidence: IV.

5. Rogozinski BM, Davids JR, Davis RB, et al: Prevalence of obesity in ambulatory children with cerebral palsy. *J Bone Joint Surg Am* 2007;89(11):2421-2426.

   Over a 10-year period, the increase in the prevalence of obesity in children with CP was similar to that of the general population. Patients at GMFCS level II were twice as likely to develop obesity as patients at level III. Level of evidence: IV.

6. Palisano RJ, Rosenbaum P, Bartlett D, Livingston MH: Content validity of the expanded and revised Gross Motor Function Classification System. *Dev Med Child Neurol* 2008;50(10):744-750.

   The expanded GMFCS classification includes validated descriptions and levels for children age 12 to 18 years.

7. World Heath Organization: *International Classification of Functioning, Disability, and Health: Short Version.* Geneva, Switzerland, World Health Organization, 2001, pp 121-160.

8. Seyler TM, Smith BP, Marker DR, et al: Botulinum neurotoxin as a therapeutic modality in orthopaedic surgery: More than twenty years of experience. *J Bone Joint Surg Am* 2008;90(suppl 4):133-145.

   The history, mechanism of action, techniques, and current indications for using botulinum toxin in orthopaedics are discussed.

9. Newman CJ, Kennedy A, Walsh M, O'Brien T, Lynch B, Hensey O: A pilot study of delayed versus immediate serial casting after botulinum toxin injection for partially reducible spastic equinus. *J Pediatr Orthop* 2007;27(8):882-885.

   Delayed casting after botulinum toxin injection for spastic equinus led to better ankle range of motion after 3 and 6 months, compared with immediate casting. Level of evidence: II.

10. Gooch JL, Oberg WA, Grams B, Ward LA, Walker ML: Complications of intrathecal baclofen pumps in children. *Pediatr Neurosurg* 2003;39(1):1-6.

11. Motta F, Stignani C, Antonello CE: Effect of intrathecal baclofen on dystonia in children with cerebral palsy and the use of functional scales. *J Pediatr Orthop* 2008;28(2):213-217.

    Dystonic symptoms were significantly improved when ITB was used in patients with GMFCS level V involvement, as measured by two individual movement scales. Level of evidence: IV.

12. Shilt JS, Lai LP, Cabrera MN, Frino J, Smith BP: The impact of intrathecal baclofen on the natural history of scoliosis in cerebral palsy. *J Pediatr Orthop* 2008;28(6):684-687.

    The progression of scoliosis in children with severe CP did not significantly differ based on whether they had received ITB treatment. Level of evidence: III.

13. Simpson DM, Blitzer A, Brashear A, et al: Assessment: Botulinum neurotoxin for the treatment of movement disorders (an evidence-based review). Report of the Therapeutics and Technology Assessment Subcommittee of the American Academy of Neurology. *Neurology* 2008;70(19):1699-1706.

    This is a comprehensive review of the available evidence for the use of botulinum neurotoxin in movement disorders.

14. Albright L: Neurosurgical treatment of dystonia, in Gage JR, ed: *The Identification and Treatment of Gait Problems in Cerebral Palsy.* London, England, Mac-Keith Press, 2009, pp 429-438.

    The treatment goals and options are summarized for focal dystonia, hemidystonia, and generalized dystonia.

15. Westberry DE, Davids JR, Shaver JC, Tanner SL, Blackhurst DW, Davis RB: Impact of ankle-foot orthoses on static foot alignment in children with cerebral palsy. *J Bone Joint Surg Am* 2007;89(4):806-813.

The use of an AFO did not lead to radiographic correction or improvement in overall segmental alignment of the foot and ankle in children with CP. Level of evidence: IV.

16. Davids JR, Rowan F, Davis RB: Indications for orthoses to improve gait in children with cerebral palsy. *J Am Acad Orthop Surg* 2007;15(3):178-188.

In a comprehensive review of the use of orthotic devices in patients with CP, the most common types of foot and ankle deformities are discussed, as well as treatment goals and indications for specific types of orthotic devices.

17. Smith PA, Hassani S, Graf A, et al: Brace evaluation in children with diplegic cerebral palsy with a jump gait pattern. *J Bone Joint Surg Am* 2009;91(2):356-365.

A comparison of the use of hinged and dynamic AFOs in children with jump gait found that both brace designs improved gait as measured by gait analysis. Level of evidence: II.

18. Bower E, Michell D, Burnett M, Campbell MJ, McLellan DL: Randomized controlled trial of physiotherapy in 56 children with cerebral palsy followed for 18 months. *Dev Med Child Neurol* 2001;43(1):4-15.

19. Weindling , AM, Cunningham CC, Glenn SM, Edwards RT, Reeves DJ: Additional therapy for young children with spastic cerebral palsy: A randomised controlled trial. *Health Technol Assess* 2007;11(16):1-71.

In a multicenter randomized controlled study, interventions including additional therapeutic sessions and visits by a family support worker did not lead to significant overall improvement in the motor or general development of children with CP.

20. Eek MN, Tranberg R, Zügner R, Alkema K, Beckung E: Muscle strength training to improve gait function in children with cerebral palsy. *Dev Med Child Neurol* 2008;50(10):759-764.

Directed muscle strength training led to improvements in muscle strength and overall gait.

21. Mäenpää H, Salokorpi T, Jaakkola R, et al: Follow-up of children with cerebral palsy after selective posterior rhizotomy with intensive physiotherapy or physiotherapy alone. *Neuropediatrics* 2003;34(2):67-71.

22. Trost JP, Schwartz MH, Krach LE, Dunn ME, Novacheck TF: Comprehensive short-term outcome assessment of selective dorsal rhizotomy. *Dev Med Child Neurol* 2008;50(10):765-771.

At a mean 18-month follow-up after selective dorsal rhizotomy, patients had improvement related to spasticity, overall gait, oxygen cost, and functional mobility. Level of evidence: IV.

23. Nordmark E, Josenby AL, Lagergren J, Andersson G, Strömblad LG, Westbom L: Long-term outcomes five years after selective dorsal rhizotomy. *BMC Pediatr* 2008;8:54.

A retrospective review found that reduction in muscle tone was maintained 5 years after selective dorsal rhizotomy. Significant improvement in passive range of motion was identified, as well as functional outcomes as measured by the Gross Motor Function Measure and Pediatric Evaluation Disability Inventory.

24. Golan JD, Hall JA, O'Gorman G, et al: Spinal deformities following selective dorsal rhizotomy. *J Neurosurg* 2007;106(suppl 6):441-449.

The incidence of spine deformity after selective dorsal rhizotomy was analyzed retrospectively in 98 patients. Commonly identified radiographic deformities included mild scoliosis (44.8%) and spondylolisthesis (19.15%). None of the patients experienced clinically significant deficits.

25. Lofterød B, Terjesen T: Results of treatment when orthopaedic surgeons follow gait-analysis recommendations in children with CP. *Dev Med Child Neurol* 2008; 50(7):503-509.

In 55 children with ambulatory CP, preoperative clinical evaluation and gait analysis recommendations were compared to determine appropriate surgical plans. A significant number of plans were altered because of the findings of gait analysis.

26. Westwell M, Ounpuu S, DeLuca P: Effects of orthopedic intervention in adolescents and young adults with cerebral palsy. *Gait Posture* 2009;30(2):201-206.

Preoperative and postoperative gait analyses were used to determine the overall effect of multilevel surgery in patients with CP after skeletal maturity. The surgical results were found to be similar to those of younger patients with CP.

27. McCarthy JJ, D'Andrea LP, Betz RR, Clements DH: Scoliosis in the child with cerebral palsy. *J Am Acad Orthop Surg* 2006;14(6):367-375.

This is a review of the incidence, natural history, assessment, and management of scoliosis in children with CP.

28. Mercado E, Alman B, Wright JG: Does spinal fusion influence quality of life in neuromuscular scoliosis? *Spine (Phila Pa 1976)* 2007;32(suppl 19):S120-S125.

The current literature related to spine fusion in neuromuscular scoliosis is systematically reviewed. Level IV evidence exists for improvement in quality of life in children with CP after spine fusion for scoliosis.

29. Soo B, Howard JJ, Boyd RN, et al: Hip displacement in cerebral palsy. *J Bone Joint Surg Am* 2006;88(1):121-129.

The incidence of hip displacement in CP is reported by analysis of the Victorian Cerebral Palsy Register. An overall rate of 35% was identified in the cohort, with the incidence showing a linear relationship with the level of gross motor function. Level of evidence: II.

30. Presedo A, Oh CW, Dabney KW, Miller F: Soft-tissue releases to treat spastic hip subluxation in children with cerebral palsy. *J Bone Joint Surg Am* 2005;87(4):832-841.

Soft-tissue release about the hip was done in 65 children with a mean age of 4.4 years. The patients were followed until a mean age of 10.8 years. Hip dislocation was prevented in 67%. The results were more favorable in patients with spastic diplegia and patients who were ambulatory.

31. Graham HK, Boyd R, Carlin JB, et al: Does botulinum toxin a combined with bracing prevent hip displacement in children with cerebral palsy and "hips at risk"? A randomized, controlled trial. *J Bone Joint Surg Am* 2008;90(1):23-33.

Botulinum injections followed by use of a variable hip abduction orthotic device did not result in improvement in hip displacement. Progressive hip displacement continued to occur, in comparison with untreated patients.

32. Krebs A, Strobl WM, Grill F: Neurogenic hip dislocation in cerebral palsy: Quality of life and results after hip reconstruction. *J Child Orthop* 2008;2(2):125-131.

This review of the results of hip reconstruction in children with CP found that radiographic improvement of the hip was achieved, although functional abilities such as sitting or standing did not change significantly. Quality-of-life improvement was most evident in patients who had preoperative pain.

33. Hogan KA, Blake M, Gross RH: Subtrochanteric valgus osteotomy for chronically dislocated, painful spastic hips. *J Bone Joint Surg Am* 2006;88(12):2624-2631.

The surgical technique and results for subtrochanteric valgus osteotomy are reviewed in 24 patients (31 hips). The clinical results, such as care of the child and diminished pain, were good, but the rate of complications was 63%. Level of evidence: IV.

34. Muthusamy K, Chu HY, Friesen RM, Chou PC, Eilert RE, Chang FM: Femoral head resection as a salvage procedure for the severely dysplastic hip in nonambulatory children with cerebral palsy. *J Pediatr Orthop* 2008;28(8):884-889.

A retrospective review of femoral head resection for treatment of a severely dysplastic hip found good clinical results despite a 41% rate of heterotopic ossification. Level of evidence: IV.

35. Davids JR, Ounpuu S, DeLuca PA, Davis RB III: Optimization of walking ability of children with cerebral palsy. *Instr Course Lect* 2004;53:511-522.

36. Karol LA, Chambers C, Popejoy D, Birch JG: Nerve palsy after hamstring lengthening in patients with cerebral palsy. *J Pediatr Orthop* 2008;28(7):773-776.

Nerve palsy occurred in 9.6% of patients undergoing hamstring lengthening. Children who were older, noncommunicative, or nonambulatory or who were receiving epidural pain management were at a statistically significant higher risk for postoperative palsy. Level of evidence: IV.

37. Stout JL, Gage JR, Schwartz MH, Novacheck TF: Distal femoral extension osteotomy and patellar tendon advancement to treat persistent crouch gait in cerebral palsy. *J Bone Joint Surg Am* 2008;90(11):2470-2484.

Patellar tendon advancement performed in conjunction with distal femoral extension osteotomy led to improved results compared with distal femoral extension osteotomy alone. Level of evidence: III.

38. Turriago CA, Arbeláez MF, Becerra LC: Talonavicular joint arthrodesis for the treatment of pes planus valgus in older children and adolescents with cerebral palsy. *J Child Orthop* 2009;3(3):179-183.

Retrospective analysis of the results of talonavicular arthrodesis for valgus deformity of the foot in CP found functional and cosmetic improvement. Pseudoarthrosis was the most frequent complication.

39. Park KB, Park HW, Lee KS, Joo SY, Kim HW: Changes in dynamic foot pressure after surgical treatment of valgus deformity of the hindfoot in cerebral palsy. *J Bone Joint Surg Am* 2008;90(8):1712-1721.

Extra-articular subtalar arthrodesis was compared with lateral column lengthening for the treatment of severe valgus deformity of the foot in patients with CP. Lateral column lengthening led to greater improvement toward normal foot pressure distribution. Level of evidence: III.

40. Bishay SN, El-Sherbini MH, Lotfy AA, Abdel-Rahman HM, Iskandar HN, El-Sayed MM: Great toe metatarsophalangeal arthrodesis for hallux valgus deformity in ambulatory adolescents with spastic cerebral palsy. *J Child Orthop* 2009;3(1):47-52.

First metatarsophalangeal arthrodesis stabilized with percutaneous Kirschner wires resulted in improved radiographic and clinical alignment for the treatment of hallux valgus deformity.

41. Schaefer MK, McCarthy JJ, Josephic K: Effects of early weight bearing on the functional recovery of ambulatory children with cerebral palsy after bilateral proximal femoral osteotomy. *J Pediatr Orthop* 2007;27(6):668-670.

Early ambulation and weight bearing after proximal femoral osteotomy resulted in an earlier return to baseline walking and reduction in pain during the early postoperative period.

Chapter 11
Myelomeningocele

A. Noelle Larson, MD   B. Stephens Richards, MD

Introduction

Myelomeningocele is among the most challenging pediatric orthopaedic conditions to treat. Malformation of the central nervous system with exposed neural elements results in paralysis distal to the level of the lesion. Orthopaedic surgeons commonly manage the associated spine, foot, and lower extremity deformities as well as fractures and wounds. Patients are best treated by a multidisciplinary team that can manage orthopaedic, neurologic, and urologic concerns. The goals of treatment are to improve mobility, optimize neurologic outcomes, and allow the child to develop into a healthy, well-functioning, independent adult.

Terminology

Myelomeningocele, meningocele, lipomeningocele, and caudal regression syndrome are the spinal dysraphisms. Patients with myelomeningocele have exposed and malformed neural elements, with sensory and motor defects distal to the level of the lesion. Spina bifida is a commonly used synonym for myelomeningocele; the term refers to the incomplete posterior elements of the spine that failed to close around the spinal cord or neural elements.

Patients with meningocele have only exposed meninges, and the neural elements are preserved. A lipomeningocele is a lipoma associated with a meningocele, with limited involvement of the neural elements. Thus, patients with myelomeningocele typically are more severely affected than patients with meningocele or lipomeningocele. Caudal regression syndrome is a severe congenital abnormality characterized by partial or complete absence of the sacrum and lumbar spine, with their accompanying neural elements; it is commonly associated with genitourinary and visceral malformations.

Neural tube defect is a more general term than spinal dysraphism; it includes encephalocele and anencephaly as well as myelomeningocele. The term open neural tube defect implies communication between neural elements and the environment, whereas in a closed defect all neural elements are covered by skin.[1]

Etiology and Epidemiology

Myelomeningocele results either from a failure of the neural tube to close at approximately 26 to 28 days of gestation or from a later pathologic reopening of the neural tube. An increased prevalence of neural tube defects among first-degree relatives of patients with myelomeningocele suggests a genetic etiology. Numerous genes in the folic acid pathway and candidate genes are being investigated based on animal studies.[1-3]

Folate deficiency has been directly associated with neural tube defects. Because folate supplementation should be initiated before conception, the US Department of Agriculture has mandated low-level folate fortification of all cereal grain foods since 1998.[4] In addition, all pregnant women are encouraged to take 0.4 to 0.8 mg of folate daily and to avoid medications that affect folate metabolism, such as valproate and carbamazepine. Women who have had an earlier pregnancy with a neural tube defect or have a first-degree relative with a neural tube defect are encouraged to take 4 mg of folate daily.

The reported incidence of myelomeningocele ranges from 1 to 5 per 10,000 live births, but it varies greatly by region and ethnicity.[5] In the United States, myelomeningocele historically has been more common in children of Hispanic descent than in those of European or Asian descent, although a similar prevalence in white and Hispanic populations was recently reported.[5,6] Girls are more frequently affected than boys.

The incidence of spina bifida has decreased 23% among newborns in the United States since folate fortification was mandated.[5] In addition, the increasing use of prenatal ultrasonography and maternal serum α-fetoprotein screening has led to elective termination of some affected pregnancies.

Neither Dr. Larson nor any immediate family member has received anything of value from or owns stock in a commercial company or institution related directly or indirectly to the subject of this chapter. Dr. Richards or an immediate family member serves as a board member, owner, officer, or committee member of the Pediatric Orthopaedic Society of North America; has received royalties from WB Saunders; has received research or institutional support from Medtronic Sofamor Danek; and holds stock or stock options in Pfizer.

2: Basic Science

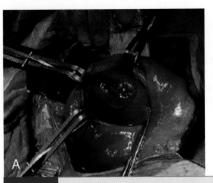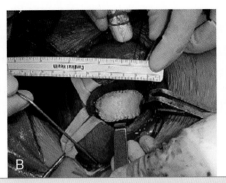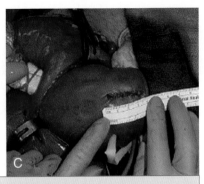

Figure 1   Photographs showing prenatal repair of a myelomeningocele defect. **A,** Exposure of the fetal defect. **B,** Repair with decellularized dermal matrix patch. **C,** Primary closure of the defect. (Reproduced with permission from Hirose S, Farmer DL: Fetal surgery for myelomeningocele. *Clin Perinatol* 2009;36:431-438. Http://www.sciencedirect.com/ science/journal/ 00955108.)

Perinatal and Neurosurgical Considerations

A two-hit hypothesis has been proposed to explain the in utero development of neural element injury: the neural elements are first damaged by neural tube malformation, and subsequently they are injured by exposure to amniotic fluid or meconium.[7] In utero surgical repair of the defect has been undertaken in an effort to improve outcomes (**Figure 1**). In preliminary results, open fetal repair of the spina bifida defect was found to lead to lower rates of hydrocephalus and hindbrain herniation (the Chiari type II malformation) in comparison with historical control subjects.[8-10] No significant difference in neurologic function has been found.[10,11] A recent study of patients who underwent intrauterine myelomeningocele repair found better motor function and ambulation than was expected based on lesion level, but there was no control group for comparison.[8] The procedure is controversial because the mother and fetus are placed at risk to treat a nonfatal condition. In utero repair can result in a precipitous delivery and associated complications of prematurity, including intraventricular hemorrhage and respiratory distress syndrome.[12,13] A prospective randomized controlled study is under way to assess the outcomes of intrauterine repair of myelomeningocele.[14]

When myelomeningocele is identified prenatally, a planned cesarean section is indicated so that trauma to the exposed neural elements can be minimized during delivery. The standard of care is early closure of the defect, typically within 24 hours of birth. Outcomes were found to improve if the defect was closed immediately after the birth.[15]

Associated central nervous system anomalies are common in patients with myelomeningocele, including Chiari type II deformity, tethered cord, diastematomyelia, and syringomyelia, in addition to hydrocephalus. Further neurosurgical intervention frequently is required after the defect is closed. Although only 35% of patients require shunt placement at the same time as defect closure, 86% eventually require shunt placement, and 95% of these patients undergo at least one shunt revision.[16,17]

Myelomeningocele is a complex and dynamic multi-system disease. Not all children have symmetric involvement of the limbs. Late deterioration of neurologic function (functional status, muscle tone, or cognition) is common and requires a diligent search for the underlying cause. For a patient with a history of hydrocephalus, shunt dysfunction is the most likely cause, followed by a symptomatic tethering of the spinal cord. A long-term natural history study found that 32% of patients required detethering of the cord at the initial surgical site.[18] On imaging studies, all patients with myelomeningocele may have a low-lying cord consistent with tethering. However, surgical intervention is indicated only with back pain, changing neurologic status, or, for some patients, a rapid progression of scoliosis. Repeated surgeries for cord detethering sometimes are indicated and may lead to improvement in symptoms, particularly back pain.[19,20]

Mortality, Function, and Quality of Life

Since the 1970s, early neural tube defect closure and the treatment of hydrocephalus have led to a markedly decreased mortality associated with myelomeningocele. Clean intermittent catheterization has eliminated much of the associated kidney disease. Some patients with spina bifida now survive well into adulthood. A recent 25-year study found a 24% mortality rate before age 25 years.[18] Patients with spina bifida were found to be as satisfied with their overall quality of life as individuals with normal neurologic function, although their health and physical quality-of-life measures were lower.[21,22]

Many patients with myelomeningocele are able to advance academically. A 25-year outcome study found that 85% of patients with spina bifida had attended or graduated from high school or college.[18] However, 80% of the patients had persistent incontinence, which for many inhibited normal social functioning.[18,23] Unemployment, social isolation, and dependence on first-degree family members are common among patients in their third decade. Now that most children with spina bifida are living into adulthood, the challenge is to provide a psychosocial support network that will allow them to live a full adult life. In addition, the availability of coordinated medical care for adults with myelomeningocele needs to be improved.

Some studies suggest that disabilities in patients with myelomeningocele are related to the associated hydrocephalus rather than to the defect itself. A patient without hydrocephalus can be expected to have average intelligence.[24,25] Patients with hydrocephalus have a shorter stride and slower gait than patients without hydrocephalus.[26] Adult patients with shunted hydrocephalus have impaired upper extremity coordination in comparison with normal control subjects.[27]

The prognosis for ambulation is associated with the level of the spine lesion. With extensive bracing above the hip, children with thoracic-level disease may become household ambulators, but adult patients typically are nonambulatory. Although neurologic involvement typically is the primary factor limiting ambulation, 70% of patients with thoracic-level myelomeningocele have associated orthopaedic abnormalities, including clubfoot, kyphosis, hip dislocation, or knee flexion contractures. Children with upper lumbar–level disease may be able to walk with braces or reciprocating gait orthoses, but many adults with this condition prefer the efficiency of a wheelchair. These patients are at risk for hip dislocation because of overpulling of the hip flexors and adductors, with flaccid hip extensors and abductors. Many patients with lower lumbar–level disease are ambulatory with the use of ankle-foot or knee-ankle-foot orthoses. Patients with grade IV or V quadriceps strength usually are community ambulators, and patients with grade IV or V gluteal strength and functional tibialis anterior strength may be able to walk without braces. Patients with sacral-level disease may be ambulatory with or without ankle-foot orthoses. All patients with myelomeningocele are at risk for skin complications of the feet.

Treatment of Patients With Myelomeningocele

A patient with myelomeningocele is best cared for by a coordinated team of practitioners, with consultation from specialists in urology, gastroenterology, orthopaedics, neurosurgery, and social services. Early multisystem intervention leads to improved outcomes related to schooling and ambulation.[28] A multidisciplinary care team can coordinate problem solving and surgical interventions, thereby reducing the strain on the primary caregivers.

Spine

A patient may have scoliosis, kyphosis, or lumbar hyperlordosis. A recent study correlated the level of the lesion with the likelihood of a spine deformity.[29]

Thoracic-level lesions were found to be highly associated with scoliosis, kyphosis, and hyperlordosis, but lesions at the L5 level or lower were not commonly associated with a spine deformity.[29]

Nonsurgical management of a spine deformity includes careful observation and adjustments in seating for a nonambulatory child. Bracing or casting can be used to treat certain scoliotic deformities but typically is not indicated for kyphosis. One study found a benefit to bracing for a small group of children with a scoliotic curve of less than 45°.[30,31] However, bracing may impede function in a patient who is ambulatory.

The surgical indications for a patient who is nonambulatory include worsening sitting balance and skin compromise refractory to seating modifications. Improved sitting balance was the only functional benefit of coronal plane correction, and no improvement in self-perception was reported.[32] Preventing the development of a large curve in adulthood has been promoted as a means of preventing pulmonary complications, although the efficacy of this approach has not been documented. Patients with a thoracic-level lesion are known to have decreased respiratory muscle strength, but the isolated impact of spine curvature on pulmonary function has not been well studied.[33] Lumbar curvature is a relative contraindication to surgical treatment in a child who is ambulatory because flexibility of the lumbar spine is critical for the child's ambulation. Other relative contraindications include an extensive absence of posterior elements, a rigid three-dimensional deformity, and poor skin condition over the area of repair.

Before any surgical spine correction, it should be recognized that patients with myelomeningocele have a high concomitant rate of neurologic abnormalities. A preoperative neurosurgical consultation should be obtained to rule out the presence of symptomatic syrinx, tethered cord, shunt dysfunction, diastematomyelia, or Chiari type II malformation. MRI is helpful in revealing these abnormalities, although almost all patients with spina bifida have evidence of a tethered cord on MRI. If cord resection is required for treatment of a complex spine deformity, some authors recommend externalization of the shunt to monitor cerebrospinal fluid flow.[34,35] Resecting the lumbar cistern may alter the flow of cerebrospinal fluid and lead to an acute insufficiency of cerebrospinal fluid flow, acute hydrocephalus, or a dural leak from excessive pressure. The limited available information from general surgical studies suggests that shunt externalization also should be done if the surgical site is grossly contaminated.[36,37] The patient's nutritional status, skin integrity, and medical condition should be optimized before surgery. Preoperative and intraoperative traction can be considered for rigid, severe deformities, but it is not used regularly. The use of preoperative antibiotics targeted at gram-negative genitourinary tract flora is recommended.[38]

Complications are common after surgical treatment of a spine deformity; they include pneumonia, urinary

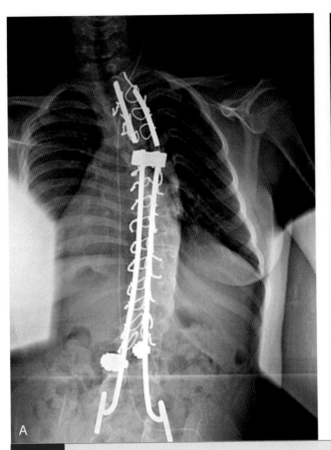
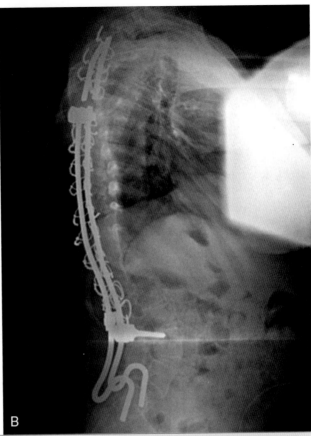

Figure 2   Standing PA (**A**) and lateral (**B**) radiographs showing failure of 3/16-inch–diameter rods in a 13-year-old girl with lumbar-level myelomeningocele, 6 years after anterior release and posterior fusion for scoliosis. Revision surgery was performed using larger diameter rods. (Reproduced with permission of the Texas Scottish Rite Hospital for Children, Dallas, TX.)

tract or other infection, wound breakdown, pseudarthrosis, implant failure, and progression of the deformity. A relatively large spine rod (1/4-inch diameter) should be used to maintain the correction, as failure of a solid fusion can lead to rod fatigue and breakage (**Figure 2**). Vigilant postoperative care is essential, with diligent pulmonary care and particular attention to keeping the wound clean and dry. After fusion extending to the pelvis, the realignment of the pelvis may cause new pressure areas to develop. Wheelchair seating changes should be made during the early postoperative period to avoid pressure ulcers.

Scoliosis

Scoliosis affects as many as 50% of children with myelomeningocele.[39] Curvature can appear in a child as old as 15 years, and progression is typical of curves greater than 20°.[39] Routine clinical and radiographic screening for scoliosis is recommended. Patients may have vertebral malformations that contribute to scoliosis resembling a congenital curve. Alternatively, the curvature may resemble an idiopathic or a neuromuscular-type deformity. Curves may result from tethering of the spinal cord, and rapid progression of scoliosis has been considered an indication for cord untethering.[40] De-

creased motor function and thoracic-level involvement are most commonly associated with scoliosis. Curves are less common in children with a sacral-level lesion.

Instrumented fusion to the pelvis generally is recommended, although successful fusion to the lower lumbar spine was reported with the use of an anterior-posterior approach.[41] In an ambulatory patient, surgery can be postponed until the curve worsens significantly because spine fusion may compromise the ability to walk. Surgery also may be delayed to maximize pulmonary function and thoracic growth before fusion.

Kyphosis and Hyperlordosis

As many as 20% of patients with myelomeningocele have severe lumbar kyphosis (gibbus deformity).[42] The indications for kyphectomy include chronic skin ulceration over the kyphotic segments and persistent difficulty with sitting balance. Patients often are quite satisfied with their appearance after a successful correction of congenital kyphosis. The risk of complications is high, however. A recent study found a 90% complication rate in nine patients with myelomeningocele who underwent kyphectomy and cord resection; two patients required shunt revision, possibly because of altered cerebrospinal fluid dynamics.[34] Another study found that removal of implants was frequently required.[43] Anterior placement of a tibial strut autograft was reported to increase the likelihood of a successful outcome.[44]

Hyperlordosis can cause seating difficulties, and it interferes with self-catheterization in patients without an appendicovesicostomy. Anterior and posterior release, osteotomy, and spinal fusion may be undertaken to treat these significant functional impairments.

Hip

Patients with myelomeningocele may have hip contractures, subluxation, or frank dislocation. Hip pain is uncommon in patients with myelomeningocele. An abduction, external rotation, and flexion contracture is common if the patient has an upper level lesion. If stretching exercises and physical therapy fail to improve contractures in a young child, a soft-tissue release of the abductors, flexors, and external rotators can be done to facilitate bracing and physiologic ambulation. A flexion deformity typically occurs with instability or dislocation of the hip and may be accompanied by knee flexion contractures. In an ambulatory patient with hip flexion contractures, isolated surgical treatment of knee flexion contractures will result in poor standing balance. Hip and knee flexion contractures should be treated at the same time. Nonambulatory patients typically tolerate hip flexion contractures well, and release is not required unless the contractures create functional impairment.

Progressive hip subluxation or dislocation is common in patients with a high lumbar–level lesion because of the unopposed pull of the hip adductors and flexors. The role of surgery is controversial. Recurrence of the deformity is common after surgical reduction, and hip stiffness and loss of flexion also may occur, worsening the patient's function. Gait studies in ambulatory patients found no gait differences attributable to hip dislocation, although patients without significant contractures had better ambulation.[45] Reduction of a dislocated hip can be considered for patients with a sacral-level lesion and near-normal function. Anterior open reduction with capsulorrhaphy almost always is required, often with a femoral shortening osteotomy, a pelvic osteotomy, and hip flexor and adductor tenotomies. Although closed reduction can be considered for an infant, a proximal femoral varus osteotomy also may be required. A Salter pelvic osteotomy typically is contraindicated in a hip affected by myelomeningocele because this procedure decreases acetabular coverage in the posterior direction of the dislocation. A Dega, Chiari, or Pemberton osteotomy is preferred to avoid compromising the posterior coverage. Muscle-balancing procedures, including iliopsoas release, transfer of the adductors or iliopsoas, or transfer of the external oblique muscle, can rebalance deforming forces across the hip. Enthusiasm for muscle transfer procedures has declined because the transferred muscle is weak and does little to prevent subsequent hip dislocation, especially in patients older than 5 years.[46,47]

Knee

Patients with myelomeningocele may have knee flexion or extension contractures or generalized knee instability. A congenital hyperextension contracture can be treated with splinting, but a frank dislocation requires surgical management. Knee flexion contractures can develop during growth, particularly in patients with a lower lumbar–level lesion, and can cause difficulty in ambulation. Contractures of less than 20° typically are well tolerated and can be managed with the use of knee-ankle-foot orthoses. Knee extension contractures are less common and can impede wheelchair seating. The V-Y quadricepsplasty is an effective procedure for treating an ambulatory patient, and a simple release is effective for a nonambulatory patient.

Rotational deformities of the femur and tibia are common in patients with myelomeningocele. Marked internal or external rotational deformities can inhibit ambulation and hinder brace fitting and use. Derotational osteotomy of the affected segment may be indicated for some ambulatory patients; in the tibia, it should be undertaken with caution because of the risk of delayed healing. Patients who have a stiff-kneed gait may be dependent on the hip flexors and adductors to ambulate. Correcting the foot progression angle may impede gait because a rotated foot clears the ground more easily during the swing phase. The risks of nonunion and infection associated with rotational osteotomies must be carefully weighed against the potential benefits.

Foot

More than 50% of patients with myelomeningocele are born with a foot deformity, such as talipes equinovarus, calcaneus, calcaneovalgus, calcaneovarus, or vertical talus.[48] Not all foot deformities can be attributed to muscle imbalance; some are severe congenital abnormalities. The treatment goals include obtaining a braceable plantigrade foot to facilitate ambulation and other functioning.

Calcaneal Deformity

Calcaneal deformity most commonly is associated with L4-level involvement, although it has been reported in patients with L5- or sacral-level involvement and even with a thoracic- or high lumbar–level lesion. In ambulatory patients, calcaneal deformity can lead to a crouch gait. Heel ulcerations sometimes result from the lack of protective sensation. Surgical intervention is commonly required for progressive or severe deformity. The surgical approaches have included Achilles tenodesis and tibialis anterior transfer to the heel.[49-51] A recent retrospective study found good results after tibialis anterior transfer in conjunction with the correction of associated bony deformities, although a calcaneus-type gait persisted in patients with hip abductor weakness

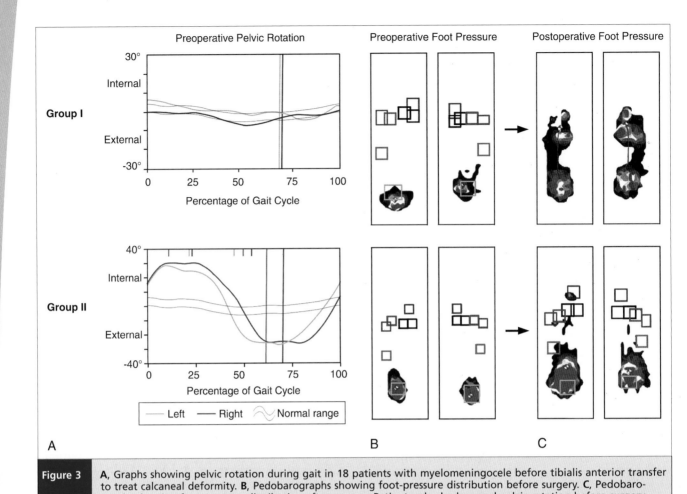

Figure 3 **A**, Graphs showing pelvic rotation during gait in 18 patients with myelomeningocele before tibialis anterior transfer to treat calcaneal deformity. **B**, Pedobarographs showing foot-pressure distribution before surgery. **C**, Pedobarographs showing foot-pressure distribution after surgery. Patients who had normal pelvic rotation before surgery (Group I) had greater improvement in foot-pressure distribution after surgery than patients with weak hip abductors and abnormal pelvic rotation (Group II). (Adapted with permission from Park KB, Park HW, Joo SY, Kim HW: Surgical treatment of calcaneal deformity in a select group of patients with myelomeningocele. *J Bone Joint Surg Am* 2008;90:2149-2159.)

who depended on pelvic rotation for ambulation[51] (Figure 3).

Clubfoot

A recent prospective study described the successful use of the Ponseti method for treating clubfoot deformity in patients with myelomeningocele. However, there was recurrence in 68% of 28 feet, most commonly in patients with a high-level lesion.[52] Most recurrences were successfully managed with repeat casting and Achilles tenotomy; only two patients required extensive soft-tissue releases. Two patients sustained an iatrogenic fracture from the casting technique. One third of the patients had to stop wearing the brace because of blister formation. In general, bracing must be used cautiously because of the risk of skin breakdown in the insensate foot.

General Treatment Considerations

Fractures

In the absence of a history of trauma, a warm, erythematous extremity in a patient with myelomeningo-cele usually represents a fracture. An infection is more likely if there are accompanying risk factors, such as pressure ulcers or a history of recent surgery. Lower extremity fractures are common, usually in the supracondylar region of the femur. Patients with myelomeningo-cele often have osteopenia or osteoporosis, which puts them at high risk for fracture.[53] Additional risk factors include nonambulatory status and a recent period of immobilization after osteotomies. Any period of immobilization should be as short as possible. Examination of the patient should be gentle and undertaken with minimal force to avoid causing a fracture. A patient may have knee effusions, which may simply be the result of synovitis from chronic knee instability. The use of knee-ankle-foot orthoses can be helpful.

Pressure Sores

Altered sensation can lead to the development of pressure ulcers in patients with myelomeningocele. Sedentary patients are at risk for decubitus ulceration, and ambulatory or crawling patients are at risk for knee or foot ulceration. Patients with a spine deformity such as kyphosis may require seating accommodations to avoid ulcer formation over a gibbus deformity. Patients with fixed pelvic obliquity or urinary incontinence are at increased risk of ulceration.[38] Fusion surgeries that result in a rigid foot also increase the risk of ulceration and should be avoided whenever possible if the patient is ambulatory. Postoperative casts must be applied cautiously, and it is important to instruct the patient and caregiver in cast care. Because of their limited sensation, patients with myelomeningocele may develop Charcot arthropathy.

Latex Sensitivity

Patients with myelomeningocele are at high risk for developing hypersensitivity to latex, especially after multiple surgeries.[54] Exposure to latex should be minimized for patients with myelomeningocele, and all surgeries should be done in a latex-free environment.

Summary

Myelomeningocele is a complex disorder involving multiple organ systems. A multidisciplinary team approach is required. The treatment must address not only muscle paralysis but also the associated sensory defects, central nervous system disorders, and expected changes in functional status. With modern neurosurgical and urologic interventions, patients may be able to lead a fulfilling life. The risks of treatment should be carefully weighed, and an assessment of the functional outcome should guide any surgical plan. Orthopaedic surgeons should be aware of the clinical features of acute fracture, shunt malfunction, and newly symptomatic tethered cord. Orthopaedic surgeons have an important role in careful interventions to improve mobility, prevent wounds, and improve functional outcomes in patients with myelomeningocele.

Annotated References

1. Bassuk AG, Kibar Z: Genetic basis of neural tube defects. *Semin Pediatr Neurol* 2009;16(3):101-110.

   This excellent update on genetic and experimental studies of the etiology of neural tube defects discusses candidate genes and etiologic mechanisms.

2. Deak KL, Boyles AL, Etchevers HC, et al: SNPs in the neural cell adhesion molecule 1 gene (NCAM1) may be associated with human neural tube defects. *Hum Genet* 2005;117(2-3):133-142.

   Single-nucleotide polymorphisms in the neural cell adhesion gene were evaluated in patients with myelomeningocele.

3. Kibar Z, Torban E, McDearmid JR, et al: Mutations in VANGL1 associated with neural-tube defects. *N Engl J Med* 2007;356(14):1432-1437.

Various mutations in the *VANGL1* gene were found in 3 of 144 patients with a neural tube defect. No such mutations were found in 106 normal control subjects.

4. Quinlivan EP, Gregory JF III: Effect of food fortification on folic acid intake in the United States. *Am J Clin Nutr* 2003;77(1):221-225.

5. Centers for Disease Control and Prevention: Racial/ethnic differences in the birth prevalence of spina bifida: United States, 1995-2005. *MMWR Morb Mortal Wkly Rep* 2009;57(53):1409-1413.

   The US Centers for Disease Control and Prevention reported on the birth prevalence of spina bifida in the United States after folic acid fortification of all cereal grain products.

6. Hendricks KA, Simpson JS, Larsen RD: Neural tube defects along the Texas-Mexico border, 1993-1995. *Am J Epidemiol* 1999;149(12):1119-1127.

7. Danzer E, Ernst LM, Rintoul NE, Johnson MP, Adzick NS, Flake AW: In utero meconium passage in fetuses and newborns with myelomeningocele. *J Neurosurg Pediatr* 2009;3(2):141-146.

   Postnatal evaluation of meconium content in myelomeningocele sacs found that 79% of sacs had histiocytes with meconium, compared with 57% of sacs resected prenatally. Meconium exposure may harm exposed neural tissues.

8. Danzer E, Gerdes M, Bebbington MW, et al: Lower extremity neuromotor function and short-term ambulatory potential following in utero myelomeningocele surgery. *Fetal Diagn Ther* 2009;25(1):47-53.

   The functional ability of patients with myelomeningocele after in utero defect closure was assessed at a mean age of 5.6 years. Function was better than expected based on neurologic level, but the study included no comparison group.

9. Sutton LN: Fetal surgery for neural tube defects. *Best Pract Res Clin Obstet Gynaecol* 2008;22(1):175-188.

   Current practices for in utero closure of myelomeningocele defects are reviewed, with a preliminary report of outcomes.

10. Sutton LN, Adzick NS, Bilaniuk LT, Johnson MP, Crombleholme TM, Flake AW: Improvement in hindbrain herniation demonstrated by serial fetal magnetic resonance imaging following fetal surgery for myelomeningocele. *JAMA* 1999;282(19):1826-1831.

11. Johnson MP, Sutton LN, Rintoul N, et al: Fetal myelomeningocele repair: Short-term clinical outcomes. *Am J Obstet Gynecol* 2003;189(2):482-487.

12. Tulipan N, Bruner JP, Hernanz-Schulman M, et al: Effect of intrauterine myelomeningocele repair on central nervous system structure and function. *Pediatr Neurosurg* 1999;31(4):183-188.

13. Hamdan AH, Walsh W, Bruner JP, Tulipan N: Intrauterine myelomeningocele repair: Effect on short-term complications of prematurity. *Fetal Diagn Ther* 2004; 19(1):83-86.

14. Hirose S, Farmer DL: Fetal surgery for myelomeningocele. *Clin Perinatol* 2009;36(2):431-438, xi.

    An ongoing clinical study of fetal surgery to treat myelomeningocele defects is described.

15. Pinto FC, Matushita H, Furlan AL, et al: Surgical treatment of myelomeningocele carried out at 'time zero' immediately after birth. *Pediatr Neurosurg* 2009;45(2): 114-118.

    Fewer myelomeningocele sacs rupture and patients have improved neurologic outcomes when the defect is closed immediately after birth rather than after admission to the nursery.

16. Sin AH, Rashidi M, Caldito G, Nanda A: Surgical treatment of myelomeningocele: Year 2000 hospitalization, outcome, and cost analysis in the US. *Childs Nerv Syst* 2007;23(10):1125-1127.

    The National Inpatient Database was used to review the surgical treatment of myelomeningocele in the first year of life. Only 35% of patients had shunt placement at the time of myelomeningocele treatment. There was only one perioperative fatality (1.27%).

17. Talamonti G, D'Aliberti G, Collice M: Myelomeningocele: Long-term neurosurgical treatment and follow-up in 202 patients. *J Neurosurg* 2007;107(suppl 5):368-386.

    Mortality, the need for additional surgery, and psychosocial outcomes of a large group of patients with myelomeningocele in the second and third decades of life were evaluated in an excellent 25-year study with a mean 10-year follow-up.

18. Bowman RM, McLone DG, Grant JA, Tomita T, Ito JA: Spina bifida outcome: A 25-year prospective. *Pediatr Neurosurg* 2001;34(3):114-120.

19. Al-Holou WN, Muraszko KM, Garton HJ, Buchman SR, Maher CO: The outcome of tethered cord release in secondary and multiple repeat tethered cord syndrome. *J Neurosurg Pediatr* 2009;4(1):28-36.

    Most of 66 patients with myelomeningocele had stable or improved neurologic status after tethered cord release. Long-term neurologic outcomes were poor in younger patients.

20. Maher CO, Goumnerova L, Madsen JR, Proctor M, Scott RM: Outcome following multiple repeated spinal cord untethering operations. *J Neurosurg* 2007;106 (suppl 6):434-438.

    Repeat spinal cord untetherings were reviewed in 22 patients with at least two earlier untethering procedures. Multiple surgeries were associated with increased risk of complications and less improvement in symptoms. Improvement in pain was the most predictable outcome.

21. Barf HA, Post MW, Verhoef M, Jennekens-Schinkel A, Gooskens RH, Prevo AJ: Life satisfaction of young adults with spina bifida. *Dev Med Child Neurol* 2007; 49(6):458-463.

    In 179 Dutch adult patients with spina bifida, overall life satisfaction was similar to that of normal adult control subjects (a 24% rate of dissatisfaction) but was lower for self-care and partnerships.

22. Danielsson AJ, Bartonek A, Levey E, McHale K, Sponseller P, Saraste H: Associations between orthopaedic findings, ambulation and health-related quality of life in children with myelomeningocele. *J Child Orthop* 2008; 2(1):45-54.

    Physical quality-of-life scores were significantly lower in 38 patients with spina bifida than in normal control subjects.

23. Verhoef M, Post MW, Barf HA, van Asbeck FW, Gooskens RH, Prevo AJ: Perceived health in young adults with spina bifida. *Dev Med Child Neurol* 2007; 49(3):192-197.

    The Medical Outcomes Study Short Form-36 Health Survey was used to study 179 Dutch adult patients with spina bifida. The emotional health score was similar to that of population control subjects, but the physical health score was significantly lower.

24. Barf HA, Verhoef M, Jennekens-Schinkel A, Post MW, Gooskens RH, Prevo AJ: Cognitive status of young adults with spina bifida. *Dev Med Child Neurol* 2003; 45(12):813-820.

25. Nejat F, Kazmi SS, Habibi Z, Tajik P, Shahrivar Z: Intelligence quotient in children with meningomyeloceles: A case-control study. *J Neurosurg* 2007;106(suppl 2): 106-110.

    Fifty children with myelomeningocele had a mean intelligence test score of 96 (range, 73 to 134), and 50 normal control group subjects had a mean score of 105 (range, 70 to 128). No association was found between shunt placement and test score.

26. Battibugli S, Gryfakis N, Dias L, et al: Functional gait comparison between children with myelomeningocele: Shunt versus no shunt. *Dev Med Child Neurol* 2007; 49(10):764-769.

    Patients without a shunt walked more quickly and with a longer stride than patients with a shunt.

27. Dennis M, Salman MS, Jewell D, et al: Upper limb motor function in young adults with spina bifida and hydrocephalus. *Childs Nerv Syst* 2009;25(11):1447-1453.

    Young adults with myelomeningocele and shunted hydrocephalus were found to have impaired upper extremity function in comparison with age-matched control subjects.

28. Rüdeberg A, Donati F, Kaiser G: Psychosocial aspects in the treatment of children with myelomeningocele: An assessment after a decade. *Eur J Pediatr* 1995;154(9, suppl 4):S85-S89.

29. Glard Y, Launay F, Viehweger E, Hamel A, Jouve JL, Bollini G: Neurological classification in myelomeningocele as a spine deformity predictor. *J Pediatr Orthop B* 2007;16(4):287-292.

A review of 210 patients with myelomeningocele found that a higher neurologic level is associated with a greater likelihood of spine deformity.

30. Müller EB, Nordwall A: Brace treatment of scoliosis in children with myelomeningocele. *Spine (Phila Pa 1976)* 1994;19(2):151-155.

31. Müller EB, Nordwall A, Odén A: Progression of scoliosis in children with myelomeningocele. *Spine (Phila Pa 1976)* 1994;19(2):147-150.

32. Wai EK, Young NL, Feldman BM, Badley EM, Wright JG: The relationship between function, self-perception, and spinal deformity: Implications for treatment of scoliosis in children with spina bifida. *J Pediatr Orthop* 2005;25(1):64-69.

In a survey of 80 patients with spina bifida and scoliosis, no association was found between functional ability and spine deformity, with the exception of sitting balance.

33. Ronchi CF, Antunes LC, Fioretto JR: Respiratory muscular strength decrease in children with myelomeningocele. *Spine (Phila Pa 1976)* 2008;33(3):E73-E75.

Decreased respiratory muscle strength was found in children with myelomeningocele compared with normal control subjects, regardless of lesion level. Children with upper level myelomeningocele had poorer respiratory muscle strength than those with a lower level lesion.

34. Ko AL, Song K, Ellenbogen RG, Avellino AM: Retrospective review of multilevel spinal fusion combined with spinal cord transection for treatment of kyphoscoliosis in pediatric myelomeningocele patients. *Spine (Phila Pa 1976)* 2007;32(22):2493-2501.

Nine patients with thoracic-level myelomeningocele were treated with spinal cord transection and spine fusion for kyphoscoliosis. The authors recommend that shunt function be optimized before spinal cord transection and that the shunt be externalized perioperatively to carefully observe cerebrospinal fluid dynamics.

35. Winston K, Hall J, Johnson D, Micheli L: Acute elevation of intracranial pressure following transection of non-functional spinal cord. *Clin Orthop Relat Res* 1977;128:41-44.

36. Li G, Dutta S: Perioperative management of ventriculoperitoneal shunts during abdominal surgery. *Surg Neurol* 2008;70(5):492-497.

No ventriculoperitoneal shunt infections developed after clean or clean-contaminated abdominal surgery. The authors recommend shunt externalization if gross contamination is present.

37. Pittman T, Williams D, Weber TR, Steinhardt G, Tracy T Jr: The risk of abdominal operations in children with ventriculoperitoneal shunts. *J Pediatr Surg* 1992;27(8):1051-1053.

38. Leibold S, Keefover-Hicks A, Wilson C, et al: Identifying nursing interventions related to spinal fusion surgery in the child with spina bifida. *Int J Nurs Intellect Dev Disabil* 2009;5(1). http://journal.ddna.org/archives. Accessed February 10, 2010.

Preoperative and postoperative factors specific to the care of patients with spina bifida undergoing spine fusion are reviewed.

39. Trivedi J, Thomson JD, Slakey JB, Banta JV, Jones PW: Clinical and radiographic predictors of scoliosis in patients with myelomeningocele. *J Bone Joint Surg Am* 2002;84-A(8):1389-1394.

40. Sarwark JF, Weber DT, Gabrieli AP, McLone DG, Dias L: Tethered cord syndrome in low motor level children with myelomeningocele. *Pediatr Neurosurg* 1996;25(6): 295-301.

41. Wild A, Haak H, Kumar M, Krauspe R: Is sacral instrumentation mandatory to address pelvic obliquity in neuromuscular thoracolumbar scoliosis due to myelomeningocele? *Spine (Phila Pa 1976)* 2001;26(14):E325-E329.

42. Carstens C, Koch H, Brocai DR, Niethard FU: Development of pathological lumbar kyphosis in myelomeningocele. *J Bone Joint Surg Br* 1996;78(6):945-950.

43. Niall DM, Dowling FE, Fogarty EE, Moore DP, Goldberg C: Kyphectomy in children with myelomeningocele: A long-term outcome study. *J Pediatr Orthop* 2004;24(1):37-44.

44. Odent T, Arlet V, Ouellet J, Bitan F: Kyphectomy in myelomeningocele with a modified Dunn-McCarthy technique followed by an anterior inlayed strut graft. *Eur Spine J* 2004;13(3):206-212.

45. Gabrieli AP, Vankoski SJ, Dias LS, et al: Gait analysis in low lumbar myelomeningocele patients with unilateral hip dislocation or subluxation. *J Pediatr Orthop* 2003; 23(3):330-334.

46. Sherk HH, Ames MD: Functional results of iliopsoas transfer in myelomeningocele hip dislocations. *Clin Orthop Relat Res* 1978;137:181-186.

47. Stillwell A, Menelaus MB: Walking ability after transplantation of the iliopsoas: A long-term follow-up. *J Bone Joint Surg Br* 1984;66(5):656-659.

48. Sharrard WJ, Grosfield I: The management of deformity and paralysis of the foot in myelomeningocele. *J Bone Joint Surg Br* 1968;50(3):456-465.

49. Oberlander MA, Lynn MD, Demos HA: Achilles tenodesis for calcaneus deformity in the myelodysplastic child. *Clin Orthop Relat Res* 1993;292:239-244.

50. Westin GW, Dingeman RD, Gausewitz SH: The results of tenodesis of the tendo achillis to the fibula for paralytic pes calcaneus. *J Bone Joint Surg Am* 1988;70(3): 320-328.

2: Basic Science

51. Park KB, Park HW, Joo SY, Kim HW: Surgical treatment of calcaneal deformity in a select group of patients with myelomeningocele. *J Bone Joint Surg Am* 2008;90(10):2149-2159.

Ambulatory patients with myelomeningocele were treated with tibialis anterior transfer for calcaneal foot deformity. Patients with excessive pelvic rotation on preoperative gait studies had less improvement in foot pressures than patients with normal preoperative pelvic movement.

52. Gerlach DJ, Gurnett CA, Limpaphayom N, et al: Early results of the Ponseti method for the treatment of clubfoot associated with myelomeningocele. *J Bone Joint Surg Am* 2009;91(6):1350-1359.

The Ponseti method was used to successfully treat 28 clubfeet in patients with myelomeningocele. These patients had a higher rate of relapse (68%) than patients with idiopathic clubfeet (26%). Most of the relapses were treated with casting and Achilles tenotomy.

53. Apkon SD, Fenton L, Coll JR: Bone mineral density in children with myelomeningocele. *Dev Med Child Neurol* 2009;51(1):63-67.

Osteopenia and osteoporosis were found to be common in patients with myelomeningocele, especially in nonambulatory patients.

54. Dormans JP, Templeton JJ, Edmonds C, Davidson RS, Drummond DS: Intraoperative anaphylaxis due to exposure to latex (natural rubber) in children. *J Bone Joint Surg Am* 1994;76(11):1688-1691.

Chapter 12

Lower Extremity and Spine Arthrogrypotic Syndromes

Christine Ho, MD

Introduction

The term arthrogryposis is used to describe a spectrum of diseases involving multiple congenital joint contractures. This condition is generally described in chapter 14, and its lower extremity and spine manifestations are discussed in this chapter. A patient with arthrogryposis multiplex congenita (AMC), also known as amyoplasia, has characteristic external rotation and flexion contractures of the hips, contractures of the knees, and equinovarus or vertical talus deformities of the foot. The phenotypic spectrum of disease is varied. Arthrogryposis often is difficult to treat.

Incidence and Etiology

Arthrogryposis occurs in 1 of 3,000 live births, and AMC occurs in 1 of 10,000 live births.[1] The term arthrogryposis does not represent a specific diagnosis, however. There are probably a multitude of etiologies, including a failure of muscular development; a lack of normal, mobile skin and connective tissue; and contracted, thick, fibrous soft tissue. The etiology of an individual patient's arthrogryposis is rarely identifiable. However, genetic mutations involving the contractile apparatus of fast-twitch myofibers have been identified in some patients with distal arthrogryposis. The pathophysiology of this condition is not well defined, although decreased fetal movement has been implicated. In animal models, paralyzing agents such as curare were found to produce fetal akinesia, leading to multiple congenital contractures.[2,3]

Associations have been reported between arthrogryposis and hyperthermia, oligohydramnios, neural tube defects, anterior horn cell dysfunction, myopathic disorders, and teratogens.[1,4-11] The presence of maternal antibodies directed to the fetal isoform of the muscle acetylcholine receptor was found in asymptomatic mothers of children with AMC.[12,13] A recent study compared the maternal antibodies in the sera of mothers of children with AMC who did or did not have central nervous system involvement; significantly more reactivity to undefined muscle and neuronal antigens was found in the antibodies of mothers whose children had central nervous system involvement.[14]

Many conditions with arthrogrypotic features are associated with a genetic abnormality. Distal arthrogryposis type I can be inherited in an autosomal dominant pattern; Escobar multiple pterygium syndrome, in an autosomal recessive pattern; and X-linked arthrogryposis type I, in an X-linked recessive pattern. Sporadic mutation and mitochondrial inheritance also occur. Classic AMC is clearly identifiable, and further genetic testing generally is not required (Figure 1). If the underlying cause is in doubt, however, it is critical to determine whether the child's condition has a genetic component. A genetic etiology may affect both the management of the child's deformities and the parents' decision regarding future pregnancies. Although classic AMC is considered sporadic, with no specific etiology, there is a 5% to 8% risk that any siblings also will have AMC.[1] A genetic evaluation of lymphocytes and fibroblast skin testing may be necessary to identify possible mosaicism.

Classification

An arthrogrypotic condition generally is classified by group. Group I disorders involve the limbs only. Classic AMC and distal arthrogryposis diagnoses such as Freeman-Sheldon syndrome and Beal syndrome are included in group I. The 10 subtypes of distal arthrogryposis are described in chapter 14. The group II disorders involve both the limbs and other body areas; there may be craniofacial, vertebral, or cardiac abnormalities. Multiple pterygium syndrome, some skeletal dysplasias, and Larsen syndrome are included in group II. The group III disorders involve both the limbs and the central nervous system. Myelomeningocele, sacral agenesis, and congenital muscular dystrophy are group III disorders.

Neither Dr. Ho nor any immediate family member has received anything of value from or owns stock in a commercial company or institution related directly or indirectly to the subject of this chapter.

2: Basic Science

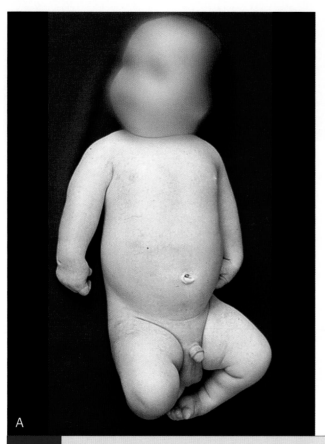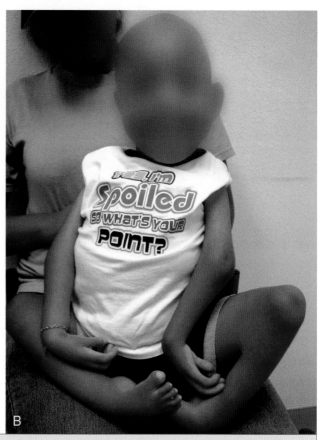

Figure 1 Photographs of an infant (**A**) and a child (**B**) with AMC, showing the classic characteristics of bilaterally symmetric lower extremity deformities with equinovarus foot deformities, knee flexion contractures, and flexed, abducted, and externally rotated hips.

Evaluation

The initial evaluation of a child with arthrogryposis should include both a family history and a thorough history of the pregnancy and delivery. Careful examination of the child's neurologic and musculoskeletal systems is necessary for identifying central nervous system involvement. Neurologic involvement negatively affects the prognosis. Joint range of motion and functional muscle group activity, such as hip and knee flexion and extension, also should be assessed, and radiographs of the spine and affected joints should be obtained. Genetic testing is required only if there is a suspicion that the child's condition has a genetic component.

Prognosis

Most patients with classic arthrogryposis do not have central nervous system or chromosomal involvement, and they usually have a good long-term prognosis. Most adult patients with arthrogryposis function well, although many have some level of financial dependence.[15] Patients with arthrogryposis had normal scores on the happiness domain of the Pediatric Outcomes Data Collection Instrument at an average 12-year follow-up after knee releases, and the scores were found not to decline with the length of follow-up.[16] These patients have normal intelligence and often are able to manipulate their environment to allow independent self-care and wheelchair mobility. The prognosis is more guarded for patients with central nervous system or chromosomal involvement, consistent with the severity of the underlying disease.

Principles of Treatment

It is important for the orthopaedic surgeon to communicate realistic goals to the parents of a child with arthrogryposis because the child will have less ability to participate in ambulatory and other physical activities than normal age- and sex-matched peers.[17] The child's range of motion may improve with treatment, but the lack of adequate musculature may preclude long-term gains in function. In addition, a lack of adequate soft-tissue coverage may prevent the child from gaining full range of motion, and long-standing bony deformities eventually may obliterate the articular joint surface. Ambulatory ability may improve in the short term but decline as the patient grows larger and reaches skeletal maturity, with contracture recurrence.[16] Although parents often focus on the desirability of achieving ambulation, many patients lead full and active lives with wheelchair mobility. Surgical intervention can be beneficial if there is a focused objective, such as improving the functional position and motion of the upper extremities to facilitate independent self-care, keyboard use, and wheelchair mobility. Long-term functional independence is better correlated with a patient's personality, education, and coping skills than with the extent of deformity or physical functioning.[15]

Treatment of Lower Extremity Arthrogrypotic Deformities

Hip

Hip contractures are present in 50% to 85% of patients with arthrogryposis, usually from birth. Hip contractures occur in conjunction with dislocation in 15% to 30% of patients.[18] The typical hip contracture involves flexion, abduction, and/or external rotation deformity. A flexion contracture can lead to compensatory lumbar lordosis; surgical release is rarely necessary, however.

Unilateral hip dislocation should be reduced to avoid pelvis obliquity and secondary scoliosis. Historically, reduction of dislocated arthrogrypotic hips has led to high rates of recurrent dislocation, stiffness, osteonecrosis, and persistent deformity. However, a long-term follow-up study found that dislocated arthrogrypotic hips were generally painless and stable after open reduction with any necessary pelvic or femoral osteotomies.[19] Patients whose unilateral hip dislocation was treated with anterolateral open reduction had function in the treated hip comparable to that of the contralateral hip, although the treated hip was stiffer. Arthrogrypotic hip dislocation generally cannot be reduced by closed means, but the medial open approach, which minimizes soft-tissue dissection, has had favorable results.[18,20,21] Medial open reduction is limited by inability to perform femoral shortening, varus derotational osteotomy, or pelvis osteotomy through the same incision. Open reduction is technically less difficult before the child begins walking and therefore ideally should be done before age 9 months. A femoral shortening osteotomy may be needed concurrently with the open reduction to reduce the risk of osteonecrosis. Osteonecrosis was reported in 70% of hips after open reduction through an extensive anterolateral approach with circumferential capsular release.[22] The high incidence of osteonecrosis was attributed to the patients' relatively advanced age at surgery (average, 31.5 months) and extreme flexion and abduction hip positioning during presurgical Pavlik harness use. Another study reported that in younger children (average age, 9.7 months), osteonecrosis occurred in 1 of 14 hips (7%).[21] A 16% rate of osteonecrosis was reported when a medial approach was used (average patient age, 8.9 months).[18]

The patient usually has multiple joint contractures, and a hyperextended or anteriorly dislocated knee should be corrected before the hip to facilitate spica casting.

The treatment of bilateral arthrogrypotic hip dislocations is controversial. Bilateral dislocations often are stable and symmetric, with a balanced pelvis. Formerly the recommendation was to avoid open reduction of bilaterally dislocated hips because of the risk of stiffness and pain, but recent studies are more optimistic. Successful single-stage, bilateral medial open reduction has resulted in mobile hips and satisfactory hip development.[18] At 4-year follow-up, four children (average age, 23 months) had generally good results after anterolateral open reduction of bilateral hip dislocations, and open reduction at a young age was recommended.[23]

Knee

Knee deformity was found in 48% to 85% of patients with arthrogryposis.[24,25] Knee flexion contracture may be the most disabling deformity in arthrogryposis; even relatively mild knee contractures can prevent motion and anatomic limb alignment. The quadriceps extensor mechanism often is poorly defined or absent in a patient with a knee contracture. These contractures are difficult to treat, and multiple surgical techniques have been proposed. Recurrence is common regardless of the technique.[25] Stretching casts may be beneficial for a neonate, although care must be taken to avoid posterior dislocation.[26-28] Distal femoral anterior physeal stapling may be useful for a mild deformity, but it produces a secondary distal femoral deformity, and a recurrence is likely after implant removal.[29] Distal femoral extension osteotomies lead to rapid remodeling and recurrence of the deformity more frequently than other surgical treatments.[25,30] Remodeling at the rate of 1° per month has been reported,[30] and therefore it may be advisable to delay osteotomies until the child reaches skeletal maturity.[25,31] An external fixator can be used to gradually correct the deformity through the joint, but the technique is demanding, the risk of complications is high, and recurrence of the deformity can be expected.[32,33]

Posterior fossa releases can be used to release all pathologic soft-tissue structures (the hamstring tendons, posterior capsule, and posterior cruciate ligament).[25,34] However, this procedure requires the surgeon to decide between maintaining a stiff, stable joint and creating a flexible but potentially unstable joint. A femoral shortening osteotomy may be necessary to gain full extension and prevent a catastrophic traction injury to the sciatic nerve. A long-term follow-up study of patients with arthrogryposis found that knee releases improved function in the short term but that ambulation and functional outcomes declined as the length of follow-up increased; most adult patients needed to use a wheelchair in the community.[16] Patient counseling must emphasize that the ambulatory ability achieved with surgery may not be permanent.

Patients with extension contractures were found to have better long-term ambulatory ability and

2: Basic Science

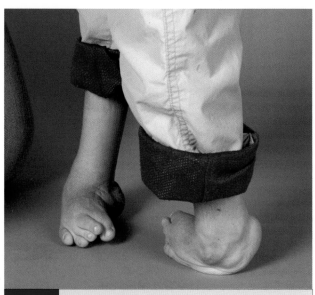

| Figure 2 | Photograph showing a recurrent arthrogrypotic clubfoot deformity, 3 years after bilateral posteromedial releases. |

functional outcomes than patients with flexion contractures,[16,35] although sitting comfortably may be difficult. Passive stretching, serial casting, and braces are used for infants with knee extension contractures. If nonsurgical treatments fail, quadricepsplasty can increase the arc of motion of the knee joint. Care must be taken during this procedure to preserve knee extension power and avoid overlengthening the muscle.

Foot and Ankle

The typical foot deformity in a patient with arthrogryposis is a rigid clubfoot, which has been considered resistant to casting (**Figure 2**). Recurrence is likely after extensive soft-tissue releases, however, leading to multiple repeat surgical procedures, extensive scarring and stiffness, and often a talectomy. Correction using a circular external fixator is technically demanding and has a high complication rate. The use of Ponseti casting has become popular for feet that were earlier believed to be uncorrectable without surgery. Ponseti casting for distal arthrogrypotic clubfoot in 12 infants younger than 6 months had encouraging results; initial correction was achieved in all 24 feet with the use of an average of 7 casts.[36] In 4 of the feet, a relapse was successfully treated with repeat casting and/or tenotomy; soft-tissue releases were required in 2 feet. In another study, the use of a modified Ponseti method achieved plantigrade, braceable feet in all patients with classic quadrimelic arthrogryposis.[37] This success was attributed to a percutaneous Achilles tenotomy performed before Ponseti casting, although 50% of the feet required repeat tenotomy and 20% required soft-tissue releases.

Congenital vertical talus is less common than clubfoot in patients with arthrogryposis but often requires surgical release to achieve a plantigrade foot. Congeni-

tal vertical talus is most severe in patients whose arthrogryposis resulted from an underlying syndrome, neurologic involvement, or severe involvement of the gastrointestinal, pulmonary, genitourinary, or cardiovascular system. The deformity in these feet often is severe and resistant to treatment. Congenital vertical talus tends to be relatively mild and amenable to one-stage surgical release in patients with distal arthrogryposis, compared with patients who have syndromic arthrogryposis or associated neurologic or visceral involvement. This deformity generally does not occur in patients with AMC.[38]

Treatment of Spine Deformities

The reported prevalence of scoliosis in patients with arthrogryposis is as high as 66%.[39] Especially in nonambulatory patients, the typical deformity is a single paralytic curve associated with pelvic obliquity. Bracing is less effective than it is for idiopathic scoliosis. However, bracing can be considered for a patient younger than 8 years, in an attempt to postpone surgery, or for an ambulatory patient with a curve of less than 30°. Bracing was found to be ineffective in nonambulatory patients with a curve of more than 30°.[39] Combined anterior and posterior spine fusion was the most effective means of achieving curve correction with a relatively low risk of loss of correction.[39]

Summary

The treatment of arthrogryposis can be challenging. The frequent recurrence of deformities after surgical correction has led to the "evil reputation"[40] of arthrogryposis among orthopaedic surgeons. Communicating realistic goals to the patient and parents is of utmost importance. Surgical planning must take into account the limited number of functional muscle units and the lack of normal joint motion, and care must be taken to ensure that surgery does not leave the patient with diminished function. Combining upper extremity and lower extremity procedures can minimize the risk associated with anesthesia and allow simultaneous rehabilitation. The results of surgical deformity correction are not always maintained over time, however. The normal intelligence of AMC patients allows them to develop inventive, resourceful ways to fully use any increased motion or improved limb position resulting from surgery. Many adult patients function as independent, productive members of society.

Annotated References

1. Hall JG: Arthrogryposis multiplex congenita: Etiology, genetics, classification, diagnostic approach, and general aspects. *J Pediatr Orthop B* 1997;6(3):159-166.

2. Drachman DB, Coulombre AJ: Experimental clubfoot and arthrogryposis multiplex congenita. *Lancet* 1962; 2(7255):523-526.

3. Moessinger AC: Fetal akinesia deformation sequence: An animal model. *Pediatrics* 1983;72(6):857-863.

4. Reid CO, Hall JG, Anderson C, et al: Association of amyoplasia with gastroschisis, bowel atresia, and defects of the muscular layer of the trunk. *Am J Med Genet* 1986;24(4):701-710.

5. Edwards MJ: Hyperthermia as a teratogen: A review of experimental studies and their clinical significance. *Teratog Carcinog Mutagen* 1986;6(6):563-582.

6. Rodríguez JI, Palacios J: Pathogenetic mechanisms of fetal akinesia deformation sequence and oligohydramnios sequence. *Am J Med Genet* 1991;40(3):284-289.

7. Banker BQ: Neuropathologic aspects of arthrogryposis multiplex congenita. *Clin Orthop Relat Res* 1985;194:30-43.

8. Sarnat HB: New insights into the pathogenesis of congenital myopathies. *J Child Neurol* 1994;9(2):193-201.

9. Sung SS, Brassington AM, Grannatt K, et al: Mutations in genes encoding fast-twitch contractile proteins cause distal arthrogryposis syndromes. *Am J Hum Genet* 2003;72(3):681-690.

10. Witters I, Moerman P, Fryns JP: Fetal akinesia deformation sequence: A study of 30 consecutive in utero diagnoses. *Am J Med Genet* 2002;113(1):23-28.

11. Hall JG, Reed SD: Teratogens associated with congenital contractures in humans and in animals. *Teratology* 1982;25(2):173-191.

12. Riemersma S, Vincent A, Beeson D, et al: Association of arthrogryposis multiplex congenita with maternal antibodies inhibiting fetal acetylcholine receptor function. *J Clin Invest* 1996;98(10):2358-2363.

13. Vincent A, Newland C, Brueton L, et al: Arthrogryposis multiplex congenita with maternal autoantibodies specific for a fetal antigen. *Lancet* 1995;346(8966): 24-25.

14. Dalton P, Clover L, Wallerstein R, et al: Fetal arthrogryposis and maternal serum antibodies. *Neuromuscul Disord* 2006;16(8):481-491.

   Evidence of reactivity of maternal antibodies to fetal muscle and neuronal antigens in babies with AMC supports the hypothesis that maternal antibodies are a cause of AMC.

15. Carlson WO, Speck GJ, Vicari V, Wenger DR: Arthrogryposis multiplex congenital: A long-term follow-up study. *Clin Orthop Relat Res* 1985;194:115-123.

16. Ho CA, Karol LA: The utility of knee releases in arthrogryposis. *J Pediatr Orthop* 2008;28(3):307-313.

   An evaluation of 32 patients with arthrogryposis at an average 12-year follow-up after surgical knee releases found that, although function improved in the short term, function and outcomes all declined as patients aged, as measured using the Pediatric Outcomes Data Collection Instrument, Functional Mobility Scale, Pediatric Evaluation of Disability Inventory, and Functional Independence Measure for Children (WeeFIM). Level of evidence: IV.

17. Dillon ER, Bjornson KF, Jaffe KM, Hall JG, Song K: Ambulatory activity in youth with arthrogryposis: A cohort study. *J Pediatr Orthop* 2009;29(2):214-217.

   Thirteen ambulatory children with AMC or distal arthrogryposis were found to have significantly less ambulatory activity than 13 age- and sex-matched control subjects. Level of evidence: II.

18. Szőke G, Staheli LT, Jaffe K, Hall JG: Medial-approach open reduction of hip dislocation in amyoplasia-type arthrogryposis. *J Pediatr Orthop* 1996;16(1):127-130.

19. Yau PW, Chow W, Li YH, Leong JC: Twenty-year follow-up of hip problems in arthrogryposis multiplex congenita. *J Pediatr Orthop* 2002;22(3):359-363.

20. Gruel CR, Birch JG, Roach JW, Herring JA: Teratologic dislocation of the hip. *J Pediatr Orthop* 1986;6(6):693-702.

21. Staheli LT, Chew DE, Elliott JS, Mosca VS: Management of hip dislocations in children with arthrogryposis. *J Pediatr Orthop* 1987;7(6):681-685.

22. Akazawa H, Oda K, Mitani S, Yoshitaka T, Asaumi K, Inoue H: Surgical management of hip dislocation in children with arthrogryposis multiplex congenita. *J Bone Joint Surg Br* 1998;80(4):636-640.

23. Asif S, Umer M, Beg R, Umar M: Operative treatment of bilateral hip dislocation in children with arthrogryposis multiplex congenita. *J Orthop Surg (Hong Kong)* 2004;12(1):4-9.

24. Gibson DA, Urs ND: Arthrogryposis multiplex congenita. *J Bone Joint Surg Br* 1970;52(3):483-493.

25. Thomas B, Schopler S, Wood W, Oppenheim WL: The knee in arthrogryposis. *Clin Orthop Relat Res* 1985; 194:87-92.

26. Murray C, Fixsen JA: Management of knee deformity in classical arthrogryposis multiplex congenita (amyoplasia congenita). *J Pediatr Orthop B* 1997;6(3):186-191.

27. Ooishi T, Sugioka Y, Matsumoto S, Fujii T: Congenital dislocation of the knee: Its pathologic features and treatment. *Clin Orthop Relat Res* 1993;287:187-192.

2: Basic Science

28. Södergård J, Ryöppy S: The knee in arthrogryposis multiplex congenita. *J Pediatr Orthop* 1990;10(2):177-182.

29. Kramer A, Stevens PM: Anterior femoral stapling. *J Pediatr Orthop* 2001;21(6):804-807.

30. DelBello DA, Watts HG: Distal femoral extension osteotomy for knee flexion contracture in patients with arthrogryposis. *J Pediatr Orthop* 1996;16(1):122-126.

31. Drummond DS, Siller TN, Cruess RL: Management of arthrogryposis multiplex congenita. *Instr Course Lect* 1974;23:79-95.

32. Damsin JP, Ghanem I: Treatment of severe flexion deformity of the knee in children and adolescents using the Ilizarov technique. *J Bone Joint Surg Br* 1996;78(1):140-144.

33. Brunner R, Hefti F, Tgetgel JD: Arthrogrypotic joint contracture at the knee and the foot: Correction with a circular frame. *J Pediatr Orthop B* 1997;6(3):192-197.

34. Heydarian K, Akbarnia BA, Jabalameli M, Tabador K: Posterior capsulotomy for the treatment of severe flexion contractures of the knee. *J Pediatr Orthop* 1984;4(6):700-704.

35. Fucs PM, Svartman C, de Assumpção RM, Lima Verde SR: Quadricepsplasty in arthrogryposis (amyoplasia): Long-term follow-up. *J Pediatr Orthop B* 2005;14(3):219-224.

    Five of eight patients with 11 AMC knee hyperextension deformities had a satisfactory outcome at an average 11-year follow-up after quadricepsplasty, as measured by gait pattern, range of motion, and orthotic requirements. Level of evidence: IV.

36. Boehm S, Limpaphayom N, Alaee F, Sinclair MF, Dobbs MB: Early results of the Ponseti method for the treatment of clubfoot in distal arthrogryposis. *J Bone Joint Surg Am* 2008;90(7):1501-1507.

    Good short-term results were reported when the Ponseti method was used for the initial treatment of clubfeet in infants with distal arthrogryposis. The Ponseti method has potential for the nonsurgical treatment of a deformity that traditionally has been surgically treated. Level of evidence: IV.

37. van Bosse HJ, Marangoz S, Lehman WB, Sala DA: Correction of arthrogrypotic clubfoot with a modified Ponseti technique. *Clin Orthop Relat Res* 2009;467(5):1283-1293.

    The use of a modified Ponseti technique achieved plantigrade, braceable feet in 10 infants (19 feet) with AMC, although most were found to require surgical intervention (Achilles tendon lengthening, posterior release) at short-term follow-up. Level of evidence: IV.

38. Aroojis AJ, King MM, Donohoe M, Riddle EC, Kumar SJ: Congenital vertical talus in arthrogryposis and other contractural syndromes. *Clin Orthop Relat Res* 2005;434:26-32.

    Based on etiology and associated syndromes, 229 patients with arthrogryposis who had congenital vertical talus were classified into five groups. Successful outcomes were found in patients whose congenital vertical talus was related to distal arthrogryposis or an unclassifiable contractural syndrome. Level of evidence: IV.

39. Yingsakmongkol W, Kumar SJ: Scoliosis in arthrogryposis multiplex congenita: Results after nonsurgical and surgical treatment. *J Pediatr Orthop* 2000;20(5):656-661.

40. Williams P: The management of arthrogryposis. *Orthop Clin North Am* 1978;9(1):67-88.

Upper Extremity

SECTION EDITOR:
DONALD S. BAE, MD

Chapter 13

Congenital Upper Extremity Differences

Charles A. Goldfarb, MD

Introduction

The incidence of congenital upper extremity differences is difficult to estimate but is approximately 1 in 500 to 1,000 live births.[1-4] Upper limb embryology is better understood now than 20 years ago, and recent advances in understanding the genetics of common abnormalities should lead to exciting future developments. The upper extremity emerges as a limb bud at 4 weeks of gestation, achieves its final form by 8 weeks, then doubles in size before birth. Limb formation requires a complex interaction among three axes of development: proximal-distal, preaxial-postaxial or anterior-posterior (radioulnar), and dorsal-ventral. The interaction between the apical ectodermal ridge and the underlying mesoderm of the progress zone is key to understanding proximal-distal development. Fibroblast growth factors key the interchange between these areas to allow the limb to grow distally. The zone of polarizing activity emits the sonic hedgehog morphogen, which is the key to radioulnar development of the limb. Finally, *Wnt-7a* controls normal development of the dorsal and palmar hand and digits. There is a continuous interplay between these signaling centers during early limb growth.[4]

The Shoulder

Congenital Pseudarthrosis of the Clavicle

Congenital pseudarthrosis of the clavicle is an uncommon, typically isolated condition that usually appears in childhood or adolescence. The accepted explanation for its development is that the pressure exerted by the subclavian artery causes a failure of the normal fusion of the primary growth centers of the central clavicle. Most patients are asymptomatic, with normal upper extremity motion, and observation of the condition

usually is appropriate. The most common symptoms are pain and an aesthetic abnormality related to the prominence of the clavicle.[5] Surgery is considered for a patient with symptoms. Resection of the pseudarthrosis with bone grafting and rigid stabilization generally alleviates the symptoms.[6] In a younger patient, a primary repair of the two clavicular segments may be possible after subperiosteal exposure. The optimal management has not been determined, and further long-term outcome studies are needed.

Sprengel Deformity

Sprengel deformity is a congenital failure of the scapula to descend (**Figure 1**). This condition sometimes is associated with scoliosis, torticollis, Klippel-Feil syndrome, a chest wall defect, or a pulmonary or renal disorder. The diagnosis is clinical, with confirmation by plain radiography. CT that includes the cervical spine can reveal the presence of an omovertebral bone (a bony connection between the superomedial scapula and the cervical spine, which is present in as many as 50% of patients) or other associated abnormalities.

Surgical intervention may be considered for functional or aesthetic reasons. Functional improvement

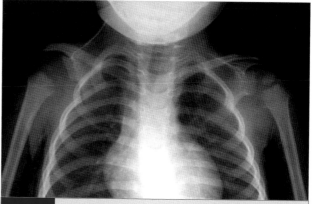

Figure 1 AP radiograph showing Sprengel deformity. The position of the right scapula is cephalad in comparison with the normal left scapula, and the glenoid is rotated. (Reproduced with permission of Charles A. Goldfarb, MD.)

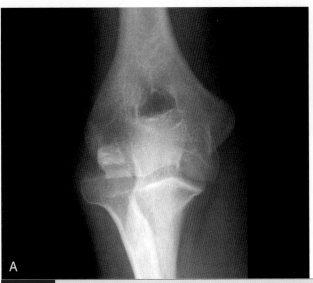
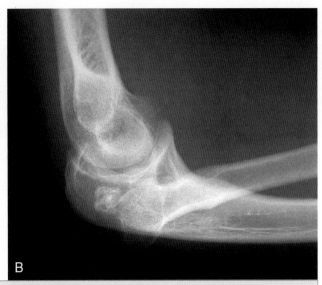

Figure 2 AP (**A**) and lateral (**B**) radiographs of a typical congenital dislocation of the radial head. The flattening of the capitellum suggests a long-standing abnormal relationship between the radial head and the capitellum. The abnormal shape of the radial head can be seen in **B**. (Reproduced with permission of Charles A. Goldfarb, MD.)

after surgery is most likely if the patient has shoulder forward flexion or abduction of less than 120°. The high-riding scapula often is quite noticeable, and its clinical appearance can be markedly improved by surgery, with the potential for improving scapulothoracic and global shoulder motion. A mild or moderate limitation is treated with range-of-motion therapy or resection of the superomedial angle of the scapula, with no attempt to further treat the scapula. A prominent scapula with an associated decrease in glenohumeral range of motion is treated by detachment of the scapular muscular attachments, caudad stabilization of the scapula to improve the anatomic position, and reattachment of the musculature.[7] Three additional surgical steps should be considered: excision of the superomedial angle to further improve the aesthetic outcome; excision of any bony or fibrous omovertebral connection to improve the correction; and, for a patient older than approximately 8 years, clavicular osteotomy (typically with morcellation through a small incision) to minimize the risk of brachial plexus palsy.[8,9]

The Elbow and Forearm

Congenital Radial Head Dislocation

Congenital radial head dislocation often is overlooked in younger children because it leads only to mild functional limitations and rarely causes pain. In a young child, the lateral or posterolateral prominence of the radial head at the elbow may be noticeably asymmetric or painful. Because the radial head is not ossified, radiographs may not clearly indicate the diagnosis.

Symptoms related to radial head dislocation become more specific during adolescence. Patients most com-

monly have discomfort related to the radial head at the lateral or posterolateral elbow. Some patients also have range-of-motion restrictions that are bothersome but rarely are functionally limiting. A posterior dislocation may limit elbow extension, and an anterior dislocation may limit elbow flexion. Posterior or anterior dislocation causes loss of forearm rotation of as much as half the typical arc; this rotational loss is well tolerated, however. Radiographs are sufficient for confirming the diagnosis and can be useful for ruling out a forearm synostosis. The classic radiographic findings include an irregular capitellum and a dome-shaped radial head with loss of the normal central concavity (**Figure 2**). It can be difficult to distinguish between a congenital and an acquired dislocation.[10]

Technically successful reduction and reconstruction procedures have been reported in patients younger than 2 years,[11,12] but evidence is lacking for any long-term benefits, including improved function. Radial head excision may be the only satisfactory option for an older adolescent with pain at a palpable radial head dislocation and radial head dysplasia on radiographs. Although radial head excision for congenital dislocation has uncertain long-term benefits, pain and motion usually are improved in the short term.[13]

One concern with radial head excision is valgus instability related to the loss of the radial head buttress and possible deterioration of the medial elbow; there is, however, little clinical evidence on this issue. Proximal migration of the radius also can occur after radial head excision, leading to ulnocarpal impaction. This complication is uncommon, but patients should be informed of the risk before considering radial head excision.

Proximal Radioulnar Synostosis

Proximal radioulnar synostosis typically is sporadic (without known genetic inheritance), is bilateral in more than 50% of patients, and is caused by a failure of radius and ulna separation during development. Although the forearm can be fixed in any position, a position of extreme rotation causes the greatest functional limitation. Because the functional limitations typically are noticed as the child's functional demands increase, the synostosis may not be observed until school age. Children who have noticeably absent forearm rotation at an earlier age may have cartilaginous synostosis. Radiographs can confirm the diagnosis and allow the radiocapitellar joint to be examined to rule out an associated radial head dislocation.

Proximal radioulnar synostosis is a painless condition. Surgery is performed to correct functional limitations, which typically occur with supination or pronation of more than 60°. Surgery is considered for a less severe bilateral deformity. Rotational osteotomies using different techniques have been successful in improving function. A neutral position or slight pronation is the generally accepted goal; this positioning facilitates the use of a keyboard. Two-stage osteoclasis through both bones without hardware fixation, osteotomy through the fusion mass with fixation, and osteotomies through both bones secured with intramedullary fixation have been successful.[14-18] Although the osteoclasis procedure had long-term satisfactory results,[15] ulnar healing was problematic, particularly with a proximal osteotomy or in a patient older than 9 years. All procedures for restoration of forearm rotation have a high failure rate, even in young children, although the free vascularized fascio-fat graft has been successful in some patients.[19]

Madelung Deformity

The understanding of the etiology and ideal treatment of Madelung deformity has grown during the past several years. The basic abnormality is a failure of the volar ulnar growth plate of the distal radius, which leads to an increased radial inclination, palmar subluxation of the carpus, and prominence of the dorsodistal ulna (Figure 3). Although it has not been determined whether the growth arrest is primary or is secondary to a tethering caused by the Vickers ligament,[20] many now believe the thickening of the ligament is secondary. Many patients with Madelung deformity have Leri-Weill dyschondrosteosis and are affected in an autosomal dominant fashion through the *SHOX* gene.[21,22] A comprehensive study of patients with Madelung deformity defined and evaluated key radiographic measurement tools.[23] With the ulna as the key reference, ulnar tilt, lunate subsidence, and palmar carpal displacement were found to be reliable tools for assessing the severity of the deformity. In a study of 26 patients (46 extremities), Madelung deformity was found to range from involvement of the distal radius only to shortening of the entire radius and forearm.[21] Patients with Madelung deformity acquired as a result of growth arrest after

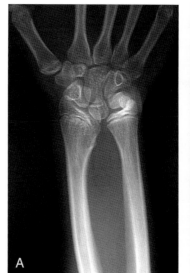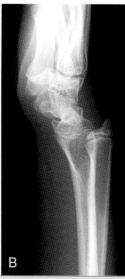

Figure 3   Madelung deformity. **A**, AP radiograph showing the classic V-shaped appearance of the carpus and the loss of volar ulnar support in the distal radius. **B**, Lateral radiograph showing volar subluxation of the carpus and hand, in comparison with the normally positioned ulna. (Reproduced with permission of Charles A. Goldfarb, MD.)

fracture or infection may have symptoms of ulnocarpal impaction.

Surgery is considered for correction of the deformity if the symptoms are not relieved with nonsurgical intervention. A dome osteotomy of the distal radius, with excision of the Vickers ligament and physiolysis, led to a good functional and aesthetic outcome and relief of pain in 26 wrists.[24] A reduction osteotomy of the ulna can be successful for adult patients, especially those with pain and a prominent dorsodistal ulna.[25]

Radial Longitudinal Deficiency

Radial longitudinal deficiency results from a failure of formation of the radial hand, forearm, and arm. The condition originally was classified by the extent of radius absence, but the classification has been extended distally to include carpal deficiency and hypoplastic thumb as well as a more severe deficiency affecting the proximal arm.[26] Radial longitudinal deficiency often occurs with disorders such as thrombocytopenia–absent radius syndrome, Holt-Oram syndrome, Fanconi anemia, and vertebral-anal-cardiac-tracheal-esophageal-renal-limb (VACTERL) association. The initial evaluation of a child with radial longitudinal deficiency may include spinal radiography, cardiac and renal ultrasonography, and a complete blood count. A chromosomal challenge test can be useful for identifying Fanconi anemia, which typically appears in late childhood and can be fatal if diagnosis is delayed.[27]

Wrist radial deviation is the most common clinical manifestation of radial longitudinal deficiency. It can be corrected using the centralization procedure, in which

3: Upper Extremity

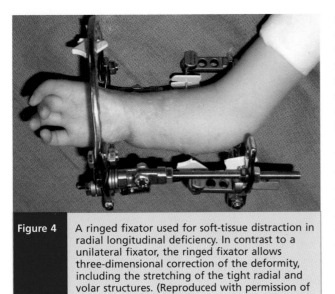

Figure 4	A ringed fixator used for soft-tissue distraction in radial longitudinal deficiency. In contrast to a unilateral fixator, the ringed fixator allows three-dimensional correction of the deformity, including the stretching of the tight radial and volar structures. (Reproduced with permission of Charles A. Goldfarb, MD.)

the hand and wrist are aligned onto the distal ulna to improve their appearance and possibly function. This procedure is not universally accepted because recurrence is common and centralization may not improve function.[28-30] The use of an external fixator for soft-tissue distraction recently has been promoted for better balancing the hand on the ulna (**Figure 4**). Although the short-term results are promising, the long-term outcomes are unknown.[31-33] For patients with a deficient thumb, the pollicization procedure is highly successful for improving both function and appearance.

The Hand

Central Deficiency

Central deficiency also is known as cleft hand. The condition most commonly affects the long finger ray but in its most severe form can affect the entire central hand, leaving the patient with a single digit or a single digit with a thumb. The most common associated abnormalities are cleft foot, cleft lip or palate, and syndactyly. Hand function often is quite good, but the appearance of the hand can be markedly abnormal. The quality of the first web space, which is a key to hand function, is the basis of a useful classification system that also can guide treatment.[34] The Snow-Littler procedure closes the cleft and uses the extra skin to reconstruct the first web space, leading to improved function and appearance.[35,36] A lack of extension of the ring finger may persist after reconstruction, probably because of a deficiency in the intrinsic musculature adjacent to the cleft.

Syndactyly

Syndactyly results from a failure of the normal regression of the cutaneous webbing between the digits, most commonly between the long and ring fingers. Syndac-

tyly and polydactyly are considered the most common congenital hand abnormalities. Syndactyly is classified on the basis of partial or complete web space involvement, cutaneous or complex bony involvement, and association with a syndrome. Acrocephalosyndactyly, also known as Apert syndrome, is the most common associated syndrome. Reconstruction of these hand abnormalities can be quite challenging.

The treatment of syndactyly entails re-creating the web space. The key component is restoration of the commissure, which must be reconstructed with native skin or a flap; skin grafting in this area inevitably leads to recurrence and narrowing of the web. Skin grafts are commonly used to fill deficits along the digits. Although skin grafts are well tolerated and initially provide a satisfactory aesthetic outcome, they tend to darken over time. There is increasing interest in graftless syndactyly reconstruction, which simplifies the initial reconstruction and avoids concerns related to skin grafting. The dorsal metacarpal artery flap or a variant is most commonly used to resurface the commissure, and digit closure is facilitated by defatting and loosely closing the zigzag flaps along the fingers.[37-41] Regardless of the technique, the patient must be advised of the risk of scar contracture and web creep. Syndactyly between the ring and small fingers or the thumb and the index finger may lead to deformity because of differential growth between the digits. Therefore, border digit syndactyly is treated at age 4 to 6 months. Other types of syndactyly can be treated with elective reconstruction, typically at age 18 to 24 months.

Polydactyly

Ulnar polydactyly, also called postaxial polydactyly, most commonly is caused by an autosomal dominant inheritance pattern and is most common among African Americans. The extra digit usually arises adjacent to the metacarpophalangeal joint. The treatment is elective surgical excision. Radial polydactyly is more common among Caucasian children; it is more challenging to treat than ulnar polydactyly. Radial polydactyly sometimes is called split thumb, but this term is not technically accurate; both thumbs are small, although their appearance varies. The treatment of radial polydactyly is based on maintaining the dominant thumb (typically, the ulnar thumb) while restoring alignment and stability. It is preferable to maintain the ulnar thumb so that the crucial ulnar collateral ligament of the metacarpophalangeal joint can be maintained; the less important radial collateral ligament can be reconstructed.[34] A more complex reconstruction may be considered if the ulnar thumb is less than 70% of the size of the contralateral thumb. The Bilhaut-Cloquet procedure combines the two thumbs to create a larger thumb. In the originally described procedure, the two thumbs are combined centrally; however, a median nail ridge, physeal abnormalities with altered growth, or poor joint motion may result. In a variation of the procedure used for Wassel type II or III thumb polydactyly, more than half of one thumb is retained and is supplemented with the lateral aspect of the other thumb. This technique augments the thumb while avoiding the complications of the traditional procedure.[42] This concept has been applied to more proximal thumb polydactyly (Wassel types III, IV, and VII), with similarly satisfactory results.[43] The most commonly noted abnormalities are decreased nail width and interphalangeal joint angulation; patients report a satisfactory subjective outcome. Interphalangeal joint angulation can be controlled during the surgical intervention by using adjunct procedures such as osteotomy or tendon centralization.

Trigger Thumb and Trigger Finger

Pediatric trigger thumb is a common hand abnormality. The prevalence is approximately 3 children per 1,000 at age 1 year.[44] It is now well established that trigger thumb is not congenital but is acquired during the first years of life. The most recent of several investigations found no trigger thumb in more than 1,000 newborns.[44] To establish the natural history of pediatric trigger thumb, 71 nonsurgically treated thumbs were followed for at least 2 years; the condition resolved spontaneously in 45 thumbs at an average of 48 months, and the flexion contracture improved in 22 additional thumbs during the study period. Importantly, the resolution was described as a neutral flexion-extension position, regardless of the extent of hyperextension on the contralateral side. Release of the A1 pulley can be considered; this procedure has an excellent clinical outcome in children, with expectation of full motion recovery and minimal complications.

Trigger finger is much less common than trigger thumb, with less straightforward treatment. Nonsurgical intervention is rarely successful, and release of the A1 pulley alone may not be sufficient. A standardized treatment plan consisting of A1 pulley release and excision of a single slip of the flexor digitorum superficialis was effective in more than 90% of patients.[45] Fifty percent of the patients had triggering at the flexor digitorum superficialis decussation site before the slip excision.

Summary

Congenital abnormalities of the upper extremity are uncommon, and treatments have been slow to advance. Unilateral functional limitation is well tolerated because of the ability to compensate by using the contralateral extremity. Physical appearance is culturally important, and aesthetic aspects of the deformity therefore must be considered.

Annotated References

1. Birch-Jensen A: *Congenital Deformities of the Upper Extremities*. Odense, Denmark, Det Danske Forlag, 1949.

2. Woolf R, Broadbent T, Woolf C: Practical genetics of congenital hand abnormalities, in Littler J, Cramer L, Smith J, eds: *Symposium on Reconstructive Hand Surgery*. St Louis, MO: Mosby, 1974, vol 9, pp 141-143.

3. Lamb DW, Wynne-Davies R, Soto L: An estimate of the population frequency of congenital malformations of the upper limb. *J Hand Surg Am* 1982;7(6):557-562.

4. Sammer DM, Chung KC: Congenital hand differences: Embryology and classification. *Hand Clin* 2009;25(2):151-156.
   This general review of congenital hand differences includes a discussion of classification and etiology.

5. Shalom A, Khermosh O, Wientroub S: The natural history of congenital pseudarthrosis of the clavicle. *J Bone Joint Surg Br* 1994;76(5):846-847.

6. Beals RK, Sauser DD: Nontraumatic disorders of the clavicle. *J Am Acad Orthop Surg* 2006;14(4):205-214.
   Congenital abnormalities of the clavicle, including congenital pseudarthrosis, are comprehensively reviewed.

7. Woodward J: Congenital elevation of the scapula: Correction by release and transplantation of muscle origins. *J Bone Joint Surg Am* 1961;43:219-228.

8. Borges JL, Shah A, Torres BC, Bowen JR: Modified Woodward procedure for Sprengel deformity of the shoulder: Long-term results. *J Pediatr Orthop* 1996;16(4):508-513.

9. Greitemann B, Rondhuis JJ, Karbowski A: Treatment of congenital elevation of the scapula: 10 (2-18) year follow-up of 37 cases of Sprengel's deformity. *Acta Orthop Scand* 1993;64(3):365-368.

10. Kim HT, Conjares JN, Suh JT, Yoo CI: Chronic radial head dislocation in children: Part 1. Pathologic changes preventing stable reduction and surgical correction. *J Pediatr Orthop* 2002;22(5):583-590.

11. Sachar K, Mih AD: Congenital radial head dislocations. *Hand Clin* 1998;14(1):39-47.

12. Kim HT, Park BG, Suh JT, Yoo CI: Chronic radial head dislocation in children: Part 2. Results of open treatment and factors affecting final outcome. *J Pediatr Orthop* 2002;22(5):591-597.

13. Campbell CC, Waters PM, Emans JB: Excision of the radial head for congenital dislocation. *J Bone Joint Surg Am* 1992;74(5):726-733.

14. Lin HH, Strecker WB, Manske PR, Schoenecker PL, Seyer DM: A surgical technique of radioulnar osteoclasis to correct severe forearm rotation deformities. *J Pediatr Orthop* 1995;15(1):53-58.

15. Dalton JF IV, Manske PR, Walker JC, Goldfarb CA: Ulnar nonunion after osteoclasis for rotational deformities of the forearm. *J Hand Surg Am* 2006;31(6):973-978.

3: Upper Extremity

By evaluating all patients treated with an osteoclasis procedure for forearm deformity, the authors concluded that the two-stage technique, without hardware, is safe and effective. There is a risk of nonunion of the ulna in older children or those with more proximal osteotomies.

16. Ogino T, Hikino K: Congenital radio-ulnar synostosis: Compensatory rotation around the wrist and rotation osteotomy. *J Hand Surg Br* 1987;12(2):173-178.

17. Hung NN: Derotational osteotomy of the proximal radius and the distal ulna for congenital radioulnar synostosis. *J Child Orthop* 2008;2(6):481-489.

    A surgical procedure for treating congenital radioulnar synostosis using osteotomy through both bones, intramedullary fixation with Kirschner wires, and derotation is described as simple and safe. Of 34 patients, 79% had a good or excellent result.

18. Murase T, Tada K, Yoshida T, Moritomo H: Derotational osteotomy at the shafts of the radius and ulna for congenital radioulnar synostosis. *J Hand Surg Am* 2003;28(1):133-137.

19. Kanaya F, Ibaraki K: Mobilization of a congenital proximal radioulnar synostosis with use of a free vascularized fascio-fat graft. *J Bone Joint Surg Am* 1998;80(8):1186-1192.

20. Vickers D, Nielsen G: Madelung deformity: surgical prophylaxis (physiolysis) during the late growth period by resection of the dyschondrosteosis lesion. *J Hand Surg Br* 1992;17(4):401-407.

21. Zebala LP, Manske PR, Goldfarb CA: Madelung's deformity: A spectrum of presentation. *J Hand Surg Am* 2007;32(9):1393-1401.

    A large number of patients with Madelung deformity were evaluated. Most had a dyschondrosteosis with associated short forearm segments and short stature. Many patients had deformity throughout the radius, not simply at the distal radius.

22. Leri-Weill dyschondrosteosis, in *Online Mendelian Inheritance in Man.* Baltimore, MD, Johns Hopkins University. http://www.ncbi.nlm.nih.gov/omim. Accessed December 15, 2009.

23. McCarroll HR Jr, James MA, Newmeyer WL III, Molitor F, Manske PR: Madelung's deformity: Quantitative assessment of x-ray deformity. *J Hand Surg Am* 2005; 30(6):1211-1220.

    Five measures for Madelung deformity were evaluated by four raters using 48 radiographs. Ulnar tilt, lunate subsidence, and palmar carpal displacement were found to be reliable and reproducible measurements. The ulna was used as the key for measurement perspective.

24. Harley BJ, Brown C, Cummings K, Carter PR, Ezaki M: Volar ligament release and distal radius dome osteotomy for correction of Madelung's deformity. *J Hand Surg Am* 2006;31(9):1499-1506.

The dome osteotomy technique is described (with physiolysis) for distal radius correction of Madelung deformity. Radiographic and clinical outcomes were improved.

25. Bruno RJ, Blank JE, Ruby LK, Cassidy C, Cohen G, Bergfield TG: Treatment of Madelung's deformity in adults by ulna reduction osteotomy. *J Hand Surg Am* 2003;28(3):421-426.

26. James MA, Green HD, McCarroll HR Jr, Manske PR: The association of radial deficiency with thumb hypoplasia. *J Bone Joint Surg Am* 2004;86-A(10):2196-2205.

27. Goldfarb CA, Manske PR, Busa R, Mills J, Carter P, Ezaki M: Upper-extremity phocomelia reexamined: A longitudinal dysplasia. *J Bone Joint Surg Am* 2005; 87(12):2639-2648.

    A type V radioulnar longitudinal deficiency was identified in patients previously diagnosed with phocomelia. Extensions of the classification scheme for radial and ulnar longitudinal deficiency incorporate these severe deficiencies.

28. Geck MJ, Dorey F, Lawrence JF, Johnson MK: Congenital radius deficiency: Radiographic outcome and survivorship analysis. *J Hand Surg Am* 1999;24(6):1132-1144.

29. Damore E, Kozin SH, Thoder JJ, Porter S: The recurrence of deformity after surgical centralization for radial clubhand. *J Hand Surg Am* 2000;25(4):745-751.

30. Goldfarb CA, Klepps SJ, Dailey LA, Manske PR: Functional outcome after centralization for radius dysplasia. *J Hand Surg Am* 2002;27(1):118-124.

31. Goldfarb CA, Murtha YM, Gordon JE, Manske PR: Soft-tissue distraction with a ring external fixator before centralization for radial longitudinal deficiency. *J Hand Surg Am* 2006;31(6):952-959.

    This is one of several recent articles describing the indications, technique, and early outcomes of using a circular frame in precentralization distraction. An easier centralization with better balancing is described when the fixator is used before centralization.

32. Sabharwal S, Finuoli AL, Ghobadi F: Pre-centralization soft tissue distraction for Bayne type IV congenital radial deficiency in children. *J Pediatr Orthop* 2005;25(3):377-381.

    This is a second report of a circular frame use for precentralization distraction in radial longitudinal deficiency.

33. Taghinia AH, Al-Sheikh AA, Upton J: Preoperative soft-tissue distraction for radial longitudinal deficiency: An analysis of indications and outcomes. *Plast Reconstr Surg* 2007;120(5):1305-1314.

    This review article suggests the use of a unilateral frame for precentralization distraction in severe and neglected radial deficiency.

34. Manske PR, Halikis MN: Surgical classification of central deficiency according to the thumb web. *J Hand Surg Am* 1995;20(4):687-697.

35. Rider MA, Grindel SI, Tonkin MA, Wood VE: An experience of the Snow-Littler procedure. *J Hand Surg Br* 2000;25(4):376-381.

36. Goldfarb CA, Chia B, Manske PR: Central ray deficiency: Subjective and objective outcome of cleft reconstruction. *J Hand Surg Am* 2008;33(9):1579-1588.

    The Snow-Littler procedure had satisfactory results when used to reconstruct the hand in patients with central deficiency affecting only the long finger ray and thumb web space, although most patients required multiple surgeries.

37. Sherif MM: V-Y dorsal metacarpal flap: A new technique for the correction of syndactyly without skin graft. *Plast Reconstr Surg* 1998;101(7):1861-1866.

38. Aydin A, Ozden BC: Dorsal metacarpal island flap in syndactyly treatment. *Ann Plast Surg* 2004;52(1):43-48.

39. Wafa AM: Hourglass dorsal metacarpal island flap: A new design for syndactylized web reconstruction. *J Hand Surg Am* 2008;33(6):905-908.

    A new technique is described for creating a commissural flap for syndactyly reconstruction. The flap can help resurface the commissure and minimize the need for skin grafting.

40. Greuse M, Coessens BC: Congenital syndactyly: Defatting facilitates closure without skin graft. *J Hand Surg Am* 2001;26(4):589-594.

41. Withey SJ, Kangesu T, Carver N, Sommerlad BC: The open finger technique for the release of syndactyly. *J Hand Surg Br* 2001;26(1):4-7.

42. Baek GH, Gong HS, Chung MS, Oh JH, Lee YH, Lee SK: Modified Bilhaut-Cloquet procedure for Wassel type-II and III polydactyly of the thumb. *J Bone Joint Surg Am* 2007;89(3):534-541.

    Seven patients were followed for more than 4 years after a modified Bilhaut procedure for type II or III radial polydactyly. The aesthetic and functional outcomes were satisfactory.

43. Tonkin MA, Bulstrode NW: The Bilhaut-Cloquet procedure for Wassel types III, IV and VII thumb duplication. *J Hand Surg Eur Vol* 2007;32(6):684-693.

    Five patients with type III, IV, or VI radial polydactyly were treated with the Bilhaut procedure. The reported results were good, with minimal nail ridging.

44. Kikuchi N, Ogino T: Incidence and development of trigger thumb in children. *J Hand Surg Am* 2006;31(4):541-543.

    No congenital trigger thumbs were noted at birth in an assessment of 1,116 newborns. The incidence was 3.3 per 1,000 at 1-year follow-up.

45. Bae DS, Sodha S, Waters PM: Surgical treatment of the pediatric trigger finger. *J Hand Surg Am* 2007;32(7):1043-1047.

    Eighteen patients (23 trigger thumbs) were treated with A1 pulley release and flexor digitorum superficialis slip excision. Seventeen of the patients or families were satisfied with this standardized approach, which treats the common finding of triggering at the flexor digitorum superficialis decussation.

3: Upper Extremity

Chapter 14

Arthrogryposis and Cerebral Palsy in the Upper Extremity

Ann E. Van Heest, MD

Introduction

Arthrogryposis and cerebral palsy are common neuromuscular disorders that cause deformities of the elbow, forearm, wrist, and hand. There have been advances in understanding the pathology of these disorders and in treating their upper extremity manifestations.

Arthrogryposis

Arthrogryposis is defined as multiple congenital contractures affecting two or more areas of the body. In contrast, isolated congenital contractures affect only a single area of the body; the most common type is talipes equinovarus. In the past, arthrogryposis sometimes was a diagnostic term, but more recently the term has been used only to describe the presence of multiple congenital contractures.[1] More than 300 disorders can be characterized by a clinical finding of arthrogryposis. Inheritance patterns, clinical manifestations, natural history, and treatment recommendations vary by disorder. A specific diagnosis therefore is imperative for a child who has multiple congenital contractures.

Arthrogryposis is classified as amyoplasia, a distal arthrogryposis, or another syndromic arthrogryposis primarily on the basis of the child's history and physical examination (Figure 1). Orthopaedic surgeons most commonly encounter amyoplasia and the various types of distal arthrogryposis. The other syndromic types of arthrogryposis are rarely treated by orthopaedic surgeons; their etiology usually involves a specific underlying central nervous system pathology or a progressive neurologic disorder.

Amyoplasia

The most common type of arthrogryposis is amyoplasia, which formerly was referred to as classic arthrogryposis.[2] The word amyoplasia is translated as "no mus-

cle growth."[3] A child with amyoplasia has some or all characteristic features, usually symmetrically: internally rotated shoulders, extended elbows, flexed wrists, thumb-in-palm deformity, stiff digits, dislocated hips, extended knees, and severe equinovarus (Figure 2). Many patients have midfacial hemangioma. More than 80% of patients in some studies had symmetric involvement of the upper and lower limbs; the other patients had only upper or lower limb involvement or asymmetric involvement.[4]

Treatment of the upper extremity begins shortly after the child's birth. Both the parents and physical or occupational therapists help the child with passive range-of-motion exercises, and splints are used during the night and naps for stretching to increase the range of motion, particularly wrist extension. Most of the 38 children in one study responded to these conservative measures, although some subsequently had surgery to improve range of motion and function in the elbow (24%), wrist (16%), or hands (8%).[4] The primary goal of upper extremity treatment throughout childhood is to develop adaptive use patterns that will allow independence in activities of daily living. The interventions are focused on improving both muscle strength and range of motion. Surgical intervention may be

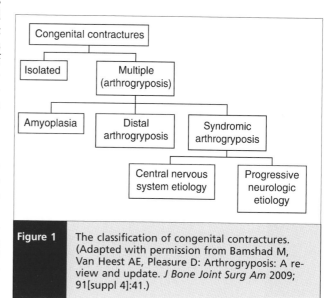

Figure 1 The classification of congenital contractures. (Adapted with permission from Bamshad M, Van Heest AE, Pleasure D: Arthrogryposis: A review and update. *J Bone Joint Surg Am* 2009; 91[suppl 4]:41.)

Neither Dr. Van Heest nor any immediate family member has received anything of value from or owns stock in a commercial company or institution related directly or indirectly to the subject of this chapter.

3: Upper Extremity

recommended for fixed joint contractures that interfere with independence in activities of daily living.

Elbow

An elbow extension contracture may prevent the child from bringing the hand to the mouth for self-feeding. A

posterior elbow capsulotomy with lengthening of the triceps was found to be effective in improving hand-to-mouth function.[5] At a 3-year follow-up after this procedure, 22 of 23 children had an improved arc of movement, with the ability to bring the hand to the mouth. In contrast to the findings of earlier studies, none of the children required a subsequent tendon transfer for elbow flexion.

Wrist

A dorsal carpal wedge osteotomy may be indicated for a school-age child with a fixed flexion posture that precludes higher level hand functions such as writing or computer use.[6] The surgery is contraindicated for a child who has significant elbow stiffness and requires wrist flexion for hand-to-mouth feeding. The dorsal carpal wedge osteotomy uses a wedge resection of bone from the midcarpal joint if a midcarpal coalition is present, as is common in children with amyoplasia and wrist stiffness (**Figure 3**). Transferring the extensor carpi ulnaris to the extensor carpi radialis brevis during the procedure can help a child with significant concomitant ulnar deviation. Children treated with this procedure gain wrist extension for improved hand positioning (**Figure 4**).

Hand

The most common manifestation of amyoplasia in the hand is thumb-in-palm deformity with stiff digits. Surgical treatment of the stiff digits has not been successful. Most children with extremely stiff digits adapt by using a side-to-side movement of the intrinsic muscles to pinch and grasp small objects. Thumb-in-palm deformity can be surgically treated with z-plasty and partial adductor release in the first web. Care must be taken to avoid extensive releases that could diminish strength.

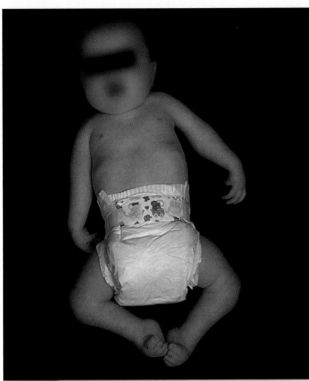

Figure 2   Photograph of a child with amyoplasia, showing the characteristic symmetric internally rotated shoulders, extended elbows, flexed wrists, thumb-in-palm deformity, stiff digits, abducted and externally rotated hips, flexed knees, and severe equinovarus feet.

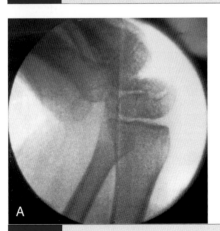 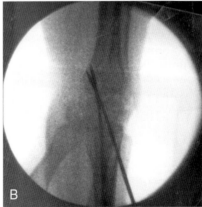 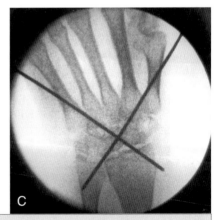

A   B   C

Figure 3   Fluoroscopic views of a dorsal carpal wedge osteotomy. **A**, The osteotomy is done at the midcarpal joint with resection of a dorsal wedge of carpus, sparing the radial carpal articulation to preserve motion. **B**, After the wedge of carpus is resected and the osteotomy site is closed, two pins hold the wrist in neutral to slight extension. **C**, The pins are placed in a retrograde manner, starting in the metacarpals, crossing the carpal osteotomy site, and secured in the radius or ulna. The wrist is immobilized with a short arm cast and pins. After 4 weeks the cast is removed, and the pins are pulled.

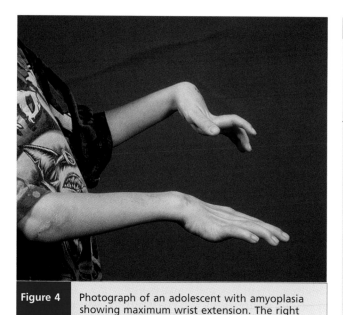

Figure 4 Photograph of an adolescent with amyoplasia showing maximum wrist extension. The right wrist has been treated with a dorsal carpal wedge osteotomy. Before surgery, the appearance of the right wrist was similar to that of the left wrist, which has not yet been treated.

Table 1

The Classification of Distal Arthrogryposis

Currently Used Term	Alternative Term or Description	Online Mendelian Inheritance in Man Identifier
DA1	Distal arthrogryposis type 1	108120
DA2A	Freeman-Sheldon syndrome	193700
DA2B	Sheldon-Hall syndrome	601680
DA3	Gordon syndrome	114300
DA4	Scoliosis	609128
DA5	Ophthalmoplegia, ptosis	108145
DA6	Sensorineural hearing loss	108200
DA7	Trismus pseudo-camptodactyly	158300
DA8	Autosomal dominant multiple pterygium syndrome	178110
DA9	Congenital contractural arachnodactyly	121050
DA10	Congenital plantar contractures	187370

(Adapted from Bamshad M, Van Heest AE, Pleasure D: Arthrogryposis: A review and update. *J Bone Joint Surg Am* 2009;91[suppl 4]:43.)

Distal Arthrogryposis

The most significant recent advances in understanding distal arthrogryposis have involved classification and etiology. Ten types have been identified and are included in the Online Mendelian Inheritance in Man database[1] (Table 1). The prototypic distal arthrogryposis, termed DA1, is characterized by camptodactyly and clubfeet of highly variable severity. Type DA2 has two subtypes, DA2A and DA2B. DA2A, commonly called Freeman-Sheldon or whistling face syndrome, is characterized by distinctive facial features, including a small oral orifice and an H-shaped chin dimple, as well as camptodactyly, clubfeet, and scoliosis. DA2B, commonly called Sheldon-Hall syndrome, is similar to DA1, with the addition of distinctive facial features including a small mouth, prominent nasolabial folds, and downslanting palpebral fissures. DA2B probably is the most common of the distal arthrogryposis disorders. Both DA2A and DA2B have mutations in *MYH3,* a gene that encodes fast-twitch myofibers. Mutation analysis of this gene is commonly used in research laboratories pursuing the molecular basis of distal arthrogryposis, although it is not yet available for clinical use.

Cerebral Palsy

Cerebral palsy is a primary central nervous system disorder with secondary upper extremity manifestations including joint malpositioning, muscle imbalance, and functional impairment (Table 2). Fixed skeletal deformities develop over time if these secondary manifestations are not treated. The most common upper extremity deformities in spastic hemiplegia due to cerebral palsy involve shoulder internal rotation, elbow flexion, forearm pronation, wrist flexion–ulnar deviation, finger clenching (flexor spasticity), and thumb-in-palm deformity. However, cerebral palsy has many different clinical manifestations; a review of 367 children with cerebral palsy reported significant variation in hand deformity patterns and functional impairments.[7]

The treatment of the upper extremity focuses on balancing muscle forces to improve joint positioning, thereby improving function and preventing fixed deformities. The current emphasis is on improving the use of the upper extremity so the patient can use hand-controlled mobility and communication devices. Treating the upper extremity does not cure cerebral palsy but simply lessens the impairment it causes.

Nonsurgical Treatment

For a patient with a hand deformity, alternatives or adjuncts to hand surgery should be discussed with a multispecialty team before a surgical intervention is undertaken. For a patient with a more general tone disorder, consultation or evaluation from a rehabilitation physician, neurologist, or neurosurgeon may be appropriate,

3: Upper Extremity

Table 2

The Treatment of Cerebral Palsy by Level of Deformity

Level	Description	Treatment
Primary	Disorder of movement and posture due to a defect or lesion of the immature central nervous system	Generally not correctible
Secondary	Peripheral manifestations: joint malpositioning, muscle imbalance, functional impairment	Tone-reducing medications Therapy (constraint, bimanual) Splints Surgery
Tertiary	Fixed deformities: skeletal deformity, joint contractures, muscle contractures	Early intervention for prevention Surgical salvage procedures

with consideration of the advantages and disadvantages of using tone-reducing medications such as diazepam or baclofen, tone-reducing injections such as botulinum toxin or phenol, and tone-reducing neurosurgical interventions such as baclofen pump placement or selective dorsal rhizotomy. A patient with quadriplegia and overall tone control difficulty should receive medications or neurosurgical intervention, and the use of the upper extremities should be allowed to stabilize before any orthopaedic intervention. Selective dorsal rhizotomy was found to have an indirect tone-reducing effect on the upper extremities in addition to its direct effect on the lower extremities.[8,9]

Botulinum Toxin Injections

Botulinum toxin type A injections are effective in reducing spasticity in the injected muscles and improving function for patients with focal muscle tone imbalance. Botulinum blocks the local release of acetylcholine at the neuromuscular junction. The action lasts approximately 3 to 4 months, during which the strength of the antagonist muscles and the possible benefits of surgery can be assessed. The antagonist muscles can be strengthened and the spastic muscles can be stretched during this period, with the benefit lasting beyond the medication's direct effect. For a child with mild involvement, the use of botulinum injections may obviate the need for surgical intervention. A recent meta-analysis found that coupling botulinum injections with an upper limb training program can have beneficial effects, including improvement in hand function.[10]

Constraint-Induced Movement Therapy

A child with hemiplegic cerebral palsy has significantly better motor function of the hand on the unaffected side than on the affected side. Many daily activities can be done without using the affected hand, and over the years the affected hand may develop progressive learned disuse. Constraint-induced movement therapy (CIMT) was designed to counteract learned disuse of the affected side. The concept was first developed for adult patients with stroke[11] and was adapted for children with spastic hemiplegic cerebral palsy. In CIMT,

the affected limb is taught new motor skills through intensive therapy accompanied by immobilization of the unaffected hand. A meta-analysis concluded that the efficacy or utility of CIMT could not be determined because the studies used different types and lengths of immobilization as well as different types and intensities of therapy during the immobilization period.[12] The reported types of immobilization included a nonremovable cast, a removable cast, a sling, a splint, and a glove. The length of immobilization ranged from several to 24 hours a day and from 2 weeks to several months.

Hand function was assessed in 21 children treated with CIMT using a restraint glove for 2 hours a day for 2 months and 20 children who did not receive CIMT.[13] The children treated with CIMT had significantly improved hand function at the end of the treatment period and 6 months later, as measured by the Assisting Hand Assessment.[14] CIMT has been criticized because it does not teach bimanual functioning, which more realistically simulates daily use of the hands. The prolonged immobilization may have a deleterious effect on the unaffected hand, which is mildly involved in most children with cerebral palsy.

Surgical Treatment

Elbow flexion, forearm pronation, wrist flexion–ulnar deviation, and thumb-in-palm deformities are most commonly encountered in spastic hemiplegic cerebral palsy. These deformities lead to upper extremity dysfunction. Each deformity is assessed separately and is subsequently integrated into an overall treatment plan. Multiple simultaneous procedures may be necessary to allow the patient to effectively position the arm and pinch, grasp, or release objects. The surgical treatment of the upper extremity for a child with cerebral palsy is governed by three principles: release or lengthening of spastic deforming muscles; tendon transfers to augment weak or absent muscle functions; and stabilization of unstable joints (Table 3).

Elbow Flexion Deformity

Brachialis and biceps lengthening is the most common treatment for elbow flexion deformity. An alternative

Table 3

Surgical Principles for Treating Cerebral Palsy

Deformity	Treatment	Example
Spastic muscles	Lengthening or release of origin or insertion	Adductor pollicus origin release
Absent muscle function	Transfer of tendons to augment function	Tendon transfer from flexor carpi ulnaris to extensor carpi radialis
Unstable joints	Capsulodesis or arthrodesis	Thumb metacarpophalangeal joint capsulodesis

procedure includes incising of the lacertus fibrosus with fractional lengthening of the brachialis aponeurosis and denuding of the peritendinous adventitia from the biceps tendon to remove afferent nerve fibers and receptors.[15] Forty-two such procedures in 40 children with spastic elbow flexion deformity from cerebral palsy yielded average improvement in elbow flexion posture angle from 104° to 55° and improvement in active extension from 43° to 44°. This procedure deviates from the original elbow flexor lengthening of the elbow, which includes lengthening of all primary elbow flexors.[16]

Forearm Pronation Deformity

Forearm pronation deformity can be treated with pronator teres release, pronator teres rerouting, or pronator quadratus release. In a comparison of pronator rerouting and release, 41 children (average age, 7.25 years) were assessed 21 months after rerouting, and 16 children (average age, 4.25 years) were assessed 94 months after release.[17] The average gain in supination was 78° after rerouting and 54° after release. Both procedures provided increased supination, although rerouting led to slightly greater supination. A cadaver study compared the biomechanics of pronator teres rerouting, brachioradialis transfer, and flexor carpi ulnaris transfer for improving supination. Transfer of the flexor carpi ulnaris to the extensor carpi radialis brevis was most effective.[18]

Wrist Flexion Deformity

Several studies assessed wrist function after tendon transfer surgery. At an average 4-year follow-up (range, 1 to 9 years), 16 children treated with a tendon transfer from the flexor carpi ulnaris to the extensor carpi radialis longus had an average final resting position of 9° of extension.[19] Fourteen patients reported improved function, and all 16 reported improved cosmesis. At an average 4-year follow-up after selective release of the flexor origin done concomitantly with transfer of the flexor carpi ulnaris, all 35 patients had improved mo-

bility of the forearm, wrist, and hand as well as improved appearance of the hand and forearm.[20] Timed forced unilateral use of the arm was not found to improve after tendon transfer surgery, although wrist flexion deformity was significantly improved.[21] Wrist arthrodesis may be indicated for a skeletally mature patient with no finger control and the ability to use the hand only as a paperweight; a recent study reported a 98% union rate after dorsal plating.[22]

Thumb-in-Palm Deformity

Thumb-in-palm deformity is one of the most complex cerebral palsy deformities to treat. The carpometacarpal, metacarpophalangeal, and interphalangeal joints of the thumb are balanced by nine muscles. Release or slide of the thumb adductor, a tendon transfer to augment thumb extension and abduction, and stabilization of the metacarpophalangeal joint are commonly used to control the position of the thumb. Of 33 children with hemiplegic cerebral palsy who underwent thumb reconstruction, 82% had improved static alignment and 61% had improved dynamic alignment.[23] A recent meta-analysis of nine studies of different surgical interventions found three primary goals: stabilization of the thumb metacarpophalangeal joint, weakening of the spastic thumb adductors, and augmentation of thumb abduction and extension.[24] The studies did not have consistent selection criteria for surgery or a standardized outcome measure, and therefore the meta-analysis reached no conclusion on the effectiveness of surgery for thumb-in-palm deformity.

Outcomes Assessment

Several instruments have been developed to measure upper extremity function in patients with cerebral palsy. In the largest study of upper extremity surgery for cerebral palsy, 134 children were followed for 25 years after 180 procedures.[25,26] On the nine-point House Upper Extremity Use Scale, arm function was found to improve from "poor passive-assist" before surgery to "fair active-assist" after surgery. Preoperative voluntary control was the most important factor for predicting improved functional use of the limb. More recently, the Shriners Hospital for Children Upper Extremity Evaluation was developed for preoperative and postoperative evaluation.[27] The Assisting Hand Assessment has been validated for assessing the ability of the affected hand to assist the contralateral hand as a simulation of daily activities.[14,28] The recently validated Manual Ability Classification System for hand function may become an important tool for future research[29] (Table 4).

Sensibility Deficiency

Several recent studies disproved the belief that hand surgery should be avoided if a child has sensibility deficiencies. Impaired sensibility had no adverse effect on surgical results in 134 children, of whom 50% had impaired two-point discrimination and 75% had

3: Upper Extremity

Table 4

The Manual Ability Classification System

Level	Description
I	Handles objects easily and successfully
II	Handles most objects, but with somewhat reduced quality or speed of achievement
III	Handles objects with difficulty; needs help to prepare or modify activities
IV	Handles a limited selection of easily managed objects in adapted situations
V	Does not handle objects and has severely limited ability to perform even simple actions

(Reproduced with permission from Eliasson AC, Krumlinde-Sundholm L, Rösblad B, et al: The Manual Ability Classification System (MACS) for children with cerebral palsy: Scale development and evidence of validity and reliability. *Dev Med Child Neurol* 2006;48[7]:549-554.)

impaired stereognosis.[26] Impaired sensibility did not affect the objective outcome in 32 children treated with tendon transfers and muscle release.[30] A study of 36 patients followed for 18 months after surgery found an improvement in stereognosis associated with improved motor function (presumably resulting from improvement in functional use).[31]

Summary

The term arthrogryposis is used to describe multiple congenital joint contractures. The three types of arthrogryposis are amyoplasia, the distal arthrogryposes, and arthrogryposis as a part of other syndromic disorders. The nonsurgical options for treating arthrogryposis and cerebral palsy in the upper extremity include botulinum toxin injections and constraint therapy. Surgical treatment for an elbow flexion, forearm pronation, wrist flexion–ulnar deviation, or thumb-in-palm deformity is recommended if nonsurgical measures are not successful. Surgical reconstruction of the upper limb in cerebral palsy has been found to effectively and consistently improve but not normalize function, and to enhance appearance. Improving hand function is important for patients with neuromuscular disorders to allow greater access to computers and mobility devices. Sensibility deficiencies in the hand of a child with cerebral palsy no longer are a contraindication to surgery.

Annotated References

1. Bamshad M, Van Heest AE, Pleasure D: Arthrogryposis: A review and update. *J Bone Joint Surg Am* 2009; 91(suppl 4):40-46.

   This up-to-date assessment of arthrogryposis includes amyoplasia and distal arthrogryposes.

2. Bevan WP, Hall JG, Bamshad M, Staheli LT, Jaffe KM, Song K: Arthrogryposis multiplex congenita (amyoplasia): An orthopaedic perspective. *J Pediatr Orthop* 2007;27(5):594-600.

   This expert opinion on the orthopaedic management of amyoplasia focuses on the lower extremities.

3. Hall JG: Don't use the term "amyoplasia" loosely. *Am J Med Genet* 2002;111(3):344.

4. Sells JM, Jaffe KM, Hall JG: Amyoplasia, the most common type of arthrogryposis: The potential for good outcome. *Pediatrics* 1996;97(2):225-231.

5. Van Heest A, James MA, Lewica A, Anderson KA: Posterior elbow capsulotomy with triceps lengthening for treatment of elbow extension contracture in children with arthrogryposis. *J Bone Joint Surg Am* 2008;90(7): 1517-1523.

   Posterior capsular release and triceps lengthening without subsequent tendon transfer surgery was done in 29 elbows, with improvement in passive range of motion. Most of the children were significantly affected, and subsequent tendon transfer surgery was not indicated. Level of evidence: IV.

6. Ezaki M: Treatment of the upper limb in the child with arthrogryposis. *Hand Clin* 2000;16(4):703-711.

7. Arner M, Eliasson AC, Nicklasson S, Sommerstein K, Hägglund G: Hand function in cerebral palsy: Report of 367 children in a population-based longitudinal health care program. *J Hand Surg Am* 2008;33(8):1337-1347.

   A population-based Swedish study reported a wide variety of hand manifestations and function in 367 children with cerebral palsy.

8. Beck AJ, Gaskill SJ, Marlin AE: Improvement in upper extremity function and trunk control after selective posterior rhizotomy. *Am J Occup Ther* 1993;47(8):704-707.

9. Loewen P, Steinbok P, Holsti L, MacKay M: Upper extremity performance and self-care skill changes in children with spastic cerebral palsy following selective posterior rhizotomy. *Pediatr Neurosurg* 1998;29(4):191-198.

10. Sakzewski L, Ziviani J, Boyd R: Systematic review and meta-analysis of therapeutic management of upper-limb dysfunction in children with congenital hemiplegia. *Pediatrics* 2009;123(6):e1111-e1122.

    A systematic review and meta-analysis of therapeutic management of the upper limbs in children with congenital hemiplegia included botulinum toxin and constraint therapy.

11. Taub E, Uswatt G: Constraint-Induced Movement therapy: Answers and questions after two decades of research. *NeuroRehabilitation* 2006;21(2):93-95.

    This landmark article presents the first author's experience with CIMT for treating upper extremity involvement in cerebral palsy.

12. Hoare B, Imms C, Carey L, Wasiak J: Constraint-induced movement therapy in the treatment of the upper limb in children with hemiplegic cerebral palsy: A Cochrane systematic review. *Clin Rehabil* 2007;21(8): 675-685.

    A Cochrane systematic review of CIMT concluded that its efficacy or utility could not be determined because the studies used different types and intensities of therapy as well as different types and lengths of immobilization.

13. Eliasson AC, Krumlinde-Sundholm L, Shaw K, Wang C: Effects of constraint-induced movement therapy in young children with hemiplegic cerebral palsy: An adapted model. *Dev Med Child Neurol* 2005;47(4): 266-275.

    A comparison of CIMT in 21 children (using a restraint glove for 2 hours a day for 2 months) and 20 children who did not receive therapy found that the treated children had significantly improved hand function at the end of the treatment period and 6 months later.

14. Krumlinde-Sundholm L, Eliasson AC: Development of the Assisting Hand Assessment: A Rasch-Built measure intended for children with unilateral upper limb impairments. *Scand J Occup Ther* 2003;10:16-26.

15. Manske PR, Langewisch KR, Strecker WB, Albrecht MM: Anterior elbow release of spastic elbow flexion deformity in children with cerebral palsy. *J Pediatr Orthop* 2001;21(6):772-777.

16. Mital MA: Lengthening of the elbow flexors in cerebral palsy. *J Bone Joint Surg Am* 1979;61(4):515-522.

17. Strecker WB, Emanuel JP, Dailey L, Manske PR: Comparison of pronator tenotomy and pronator rerouting in children with spastic cerebral palsy. *J Hand Surg Am* 1988;13(4):540-543.

18. Cheema TA, Firoozbakhsh K, De Carvalho AF, Mercer D: Biomechanic comparison of 3 tendon transfers for supination of the forearm. *J Hand Surg Am* 2006; 31(10):1640-1644.

    The biomechanics of pronator teres rerouting, brachioradialis transfer, and flexor carpi ulnaris transfer were compared for improving supination. Transfer of the flexor carpi ulnaris to the extensor carpi radialis brevis was most effective.

19. Wolf TM, Clinkscales CM, Hamlin C: Flexor carpi ulnaris tendon transfers in cerebral palsy. *J Hand Surg Br* 1998;23(3):340-343.

20. El-Said NS: Selective release of the flexor origin with transfer of flexor carpi ulnaris in cerebral palsy. *J Bone Joint Surg Br* 2001;83(2):259-262.

21. Van Heest AE, Ramachandran V, Stout J, Wervey R, Garcia L: Quantitative and qualitative functional evaluation of upper extremity tendon transfers in spastic hemiplegia caused by cerebral palsy. *J Pediatr Orthop* 2008;28(6):679-683.

    Thirteen patients underwent tendon transfer surgery at a mean age of 10.8 years. At a mean 3.6-year follow-up, there was no significant change in timed testing with the pediatric Jebsen hand test. Elbow, forearm, wrist, and finger position significantly improved, but there was no significant change in thumb position.

22. Van Heest AE, Strothman D: Wrist arthrodesis in cerebral palsy. *J Hand Surg Am* 2009;34(7):1216-1224.

    In 41 wrists (34 patients) treated for severe spastic wrist flexion deformities using wrist arthrodesis with dorsal plating, the union rate was 98%. Patients had improved appearance, ease of daily care, and hygiene. Fracture before plate removal was the most common complication.

23. Davids JR, Sabesan VJ, Ortmann F, et al: Surgical management of thumb deformity in children with hemiplegic-type cerebral palsy. *J Pediatr Orthop* 2009; 29(5):504-510.

    The surgical management of thumb deformity is presented, with a comprehensive description of procedures for rebalancing thumb position in children with hemiplegia caused by cerebral palsy.

24. Smeulders M, Coester A, Kreulen M: Surgical treatment for the thumb-in-palm deformity in patients with cerebral palsy. *Cochrane Database Syst Rev* 2005;4: CD004093.

    This meta-analysis of nine studies of different surgical interventions for thumb-in-palm deformity found no consistent selection criteria for surgery and no standard outcomes. Therefore, no conclusion was reached on the effectiveness of surgery.

25. House JH, Gwathmey FW, Fidler MO: A dynamic approach to the thumb-in palm deformity in cerebral palsy. *J Bone Joint Surg Am* 1981;63(2):216-225.

26. Van Heest AE, House JH, Cariello C: Upper extremity surgical treatment of cerebral palsy. *J Hand Surg Am* 1999;24(2):323-330.

27. Davids JR, Peace LC, Wagner LV, Gidewall MA, Blackhurst DW, Roberson WM: Validation of the Shriners Hospital for Children Upper Extremity Evaluation (SHUEE) for children with hemiplegic cerebral palsy. *J Bone Joint Surg Am* 2006;88(2):326-333.

    The Shriners Hospital for Children Upper Extremity Evaluation is commonly used for comprehensive assessment of upper extremity function before and after interventions.

28. Krumlinde-Sundholm L, Holmefur M, Kottorp A, Eliasson AC: The Assisting Hand Assessment: Current evidence of validity, reliability, and responsiveness to change. *Dev Med Child Neurol* 2007;49(4):259-264.

    The Assisting Hand Assessment is a well-established upper extremity functional outcome measure that assesses not only the affected hand but also its bimanual functioning with the contralateral side.

29. Eliasson AC, Krumlinde-Sundholm L, Rösblad B, et al: The Manual Ability Classification System (MACS) for

3: Upper Extremity

children with cerebral palsy: Scale development and evidence of validity and reliability. *Dev Med Child Neurol* 2006;48(7):549-554.

The Manual Ability Classification System is a scale that reliably classifies the extent of upper extremity involvement in cerebral palsy.

30. Eliasson AC, Ekholm C, Carlstedt T: Hand function in children with cerebral palsy after upper-limb tendon transfer and muscle release. *Dev Med Child Neurol* 1998;40(9):612-621.

31. Dahlin LB, Komoto-Tufvesson Y, Sälgeback S: Surgery of the spastic hand in cerebral palsy: Improvement in stereognosis and hand function after surgery. *J Hand Surg Br* 1998;23(3):334-339.

3: Upper Extremity

Chapter 15

Brachial Plexus Birth Palsy

Roger Cornwall, MD

Introduction

Although brachial plexus birth palsy (BPBP) has been a recognized condition for centuries, many questions persist related to the evaluation and treatment of the primary neurologic injury as well as the pathophysiology and optimal treatment of secondary musculoskeletal deformities. Research and clinical innovations during the past 5 years have advanced the understanding of BPBP and improved the ability to treat it.

Epidemiology and Natural History

The cause of BPBP is presumed to be a traction injury to the brachial plexus during a difficult birth. Factors such as shoulder dystocia, macrosomia, and instrumented delivery therefore would be expected to increase the risk of BPBP. A study of more than 11 million births in the United States identified 17,334 brachial plexus injuries (an incidence of 1.5 per 1,000 live births).[1] The risk of BPBP was increased 100-fold by shoulder dystocia, 14-fold by macrosomia (birth size larger than 4.5 kg), and ninefold by forceps delivery. However, only 46% of the infants with brachial plexus injury in this study were documented to have one of these known risk factors.

The natural history of BPBP is less favorable than is generally believed. However, true natural history studies of BPBP are lacking, and the true natural history is unlikely to be elucidated because such studies would require withholding treatment that has become accepted as important for an optimal outcome. A systematic review of 76 studies found that none of the studies met all four established criteria for a natural history study, and only two studies met two of the criteria.[2] These two studies found that 20% to 30% of children with BPBP had residual neurologic deficits.

Neither Dr. Cornwall nor any immediate family member has received anything of value from or owns stock in a commercial company or institution related directly or indirectly to the subject of this chapter.

Rehabilitation

Occupational and physical therapy is the cornerstone of the initial treatment of BPBP, and it is the only treatment most children require. The goals of therapy are to maintain passive joint range of motion while awaiting neurologic recovery and, after neurologic recovery, to improve function and motor skills development.

Improvements in understanding and evaluating normal and abnormal pediatric upper extremity movement could lead to advancements in the rehabilitative treatment of children with BPBP. In a study of 16 children with unilateral brachial plexus injury, the movements of both upper limbs were evaluated using a magnetic three-dimensional tracking system.[3] A greater scapulothoracic contribution and a smaller glenohumeral contribution to forward elevation was found on the involved side than on the normal side, especially in children with greatly impaired global active elevation. A study of 30 children with BPBP found only moderate agreement between a therapist's estimate of active joint movement and measurements of active joint movement using two-dimensional motion analysis.[4] These study results suggest that increased use of upper extremity motion analysis could improve the understanding and evaluation of joint motion in children with BPBP.

Rehabilitative interventions such as botulinum toxin type A injection and constraint-induced movement therapy increasingly are used with physical and occupational therapy to treat some pediatric neurologic disorders, and recent studies have reported their use in treating BPBP. Although brachial plexus injury, as a peripheral nerve injury, does not result in muscle spasticity, botulinum toxin has been used to facilitate motor learning in muscles recovering from BPBP by temporarily weakening the antagonists. An uncontrolled study of eight children who received botulinum toxin injections into the triceps, pectoralis major, and/or latissimus dorsi muscles found improvement in the function of the opposing reinnervating muscles immediately after injection and at 4-month follow-up.[5] Similarly, four patients with biceps-triceps cocontraction had improved active elbow flexion 18 months after a single botulinum toxin injection into the triceps muscle.[6] The indications for botulinum toxin injection in children with BPBP require further elucidation. The use of constraint-induced movement therapy has been

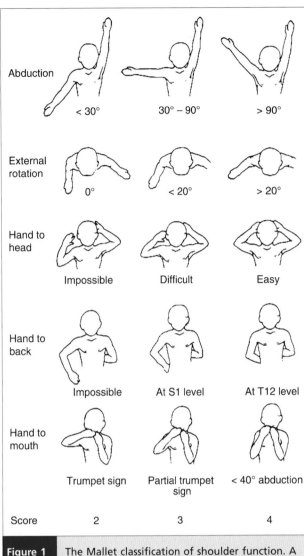

| Score | 2 | 3 | 4 |

Figure 1 The Mallet classification of shoulder function. A score of 0 is assigned for no movement in the plane, and a score of 5 is assigned for full movement. Trumpet sign = shoulder abduction during the attempt to bring hand to mouth. (Adapted with permission from Aydin A, Ozkan T, Onel D: Does preoperative abduction value affect functional outcome of combined muscle transfer and release procedures in obstetrical palsy patients with shoulder involvement? *BMC Musculoskelet Disord* 2004;5:25.)

reported only in individual children with BPBP, and its potential benefit has yet to be defined.[7]

Primary Nerve Reconstruction

Clinical Indications

Although nonsurgical therapy remains the first line of treatment for BPBP, some children with severe injury can benefit from surgical exploration and reconstruction of the injured brachial plexus. There is little controversy as to the importance of exploration and recon-

struction in children with global (C5-T1) plexus injury, but the indications for and timing of nerve surgery for upper plexus injury remain unclear. Early reports focused on the timing of biceps functional recovery as a predictor of overall functional recovery, with some authors recommending surgery for children without biceps function by age 3 months. However, this criterion cannot be used as the sole indication for surgical exploration. A long-term follow-up study of 22 patients who lacked biceps function at age 3 months but did not undergo primary nerve reconstruction found that 55% ultimately had good global shoulder function, as assessed using the Mallet scale[8] (**Figure 1**). A study of 209 patients found that active movement significantly improved with or without nerve surgery in children who did not have biceps function at age 3 months.[9] Surgical decision making therefore requires evaluating the entire limb of the individual child.

Preoperative Evaluation

The necessity for relying on the clinical indications for primary nerve surgery stems from the limited ability of ancillary diagnostic testing to precisely characterize the severity of brachial plexus injury. MRI of the brachial plexus and cervical spine before surgical exploration in 31 infants with BPBP was found to have high specificity but low sensitivity for nerve root avulsion. MRI was able to determine the side of an extraforaminal injury but not the involved nerve roots or the degree of nerve root injury.[10] Magnetic resonance neurography may better show extraforaminal nerve root pathology, and it was found to be better correlated with clinical examination findings than electrodiagnostic testing.[11] Electromyographic interference pattern and clinical muscle assessment were found to be poorly correlated in 41 infants with BPBP, with electromyography overestimating the extent of functional muscle recovery.[12] Ongoing investigation will further define the usefulness of diagnostic imaging and electrodiagnostic testing as adjuncts to physical examination in determining the indications for primary nerve surgery.

Results

Controversies remain as to the surgical indications and timing for patients with BPBP. Nonetheless, it is now possible to evaluate the long-term results of primary nerve reconstruction in large groups of patients. A retrospective study evaluated outcomes in 124 patients who underwent surgical plexus exploration between 1971 and 1997.[13] The 11 surgeons used a wide variety of surgical strategies, the most common of which was direct neurorrhaphy. At a mean 13.3-year follow-up, two thirds of the patients were satisfied with the results of surgery. One third of the patients had persistent pain, however, and one third needed help with activities of daily living. A clear correlation was found between the patient's outcome and the number of nerve roots involved in the initial injury; only 37% of children with C5-6 injury had good shoulder function as measured using the Mallet scale. A study of a heterogeneous group of 100 patients found similar results at a mean 7.1-year follow-up.[14] A study of 73 children with surgically treated global plexus injury found even worse results at the shoulder, presumably because of the transfer of ruptured upper nerve roots to the avulsed lower roots to gain hand function. At 8-year follow-up, 76% of children had hand function described as useful.[15]

These studies are limited by the heterogeneity of the surgical procedures for primary brachial plexus repair or reconstruction. A recent study of 108 patients specifically considered the role of neurolysis alone by comparing it to neuroma resection and nerve grafting.[16] At 4-year follow-up, the patients treated with grafting had significant improvement in muscle function, but the patients treated with neurolysis had no improvement. This result argues for the abandonment of neurolysis alone. The usefulness of the long-term studies of nerve surgery for BPBP is further limited because many patients also underwent secondary musculoskeletal procedures. Nonetheless, the studies reveal a lack of uniformly good results after brachial plexus exploration and repair, and they have set the stage for continuing surgical innovation.

Nerve Transfers

Conventional nerve reconstruction with excision of the neuroma and interposition of cable nerve grafts has several limitations. The technique requires intact nerve roots for use as donor nerves, a long regeneration time (because of the proximal level of the neurorrhaphy), and graft navigation by the regenerating axons. As an attractive alternative, functioning motor nerves can be transferred to the motor nerves of paralyzed muscles. Such transfers can use extraplexal sources if intraplexal donor nerves are not available, and direct neurorrhaphy can be used at a site closer to the target muscle. The more distal location of the neurorrhaphy allows a shorter regeneration time, faster recovery, and a longer window of time for awaiting spontaneous recovery before motor end plate degeneration becomes a concern.

As for a tendon transfer, the donor nerve must be functioning, expendable, suitably sized, and capable of reaching the recipient nerve. The three typical nerve transfers for upper plexus injuries are spinal accessory nerve to suprascapular nerve, triceps branch of the radial nerve to deltoid branch of axillary nerve, and ulnar nerve motor fascicle to biceps branch of musculocutaneous nerve. The use of these transfers and many others has been well documented in adult brachial plexus and peripheral nerve injuries. The transfer of the spinal accessory to the suprascapular nerve has been widely used in BPBP in conjunction with conventional neuroma resection and grafting.[17] However, the use of multiple nerve transfers instead of brachial plexus exploration, neuroma resection, and nerve grafting has yet to be studied systematically in infants with BPBP.[18]

Secondary Shoulder Deformities

Contracture and Glenohumeral Dysplasia

Internal rotation contracture of the shoulder is a well-recognized sequela of unresolved upper trunk palsy and is associated with glenohumeral dysplasia, subluxation, and dislocation. Morbidity associated with acquired shoulder abnormalities in BPBP has not been reported for adults. Although the existence of progressive glenohumeral dysplasia has been documented for more than a decade, recent research has revealed an early onset of severe dysplasia and has attempted to determine the etiology of dysplasia and contracture.

Dislocation of the glenohumeral joint in infancy was previously considered to be rare, but two recent studies documented a higher incidence than was believed to exist. One study is a review of the treatment of 134 consecutive infants referred to a brachial plexus center in the United States.[19] All patients underwent physical examination. Shoulders with any clinical sign of posterior shoulder dislocation (rapid loss of passive external rotation, asymmetric axillary skin folds, apparently shortened humeral segment, or palpable clunking during shoulder manipulation) received ultrasonographic imaging. Eight percent were found to have a posterior dislocation; the mean age was 6 months, and the youngest age was 3 months. The ultrasonographic method used to detect posterior glenohumeral dislocation was similar to the method for detecting hip dysplasia in infants. The findings of the first study were confirmed by a more recent population-based study conducted in Sweden, which found a 7.3% incidence of glenohumeral dislocation among infants with BPBP.[20] In clinical practice, the early age at which glenohumeral dislocation develops warrants vigilance in physical examination and imaging of infants with BPBP to allow early detection and treatment.

The shoulder internal rotation contracture and glenohumeral dysplasia are believed to result from muscle imbalance between the functional internal rotators and the paralyzed external rotators, which applies a posteriorly subluxating force on the glenohumeral articulation. This theory was supported by a recent MRI study that found a correlation between relative muscle atrophy and dysplasia severity.[21] In 74 patients, the cross-sectional areas of the pectoralis major, subscapularis, and infraspinatus–teres minor muscles were evaluated on MRI of the shoulder. Glenohumeral dysplasia was graded using the Waters-Jaramillo scale (**Table 1**). The ratio of the pectoralis major cross-sectional area to that of the external rotators was higher in affected than unaffected shoulders, and the ratio increased as the severity of glenohumeral deformity increased. The study thus supported an association between muscle imbalance and glenohumeral deformity. The precise relationship between shoulder girdle muscular atrophy and glenohumeral dysplasia and dysfunction is difficult to define, however. A similar study used MRI to evaluate the cross-sectional area and volume of muscles about

Table 1	
The Waters-Jaramillo Scale for Assessing Glenohumeral Dysplasia	
Grade	**Description**
I	Normal glenoid (less than 5° difference in retroversion compared with the normal, contralateral side)
II	Minimal deformity (more than 5° difference in retroversion compared with the normal, contralateral side)
III	Moderate deformity (posterior subluxation of the humeral head, defined as less than 35% of the head anterior to the bisecting line)
IV	Severe deformity (false glenoid)
V	Severe flattening of the humeral head and glenoid, with progressive or complete dislocation of the head
VI	Dislocation of the glenohumeral joint in infancy
VII	Growth arrest of the proximal aspect of the humerus

the shoulder and attempted to correlate these measures with glenohumeral dysplasia, passive external rotation, and global shoulder function (using the Mallet scale).[22] Atrophy of the infraspinatus and subscapularis was correlated with glenohumeral dysplasia but not with passive external rotation or Mallet score. The interplay between denervation, muscle atrophy, and musculoskeletal growth probably is complex.

Uncertainty as to the precise etiology of glenohumeral contracture and dysplasia has led to attempts to develop animal models of neonatal brachial plexus injury. In one such model, infraclavicular upper trunk neurotomy in neonatal rats led to internal rotation contractures and glenohumeral dysplasia closely resembling those of humans.[23] The ability to create glenohumeral dysplasia in animals was confirmed by a recent study that induced shoulder paralysis in neonatal mice by injecting botulinum toxin into the subscapularis.[24] Shoulder internal rotation contractures and glenohumeral dysplasia resulted despite the physiologic dissimilarity between this method of paralysis and that of upper trunk brachial plexus injury. There also were elbow flexion contractures similar to those in humans, despite the injection of the paralytic agent into the supraspinatus muscle. The soft-tissue contractures improved when the botulinum injections ceased, but the skeletal deformities were permanent. Once again, the relationships between denervation, muscle dysfunction, and glenohumeral dysplasia were confirmed as complex and remaining to be fully defined.

Shoulder Contracture Release and Tendon Transfers

A variety of surgical procedures have been described and modified over many decades for releasing the shoulder internal rotation contracture and augmenting external rotation strength. The procedures typically involve lengthening or sectioning internal rotators (such as the subscapularis and/or pectoralis major) and transferring functioning muscles (such as the latissimus dorsi and/or teres major) to the posterior or posterosuperior rotator cuff to augment external rotation and abduc-

tion function. Global shoulder function improves in the short and medium term but tends to deteriorate over time.

As awareness of glenohumeral dysplasia has increased during the past decade, studies have evaluated the effect of surgical procedures on glenohumeral dysplasia progression. A 2005 study evaluated 25 children after latissimus dorsi and teres major tendon transfers, with or without lengthening of the subscapularis or pectoralis major.[25] At 2-year follow-up, global shoulder function improved, as indicated by a 5-point increase in the Mallet scale. This result is consistent with earlier reports. However, MRI or CT revealed only modest improvements in glenoid retroversion and glenohumeral subluxation. The authors concluded that muscle-rebalancing surgery only halts the progression of dysplasia and does not allow substantial remodeling. Another study found a complete lack of glenohumeral remodeling at 1-year follow-up of 23 children treated with a similar combination of procedures.[26] However, a study of 33 children who underwent arthroscopic release of the subscapularis, with or without latissimus dorsi transfer, found substantial glenohumeral remodeling in 12 of the 15 children for whom preoperative and 2-year follow-up MRI was available.[27] In a retrospective study of 109 patients who underwent open subscapularis release and teres major transfer, CT of 39 patients at least 1 year after surgery revealed glenoid retroversion that was positively correlated with age at the time of surgery.[28] Children who were younger than 4 years had normal glenoid retroversion at follow-up, and children who were younger than 2 years had no glenohumeral subluxation. These two studies, in contrast to the first two studies, suggest that remodeling is possible.

The finding of potential for remodeling has been validated by several recent studies. Of 23 patients who underwent subscapularis–pectoralis major lengthening and latissimus dorsi–teres major transfer with the addition of open glenohumeral reduction, 83% had glenohumeral remodeling at 2-year follow-up, with significant improvement in both glenoid retroversion and

3: Upper Extremity

glenohumeral subluxation.[29] A study of 44 children who underwent arthroscopic subscapularis release, with or without external rotation tendon transfer, found significant remodeling on MRI at 1-year follow-up.[30] These reports draw attention to the adaptation of surgical technique to emphasize obtaining appropriate glenohumeral articular alignment, in addition to extra-articular muscle balance. The maximum patient age at which remodeling can occur is unknown, as is the severity of glenohumeral deformity that can remodel. Nonetheless, the possibility of restoring normal skeletal structure with early surgery underscores the importance of early detection of glenohumeral dysplasia.

Surgical treatment of the internal rotation contracture can lead to complications, especially with regard to achieving optimal balance between internal and external rotation. Several studies of open and arthroscopic techniques have called attention to the postoperative loss of active internal rotation function.[26,27,31-33] The resulting "severe, functionally disturbing" external rotation contracture can require internal rotation humeral osteotomy to restore midline function.[33] To avoid this complication, the surgeon should consider a partial release of the subscapularis tendon or less aggressive musculotendinous lengthening. Conversely, the internal rotation contracture may recur after release and tendon transfers. A recent report described improvement in active external rotation after revision subscapularis lengthening with transfer of the lower trapezius muscle to the infraspinatus tendon.[34]

Humeral Osteotomy

External rotation osteotomy of the humerus was commonly used to improve external rotation before soft-tissue and articular procedures became popular for shoulder internal rotation contracture. Osteotomy still has a role, most often for a child who has advanced glenohumeral deformity or insufficient power in the muscles needed for transfer. At a minimum 2-year follow-up, 27 patients who underwent humeral external rotation osteotomy had a 5-point improvement in global shoulder function on the Mallet scale, with few complications.[35] The authors concluded that the treatment is effective for children with advanced dysplasia that precludes tendon transfer surgery. The extent of dysplasia that precludes successful tendon transfer surgery is unknown, however. Moreover, the results of humeral osteotomy tend to worsen over time. Seventeen children who underwent low humeral osteotomy had a progressive loss of abduction during the minimum 8-year follow-up period.[36] The loss of abduction may not be the result of failure of the surgical realignment but rather of the progression of glenohumeral deformity. This has led some investigators to believe that early dysplasia detection and intervention are essential so that the opportunity to restore glenohumeral alignment and muscle balance about the shoulder can be seized.

Distal Extremity Deformities

Supination Contracture
Limitations of passive and active forearm rotation can occur with BPBP, especially if the lower trunk is involved. In 56 children with unresolved BPBP, active or passive forearm pronation was limited in 48 or 22 children, respectively, and active or passive supination was limited in 36 or 9 children, respectively.[37] These limitations were more common in children with global brachial plexus injury, but they were not correlated with the timing of biceps recovery. A dichotomy was noted between initial weakness in supination and long-term weakness in pronation, which is more common. The cause of the supination contracture therefore remains to be elucidated.

Impaired active supination in a supple forearm can be treated with tendon transfers. However, correction of the supination deformity frequently requires forearm osteotomy because of the fixed nature of the contracture. Several recent studies described the short-term results of forearm osteotomy techniques for this condition. A combined proximal ulna and distal radius osteotomy in 12 patients led to a change in forearm position from an average 76° of supination before surgery to an average 2° of pronation at an average 16-month follow-up.[38] Distal ulna and midshaft radius osteotomy in 14 patients led to an average correction from 80° of supination to 24° of pronation at a minimum 6-month follow-up.[39] Similar results have been achieved with the use of radius osteotomy alone,[40] although supination contracture can recur in as many as 40% of children treated in early childhood.[41] The less common pronation deformity can be treated with pronator teres rerouting, provided that passive supination is adequate. In 14 children at a minimum 8-month follow-up, this procedure improved active supination from 5° to 75° without a loss of active pronation.[42]

Hand Functional Impairment
Functional and sensory impairment of the hand is common after global brachial plexus injury, and it should not be overlooked. However, secondary reconstructive procedures are more limited in the hand than in the more proximal parts of the limb because of the relative distance from the hand to extraplexal donor nerves and muscles for transfer to restore motor function. It is therefore imperative that the strategies used during primary nerve surgery aim to provide innervation of the lower trunk. A retrospective review of 25 patients who underwent primary brachial plexus exploration and nerve grafting and transfers illustrates this point.[43] Surgery done before 1995 did not include an attempt to reconstruct the lower trunk; only 3 of the 8 patients had good hand function after surgery, as measured using the Raimondi scale. Later surgery included reconstruction of the lower trunk as a priority; 8 of the 14 patients had good or very good hand function after sur-

gery. In a similar study, useful hand function (defined as grade 3 or higher on the Raimondi scale) was gained in 9 of 13 patients who had lower trunk reconstruction but only in 1 of 3 patients who did not have lower trunk reconstruction.[44]

Secondary reconstruction of motor function in the hand is challenging. The most frequently performed tendon transfers are to improve wrist extension. Restoration of finger flexion is more difficult. A recent study reported some success after free-functioning gracilis muscle transfer for restoring flexor digitorum profundus function in four children older than 6 years.[45] All of the children had undergone earlier primary nerve surgery without attempted reconstruction of the lower trunk.

Long-term sensory impairment is not uncommon in the hand, even after isolated upper plexus injury. Hand sensation was tested using Semmes-Weinstein monofilaments in 95 children with BPBP who were older than 6 years.[46] Impaired sensation was detected in 7 of 64 patients with a C5-6 injury, 5 of 19 with a C5-7 injury, and 4 of 12 with a C5-T1 injury. These findings are consistent with those of a study of 105 patients, in whom sensation was found to be correlated with the number of involved nerve roots. Only 69% of patients with C5-6 injury had normal sensation.[47]

Outcomes and Quality of Life

Most of the clinical research on BPBP has used provider-based measures of function. However, the trend in clinical research is to emphasize the impact of disease and its treatment on patient-rated outcomes and quality of life. The Pediatric Outcomes Data Collection Instrument (PODCI) has been found to be sensitive to several diseases and treatments in children, and it has now been studied in children with BPBP. A prospective study of 23 children with unresolved BPBP found significant differences from age-matched control subjects in upper extremity function, sports participation, and global function.[48] A subsequent study of 150 children with BPBP who were age 2 to 5 years found that they significantly differed from age-matched normative control subjects in global function, upper extremity function, sports and physical functioning, mobility, comfort and pain, and happiness.[49] When the children's PODCI scores were compared with the Mallet classification of global shoulder function, the Toronto Test score, and the Active Movement Scale, the PODCI global function score was best correlated with the Mallet score in children age 2 to 5 years and with the Toronto Test score in children age 6 to 10 years.

The PODCI was found to be sensitive to the effects of shoulder external rotation tendon transfers. A prospective study of 23 children found significant improvement in PODCI global function, upper extremity function, and sports participation scores after shoulder tendon transfers.[50] Active range of motion in abduction and external rotation also improved significantly but was not correlated with improved PODCI scores.

Another patient-based outcome measure, the Pediatric Evaluation of Disability Inventory (PEDI), has been studied in children with BPBP.[51] In a review of 45 children, the 15 children with hand impairment were found to have significantly lower PEDI scores than the 30 without hand impairment. Only the children with hand impairment scored more than 2 standard deviations below the normative mean. Although there is no ideal patient-based outcomes instrument specifically designed for patients with BPBP, the PODCI and PEDI are useful in evaluating the effects of treatment and the impact of BPBP on patients' quality of life.

The parents of children with BPBP often have questions about future sports participation, upper extremity size differences, and overall musculoskeletal development. When a questionnaire was used to investigate sports participation in 85 children, sports participation rates and levels of competition were found to be similar to published norms, despite the children's lower PODCI scores.[52] Upper extremity size difference was evaluated in a study of 45 children.[53] The affected limb segments were found to be approximately 95% the length of the contralateral limb segments, and this size difference was considered very or extremely important to 37% of patients or families. An investigation of the effects of BPBP on remote musculoskeletal development in 111 children with BPBP who required nerve surgery found no limb-length discrepancies and an incidence of scoliosis similar to that of the general public.[54]

Summary

BPBP is not a challenge of the past, and its natural history is not as favorable as once thought. The decision to surgically explore the brachial plexus must be preceded by careful clinical assessment, with judicious use and interpretation of ancillary tests. Traditional neuroma excision and grafting in the future may be replaced by nerve transfers as the most effective option for nerve reconstruction. In children with unresolved BPBP, glenohumeral dysplasia can occur early in infancy. Shoulder function can be improved by surgical intervention aimed at restoring articular congruity and muscle balance, but early detection of glenohumeral dysplasia and dislocation is recommended before such surgery. Surgical release of the internal rotation contracture, whether open or arthroscopic, risks a loss of internal rotation function. Humeral osteotomy has a role in improving shoulder function in the presence of severe glenohumeral deformity. Supination contracture is often fixed and requires forearm osteotomy for correction, although some deformity may recur over time. Restoring hand function in a child with global plexus injury requires attention to the lower trunk during primary nerve reconstruction. Validated patient-based outcomes instruments can be used to assess the impact of BPBP on overall health and the effects of treatments on patient outcome. Research into BPBP, if it continues at the pace of the past 5 years, has the ability to continue to advance the understanding and treatment of this complex condition.

Annotated References

1. Foad SL, Mehlman CT, Ying J: The epidemiology of neonatal brachial plexus palsy in the United States. *J Bone Joint Surg Am* 2008;90(6):1258-1264.

   A review of 11 million records in the Kids' Inpatient Database for 1997, 2000, and 2003 found that the incidence of BPBP was 1.51 per 1,000. Associated risk factors were examined. Level of evidence: II.

2. Pondaag W, Malessy MJ, van Dijk JG, Thomeer RT: Natural history of obstetric brachial plexus palsy: A systematic review. *Dev Med Child Neurol* 2004;46(2):138-144.

3. Duff SV, Dayanidhi S, Kozin SH: Asymmetrical shoulder kinematics in children with brachial plexus birth palsy. *Clin Biomech (Bristol, Avon)* 2007;22(6):630-638.

   The shoulder kinematics of children with BPBP were compared to those of control subjects. Level of evidence: III.

4. Bialocerkowski AE, Galea M: Comparison of visual and objective quantification of elbow and shoulder movement in children with obstetric brachial plexus palsy. *J Brachial Plex Peripher Nerve Inj* 2006;1:5.

   There was poor correlation between Active Movement Scale assessments as determined by therapists and by motion analysis. Level of evidence: II.

5. DeMatteo C, Bain JR, Galea V, Gjertsen D: Botulinum toxin as an adjunct to motor learning therapy and surgery for obstetrical brachial plexus injury. *Dev Med Child Neurol* 2006;48(4):245-252.

   A small, uncontrolled study found motor improvement in reinnervating muscles after botulinum injections in antagonists. Level of evidence: IV.

6. Heise CO, Gonçalves LR, Barbosa ER, Gherpelli JL: Botulinum toxin for treatment of cocontractions related to obstetrical brachial plexopathy. *Arq Neuropsiquiatr* 2005;63(3A):588-591.

   A small, uncontrolled study found improved biceps function after botulinum toxin injection into the cocontracting triceps. Level of evidence: IV.

7. Buesch FE, Schlaepfer B, de Bruin ED, Wohlrab G, Ammann-Reiffer C, Meyer-Heim A: Constraint-induced movement therapy for children with obstetric brachial plexus palsy: Two single-case series. *Int J Rehabil Res* 2009.

   The use of constraint therapy was reported in two patients with BPBP.

8. Smith NC, Rowan P, Benson LJ, Ezaki M, Carter PR: Neonatal brachial plexus palsy: Outcome of absent biceps function at three months of age. *J Bone Joint Surg Am* 2004;86-A(10):2163-2170.

9. Fisher DM, Borschel GH, Curtis CG, Clarke HM: Evaluation of elbow flexion as a predictor of outcome in obstetrical brachial plexus palsy. *Plast Reconstr Surg* 2007;120(6):1585-1590.

   A retrospective study found that elbow flexion at 3-month follow-up was a poor single predictor of upper limb motor recovery in 209 children with BPBP. Level of evidence: III.

10. Medina LS, Yaylali I, Zurakowski D, Ruiz J, Altman NR, Grossman JA: Diagnostic performance of MRI and MR myelography in infants with a brachial plexus birth injury. *Pediatr Radiol* 2006;36(12):1295-1299.

    In 31 infants, MRI before surgical exploration had low sensitivity but high specificity for nerve root avulsions. The nature of extraforaminal injury could not be delineated.

11. Smith AB, Gupta N, Strober J, Chin C: Magnetic resonance neurography in children with birth-related brachial plexus injury. *Pediatr Radiol* 2008;38(2):159-163.

    In 11 patients with BPBP, magnetic resonance neurography was better correlated with physical examination than with electrodiagnostic testing. Level of evidence: IV.

12. Heise CO, Siqueira MG, Martins RS, Gherpelli JL: Clinical-electromyography correlation in infants with obstetric brachial plexopathy. *J Hand Surg Am* 2007;32(7):999-1004.

    Electromyography overestimated function and was poorly correlated with clinical motor function examination in 41 infants with BPBP.

13. Kirjavainen M, Remes V, Peltonen J, et al: Long-term results of surgery for brachial plexus birth palsy. *J Bone Joint Surg Am* 2007;89(1):18-26.

    A long-term, retrospective, population-based study of 124 children who underwent primary nerve surgery for BPBP found that one third had pain and one third needed help with activities of daily living.

14. Birch R, Ahad N, Kono H, Smith S: Repair of obstetric brachial plexus palsy: Results in 100 children. *J Bone Joint Surg Br* 2005;87(8):1089-1095.

    A study of 100 children found that surgery for BPBP led to good results in 24% to 57% of grafted nerve roots. Level of evidence: IV.

15. Haerle M, Gilbert A: Management of complete obstetric brachial plexus lesions. *J Pediatr Orthop* 2004;24(2):194-200.

16. Lin JC, Schwentker-Colizza A, Curtis CG, Clarke HM: Final results of grafting versus neurolysis in obstetrical brachial plexus palsy. *Plast Reconstr Surg* 2009;123(3):939-948.

The results of nerve grafting and neurolysis were compared in a retrospective study of 108 patients who underwent primary nerve surgery. At 4-year follow-up, the patients with neurolysis had no improvement in upper or global plexus injury.

17. Ruchelsman DE, Ramos LE, Alfonso I, Price AE, Grossman A, Grossman JA: Outcome following spinal accessory to suprascapular (spinoscapular) nerve transfer in infants with brachial plexus birth injuries. *Hand (NY)* 2009;4(4):391-396.

    The role of transferring the spinal accessory to the suprascapular nerve as a component of brachial plexus reconstruction was investigated in 25 children. Level of evidence: IV.

18. Kozin SH: Nerve transfers in brachial plexus birth palsies: Indications, techniques, and outcomes. *Hand Clin* 2008;24(4):363-376, v.

    Current concepts in the use of nerve transfers for BPBP are reviewed. Level of evidence: V.

19. Moukoko D, Ezaki M, Wilkes D, Carter P: Posterior shoulder dislocation in infants with neonatal brachial plexus palsy. *J Bone Joint Surg Am* 2004;86-A(4):787-793.

20. Dahlin LB, Erichs K, Andersson C, et al: Incidence of early posterior shoulder dislocation in brachial plexus birth palsy. *J Brachial Plex Peripher Nerve Inj* 2007;2:24.

    A population-based study found a 7.3% incidence of shoulder dislocation among infants with BPBP. Level of evidence: II.

21. Waters PM, Monica JT, Earp BE, Zurakowski D, Bae DS: Correlation of radiographic muscle cross-sectional area with glenohumeral deformity in children with brachial plexus birth palsy. *J Bone Joint Surg Am* 2009;91(10):2367-2375.

    An MRI study correlated the muscle cross-sectional area ratios between internal and external rotators with shoulder contractures and deformity.

22. van Gelein Vitringa VM, van Kooten EO, Jaspers RT, Mullender MG, van Doorn-Loogman MH, van der Sluijs JA: An MRI study on the relations between muscle atrophy, shoulder function and glenohumeral deformity in shoulders of children with obstetric brachial plexus injury. *J Brachial Plex Peripher Nerve Inj* 2009;4(1):9.

    An MRI study of dysplastic shoulders found muscle atrophy to be greater in the subscapularis than in the abductors or external rotators.

23. Li Z, Ma J, Apel P, Carlson CS, Smith TL, Koman LA: Brachial plexus birth palsy-associated shoulder deformity: A rat model study. *J Hand Surg Am* 2008;33(3):308-312.

    A rat model of neonatal brachial plexus injury was created by extraforaminal C5-6 neurotomy.

24. Kim HM, Galatz LM, Patel N, Das R, Thomopoulos S: Recovery potential after postnatal shoulder paralysis:

An animal model of neonatal brachial plexus palsy. *J Bone Joint Surg Am* 2009;91(4):879-891.

    Botulinum toxin injection into the supraspinatus of neonatal mice was used to simulate neonatal brachial plexus injury.

25. Waters PM, Bae DS: Effect of tendon transfers and extra-articular soft-tissue balancing on glenohumeral development in brachial plexus birth palsy. *J Bone Joint Surg Am* 2005;87(2):320-325.

    In 25 children, no remodeling of glenohumeral dysplasia was found after external rotation tendon transfers, with or without contracture release.

26. Kozin SH, Chafetz RS, Barus D, Filipone L: Magnetic resonance imaging and clinical findings before and after tendon transfers about the shoulder in children with residual brachial plexus birth palsy. *J Shoulder Elbow Surg* 2006;15(5):554-561.

    In 23 children, no remodeling of glenohumeral dysplasia was found after external rotation tendon transfers, with or without contracture release.

27. Pearl ML, Edgerton BW, Kazimiroff PA, Burchette RJ, Wong K: Arthroscopic release and latissimus dorsi transfer for shoulder internal rotation contractures and glenohumeral deformity secondary to brachial plexus birth palsy. *J Bone Joint Surg Am* 2006;88(3):564-574.

    In 33 children with BPBP, global shoulder function improved and glenohumeral remodeling occurred after arthroscopic contracture release, with or without concomitant external rotation tendon transfers, but there was loss of internal rotation function.

28. El-Gammal TA, Saleh WR, El-Sayed A, Kotb MM, Imam HM, Fathi NA: Tendon transfer around the shoulder in obstetric brachial plexus paralysis: Clinical and computed tomographic study. *J Pediatr Orthop* 2006;26(5):641-646.

    In 39 children, glenohumeral remodeling occurred after subscapularis release, with or without concomitant external rotation tendon transfers, if the surgery was performed before age 2 years.

29. Waters PM, Bae DS: The early effects of tendon transfers and open capsulorrhaphy on glenohumeral deformity in brachial plexus birth palsy: Surgical technique. *J Bone Joint Surg Am* 2009;91(suppl 2):213-222.

    A review of 23 patients with glenohumeral dysplasia and BPBP found that open reduction, capsulorrhaphy, contracture release, and external rotation tendon transfers had led to remodeling of the glenohumeral joint at 2-year follow-up.

30. Kozin SH, Boardman MJ, Chafetz RS, Williams GR, Hanlon A: Arthroscopic treatment of internal rotation contracture and glenohumeral dysplasia in children with brachial plexus birth palsy. *J Shoulder Elbow Surg* 2010;19(1):102-110.

    In 44 patients, arthroscopic contracture release, with or without external rotation tendon transfers, allowed remodeling of glenohumeral dysplasia. Functional improvement was greater in patients who received both the release and transfers.

31. Newman CJ, Morrison L, Lynch B, Hynes D: Outcome of subscapularis muscle release for shoulder contracture secondary to brachial plexus palsy at birth. *J Pediatr Orthop* 2006;26(5):647-651.

In 13 children with BPBP, function improved after subscapularis release without concomitant external rotation tendon transfers for shoulder contractures.

32. Kambhampati SB, Birch R, Cobiella C, Chen L: Posterior subluxation and dislocation of the shoulder in obstetric brachial plexus palsy. *J Bone Joint Surg Br* 2006; 88(2):213-219.

In 183 surgically treated shoulder contractures following BPBP, postoperative outcomes were correlated with the extent of neurologic injury, duration of dislocation, and onset of glenohumeral deformity.

33. van der Sluijs JA, van Ouwerkerk WJ, de Gast A, Nollet F, Winters H, Wuisman PI: Treatment of internal rotation contracture of the shoulder in obstetric brachial plexus lesions by subscapular tendon lengthening and open reduction: Early results and complications. *J Pediatr Orthop B* 2004;13(3):218-224.

34. Bertelli JA: Lengthening of subscapularis and transfer of the lower trapezius in the correction of recurrent internal rotation contracture following obstetric brachial plexus palsy. *J Bone Joint Surg Br* 2009;91(7):943-948.

The results of a novel trapezius transfer to restore external rotation function are described in 7 children with BPBP.

35. Waters PM, Bae DS: The effect of derotational humeral osteotomy on global shoulder function in brachial plexus birth palsy. *J Bone Joint Surg Am* 2006;88(5): 1035-1042.

A retrospective study of 43 patients with substantial glenohumeral dysplasia found that global shoulder function improved after external rotation humeral osteotomy for internal rotation contracture.

36. Al-Qattan MM, Al-Husainan H, Al-Otaibi A, El-Sharkawy MS: Long-term results of low rotation humeral osteotomy in children with Erb's obstetric brachial plexus palsy. *J Hand Surg Eur Vol* 2009;34(4): 486-492.

The long-term results are reported for humeral rotational osteotomy for shoulder contracture in children with BPBP. External rotation was preserved, but there was loss of abduction over time.

37. Sibinski M, Sherlock DA, Hems TE, Sharma H: Forearm rotational profile in obstetric brachial plexus injury. *J Shoulder Elbow Surg* 2007;16(6):784-787.

Active and passive forearm rotation was measured in 56 children with BPBP to establish the rotational profile of the forearm after injury.

38. Hankins SM, Bezwada HP, Kozin SH: Corrective osteotomies of the radius and ulna for supination contracture of the pediatric and adolescent forearm secondary to neurologic injury. *J Hand Surg Am* 2006;31(1):118-124.

The use of proximal ulna and distal radius osteotomies for correction of supination contractures is described in 12 patients with BPBP.

39. Rolfe KW, Green TA, Lawrence JF: Corrective osteotomies and osteosynthesis for supination contracture of the forearm in children. *J Pediatr Orthop* 2009;29(4): 406-410.

The use of distal ulna and diaphyseal radius osteotomies for correction of supination contractures is described in 11 patients with BPBP.

40. van Kooten EO, Ishaque MA, Winters HA, Ritt MJ, van der Sluijs HA: Pronating radius osteotomy for supination deformity in children with obstetric brachial plexus palsy. *Tech Hand Up Extrem Surg* 2008;12(1):34-37.

The use of isolated diaphyseal radius osteotomy for correction of supination contractures is described in eight patients with BPBP.

41. Yam A, Fullilove S, Sinisi M, Fox M: The supination deformity and associated deformities of the upper limb in severe birth lesions of the brachial plexus. *J Bone Joint Surg Br* 2009;91(4):511-516.

The surgical treatment of supination contractures is described in 42 patients with BPBP. There was a 40% recurrence rate of the contracture after osteotomy alone.

42. Amrani A, Dendane MA, El Alami ZF: Pronator teres transfer to correct pronation deformity of the forearm after an obstetrical brachial plexus injury. *J Bone Joint Surg Br* 2009;91(5):616-618.

The results of pronator teres transfer to correct pronation contractures are described in 14 children with BPBP.

43. Maillet M, Romana C: Complete obstetric brachial plexus palsy: Surgical improvement to recover a functional hand. *J Child Orthop* 2009;3(2):101-108.

Long-term recovery of hand function was assessed in 30 children after surgery for global brachial plexus injuries. The importance of attention to the lower trunk during neurosurgical plexus reconstruction is highlighted.

44. Pondaag W, Malessy MJ: Recovery of hand function following nerve grafting and transfer in obstetric brachial plexus lesions. *J Neurosurg* 2006;105(1, suppl) 33-40.

After surgery for global brachial plexus injuries, 69% of 33 patients recovered useful hand function.

45. Bahm J, Ocampo-Pavez C: Free functional gracilis muscle transfer in children with severe sequelae from obstetric brachial plexus palsy. *J Brachial Plex Peripher Nerve Inj* 2008;3:23.

The indications, technique, and results of free-functioning muscle transfers to restore hand function are described in four children with BPBP.

46. Palmgren T, Peltonen J, Linder T, Rautakorpi S, Nietosvaara Y: Sensory evaluation of the hands in children with brachial plexus birth injury. *Dev Med Child Neurol* 2007;49(8):582-586.

3: Upper Extremity

In a study of 95 children with BPBP, fine sensation in the hand was impaired in 11% of those with C5-6 injury, 26% of those with C5-7 injury, and 33% of those with global injury.

47. Kirjavainen M, Remes V, Peltonen J, Rautakorpi S, Helenius I, Nietosvaara Y: The function of the hand after operations for obstetric injuries to the brachial plexus. *J Bone Joint Surg Br* 2008;90(3):349-355.

In 105 patients who underwent surgery for BPBP, impairment of hand function was correlated with the distribution of root injury and the presence of root avulsions.

48. Huffman GR, Bagley AM, James MA, Lerman JA, Rab G: Assessment of children with brachial plexus birth palsy using the Pediatric Outcomes Data Collection Instrument. *J Pediatr Orthop* 2005;25(3):400-404.

A prospective study found that the PODCI was able to detect differences in function between 23 children with BPBP and normal control subjects.

49. Bae DS, Waters PM, Zurakowski D: Correlation of pediatric outcomes data collection instrument with measures of active movement in children with brachial plexus birth palsy. *J Pediatr Orthop* 2008;28(5):584-592.

A prospective evaluation found that PODCI scores were lower for 150 children with BPBP than for age-matched control subjects in all domains, most notably in the upper extremity function and sports domains.

50. Dedini RD, Bagley AM, Molitor F, James MA: Comparison of pediatric outcomes data collection instrument scores and range of motion before and after shoulder tendon transfers for children with brachial plexus birth palsy. *J Pediatr Orthop* 2008;28(2):259-264.

In 23 children who underwent external rotation tendon transfers for BPBP, improvements in PODCI scores were correlated with improved abduction but not with improved overall shoulder range of motion.

51. Ho ES, Curtis CG, Clarke HM: Pediatric Evaluation of Disability Inventory: Its application to children with obstetric brachial plexus palsy. *J Hand Surg Am* 2006; 31(2):197-202.

Self-care scores on the PEDI were found to be lower in 45 children with BPBP than in normal control subjects only if hand function was impaired by the injury.

52. Bae DS, Zurakowski D, Avallone N, Yu R, Waters PM: Sports participation in selected children with brachial plexus birth palsy. *J Pediatr Orthop* 2009;29(5):496-503.

In 85 children with brachial plexus birth injury, sports participation was similar to that of normal control subjects.

53. Bae DS, Ferretti M, Waters PM: Upper extremity size differences in brachial plexus birth palsy. *Hand (N Y)* 2008;3(4):297-303.

A study of 48 children with BPBP found that the length of the affected extremity on average was 95% of that of the opposite limb.

54. Kirjavainen MO, Remes VM, Peltonen J, et al: Permanent brachial plexus birth palsy does not impair the development and function of the spine and lower limbs. *J Pediatr Orthop B* 2009;18(6):283-288.

A study of 11 children with severe BPBP did not find an increased incidence of scoliosis or any evidence of lower limb dysfunction or length discrepancy.

Chapter 16

Transverse Deficiency in the Upper Limb

Michelle A. James, MD   Derek F. Amanatullah, MD, PhD

Introduction

Transverse deficiency (TD) is the result of an embryonic failure of limb formation. TD has an appearance similar to that of acquired amputation, and the condition formerly was known as congenital amputation.[1,2] TD is characterized by axial bone dysplasia and minimal involvement of proximal structures in the limb.[2]

TD is unilateral, occurs sporadically, and is not commonly associated with other congenital anomalies. During the past 40 years, the incidence of TD has remained between 2 and 7 per 10,000 births, and it has not varied greatly among developed countries.[3] TD occurs two to three times more often in the upper limb than in the lower limb.[3] The most common upper limb deficiency is below-elbow deficiency (BED), which occurs at the junction of the proximal one third and distal two thirds of the forearm[3] (Figure 1). Upper limb TD also can occur at the level of the wrist as a radiocarpal deficiency or at the level of the hand as a transmetacarpal deficiency or symbrachydactyly.[4] Symbrachydactyly is considered a form of TD because 93% of extremities with BED have stigmata of symbrachydactyly, such as soft-tissue nubbins, skin invaginations, or hypoplasia of the proximal radius and ulna.[5]

The cause of TD probably is a process that interrupts the vascular supply to the limb during development, such as fetal exposure to an environmental teratogen or a gene-environment interaction. Chorionic villus sampling and maternal ingestion of misoprostol have been linked to TD.[6] The association of symbrachydactyly with Poland syndrome suggests that TD has a vascular origin. The manifestations of Poland syndrome, which include ipsilateral pectoral aplasia as well as symbrachydactyly, may be caused by an early disruption of the subclavian artery.[7]

Dr. James or an immediate family member serves as a board member, owner, officer, or committee member of the American Board of Orthopaedic Surgery and the Ruth Jackson Orthopaedic Society. Dr. Amanatullah or an immediate family member has received research or institutional support from Arthrex, DePuy, Medtronic, Smith & Nephew, Stryker, Synthes, and Zimmer and holds stock or stock options in Merck and Stryker.

Like TD, longitudinal deficiency results from an embryonic failure of limb formation. The radial, ulnar, or central structures are affected. Fingers are absent in the longitudinal axis of the limb. A radial deficiency can result in thumb aplasia or hypoplasia, and a central deficiency may appear as cleft hand.[4,8]

Pediatric Prostheses

An upper limb prosthesis traditionally was used if it could be accommodated by the TD. For example, a BED at the proximal one third–distal two thirds forearm level provides sufficient space for a prosthesis to be fitted. The empiric assumption was that a TD, like an acquired amputation in an adult, causes substantial

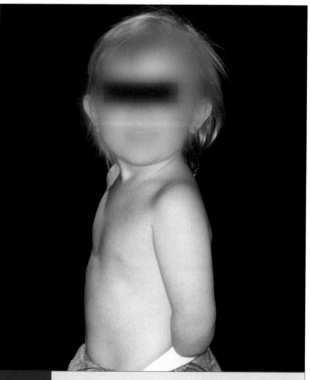

Figure 1   A child with below-elbow deficiency, which is the most common type of transverse deficiency.

Table 1

Questionnaires Used to Assess Pediatric Hand Function

Questionnaire	ICF Domain	Comments
ABILHAND-Kids	Activity	Designed for use in children with cerebral palsy
Childhood Assessment of Participation and Enjoyment	Participation	Requires a long administration time
Canadian Occupational Performance Measure	Participation	Requires specialized training for administration Requires a long administration time
Pediatric Outcomes Data Collection Instrument	Activity Participation	Well validated Requires only a short administration time Limited by a ceiling effect
Prosthetic Upper Limb Functional Index	Activity	Useful for a child who wears a prosthesis

Table 2

Functional Tests Used to Assess Pediatric Hand Function

Functional Test	ICF Domain	Comments
Assisting Hand Assessment	Activity	Designed for use in children with cerebral palsy Requires specialized training for administration Requires videotaping and review
Jebsen-Taylor Hand Function Test	Activity	Forces the use of the affected extremity
Shriners Hospital for Children Upper Extremity Evaluation	Activity	Designed for use in children with cerebral palsy Requires specialized training for administration Requires videotaping and review
Unilateral Below Elbow Test	Activity	Requires only a short administration time Requires videotaping and review
University of New Brunswick Test of Prosthetic Function	Activity	Useful for a child who wears a prosthesis

disability and diminishes a child's quality of life. A prosthesis was prescribed as soon as an infant was able to sit independently, and prosthesis use was encouraged throughout childhood, in the belief that it would lead to more effective prosthesis use and improve overall upper limb function. The use of an upper limb prosthesis was found not to be universally helpful to adults with an acquired amputation, however.[9] Early prosthesis use by children with TD has not led to better prosthesis use or overall upper limb function,[10-12] and one large study found that 49% of children with BED abandoned their prosthesis over time.[13]

Upper Limb Function and Quality of Life

The International Classification of Functioning, Disability, and Health (ICF) describes the manner in which people cope with a health condition and provides caregivers with a means of understanding and measuring outcomes from body structure, individual, and societal perspectives.[14] The ICF defines a deficiency of body structure such as TD as an impairment. Impairment is assessed by measuring parameters such as range of motion and grip and pinch strength. However, an impairment does not necessarily cause a disability (defined as a limitation in the ability to perform activities of daily living) or a restriction in participation (defined as integration of activities necessary for accomplishing a chosen life role).

Activity is assessed through the use of a questionnaire or an objective function test (Tables 1 and 2). Questionnaires such as the Pediatric Orthopaedic Data Collection Instrument (PODCI) also are used to assess participation and quality of life[11,15,16] (Table 1). Questionnaires specifically designed for children with hemiplegic cerebral palsy or children who use an upper limb prosthesis have been used to assess the function of children with TD.[17,18] Questionnaires that address participation are useful but time consuming to administer.[19-21] The Pediatric Quality of Life Inventory (PedsQL) is the only questionnaire that specifically evaluates quality of life and the psychological effect of limb absence.[22]

The Jebsen-Taylor Hand Function Test is the most widely used functional test of upper limb activity in children.[23] Because each hand is tested separately and the use of the affected limb is forced, the Jebsen-Taylor Hand Function Test is not appropriate for a child with BED. Functional tests designed for children with a unilateral neurologic condition or a prosthesis may be

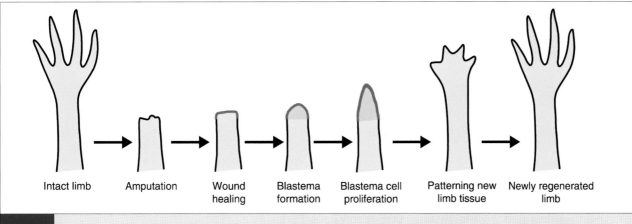

Figure 2	A schematic representation of the key morphologic events of limb regeneration: intact limb, amputation, wound healing (apical epidermal cap formation), blastema formation, blastema proliferation, patterning, and regeneration. (Adapted with permission from Whited JL, Tabin CJ: Limb regeneration revisited. *J Biol* 2009;8[1]:5.)

Labels under figure: Intact limb, Amputation, Wound healing, Blastema formation, Blastema cell proliferation, Patterning new limb tissue, Newly regenerated limb

useful for activity testing of children with TD.[18,24-26] The Unilateral Below Elbow Test (UBET) is specifically designed for evaluating children with TD, regardless of prosthesis use.[27,28]

A multicenter outcomes study used the PODCI, Prosthetic Upper Limb Functional Index (PUFI), PedsQL, and UBET (with and without the use of a prosthesis) to assess the function and quality of life of children with BED.[11] Of the 489 surveyed children, 66% wore a prosthesis, and 34% did not. Prosthesis wear was not associated with any clinically relevant differences in PODCI, PUFI, or PedsQL scores. In fact, children with BED scored at least as high as the general population on the PedsQL and had only slightly lower upper limb physical function as measured by the PODCI. Hence, children with BED were found to have close-to-normal function and quality-of-life scores.[11] On the UBET, children with BED who did not wear a prosthesis performed at least as well as those who wore a prosthesis; children who usually wore a prosthesis performed at least as well when they were not wearing the prosthesis.[11] Although prosthesis use may be helpful for achieving social acceptance or performing specialized activities, a child's function or quality of life does not appear to be improved. This factor may be the reason that half of patients with BED abandon prosthesis use over time.[11,13]

New Horizons in Prosthesis Design

Pediatric care providers tend to focus on structure and physical impairment because this is the most easily measured functional domain. In doing so, they may overestimate a child's disability, underestimate a child's quality of life, and erroneously attribute improvements in function to interventions such as prosthesis use or surgery rather than to the child's growth and development. Of the three ICF domains of function (body structure, activity, and participation), impairment of

body structure is the least relevant to quality of life. Participation is the domain of function that has the strongest association with quality of life.[11,24] The possibility of improving a child's quality of life through limb regeneration or use of an advanced prosthesis is a challenging opportunity that could lead to fulfilling the child's desire to have two hands and to achieve life priorities. Although surgical hand transplantation has been attempted, it is absolutely contraindicated in children and is controversial in adults because of ethical concerns and the long-term need for immunosuppressive therapy.[29]

Recent advances in genomics, proteomics, and molecular biology offer the potential for understanding the cellular and molecular mechanisms of limb regeneration[30-32] (Figure 2). Epithelialization within the first days after amputation and formation of the apical epidermal cap are essential for limb regeneration in vertebrates.[33,34] The next critical steps are formation and proliferation of the blastema (a group of undifferentiated and uncharacterized mesodermal cells that arise below the apical epidermal cap).[35] A denervated amputated limb does not undergo blastema proliferation, and regeneration will fail.[36-38]

In comparison with research into limb replacement, integrated engineering approaches to controlling an upper limb prosthesis may yield a more practical type of limb replacement within a shorter period of time. The traditional myoelectric upper limb prosthesis performs one action at a time, using surface electromyography signals from voluntarily activated muscles. The technology related to myoelectric prostheses continues to advance, but such a prosthesis is costly ($10,000 to $20,000) and is limited by its two-input system.[39] The targeted muscle reinnervation prosthesis has been developed to allow multiple simultaneous movements. Targeted muscle reinnervation involves cutting the cutaneous sensory nerves supplying the skin over the target muscle and reinnervating them with the afferent motor fibers of the target muscle. In this way the skin

3: Upper Extremity

becomes a representation of the amputated limb and can provide signals to the prosthesis.[40,41] In a cybernetic system, a bidirectional electrode is directly implanted into the median nerve to analyze the signal from the nerve, and an articulated hand is controlled by detecting activity from the nerve.[42] A brain-computer interface (BCI) foregoes the normal output system (the peripheral nerves or muscles). Instead, a BCI attempts to use thought, as determined via electroencephalography, to control the external environment through a robotic limb or a computer screen cursor.[43] BCI is limited by the inability to train a person to simulate a kinesthetic movement rather than image it; these two thought processes are interpreted quite differently on electroencephalography.[44] Combinations of cybernetics and BCI have been developed in which an implanted computer chip records cortical activity and correlates the data with real-time electromyography to allow stimulation of peripheral nerves or spinal tracts for the purpose of controlling movement.[45]

These new prosthesis-control technologies are creative and promising, but they remain experimental and prohibitively expensive. The current commercially available prostheses are heavy, lack durability, fail to provide meaningful sensory feedback, and are not sold in pediatric sizes.

Summary

TD of the upper limb is an uncommon condition caused by interruption of embryonic limb formation. TD causes less disability than commonly assumed. Current prostheses are not consistently useful for the treatment of TD, but recent developments in prosthetic technology are promising. Advances in molecular biology may eventually enable limb regeneration.

Annotated References

1. Swanson AB: A classification for congenital limb malformations. *J Hand Surg Am* 1976;1(1):8-22.

2. De Smet L, International Federation for Societies for Surgery of the Hand, Japanese Society for Surgery of the Hand: Classification for congenital anomalies of the hand: The IFSSH classification and the JSSH modification. *Genet Couns* 2002;13(3):331-338.

3. Ephraim PL, Dillingham TR, Sector M, Pezzin LE, Mackenzie EJ: Epidemiology of limb loss and congenital limb deficiency: A review of the literature. *Arch Phys Med Rehabil* 2003;84(5):747-761.

4. Ogino T: Clinical features and teratogenic mechanisms of congenital absence of digits. *Dev Growth Differ* 2007;49(6):523-531.

   A classification system is presented for congenital hand anomalies, with clinical features and teratogenic mechanisms of congenital absence of digits, including ulnar and radial deficiencies, cleft hand, symbrachydactyly, and constriction band syndrome.

5. Kallemeier PM, Manske PR, Davis B, Goldfarb CA: An assessment of the relationship between congenital transverse deficiency of the forearm and symbrachydactyly. *J Hand Surg Am* 2007;32(9):1408-1412.

   An investigation of the relationship between symbrachydactyly and transverse deficiency found that most patients with a diagnosis of transverse deficiency have soft-tissue nubbins, skin invaginations, or hypoplasia of the proximal radius and ulna at the end of the amputation stump.

6. Holmes LB: Teratogen-induced limb defects. *Am J Med Genet* 2002;112(3):297-303.

7. Bavinck JN, Weaver DD: Subclavian artery supply disruption sequence: Hypothesis of a vascular etiology for Poland, Klippel-Feil, and Möbius anomalies. *Am J Med Genet* 1986;23(4):903-918.

8. Goldfarb CA, Manske PR, Busa R, Mills J, Carter P, Ezaki M: Upper-extremity phocomelia reexamined: A longitudinal dysplasia. *J Bone Joint Surg Am* 2005; 87(12):2639-2648.

   A retrospective review of 60 upper extremities with phocomelia yielded evidence that these abnormalities represent a proximal continuum of radial or ulnar longitudinal dysplasia.

9. Davidson J: A survey of the satisfaction of upper limb amputees with their prostheses, their lifestyles, and their abilities. *J Hand Ther* 2002;15(1):62-70.

10. Postema K, van der Donk V, van Limbeek J, Rijken RA, Poelma MJ: Prosthesis rejection in children with a unilateral congenital arm defect. *Clin Rehabil* 1999;13(3): 243-249.

11. James MA, Bagley AM, Brasington K, Lutz C, McConnell S, Molitor F: Impact of prostheses on function and quality of life for children with unilateral congenital below-the-elbow deficiency. *J Bone Joint Surg Am* 2006; 88(11):2356-2365.

    Children with unilateral congenital BED were found to have nearly normal function and quality of life, regardless of whether they wear a prosthesis.

12. Meurs M, Maathuis CG, Lucas C, Hadders-Algra M, van der Sluis CK: Prescription of the first prosthesis and later use in children with congenital unilateral upper limb deficiency: A systematic review. *Prosthet Orthot Int* 2006;30(2):165-173.

    There is little evidence to support a relationship between the fitting of a first prosthesis in children with a congenital upper limb deficiency and rejection rates or functional outcomes. Clinical practice for introducing a prosthesis is guided by experience rather than evidence-based medicine.

13. Davids JR, Wagner LV, Meyer LC, Blackhurst DW: Prosthetic management of children with unilateral con-

genital below-elbow deficiency. *J Bone Joint Surg Am* 2006;88(6):1294-1300.

This study supports an initial prosthesis fitting before age 3 years for a child with unilateral congenital BED. Intensive training should be provided under the direction of an occupational therapist when an active terminal device is applied. A variety of prosthetic designs should be used during the child's years of growth.

14. World Health Organization: *International Classification of Functioning, Disability, and Health.* http://www.who.int/classifications/icf/en/. Accessed Sept 2009.

The ICF and the domains of body structure, activity, and participation are described.

15. Lerman JA, Sullivan E, Barnes DA, Haynes RJ: The Pediatric Outcomes Data Collection Instrument (PODCI) and functional assessment of patients with unilateral upper extremity deficiencies. *J Pediatr Orthop* 2005; 25(3):405-407.

The PODCI was used to quantify the functional abilities of patients with unilateral upper extremity deficiency. Scores from both parent and patient questionnaires were significantly lower than the normal range for upper extremity function and sports.

16. Hunsaker FG, Cioffi DA, Amadio PC, Wright JG, Caughlin B: The American Academy of Orthopaedic Surgeons outcomes instruments: Normative values from the general population. *J Bone Joint Surg Am* 2002;84-A(2):208-215.

17. Buffart LM, Roebroeck ME, van Heijningen VG, Pesch-Batenburg JM, Stam HJ: Evaluation of arm and prosthetic functioning in children with a congenital transverse reduction deficiency of the upper limb. *J Rehabil Med* 2007;39(5):379-386.

The Assisting Hand Assessment and Prosthetic Upper Extremity Functional Index and other standardized instruments provide relevant information on the functioning of children with an upper limb reduction deficiency.

18. Wright FV, Hubbard S, Naumann S, Jutai J: Evaluation of the validity of the prosthetic upper extremity functional index for children. *Arch Phys Med Rehabil* 2003; 84(4):518-527.

19. Carswell A, McColl MA, Baptiste S, Law M, Polatajko H, Pollock N: The Canadian Occupational Performance Measure: A research and clinical literature review. *Can J Occup Ther* 2004;71(4):210-222.

20. Law M, King G, King S, et al: Patterns of participation in recreational and leisure activities among children with complex physical disabilities. *Dev Med Child Neurol* 2006;48(5):337-342.

The Children's Assessment of Participation and Enjoyment was used to examine the participation of children with complex physical disabilities in day-to-day formal and informal activities. These findings can assist families and service providers in planning activities the child will enjoy and actively participate in.

21. King GA, Law M, King S, et al: Measuring children's participation in recreation and leisure activities: Construct validation of the CAPE and PAC. *Child Care Health Dev* 2007;33(1):28-39.

In a construct validation of the Children's Assessment of Participation and Enjoyment and its companion measure (Preferences for Activities of Children); intensity, enjoyment, and preference scores were significantly correlated in expected ways with environmental, family, and child variables. The predictions were supported with respect to mean score differences between boys and girls and between children in different age groups.

22. Varni JW, Burwinkle TM, Seid M, Skarr D: The PedsQL 4.0 as a pediatric population health measure: Feasibility, reliability, and validity. *Ambul Pediatr* 2003; 3(6):329-341.

23. Jebsen RH, Taylor N, Trieschmann RB, Trotter MJ, Howard LA: An objective and standardized test of hand function. *Arch Phys Med Rehabil* 1969;50(6):311-319.

24. Davids JR, Peace LC, Wagner LV, Gidewall MA, Blackhurst DW, Roberson WM: Validation of the Shriners Hospital for Children Upper Extremity Evaluation (SHUEE) for children with hemiplegic cerebral palsy. *J Bone Joint Surg Am* 2006;88(2):326-333.

The Shriners Hospital for Children Upper Extremity Evaluation was found to have clinical reliability, concurrent validity, and construct validity for assessing the upper extremity function of children with hemiplegic cerebral palsy.

25. Krumlinde-Sundholm L, Holmefur M, Kottorp A, Eliasson AC: The Assisting Hand Assessment: Current evidence of validity, reliability, and responsiveness to change. *Dev Med Child Neurol* 2007;49(4):259-264.

The Assisting Hand Assessment measures the effectiveness of hand use for bimanual activity, which may be the most important aspect of hand function for a child with a unilateral upper limb disability.

26. Burger H, Brezovar D, Marincek C: Comparison of clinical test and questionnaires for the evaluation of upper limb prosthetic use in children. *Disabil Rehabil* 2004;26(14-15):911-916.

27. Bagley AM, Molitor F, Wagner LV, Tomhave W, James MA: The Unilateral Below Elbow Test: A function test for children with unilateral congenital below elbow deficiency. *Dev Med Child Neurol* 2006;48(7):569-575.

The UBET was developed to evaluate bimanual activity function in prosthesis wearers and nonwearers. This instrument is recommended for the functional evaluation of task completion in children with unilateral congenital BED, both with and without a prosthesis.

28. Buffart LM, Roebroeck ME, Janssen WG, Hoekstra A, Hovius SE, Stam HJ: Comparison of instruments to assess hand function in children with radius deficiencies. *J Hand Surg Am* 2007;32(4):531-540.

Instruments such as the Assisting Hand Assessment and the Prosthetic Upper Extremity Functional Index provide valid and reliable results in children with a radius deficiency. Level of evidence: I.

29. Breidenbach WC, Gonzales NR, Kaufman CL, Klapheke M, Tobin GR, Gorantla VS: Outcomes of the first 2 American hand transplants at 8 and 6 years post-transplant. *J Hand Surg Am* 2008;33(7):1039-1047.

Hand transplantation surgery leads to a return of function similar to that of a hand replantation. Graft survival and quality of life after hand transplantation have far exceeded initial expectations. Allogeneic hand transplantation is considered a feasible treatment for catastrophic upper extremity loss. Level of evidence: IV.

30. Pearl EJ, Barker D, Day RC, Beck CW: Identification of genes associated with regenerative success of Xenopus laevis hindlimbs. *BMC Dev Biol* 2008;8:66.

Xenopus laevis transgenic hind limbs do not regenerate and do not form an apical epithelial cap or cone-shaped blastema after amputation. A comparison of gene expression in stage-matched *Xenopus laevis* compared with wild-type hind limb buds revealed several new targets for regeneration research.

31. Monaghan JR, Epp LG, Putta S, et al: Microarray and cDNA sequence analysis of transcription during nerve-dependent limb regeneration. *BMC Biol* 2009;7:1.

Microarray analysis and sequencing were used to investigate the basis of nerve-dependent limb regeneration in salamanders. Most of the transcriptional differences between innervated and denervated forelimbs were correlated with blastema formation.

32. Whited JL, Tabin CJ: Limb regeneration revisited. *J Biol* 2009;8(1):5.

The developmental biology of vertebrate limb regeneration is reviewed.

33. Satoh A, Graham GM, Bryant SV, Gardiner DM: Neurotrophic regulation of epidermal dedifferentiation during wound healing and limb regeneration in the axolotl (Ambystoma mexicanum). *Dev Biol* 2008;319(2):321-335.

The buttonhead-like zinc-finger transcription factor Sp9 was identified as being involved in the formation of the regenerating epithelium. Sp9 expression is induced in basal keratinocytes of the apical blastema epithelium in a pattern comparable to its expression in developing limb buds and, thus, is an important marker for dedifferentiation of the epidermis. Induction of Sp9 expression is nerve dependent.

34. Satoh A, Bryant SV, Gardiner DM: Regulation of dermal fibroblast dedifferentiation and redifferentiation during wound healing and limb regeneration in the Axolotl. *Dev Growth Differ* 2008;50(9):743-754.

In the axolotl (*Ambystoma mexicanum*), AmTwist is the ortholog of Twist, a basic helix-loop-helix transcription factor involved in the regeneration of the dermis during limb regeneration. AmTwist is expressed during the blastema stages of regeneration but is inhibited by signals from the nerve during the early stages, when dermal fibroblasts dedifferentiate to form blastema cells.

35. Sobkow L, Epperlein HH, Herklotz S, Straube WL, Tanaka EM: A germline GFP transgenic axolotl and its use to track cell fate: Dual origin of the fin mesenchyme during development and the fate of blood cells during regeneration. *Dev Biol* 2006;290(2):386-397.

Germline transmission of a transgene was used to assess cell fate during dorsal fin development in the axolotl.

36. Satoh A, James MA, Gardiner DM: The role of nerve signaling in limb genesis and agenesis during axolotl limb regeneration. *J Bone Joint Surg Am* 2009;91(suppl 4):90-98.

The developmental and molecular biology of nerve-dependent vertebrate limb regeneration is reviewed.

37. Mullen LM, Bryant SV, Torok MA, Blumberg B, Gardiner DM: Nerve dependency of regeneration: The role of Distal-less and FGF signaling in amphibian limb regeneration. *Development* 1996;122(11):3487-3497.

38. Kumar A, Godwin JW, Gates PB, Garza-Garcia AA, Brockes JP: Molecular basis for the nerve dependence of limb regeneration in an adult vertebrate. *Science* 2007; 318(5851):772-777.

The local expression of nAG after electroporation is sufficient to rescue a denervated blastema and regenerate the distal structures.

39. Page L: Cyborg-style 'iLimb' hand a big hit with Iraq veterans. *The Register.* July 18, 2007. http://www.the register.co.uk/2007/07/18/robo_hand_gets_big_hand/. Accessed Sept 2009.

40. Kuiken TA, Dumanian GA, Lipschutz RD, Miller LA, Stubblefield KA: The use of targeted muscle reinnervation for improved myoelectric prosthesis control in a bilateral shoulder disarticulation amputee. *Prosthet Orthot Int* 2004;28(3):245-253.

41. Kuiken TA, Miller LA, Lipschutz RD, et al: Targeted reinnervation for enhanced prosthetic arm function in a woman with a proximal amputation: A case study. *Lancet* 2007;369(9559):371-380.

Targeted sensory reinnervation can provide a pathway for meaningful sensory feedback, and it was found to improve prosthetic function and ease of use.

42. Warwick K, Gasson M, Hutt B, et al: The application of implant technology for cybernetic systems. *Arch Neurol* 2003;60(10):1369-1373.

43. Blankertz B, Dornhege G, Krauledat M, et al: The Berlin Brain-Computer Interface: EEG-based communication without subject training. *IEEE Trans Neural Syst Rehabil Eng* 2006;14(2):147-152.

Untrained as well as very well-trained individuals efficaciously used an electroencephalography-based BCI system independent of peripheral nervous system activity and evoked potentials.

44. Hwang HJ, Kwon K, Im CH: Neurofeedback-based motor imagery training for brain-computer interface (BCI). *J Neurosci Methods* 2009;179(1):150-156.

A neurofeedback-based motor imagery training system for an electroencephalography-based BCI was used as a training tool for motor imagery tasks in BCI applications.

45. Jackson A, Moritz CT, Mavoori J, Lucas TH, Fetz EE: The Neurochip BCI: Towards a neural prosthesis for upper limb function. *IEEE Trans Neural Syst Rehabil Eng* 2006;14(2):187-190.

The Neurochip BCI is an autonomously operating interface between an implanted computer chip and recording and stimulating electrodes in the nervous system. Spinal microstimulation controlled by cortical neurons could help compensate for damaged corticospinal projections.

3: Upper Extremity

Lower Extremity

SECTION EDITOR:
ERNEST L. SINK, MD

Chapter 17

Developmental Dysplasia of the Hip

Lori A. Karol, MD

Introduction

Developmental dysplasia of the hip (DDH) is one of the most common pediatric orthopaedic conditions, and it is an area of focus during the physical examination of newborns and infants. The diagnosis of DDH can apply to a hip that is dislocated and irreducible, unstable, or simply dysplastic but reduced within the acetabulum. The term developmental dysplasia of the hip is preferred to the term congenital dislocation of the hip because it has been thoroughly documented that in rare instances a late-presenting dislocation occurs in a child who had normal imaging results as a newborn.[1]

It is important to differentiate DDH from teratologic dislocation of the hip. Infants with DDH usually are otherwise normal, without genetic, neurologic, or muscular conditions that predispose them to joint malformation. A hip dislocation in an infant with myelomeningocele, arthrogryposis, or Larsen syndrome is considered teratologic, and the treatment is different from that of DDH.

Incidence and Etiology

The incidence of DDH varies with the severity of the disease. Dysplasia, which is defined as a reduced hip with insufficient development of the acetabulum, has an incidence of 1 in 100 newborns. Hip dislocation has an incidence of 1 in 1,000 newborns. The incidence of hip instability is between these extremes.

The etiology of DDH is multifactorial, and genetic factors have a role. A recent study of 1,649 individuals with DDH in Utah found that children of affected parents are 12 times more likely to have DDH than children of unaffected parents. The rate of DDH also is 12 times higher among siblings of individuals with DDH.[2] Girls are four times as likely as boys to have DDH, but

it is unknown whether the responsible influence is genetic or hormonal. Firstborn children are most likely to have hip dislocation or dysplasia, in theory because a primiparous mother has a smaller uterus.

The most widely recognized risk factor for DDH is a fetal breech position at birth, regardless of the method of delivery (most infants in the breech position are delivered through a cesarean section). Breech position occurs only in 2% to 3% of all births, but it is noted in 16% of infants with DDH. A frank breech position, in which both hips are flexed with extended knees, is most likely to result in a hip dislocation. In 2000, the American Academy of Pediatrics encouraged ultrasonographic or radiographic imaging of the hips of all newborn girls delivered with a breech presentation.[3]

Although infants with Larsen syndrome or another connective tissue disease do not have idiopathic DDH, many infants with a connective tissue disorder appear to be normal except for the apparent presence of DDH; the underlying connective tissue disease often is not recognized until the child reaches walking age (generally at age 1 year or later). The presence of an orthopaedic condition such as congenital knee dislocation, congenital muscular torticollis, or metatarsus adductus has been linked to coexisting DDH. Among infants in New York who had torticollis, 12.7% were found to have DDH. Only 3.7% of infants first referred to an orthopaedic surgeon for treatment of torticollis were later found to have hip dysplasia or instability through ultrasonographic studies.[4]

Diagnosis

Screening

The utility of clinical or ultrasonographic screening of all newborns for DDH has received recent attention. A US Preventive Services Task Force report suggested that the iatrogenic risks of DDH treatment outweigh the benefits of early identification.[5] Subsequent studies established the merit of clinical examination for screening, however.[6] There is support for ultrasonographic screening of at-risk infants (those who were delivered in a breech position, have a positive family history, or

Dr. Karol or an immediate family member has received nonincome support (such as equipment or services), commercially derived honoraria, or other non–research-related funding (such as paid travel) from the Journal of the American Academy of Orthopaedic Surgeons and Saunders/Mosby-Elsevier.

4: Lower Extremity

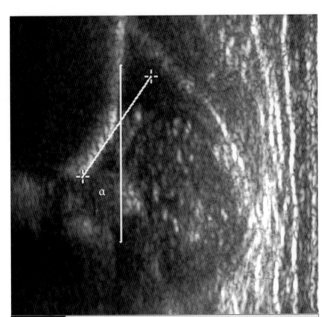

Figure 1 Coronal ultrasonogram of a frankly dislocated right hip of a 19-day-old girl. The α angle, defined as the angle between a line drawn vertically from the lateral edge of the acetabulum (the Perkin line) and a second line along the acetabulum, measures 35°; a normal α angle is greater than 60°.

have an associated orthopaedic condition).[7] Routine screening ultrasonography of all newborns is popular in Europe but has not been adopted in North America. The arguments against routine ultrasonography for newborns center on possible overtreatment of dysplastic hips that are not unstable and may resolve with time and growth if left untreated.

Physical Examination

A newborn must be calm for the clinical examination. The Ortolani maneuver is done by gently abducting the flexed hip while anteriorly lifting the greater trochanter; in a positive examination, the dislocated hip is palpably reduced. The Barlow maneuver is done by adducting the flexed hip while gently pushing posteriorly on the thigh; an unstable hip palpably dislocates posteriorly during adduction. Although the absence of an Ortolani or Barlow sign most often signifies a normal hip, an infant with a fixed, irreducible dislocation of the hip may have an apparently stable examination. Abduction may be noticeably limited in a unilateral dislocation, but the diagnosis of fixed dislocation is more difficult if the dislocation is bilateral. The Klisic sign is done by placing one finger on the greater trochanter of the femur and another on the anterosuperior iliac spine; an abnormal result is elicited if a line between the two landmarks projects inferior to the umbilicus. Ultrasonography is used to confirm the dislocation.

As the dislocation becomes fixed in an older infant, the Ortolani and Barlow signs rarely are present.

Asymmetric, limited abduction almost always is present in a unilateral dislocation. The Galeazzi sign may be present in an older infant; the apparent length of the thigh segment is shortened when the hips and knees are flexed, as a result of the posterior dislocation of the femoral head. A child with a unilateral dislocation who is walking age has a short leg gait and may toe walk on the side of the dislocation. If both hips are dislocated, the lumbar spine appears to be lordotic because of the flexion contractures of the hips; the patient sways from side to side while walking, exhibiting a Trendelenburg gait pattern caused by abductor insufficiency.

Imaging

Ultrasonography is the preferred imaging modality for diagnosing hip dysplasia, instability, or dislocation in an infant younger than 4 months. During the child's first 4 months, the femoral epiphysis is unossified, and plain radiographs therefore can be misleading. Ultrasonography clearly depicts the position of the femoral head relative to the acetabulum. Static imaging reveals the development of the acetabulum. The α angle (formed by a line along the bony acetabulum and a vertical line at the edge of the acetabulum) should be greater than 60° in the infant hip (**Figure 1**). The β angle (formed by a line extending from the lateral edge of the acetabulum to the edge of the labrum and a vertical line at the edge of the acetabulum) quantifies the depth of the acetabular labrum. Dynamic imaging can quantify the extent of instability present during the Barlow maneuver by revealing the percentage of the femoral head lying lateral to the edge of the bony acetabulum at rest and during stress. Ultrasonography is very sensitive, and it is best used in babies without clinical instability who are older than 6 weeks.

Plain radiographs are useful in a child older than 3 to 4 months. The Shenton line, drawn along the inferior aspect of the femoral neck, should not lie superior to the inferior cortex of the superior pubic ramus. Four quadrants are defined at the intersection of the Hilgenreiner line (drawn through the left and right triradiate cartilages) and the Perkin line (drawn vertically along the lateral edge of the acetabulum). The reduced hip or the medial corner of the femoral neck should be located in the inferomedial quadrant. Other findings on AP radiographs of the pelvis include delayed ossification of the proximal femoral epiphysis and dysplasia of the acetabulum, as evidenced by an increased acetabular index (**Figure 2**).

Treatment

Pavlik Harness

Treatment of an unstable or dislocated hip in a newborn begins with application of a Pavlik harness. The Pavlik harness holds the hip at 90° of flexion and inhibits hip adduction. It allows knee and ankle motion as well as abduction and greater flexion of the hip. The harness is applied by the treating physician and is adjusted every few weeks as the infant grows. The harness typically is used for at least 6 weeks after the hip becomes stable on examination. The progress of the hip customarily was monitored using plain radiographs, but recently the use of serial ultrasonograms with the infant in the harness has been promoted to monitor femoral head position, laxity, and acetabular development.

The Pavlik harness is almost universally effective in resolving laxity and dysplasia in infants who do not have a dislocated hip. It may not be necessary to treat a dysplastic but stable hip, as revealed on ultrasonography. In an infant younger than 2 months, the natural history of dysplasia is improvement, regardless of treatment[8] (Figure 3). The research literature supports observation of very young infants, and it is recommended that imaging the hips of an infant with possible DDH but a normal physical examination be deferred until age 6 weeks.[8] A Pavlik harness should be considered for treating stable dysplasia diagnosed using ultrasonography in an infant who is at least 6 weeks old. If successive ultrasonographic imaging reveals improvement of mild dysplasia, observation can be continued with frequent ultrasonographic follow-up.

Treatment with a Pavlik harness has few risks. Hip osteonecrosis has been reported but is almost nonexistent in clinical practice. Extreme positioning (forced abduction of the hips) must be avoided, and the position of the harness straps should be adjusted frequently as the infant grows. Flexion of the hip in the Pavlik harness can lead to femoral nerve palsy, in which the infant is unable to extend the knee. An older, larger infant or an infant with a frankly dislocated hip appears to be at greatest risk of femoral nerve palsy. The treatment is to discontinue using the harness until quadriceps power returns and then to carefully reinstate treatment under close observation.

The Pavlik harness may fail to reduce a dislocated hip. Prolonged use of the harness for a dislocated hip is associated with a posterior acetabular deficiency, which will make it more difficult to stabilize the hip with closed or open reduction in the future. Therefore, use

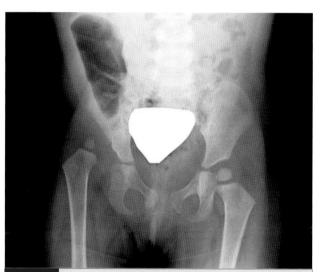

Figure 2 AP radiograph of the pelvis of a 13-month-old girl. In the dislocated right hip, the Shenton line is broken, the ossific nucleus is present but smaller than on the left side, and the acetabulum is dysplastic.

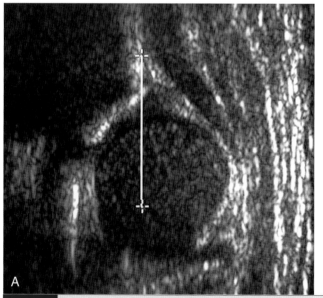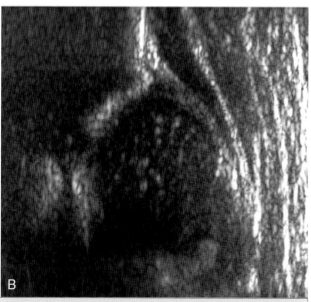

Figure 3 A, Coronal stress ultrasonogram of the left hip of a 7-week-old girl. The α angle is 52°, with mild lateralization of the femoral head. B, A repeat ultrasonogram 4 weeks later, showing resolution of the mild laxity and improvement in acetabular development.

of the Pavlik harness should be abandoned if it does not lead to reduction of the hip within 4 weeks, and plans should be made for a closed reduction. Some hips become reduced but not stable in the Pavlik harness; a short course of abduction bracing may be successful in resolving the instability. A transition to a fixed abduction orthosis is recommended for infants whose hips are dislocated but reducible (the Ortolani sign) after 3 weeks in the Pavlik harness.[9]

Closed Reduction

Closed reduction under anesthesia is done only if the hip is not reduced using the Pavlik harness or if dislocation is discovered when the infant is age 6 months or older. The upper age limit for attempting a closed reduction is ill defined but commonly is approximately 18 months. However, in France closed reduction facilitated by traction is used for children as old as 5 years.[10]

Preoperative traction for infants with DDH is controversial and currently is infrequently used. The position of traction is with the knees extended and the hips flexed and mildly abducted. Advocates of traction believe that the ability to achieve a closed reduction may be improved through a course of preoperative traction. It is unknown whether traction reduces the risk of osteonecrosis. Surgeons who do not use traction believe that the position of traction does not truly stretch the muscles that interfere with reduction (specifically, the iliopsoas).

Whether the reduction should be delayed until ossification of the femoral epiphysis also is controversial. Advocates of delaying the reduction believe that the rate of osteonecrosis is higher in infants with cartilaginous epiphyses because the cartilaginous femoral head is more compressible and, therefore, more susceptible to vascular insult.[11,12] Others find that a delay in achieving a reduced hip can lead to a need for open reduction and a secondary procedure such as acetabular osteotomy. A recent meta-analysis of six studies to evaluate the relationship between the presence of the ossific nucleus and the development of osteonecrosis failed to establish a significant correlation after either open or closed reduction of the hip.[13] It appeared that absence of the ossific nucleus was linked to a greater likelihood of osteonecrosis after closed reduction and that the osteonecrosis was more likely to be severe. However, the quality of the evidence was only moderate. The appropriate age for a closed reduction continues to be based on the surgeon's opinion rather than on evidence.

A closed reduction is done under general anesthesia. The affected hip is abducted while the greater trochanter is gently lifted anteriorly (the Ortolani maneuver). An arthrogram is used to better observe the femoral head and the acetabular labrum and to assess the depth of the reduction. A small amount of radiopaque dye is injected into the hip capsule, and the hip is manipulated without force (**Figure 4**). The safe zone (between the maximum abduction of the hip and the extent of abduction necessary to maintain the reduced

hip) is determined, with a narrow safe zone implying an unstable reduction. If the reduction cannot be achieved gently, if there is a wide dye pool medial to the femoral head, or if the reduction cannot be maintained without significant abduction, the attempt at closed reduction should be abandoned in favor of an open reduction.

After an acceptable closed reduction, a double spica cast typically is applied with the hips in a position of 90° of flexion and less-than-maximal abduction. Imaging through the spica cast confirms the reduction, and later imaging is done to confirm that the reduction has been maintained. Limited CT also can be useful to confirm the reduction, with only the CT slices necessary to observe the relationship between the femoral head and the acetabulum. If the metaphysis of the proximal femur is positioned posterior to the pubic ramus, redislocation should be suspected (**Figure 5**).

MRI can be used to confirm a maintained reduction in infants with DDH (**Figure 6**). The benefits of MRI are the lack of exposure to radiation and the potential for assessing the blood supply to the femoral epiphysis in the cast. Contrast-enhanced MRI was obtained in 28 hips by injecting intravenous gadolinium immediately after casting.[14] Of the 6 hips that had radiographic signs of osteonecrosis within 1 year of the reduction, 3 had decreased enhancement on the postoperative MRI, and 3 did not. Two of the remaining 22 hips had decreased enhancement on the postoperative MRI but did not develop osteonecrosis. Thus, the positive prediction rate was 50%, and the false-positive rate was 9%. A recent study evaluated the quality of MRI after open reduction with femoral osteotomy and internal fixation, finding that the scans were diagnostic for reduction quality.[15] The blood supply was not evaluated.

Open Reduction

Open reduction of a dislocated hip is indicated if a closed reduction cannot be achieved or maintained in a safe position, the hip becomes redislocated after closed reduction, the child is older than 18 to 24 months, or an infant has a teratologic dislocation. Two basic surgical approaches are used. An anterior open reduction is done through a bikini incision; the hip capsule is approached through the interval superficially between the sartorius and the tensor fascia lata and deeper between the rectus femoris and the gluteus medius. This approach allows direct access to the hip capsule and repair of the capsule using capsulorrhaphy. All of the impediments to reduction of the hip (the iliopsoas tendon, pulvinar, inverted labrum, inferomedial capsule, ligamentum teres, and transverse acetabular ligament) can be addressed through this incision.

A medial open reduction is done through a groin incision in the area of the adductor tendons. The Weinstein modification of the Ludloff medial approach uses the interval between the pectineus muscle and the femoral neurovascular bundle. The medial approach is quite useful in infants younger than 1 year. There is more direct

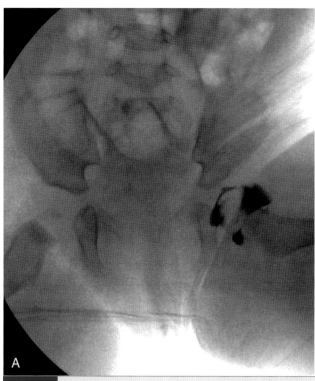
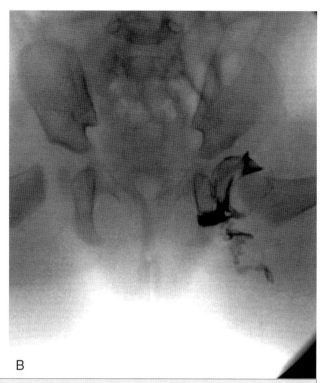

Figure 4 **A,** Arthrogram of the left hip of a 6-month-old girl after unsuccessful treatment with a Pavlik harness. The hip is reducible, and the safe zone is adequate. **B,** Arthrogram 6 weeks later, showing that the hip remains reduced and the labrum is now clearly defined.

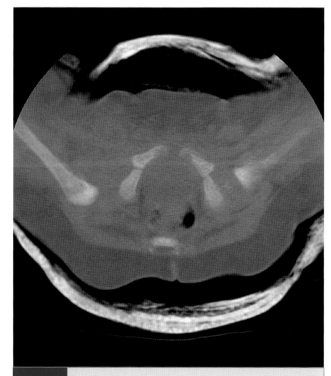

Figure 5 Limited CT of the right hip of a 7-week-old girl, showing redislocation after closed reduction and spica cast application. The femoral metaphysis is posterior to a line drawn through the triradiate cartilages.

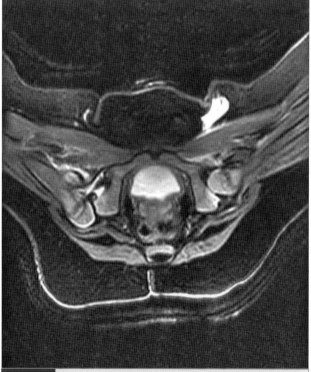

Figure 6 MRI of the hip of a 5-month-old girl after closed reduction, showing a redislocation of the right hip. Perfusion was believed to be present. Note that the femoral head can be clearly seen.

access to the impediments to reduction than with the anterior approach, but the limited visibility and exposure do not allow a capsulorrhaphy. The medial open reduction therefore is less stable than the anterior open reduction and has limited usefulness in a child of walking age. The medial approach exposes the medial femoral circumflex artery, which supplies the femoral epiphysis and therefore carries a higher risk of osteonecrosis than the anterior approach. Because of the direct approach to the medial capsule and the lack of exposure of the iliac crest, a medial open reduction entails minimal blood loss and a relatively short surgical time. These factors have led to the successful use of this approach in infants with bilateral dislocation of the hips.

The ligamentum teres usually is large and elongated in infants with DDH; it is readily found at its attachment to the femoral head and is useful in leading the surgeon to the true acetabulum. The ligamentum teres can prevent deep seating of the femoral head into the medial acetabulum, and excising it is believed to be an important step in preparing the hip for reduction into the acetabulum. A recent study described a technique for shortening and reattaching the ligamentum teres to assist in the stabilization of the femoral head as part of a medial open reduction, with favorable results.[16,17] Few surgeons have incorporated this technique into clinical practice, however.

The reduction of the hip into the acetabulum should avoid creating excessive pressure on the femoral head for fear of osteonecrosis. If force is required to reduce the hip, or if the hip has a tendency to redislocate despite a thorough release of the transverse acetabular ligament, femoral shortening should be performed to allow a gentler, more stable reduction. The femoral shaft is approached laterally, a 1- to 2-cm piece is resected, and the site is stabilized with a plate and screws. Femoral shortening has replaced preoperative traction for a child who is to undergo open reduction.

Pelvic Osteotomy

Children with a DDH dislocation have acetabular dysplasia, which is defined as a lack of anterior and lateral coverage resulting from underdevelopment of the acetabulum. Acetabular dysplasia can be present in a child with a reduced hip (this combination is the mildest manifestation of DDH). Infants and young children with acetabular dysplasia are asymptomatic; the hip typically does not become painful until adolescence or young adulthood.

In infants with hip instability or dislocation, acetabular dysplasia usually improves when the hip is reduced and stable. The younger the age at which the hip is stabilized, the greater the likelihood there is that the acetabulum will respond and develop normally. Children age 18 to 24 months or older who have a fixed dislocation of the hip generally benefit from concomitant pelvic osteotomy when they undergo open reduction. Reduction of the hip is obtained before the pelvic osteotomy through meticulous dissection, releases, and femoral

shortening. Pelvic osteotomy is used to treat the acetabular dysplasia and thereby minimize the need for future surgery (**Figure 7**). In children age 7 years or younger, the Salter and Pemberton osteotomies are popular for improving anterolateral acetabular coverage.

After a child younger than 18 to 24 months undergoes closed or open reduction of the hip, the development of the acetabulum is followed on serial radiographs. If the acetabular index is not normal when the child is 4 to 5 years old or if it does not improve on serial radiographs, pelvic osteotomy is recommended. Because the child is asymptomatic, however, the parents may be reluctant to proceed with osteotomy.

Complications

Redislocation

Redislocation can occur after either closed or open reduction of the hip in a child with DDH. Plain radiographs taken through a spica cast can be misleading, and advanced postoperative imaging with MRI or limited CT is helpful for ensuring that the hip is reduced. The treatment for a redislocated hip is removal of the cast, if femoral shortening was not done, and additional surgery for reduction. If examination of the cast reveals that the hip was inadequately positioned or immobilized, closed reduction can be attempted with an improved spica cast. Usually an open reduction will be indicated because of inability to reduce the hip or the marked instability that led to the redislocation.

Redislocation after open reduction almost always requires a repeat open reduction. Often the hip was not initially reduced deep into the true acetabulum, and deeper medial exposure of the acetabulum allows a better reduction. Repeat capsulorrhaphy is challenging but useful as part of this difficult procedure. Femoral shortening, if it was not done initially, may decrease the tendency for the hip to redislocate again. The combination of a derotational osteotomy of the femur, a pelvic procedure such as a Salter osteotomy, and a tight anterior capsulorrhaphy can uncover the hip posteriorly and increase the likelihood of a posterior dislocation. Careful assessment of the femoral rotational profile is necessary to improve the stability of the hip.

Osteonecrosis

Osteonecrosis, defined as a partial or complete loss of blood supply to the immature femoral epiphysis, is one of the most feared and least predictable complications of DDH. Osteonecrosis is always iatrogenic; it is not seen in patients with untreated DDH. Osteonecrosis occurs very rarely in patients who were treated with a Pavlik harness. The studies describing osteonecrosis secondary to Pavlik harness use included older infants with a fixed dislocation who were treated for a prolonged time.[18] Careful monitoring of the fit of the harness, with care to avoid tightening the posterior straps

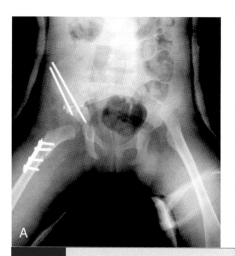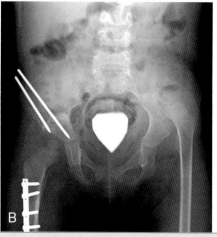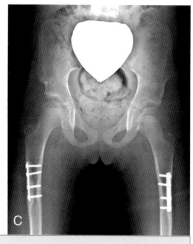

Figure 7 **A,** Radiograph of the pelvis of a 3-year-old girl with bilateral hip dislocation after the right hip was treated with an anterior open reduction, femoral shortening, and Salter osteotomy. **B,** AP standing radiograph taken 4 months later, showing the left hip before open reduction. **C,** AP standing radiograph taken at age 7 years, showing maintenance of reduction, good acetabular formation, and no evidence of osteonecrosis.

into a forced abduction position, should prevent osteonecrosis.

Osteonecrosis is more common after closed or open reduction of the hip. The signs of osteonecrosis usually appear within 1 year of the reduction; they include an absence of ossification in the femoral epiphysis, a failure of the ossific nucleus to grow, or fragmentation of the femoral epiphysis on follow-up radiographs. The radiographic appearance of the ossific nucleus is significant. Type I osteonecrosis, defined as irregular temporary ossification of the femoral epiphysis, has no known clinical significance and frequently is excluded from reports of osteonecrosis rates. In type II osteonecrosis there is a lateral arrest of the physis so that the femoral epiphysis assumes a valgus position over time, which may lead to subluxation and further dysplasia;[19] type II osteonecrosis may not be apparent for several years after a closed or open reduction. Type III osteonecrosis is a medial arrest of the proximal femoral physis and is rare. In type IV, the entire femoral head is involved; the result is an irregular, flattened femoral epiphysis and coxa breva, with relative trochanteric overgrowth over time. Patients with type IV osteonecrosis are predisposed to early degenerative arthritis.

The best treatment of osteonecrosis is prevention. A closed reduction is acceptable only if it can be obtained gently and maintained in modest, never forced, abduction. An open reduction should be accompanied by femoral shortening if there is undue pressure on the femoral head in the reduced position. Attention should be given to protecting the blood supply to the femoral head during open reduction, especially if the medial open approach is used. There is no pharmacologic treatment for osteonecrosis. If the hip becomes uncovered or the acetabulum remains dysplastic, secondary acetabular osteotomy should be considered to improve the long-term clinical outcome. In a hip with type II os-

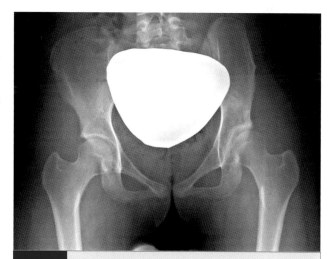

Figure 8 AP standing radiograph of the pelvis of a 13-year-old girl with left anterior groin pain. She had undergone medial open reduction followed by Pemberton osteotomy in the left hip before age 2 years. Acetabular dysplasia and lateralization, as evidenced by a reduced center-edge angle, are present.

teonecrosis, valgus deformity can be improved with a proximal femoral varus osteotomy.

Late Dysplasia

Controversy persists as to how long children with DDH should be followed radiographically. Most surgeons agree that children who have had a closed or open reduction should be followed until skeletal growth is complete. The need to follow children who were treated nonsurgically is less certain. Some children who were believed to have well-seated hips during the first decade after treatment develop symptomatic acetabular dysplasia as adolescents (**Figure 8**). It is impor-

4: Lower Extremity

tant to carefully assess the contralateral hip in children believed to have unilateral DDH. A recent study found that 40% of children treated for unilateral hip instability had subtle evidence of contralateral dysplasia at maturity.[20]

Outcomes

Long-term outcomes recently were reported for 60 patients with 80 hips that were treated with one-stage open reduction and Salter innominate osteotomy for fixed dislocation of the hip at age 1.5 to 5 years.[21] Preoperative traction was used, as the surgical procedures predated the use of femoral shortening in DDH. At 40- to 48-year follow-up, 30% of the hips had required total hip arthroplasty. At 45-year follow-up, the calculated survival rate of the hips was 54%. Bilateral DDH was the only identified poor prognostic factor. Open reduction with Salter osteotomy was found to lead to a successful result through the first 30 years, with possible deterioration thereafter.

Summary

DDH represents a spectrum of disease ranging from dysplasia to dislocation, and it is treated using a spectrum of interventions ranging from the Pavlik harness to open reduction, femoral shortening, and pelvic osteotomy. Although treatment of dysplasia in newborns may not be necessary, early treatment of instability is usually successful with closed means such as the Pavlik harness. Surgical reduction is reserved for children with later-presenting DDH and children whose hips failed to reduce with nonsurgical treatment. Osteonecrosis remains a concern after treatment. Late dysplasia requires long-term follow-up.

Annotated References

1. Gwynne Jones DP, Dunbar JD, Theis JC: Late presenting dislocation of sonographically stable hips. *J Pediatr Orthop B* 2006;15(4):257-261.

   Seven instances are described of late hip dislocations in infants who had ultrasonographically stable hips in the newborn period.

2. Stevenson DA, Mineau G, Kerber RA, Viskochil DH, Schaefer C, Roach JW: Familial predisposition to developmental dysplasia of the hip. *J Pediatr Orthop* 2009; 29(5):463-466.

   The Utah Population Database was used to identify 1,649 individuals with DDH. The relative risk of DDH in their children or siblings was 12.1.

3. American Academy of Pediatrics: Clinical practice guideline: Early detection of developmental dysplasia of the hip. Committee on Quality Improvement, Subcommittee on Developmental Dysplasia of the Hip. *Pediatrics* 2000;105(4, pt 1):896-905.

4. von Heideken J, Green DW, Burke SW, et al: The relationship between developmental dysplasia of the hip and congenital muscular torticollis. *J Pediatr Orthop* 2006;26(6):805-808.

   In 109 patients referred for treatment of congenital muscular torticollis, ultrasonographic screening revealed DDH in 3.7% who were thought to have normal hips.

5. US Preventive Services Task Force: Screening for developmental dysplasia of the hip: Recommendation statement. *Pediatrics* 2006;117(3):898-902.

6. Schwend RM, Schoenecker P, Richards BS, Flynn JM, Vitale M, Pediatric Orthopaedic Society of North America: Screening the newborn for developmental dysplasia of the hip: Now what do we do? *J Pediatr Orthop* 2007;27(6):607-610.

   This is a review of the 2007 Pediatric Orthopaedic Society of North America position statement on the usefulness of clinical examination in screening infants for DDH. Ultrasonography can be used as an adjunct in infants with risk factors or an inconclusive physical examination.

7. Mahan ST, Katz JN, Kim YJ: To screen or not to screen? A decision analysis of the utility of screening for developmental dysplasia of the hip. *J Bone Joint Surg Am* 2009;91(7):1705-1719.

   Decision analysis supported ultrasonographic screening only for infants having risk factors for DDH.

8. Rosendahl K, Dezateux C, Fosse KR, et al: Immediate treatment versus sonographic surveillance for mild hip dysplasia in newborns. *Pediatrics* 2010;125(1):e9-e16.

   Sixty-four newborns with a stable examination but mild sonographic dysplasia were observed. Repeat ultrasonograms at 6 weeks revealed improvement in most hips; only 47% were treated at follow-up.

9. Swaroop VT, Mubarak SJ: Difficult-to-treat Ortolani-positive hip: Improved success with new treatment protocol. *J Pediatr Orthop* 2009;29(3):224-230.

   Ninety-three percent of Ortolani-positive hips were successfully treated with the use of a Pavlik harness, followed by abduction orthoses if the hip failed to stabilize within 3 weeks.

10. Rampal V, Sabourin M, Erdeneshoo E, Koureas G, Seringe R, Wicart P: Closed reduction with traction for developmental dysplasia of the hip in children aged between one and five years. *J Bone Joint Surg Br* 2008; 90(7):858-863.

    Hips were successfully reduced using the Petit-Morel method of gradual closed reduction with traction (average duration, 5.4 weeks), spica casting, and pelvic osteotomy in 36 children age 1 to 5 years.

11. Segal LS, Schneider DJ, Berlin JM, Bruno A, Davis BR, Jacobs CR: The contribution of the ossific nucleus to

the structural stiffness of the capital femoral epiphysis: a porcine model for DDH. *J Pediatr Orthop* 1999;19(4): 433-437.

12. Clarke NM, Jowett AJ, Parker L: The surgical treatment of established congenital dislocation of the hip: Results of surgery after planned delayed intervention following the appearance of the capital femoral ossific nucleus. *J Pediatr Orthop* 2005;25(4):434-439.

   Osteonecrosis occurred in 7% of hips following closed reduction and 14% of hips following open reduction.

13. Roposch A, Stöhr KK, Dobson M: The effect of the femoral head ossific nucleus in the treatment of developmental dysplasia of the hip: A meta-analysis. *J Bone Joint Surg Am* 2009;91(4):911-918.

   A meta-analysis of six studies suggested that absence of ossification of the femoral epiphysis is associated with an increased incidence of significant osteonecrosis only in hips undergoing closed reduction. Level I evidence was lacking.

14. Tiderius C, Jaramillo D, Connolly S, et al: Post-closed reduction perfusion magnetic resonance imaging as a predictor of avascular necrosis in developmental hip dysplasia: A preliminary report. *J Pediatr Orthop* 2009; 29(1):14-20.

   Six of 28 hips developed radiographic osteonecrosis after closed reduction. Postreduction MRI indicated abnormal perfusion in 3 of the 6 hips.

15. Ranawat V, Rosendahl K, Jones D: MRI after operative reduction with femoral osteotomy in developmental dysplasia of the hip. *Pediatr Radiol* 2009;39(2):161-163.

16. Wenger DR, Mubarak SJ, Henderson PC, Miyanji F: Ligamentum teres maintenance and transfer as a stabilizer in open reduction for pediatric hip dislocation: Surgical technique and early clinical results. *J Child Orthop* 2008;2(3):177-185.

   The technique of ligamentum teres tenodesis is described as an adjunct in the stabilization of a dislocated hip undergoing open reduction.

17. Bache CE, Graham HK, Dickens DR, et al: Ligamentum teres tenodesis in medial approach open reduction for developmental dislocation of the hip. *J Pediatr Orthop* 2008;28(6):607-613.

   This is a second article describing the technique of ligamentum teres tenodesis as an adjunct in the stabilization of a dislocated hip undergoing open reduction.

18. Kitoh H, Kawasumi M, Ishiguro N: Predictive factors for unsuccessful treatment of developmental dysplasia of the hip by the Pavlik harness. *J Pediatr Orthop* 2009; 29(6):552-557.

   Osteonecrosis occurred in 88% of hips treated with a Pavlik harness applied at an average age of 3.9 months.

19. Oh CW, Joo SY, Kumar SJ, Macewen GD: A radiological classification of lateral growth arrest of the proximal femoral physis after treatment for developmental dysplasia of the hip. *J Pediatr Orthop* 2009;29(4):331-335.

   At an average age of 22 years, only 41% of hips with type II osteonecrosis after treatment for DDH had a satisfactory result, as graded using the Severin classification, because of residual poor acetabular coverage and subluxation. Hips with coxa valga fared the worst.

20. Song FS, McCarthy JJ, MacEwen GD, Fuchs KE, Dulka SE: The incidence of occult dysplasia of the contralateral hip in children with unilateral hip dysplasia. *J Pediatr Orthop* 2008;28(2):173-176.

   As many as 40% of contralateral hips believed to be normal in infants with DDH were mildly dysplastic at skeletal maturity.

21. Thomas SR, Wedge JH, Salter RB: Outcome at forty-five years after open reduction and innominate osteotomy for late-presenting developmental dislocation of the hip. *J Bone Joint Surg Am* 2007;89(11):2341-2350.

   Hips that had undergone anterior open reduction and Salter osteotomy when the child was age 1 to 5 years had a 54% survival rate.

Chapter 18

Hip Disorders in Adolescents and Young Adults

Young-Jo Kim, MD, PhD   Ira Zaltz, MD

Introduction

The development of hip arthritis is known to be associated with disorders of the hip including developmental dysplasia of the hip, slipped capital femoral epiphysis (SCFE), Legg-Calvé-Perthes (LCP) disease, and developmental deformity of the femoral head (pistol-grip deformity). Residual deformities associated with these developmental disorders lead to pathologic hip mechanics that may overload the hip joint and lead to acetabular labral damage and degenerative chondral changes. Diagnostic capacity and the understanding of hip deformity have been improved by the use of hip imaging techniques including specific plain radiographic views, CT, and MRI.[1] The development of techniques for hip arthroscopy, surgical dislocation, and periacetabular osteotomy is contributing to an understanding of the consequences of hip deformity and, increasingly, to the treatment of prearthritic conditions. Knowledge and treatments related to femoroacetabular impingement (FAI) and hip dysplasia in skeletally mature patients are evolving.

Clinical Evaluation

An adolescent patient with a symptomatic hip disorder may have gait disturbance, pain, walking intolerance, and mechanical symptoms referable to the hip joint, such as locking or catching. Most symptoms can be categorized as related to instability or related to FAI. Patients with a history of developmental dysplasia of the hip or instability from another etiology may report

intolerance of walking and standing or difficulty with activities that require a single-leg stance, such as dancing or running. The pain is classically located in the peritrochanteric region but can be referred to the thigh, knee, or groin. The symptoms may worsen if the acetabular labrum is damaged.

Patients with deformity of the femoral head and/or acetabulum that limits hip mobility or causes nonconcentric motion are at risk for FAI. These patients typically have groin pain that is provoked by activities involving hip flexion and rotation. Athletes with anatomically susceptible hips who are involved in a sport such as soccer, hockey, wrestling, gymnastics, or dance may be susceptible to developing impingement symptoms. Patients with a history of SCFE or LCP disease are at risk for impingement-type symptoms.

History and Examination

A thorough history is essential to the initial evaluation of an adolescent with hip pain. Determining the primary symptom is of utmost importance, as a thorough understanding of the patient's symptoms will ultimately guide treatment. Whether a patient has difficulty related to hip instability or impingement often is elucidated only through a careful history and examination. A history of developmental dysplasia of the hip, SCFE, LCP disease, malignancy, blood dyscrasia, or trauma may have affected hip development. The onset of symptoms, any specific precipitating event (such as a change in athletic training), and the nature and location of symptoms are important. The physician should question the patient about walking tolerance and duration; sports participation; peritrochanteric, groin, buttock, thigh, or knee pain; mechanical symptoms; and night pain. Often the patient has a family history of hip osteoarthritis.

The physical examination is essential to the evaluation, diagnosis, and management of an adolescent patient with a hip disorder. No single examination finding or combination of examination findings has been found highly sensitive or specific for surgically treatable anatomic abnormalities. The patient should be inspected in the standing and supine positions for limb-length discrepancy and overall development and muscular sym-

Dr. Kim or an immediate family member serves as an unpaid consultant to Siemens Health Care; has received research or institutional support from Siemens Health Care and Bayer Health Care; and owns stock or stock options in Johnson & Johnson. Dr. Zaltz or an immediate family member serves as a board member, owner, officer, or committee member of Michigan Orthopaedic Society; and has received nonincome support (such as equipment or services), commercially derived honoraria, or other non-research–related funding (such as paid travel) from DePuy, a Johnson & Johnson company.

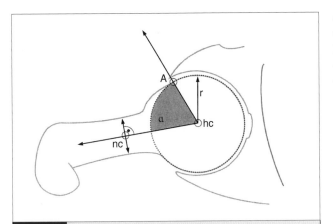

Figure 1 The α angle of Nötzli is subtended by a line drawn parallel to and through the center of the femoral neck (nc) with a line drawn to the center of the femoral head (hc) at a point (A) when the radius of curvature (r) begins to increase. (Reproduced with permission from Nötzli HP, Wyss TF, Stoecklin CH, Schmid MR, Treiber K, Hodler J: The contour of the femoral head-neck junction as a predictor for the risk of anterior impingement. *J Bone Joint Surg Br* 2002;84[4]:558.)

metry. The spine, abdomen, and pelvis should be evaluated, with specific attention to palpation of the lower abdomen, inguinal region, pubis, trochanters, and anterior hips. A complete neurovascular examination should include an assessment of hip muscle strength with a side-lying assessment of gluteal and tensor fascia lata strength. The patient's gait should be assessed for a Trendelenburg or antalgic pattern as well as the foot progression angle, and the single-leg Trendelenburg sign should be sought. Finally, the hip range of motion should be recorded with the patient supine and as relaxed as possible. Hip flexion often is overestimated; it should be tested slowly so that the examiner is able to feel resistance at the end of hip flexion. Specific motions include flexion in the sagittal plane, internal rotation at 90° of flexion, external rotation at 90° of flexion, abduction and external rotation, abduction in extension, and internal and external rotation in extension. The impingement test is a provocative test that indicates hip irritability; it is performed by passively flexing the hip in slight adduction, with simultaneous internal rotation of the hip to produce pain. Posterior impingement should be tested for by flexing, abducting, and externally rotating the hip joint. The apprehension test should be used to test for anterior instability. The test is performed by maximally externally rotating and abducting the hip and evaluating for groin pain or a subjective sensation of instability.

Radiographic Evaluation

The evaluation of an adolescent patient with a possible hip disorder begins with proper plain radiographs. Care in patient positioning and x-ray beam direction

are essential for obtaining high-quality diagnostic radiographs. The initial radiographs for assessing hip pain include AP and lateral projections of the hip. The AP projection is either standing or supine. An AP pelvic radiograph is important for assessing overall bone quality and maturation and is useful for evaluating the acetabular sourcil, femoral head shape, acetabular inclination and version, femoral head coverage, neck-shaft angle, head-neck offset, and Shenton line. In addition, the physeal plate or scar can be used to infer femoral head shape. The AP pelvic radiograph should not be rotated or tilted more than 5° to avoid interfering with the evaluation of acetabular version.[2] A good AP pelvic radiograph will show the sacrococcygeal joint 2 to 4 cm above the symphysis. The methods of lateral projection include cross-table lateral view with the leg internally rotated 15° to evaluate the anterior-lateral head-neck junction, the frog lateral view, and the Dunn lateral view (an AP projection with the leg flexed 45° to 90°, abducted 30°, and in neutral rotation). Additional radiographs may be necessary, depending on the clinical situation, and may include the abduction–internal rotation AP pelvic, false profile (oblique), and flexion false profile views. The presence of a vacuum sign on the frog lateral radiograph may indicate nonconcentric hip joint motion. False profile views are lateral radiographs of the acetabulum used to assess the extent of anterior acetabular coverage; they also can be useful in evaluating the anterior head-neck junction. Properly obtained cross-table lateral radiographs are useful for evaluating the sphericity of the femoral head and the head-neck junction. One means of assessing the sphericity of the femoral head and the head-neck junction is the α angle of Nötzli, which is obtained by drawing a circle on the femoral head, then creating an angle composed of a line from the center of the femoral head through the center of the femoral neck and a second line from the center of the femoral head to the point where the bone is outside the circle[3] (**Figure 1**). When considering an acetabular reorientation, concentricity of the hip must be assessed on an abduction–internal rotation AP pelvic radiograph and, occasionally, a flexion false profile radiograph.

CT is an established means of evaluating the hip joint. Conventional CT for intra-articular and labral evaluation has been replaced by MRI, but noncontrast three-dimensional CT has become useful for assessing complex femoral head deformities and deformities of the proximal femur, and it also is useful in planning arthroscopic surgical management of FAI. MRI is the imaging modality of choice for evaluating the acetabular labrum. Recent advances have led to improvements in the evaluation of the articular cartilage. Chondral mapping sequences can be used to assess the cartilage thickness and focal defects, and delayed gadolinium-enhanced MRI of cartilage (dGEMRIC; Magnevist, Bayer Health Care Pharmaceuticals, Wayne, NJ) is useful in the biochemical assessment of hyaline cartilage. Oblique sagittal and radial sequence images are useful for evaluating the shape and orientation of the head-neck junction.[1] The intra-articular administration of dilute gadolinium increases the sensitivity of MRI for diagnosing labral pathology.

Hip arthrography is useful if a dynamic evaluation of the hip joint is necessary, and it also is often useful if a redirectional osteotomy is being considered or certain types of impingement are being evaluated. The procedure usually is performed with the patient under anesthesia to eliminate muscle spasm and allow accurate evaluation of hip range of motion.

Acetabular Dysplasia

Acetabular dysplasia is believed to cause osteoarthritis by mechanically overloading the primary weight-bearing portions of the acetabular articular cartilage. The first natural history of this condition postulated that hips with a center-edge angle of less than 20° definitely are pathologic and lead to osteoarthritis.[4] A later study stated that hips with a center-edge angle of less than 16° develop end-stage arthritis by the sixth decade of life.[5] The time of onset of arthritis, as a function of the severity of dysplasia, has been difficult to elucidate. A tendency to rapid-onset degeneration was found in hips with radiographic subluxation.[6] However, the onset of osteoarthritis in hips without subluxation has been difficult to predict based on plain radiographs. The importance of acetabular dysplasia as a cause of hip osteoarthritis in the general population has been debated for some time. Acetabular dysplasia is more common among females than among males, and at least among females it appears to be a significant risk factor for hip osteoarthritis.[7-9]

The symptoms of hip dysplasia may be mild and intermittent, but usually they include activity-related groin pain and abductor fatigue. Patients may have a positive Trendelenburg test and apprehension sign. Patients with hip dysplasia commonly have more hip flexion and internal rotation than those with hip impingement. Radiographs reveal a decreased anterior or lateral center-edge angle and possibly a break in the Shenton line. MRI reveals a labrum that is thicker than normal and perilabral cysts.[10]

Early osteoarthritis is characterized by loss of proteoglycans, which form the negatively charged extracellular matrix of cartilage.[11,12] The recent development of dGEMRIC, which is an advanced MRI technique using the negatively charged gadolinium contrast agent gadopentetate dimeglumine, allows the loss of charge density to be measured in early osteoarthritis.[13-15] When dGEMRIC was applied to the study of early osteoarthritis in dysplastic hips, a correlation was found between the severity of dysplasia, as measured by the center-edge angle of Wiberg, and the presence of early osteoarthritis.[16] The presence of a labral tear and radiographic subluxation also were associated with advanced osteoarthritis.[17] Age was found to be a factor in the development of osteoarthritis; in patients with severely dysplastic hips, osteoarthritis sometimes was present before age 30 years. It is believed that these advanced imaging techniques will improve the understanding of osteoarthritis development in patients with hip deformities.

The current treatment recommendation is to treat only the symptomatic hip in an adolescent or young adult. An argument can be made for preventive surgery in an asymptomatic patient with subluxation and a lateral center-edge angle of less than 16° because of the likelihood that osteoarthritis eventually will develop. However, no long-term studies are available to confirm prevention or delay in osteoarthritis development after a prophylactic intervention.

In many patients, the first symptom of a dysplastic hip is a labral tear. The function of the labrum is not clearly understood, but in a dysplastic hip it acts as a mechanical stabilizer; when torn or débrided, it can exacerbate mechanical instability and hence the patient's symptoms. A labral tear was found to be present in 77% of hips with dysplasia.[18] Several osteotomy options are used, although comparison studies have not been published. The most common are the Bernese periacetabular osteotomy (PAO), variations of the triple innominate osteotomy, and other forms of the PAO with spherical cuts close to the acetabulum. The PAO is increasing in popularity. The benefits of the Bernese PAO are the ability to medialize the joint center, correct the version, leave the posterior column intact, and preserve the blood supply to the acetabular fragment.

After a safe and optimal correction is obtained, the clinical outcome of an osteotomy appears to depend upon the extent of preexisting osteoarthritis.[19] Pain relief was reported in 80% of symptomatic patients.[20,21] Using conversion to total hip arthroplasty as an end point, early failure after osteotomy was found to be best predicted using the preoperative dGEMRIC index.[16] Hip survival 10 years after osteotomy was found to be 82% to 84%,[20,21] and at long-term follow-up of approximately 20 years, survival approached 60%.[22] Predictors of poor outcome include severe dysplasia, presence of an os acetabuli, age older than 35 years, a relatively poor pain score, a positive impingement test, a limp, an advanced radiographic osteoarthritis grade, and poor joint congruency.[20-22] There has been no direct comparison of these results to the natural history of osteoarthritis.

Arthroplasty and pelvic osteotomy can achieve equivalent functional improvement.[23,24] However, the failure rate of osteotomy is higher in patients older than 40 years, who have only a 76% survival rate after 5 years.[25] To decrease the risk of early failure after osteotomy and make the procedure more cost-effective, it is important to identify significant acetabular dysplasia at a younger age, before the onset of significant osteoarthritis.[26]

The typical dysplastic hip has an anteverted proximal femur and an anteverted acetabulum. However, one in six dysplastic hips is associated with a retroverted acetabulum and also may be associated with a retroverted proximal femur or decreased head-neck offset.[27,28] The cause may be earlier surgery, such as a femoral osteotomy or an innominate pelvic osteotomy, which obligates retroversion of the acetabulum. If the patient's hip internal rotation is limited on clinical examination, the pelvic radiograph should be analyzed for acetabular retroversion, and CT or MRI should be used to look at the proximal femoral version. To avoid iatrogenic impingement, all of these deformities must be understood and considered when performing a redirectional pelvic osteotomy. These secondary deformities may be the source of residual symptoms in a seemingly well-corrected acetabular dysplasia. However, good clinical outcomes can be achieved when these deformities are taken into account.[29]

Slipped Capital Femoral Epiphysis

In severe SCFE, the metaphyseal prominence may not remodel completely and can cause limitation of range of motion, FAI, and, eventually, osteoarthritis of the joint.[30,31] In addition, there is now evidence that extensive intra-articular damage occurs even in mild or moderate SCFE.[32] The natural history of an uncorrected SCFE has been difficult to study because of the slow radiographic progression of osteoarthritis in these hips and a lack of clinical outcome data. However, the literature suggests that osteoarthritis does develop and may be related to the severity of the SCFE and the presence of osteonecrosis.[30]

In addition to the proximal femoral deformity, these hips have a retroverted femur and acetabulum.[33] Both the femoral and acetabular deformities can lead to FAI, which can cause hip pain and, eventually, osteoarthritis of the hip. Many hips with mild, symptomatic SCFE can be treated with débridement of the head-neck junction.[34] In a hip with moderate or severe SCFE and a persistent external rotation contracture, simple osteoplasty is not sufficient to correct the limitation of hip internal rotation. Traditionally, an intertrochanteric osteotomy is recommended to safely correct the proximal femoral deformity. The two types of intertrochanteric osteotomies are the Imhauser flexion and Southwick flexion-valgus techniques. When CT simulation data are used, the simpler Imhauser flexion osteotomy may produce an improvement in clinical range of motion equivalent to that of the more complex Southwick osteotomy.[35] An intertrochanteric osteotomy corrects the range-of-motion limitation and improves the hip mechanics by bringing the posteriorly slipped articular surface back into the acetabulum. However, it has been difficult to detect significant positive effects on the natural history of osteoarthritis development in these hips.[36] The possible reasons for the continued progression of osteoarthritis may be existing joint damage at the time of intertrochanteric osteotomy or residual FAI

from the metaphyseal prominence.[37] By using newer surgical dislocation techniques, it is possible to combine a femoral head-neck junction osteoplasty with an intertrochanteric osteotomy, with good results[34]

The ideal location for correcting the deformity in a stable SCFE is the head-neck junction. A safe correction at this level can be achieved in an immature hip using a modified Dunn procedure performed through a surgical dislocation approach.[38] However, femoral neck osteotomy in a healed SCFE is recognized as having the potential for serious complications and generally should be avoided.[39] Promising early results recently were reported after the modified Dunn technique was used to manage acute unstable SCFE.[38]

Legg-Calvé-Perthes Disease

A patient with LCP disease may develop osteoarthritis related to loss of femoral head sphericity and the congruence of the femoral and acetabular articulation. Over a long period of time, deteriorating hip function can lead to joint osteoarthritis.[40] When the development of radiographic osteoarthritis was studied in hips with LCP disease, hips with a round or oval femoral head did well over the long term, and some hips with aspherical congruency had satisfactory results into the fifth or sixth decade of life.[41] The worst outcome was in aspherical incongruent hips, which deteriorated by the fourth decade of life. Safe surgical dislocation of the hip, periacetabular osteotomy, and hip arthroscopy may improve the treatment of a prearthritic hip with impingement and instability from LCP disease.

If a patient with a healed LCP hip has pain and dysfunction, the primary concern is the development of osteoarthritis. However, secondary conditions, including FAI, leading to labral tears and limitation of motion or extra-articular impingement from an overgrown trochanter can be just as functionally limiting.[42] Therefore, the goal of treating a healed but symptomatic hip with LCP disease is to improve the hip's function by improving its mechanics. It is unclear whether surgical intervention alone can truly prolong the life of the joint.[43]

When treating a mature hip with LCP disease, both the deformity resulting from the disease and any earlier treatment must be considered. In mild LCP disease, the femoral head may be oval but congruent with the acetabulum. The patient may have labral symptoms at an early age because of a complex cam-type impingement (Figure 2). In addition to an aspherical femoral head, a limb-length discrepancy and trochanteric overgrowth may be present, as a result of the proximal femoral growth arrest from LCP disease or a varus osteotomy for containment. An earlier innominate pelvic osteotomy or shelf acetabuloplasty can lead to secondary impingement in adulthood, in addition to FAI caused by the femoral deformity. Both a femoral head-neck junction osteoplasty and an acetabular rim trimming may be required.

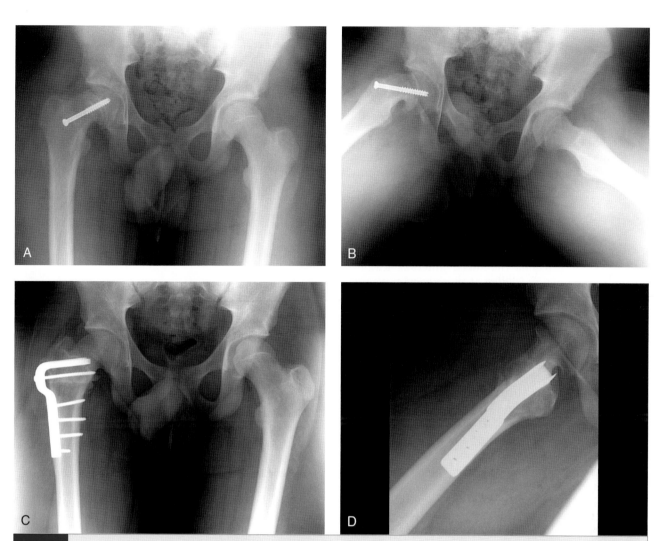

Figure 2 Preoperative AP (**A**) and frog-lateral (**B**) radiographs showing a pinned slipped capital femoral epiphysis in a 15-year-old patient. AP (**C**) and frog-lateral (**D**) radiographs after surgical dislocation, femoral neck osteochondroplasty and simultaneous flexion, and derotational intertrochanteric osteotomy.

In severe LCP disease, the femoroacetabular articulation may be incongruent. The intact round femoral head is located posteromedially in many patients.[44] This portion of the femoral head can be repositioned using a flexion valgus femoral osteotomy. It is important to reposition the femoral head in the most congruent position possible. It also is important to restore as much of the proximal femoral anatomy as possible, given the high probability that the hip eventually will require arthroplasty.

In severe LCP disease, the hip joint may be incongruent or the acetabulum may have remodeled to the point at which the articulation is congruent but dysplastic. It is important to reposition the articulation in a congruent and stable position, and doing so frequently requires both pelvic and femoral osteotomies.[29] Often these procedures are difficult, requiring direct visual inspection of the articulation through a safe surgical dislocation approach.[39]

Femoroacetabular Impingement

In adolescents and young adults, FAI caused by decreased anterior head-neck offset in the proximal femur and/or acetabular overcoverage or retroversion increasingly is being recognized as a cause of significant hip pain.[45] Mechanical impingement causes anterior labral damage and posterior contrecoup articular cartilage damage. Two types of mechanical derangement—cam and pincer—lead to articular cartilage and labral damage. In cam impingement, the aspherical anterior head-neck junction is forced into the acetabulum, causing increased mechanical stress at the labrochondral junction. The articular cartilage is damaged early at the anterosuperior labrochondral junction, even before labral damage occurs. In pincer impingement, the acetabulum is too deep globally (as in protrusio acetabuli or coxa profunda) or locally (as in anterior overcoverage) or is retroverted, causing impaction of the anterior acetabular rim on the anterior head-neck junction.

Cam and pincer impingement can coexist in a mixed-type impingement. The presence of FAI is clinically characterized as anterior groin pain exacerbated by flexion activities. The impingement test often is positive. Unlike hip dysplasia, FAI is characterized by limited hip flexion and internal rotation.

Radiographically, FAI is characterized as an increased α angle on MRI or a lateral hip radiograph;[3] acetabular overcoverage, as suggested by increased center-edge angle of Wiberg; a negative Tönnis angle; the presence of a crossover, posterior wall, or ischial sign; or protrusion of the femoral head medial to the ilioischial line.[46] Often the deformity causing the impingement is subtle, and it may be missed on radiographs.[47] Radial MRI is increasingly considered necessary for detecting the subtle anterior head-neck junction abnormality leading to impingement.

Cam-type deformity is more common in boys than in girls and is not always associated with pain or osteoarthritis.[48] Although deformity-causing FAI often is bilateral, it is not unusual for only one hip to be symptomatic.[49] The rate of osteoarthritis progression in the presence of FAI is unpredictable.[50] Therefore, prophylactic treatment has no role for a deformity that may lead to FAI. If the patient is symptomatic, multiple surgical options ranging from arthroscopy to limited open surgery and surgical dislocation allow correction of the underlying problem. The goal of surgery is to create impingement-free motion; osteochondroplasty is used, with acetabular rim trimming and labral refixation, if necessary. Although no randomized studies have been published, multiple-cohort single-surgeon studies found that patients' symptoms and quality-of-life outcome measures improve after osteochondroplasty, provided there is no evidence of extensive acetabular cartilage damage.[51-54] As expected, femoral head-neck junction osteoplasty also appears to be effective in active adolescents.[55]

Patients with a labral tear commonly have an underlying structural abnormality.[56] Simple labral débridement may improve the symptoms, even in the presence of FAI; however, better outcomes probably can be achieved by combining labral débridement with osteochondroplasty.[57] In the presence of extensive damage at the labrochondral junction, the treatment choices include labral and acetabular rim resection, labral detachment, acetabular rim resection, and labral repair. Labral repair appears to provide improved clinical outcome, regardless of whether an open or arthroscopic technique was used.[58,59] There are continuing efforts to lessen the morbidity associated with surgical treatment of FAI and to refine patient selection and treatment algorithms. Although treatment is effective in providing short- and intermediate-term symptom relief, the effect of treatment on the natural history of hip osteoarthritis is unknown.

Summary

Advances in radiologic imaging, surgical technique, and understanding of natural history have enabled the successful management of a variety of pathoanatomic hip disorders that previously were neither recognized nor routinely treated. Better cartilage imaging and an improved understanding of hip mechanics in the future will lead to refinements in the management of hip abnormalities in adolescents and young adults.

Annotated References

1. Kim YJ, Bixby S, Mamisch TC, Clohisy JC, Carlisle JC: Imaging structural abnormalities in the hip joint: Instability and impingement as a cause of osteoarthritis. *Semin Musculoskelet Radiol* 2008;12(4):334-345.

   This review article outlines the most commonly used radiographic views and signs used in assessing hip deformities.

2. Siebenrock KA, Kalbermatten DF, Ganz R: Effect of pelvic tilt on acetabular retroversion: A study of pelves from cadavers. *Clin Orthop Relat Res* 2003;407:241-248.

3. Nötzli HP, Wyss TF, Stoecklin CH, Schmid MR, Treiber K, Hodler J: The contour of the femoral head-neck junction as a predictor for the risk of anterior impingement. *J Bone Joint Surg Br* 2002;84(4):556-560.

4. Wiberg G: Studies on dysplastic acetabula and congenital subluxation of the hip joint: With special reference to the complications of osteoarthritis. *Acta Chir Scand* 1939;58(suppl):5-135.

5. Murphy SB, Ganz R, Müller ME: The prognosis in untreated dysplasia of the hip: A study of radiographic factors that predict the outcome. *J Bone Joint Surg Am* 1995;77(7):985-989.

6. Cooperman DR, Wallensten R, Stulberg SD: Acetabular dysplasia in the adult. *Clin Orthop Relat Res* 1983;175:79-85.

7. Lane NE, Lin P, Christiansen L, et al: Association of mild acetabular dysplasia with an increased risk of incident hip osteoarthritis in elderly white women: The study of osteoporotic fractures. *Arthritis Rheum* 2000;43(2):400-404.

8. Lane NE, Nevitt MC, Cooper C, Pressman A, Gore R, Hochberg M: Acetabular dysplasia and osteoarthritis of the hip in elderly white women. *Ann Rheum Dis* 1997;56(10):627-630.

9. Jacobsen S, Sonne-Holm S, Søballe K, Gebuhr P, Lund B: Hip dysplasia and osteoarthrosis: A survey of 4151 subjects from the Osteoarthrosis Substudy of the

Copenhagen City Heart Study. *Acta Orthop* 2005; 76(2):149-158.

In a population-based radiographic study, a significant relationship between acetabular dysplasia and radiographic ostearthritis was found. Subjects with acetabular dysplasia tended to develop osteoarthritis at a younger age.

10. Leunig M, Podeszwa D, Beck M, Werlen S, Ganz R: Magnetic resonance arthrography of labral disorders in hips with dysplasia and impingement. *Clin Orthop Relat Res* 2004;418:74-80.

11. Venn M, Maroudas A: Chemical composition and swelling of normal and osteoarthrotic femoral head cartilage. I. Chemical composition. *Ann Rheum Dis* 1977; 36(2):121-129.

12. Maroudas A, Venn M: Chemical composition and swelling of normal and osteoarthrotic femoral head cartilage. II. Swelling. *Ann Rheum Dis* 1977;36(5):399-406.

13. Bashir A, Gray ML, Boutin RD, Burstein D: Glycosaminoglycan in articular cartilage: In vivo assessment with delayed Gd(DTPA)(2-)-enhanced MR imaging. *Radiology* 1997;205(2):551-558.

14. Bashir A, Gray ML, Hartke J, Burstein D: Nondestructive imaging of human cartilage glycosaminoglycan concentration by MRI. *Magn Reson Med* 1999;41(5):857-865.

15. Burstein D, Velyvis J, Scott KT, et al: Protocol issues for delayed Gd(DTPA)(2-)-enhanced MRI (dGEMRIC) for clinical evaluation of articular cartilage. *Magn Reson Med* 2001;45(1):36-41.

16. Cunningham T, Jessel R, Zurakowski D, Millis MB, Kim YJ: Delayed gadolinium-enhanced magnetic resonance imaging of cartilage to predict early failure of Bernese periacetabular osteotomy for hip dysplasia. *J Bone Joint Surg Am* 2006;88(7):1540-1548.

In a cohort study comparing various clinical and radiographic preoperative factors, investigators found that preexisting hip osteoarthritis (as measured by the dGEMRIC technique) is the best predictor of a poor early outcome after periacetabular osteotomy. Level of evidence: II.

17. Jessel RH, Zurakowski D, Zilkens C, Burstein D, Gray ML, Kim YJ: Radiographic and patient factors associated with pre-radiographic osteoarthritis in hip dysplasia. *J Bone Joint Surg Am* 2009;91(5):1120-1129.

By using the dGEMRIC technique to measure osteoarthritis, severity of osteoarthritis was associated with severity of dysplasia, presence of a labral tear, and age of the patient. Level of evidence: III.

18. Ganz R, Klaue K, Vinh TS, Mast JW: A new periacetabular osteotomy for the treatment of hip dysplasias. Technique and preliminary results. *Clin Orthop Relat Res* 1988;232:26-36.

19. Trousdale RT, Ekkernkamp A, Ganz R, Wallrichs SL: Periacetabular and intertrochanteric osteotomy for the treatment of osteoarthrosis in dysplastic hips. *J Bone Joint Surg Am* 1995;77(1):73-85.

20. Matheny T, Kim YJ, Zurakowski D, Matero C, Millis M: Intermediate to long-term results following the Bernese periacetabular osteotomy and predictors of clinical outcome. *J Bone Joint Surg Am* 2009;91(9):2113-2123.

Standard clinical and radiographic preoperative factors were used in determining that intermediate-term results after periacetabular osteotomy are best predicted by patient age and preoperative joint congruency. If the patient had no risk factors for early failure, the probability of a poor intermediate-term result was approximately 14%. Level of evidence: II.

21. Troelsen A, Elmengaard B, Søballe K: Medium-term outcome of periacetabular osteotomy and predictors of conversion to total hip replacement. *J Bone Joint Surg Am* 2009;91(9):2169-2179.

Factors predicting a poor intermediate-term outcome after a periacetabular osteotomy included Tönnis grade II and III osteoarthritis. Acetabular retroversion on CT and the presence of a calcified detached labrum were identified as additional risk factors when the osteoarthritis grade was adjusted for severe dysplasia. Level of evidence: II.

22. Steppacher SD, Tannast M, Ganz R, Siebenrock KA: Mean 20-year followup of Bernese periacetabular osteotomy. *Clin Orthop Relat Res* 2008;466(7):1633-1644.

A long-term study found 60% survival 20 years after periacetabular osteotomy. Age at surgery, severity of hip pain, positive impingement sign, and osteoarthritis grade were predictors of success or failure. Level of evidence: III.

23. Hsieh PH, Huang KC, Lee PC, Chang YH: Comparison of periacetabular osteotomy and total hip replacement in the same patient: A two- to ten-year follow-up study. *J Bone Joint Surg Br* 2009;91(7):883-888.

The clinical outcomes of total hip replacement and periacetabular osteotomy in patients with bilateral dysplasia were found to be comparable 2 to 10 years after surgery, although patients preferred the osteotomy.

24. Garbuz DS, Awwad MA, Duncan CP: Periacetabular osteotomy and total hip arthroplasty in patients older than 40 years. *J Arthroplasty* 2008;23(7):960-963.

Both periacetabular osteotomy and joint arthroplasty had a good clinical outcome in a matched cohort study of patients older than 40 years, but the outcome of joint arthroplasty was superior.

25. Millis MB, Kain M, Sierra R, et al: Periacetabular osteotomy for acetabular dysplasia in patients older than 40 years: A preliminary study. *Clin Orthop Relat Res* 2009;467(9):2228-2234.

The clinical outcomes of 87 hips in patients older than 40 years were compared after periacetabular osteotomy. At a mean 5.2 years, 24% of the hips had been

4: Lower Extremity

converted to arthroplasty. The surviving hips had good symptomatic improvement.

26. Sharifi E, Sharifi H, Morshed S, Bozic K, Diab M: Cost-effectiveness analysis of periacetabular osteotomy. *J Bone Joint Surg Am* 2008;90(7):1447-1456.

    Periacetabular osteotomy is more cost-effective than arthroplasty in hips with Tönnis grade I or II osteoarthritis. Level of evidence: II.

27. Li PL, Ganz R: Morphologic features of congenital acetabular dysplasia: One in six is retroverted. *Clin Orthop Relat Res* 2003;416:245-253.

28. Clohisy JC, Nunley RM, Carlisle JC, Schoenecker PL: Incidence and characteristics of femoral deformities in the dysplastic hip. *Clin Orthop Relat Res* 2009;467(1):128-134.

    The incidence of femoral head deformity and decreased head-neck offset in hips with acetabular dysplasia is as high as 75%. Level of evidence: II.

29. Clohisy JC, Nunley RM, Curry MC, Schoenecker PL: Periacetabular osteotomy for the treatment of acetabular dysplasia associated with major aspherical femoral head deformities. *J Bone Joint Surg Am* 2007;89(7):1417-1423.

    Hips with both femoral deformity and acetabular dysplasia can be successfully treated with combined femoral and acetabular procedures. Careful intraoperative assessment is needed to minimize the risk of secondary FAI. Level of evidence: IV.

30. Carney BT, Weinstein SL, Noble J: Long-term follow-up of slipped capital femoral epiphysis. *J Bone Joint Surg Am* 1991;73(5):667-674.

31. Ross PM, Lyne ED, Morawa LG: Slipped capital femoral epiphysis long-term results after 10-38 years. *Clin Orthop Relat Res* 1979;141:176-180.

32. Leunig M, Casillas MM, Hamlet M, et al: Slipped capital femoral epiphysis: Early mechanical damage to the acetabular cartilage by a prominent femoral metaphysis. *Acta Orthop Scand* 2000;71(4):370-375.

33. Gelberman RH, Cohen MS, Shaw BA, Kasser JR, Griffin PP, Wilkinson RH: The association of femoral retroversion with slipped capital femoral epiphysis. *J Bone Joint Surg Am* 1986;68(7):1000-1007.

34. Spencer S, Millis MB, Kim YJ: Early results of treatment of hip impingement syndrome in slipped capital femoral epiphysis and pistol grip deformity of the femoral head-neck junction using the surgical dislocation technique. *J Pediatr Orthop* 2006;26(3):281-285.

    In a review of 19 patients who underwent surgical dislocation, with or without concomitant intertrochanteric osteotomy, for the treatment of pistol-grip deformity or SCFE, inferior results were found in patients with preexisting arthrosis. Level of evidence: III.

35. Mamisch TC, Kim YJ, Richolt J, et al: Range of motion after computed tomography-based simulation of intertrochanteric corrective osteotomy in cases of slipped capital femoral epiphysis: Comparison of uniplanar flexion osteotomy and multiplanar flexion, valgisation, and rotational osteotomies. *J Pediatr Orthop* 2009; 29(4):336-340.

    A retrospective study used computer-reconstructed CT data to simulate uniplanar and multiplanar osteotomies for the treatment of SCFE-related deformity. Multiplanar osteotomy is associated with a greater range of motion in the plane of abduction and internal rotation. Level of evidence: III.

36. Schai PA, Exner GU, Hänsch O: Prevention of secondary coxarthrosis in slipped capital femoral epiphysis: A long-term follow-up study after corrective intertrochanteric osteotomy. *J Pediatr Orthop B* 1996;5(3):135-143.

37. Mamisch TC, Kim YJ, Richolt JA, Millis MB, Kordelle J: Femoral morphology due to impingement influences the range of motion in slipped capital femoral epiphysis. *Clin Orthop Relat Res* 2009;467(3):692-698.

    Based on analysis of computer-simulated CT data, femoral morphology and acetabular version were found to significantly affect post-SCFE range of motion and FAI. Level of evidence: III.

38. Ziebarth K, Zilkens C, Spencer S, Leunig M, Ganz R, Kim YJ: Capital realignment for moderate and severe SCFE using a modified Dunn procedure. *Clin Orthop Relat Res* 2009;467(3):704-716.

    A retrospective review of 40 patients treated using a modified Dunn procedure for realignment of SCFE found restoration of normal capital-femoral alignment, with no osteonecrosis.

39. Rebello G, Spencer S, Millis MB, Kim YJ: Surgical dislocation in the management of pediatric and adolescent hip deformity. *Clin Orthop Relat Res* 2009;467(3):724-731.

    Complications and outcomes are described in a retrospective review of patients treated with surgical dislocation for a variety of pediatric hip disorders. Level of evidence: III.

40. McAndrew MP, Weinstein SL: A long-term follow-up of Legg-Calvé-Perthes disease. *J Bone Joint Surg Am* 1984; 66(6):860-869.

41. Stulberg SD, Cooperman DR, Wallensten R: The natural history of Legg-Calvé-Perthes disease. *J Bone Joint Surg Am* 1981;63(7):1095-1108.

42. Yoo WJ, Choi IH, Cho TJ, Chung CY, Park MS, Lee DY: Out-toeing and in-toeing in patients with Perthes disease: Role of the femoral hump. *J Pediatr Orthop* 2008;28(7):717-722.

    Nine patients with a transverse plane gait abnormality were assessed using CT and kinematic gait analysis. Location of femoral deformity was found to be associated with the direction of the transverse gait pattern. Level of evidence: III.

43. Rowe SM, Jung ST, Cheon SY, Choi J, Kang KD, Kim KH: Outcome of cheilectomy in Legg-Calve-Perthes disease: Minimum 25-year follow-up of five patients. *J Pediatr Orthop* 2006;26(2):204-210.

This is a retrospective review of five patients treated with cheilectomy for hinge abduction associated with LCP disease.

44. Kim HT, Wenger DR: Surgical correction of "functional retroversion" and "functional coxa vara" in late Legg-Calvé-Perthes disease and epiphyseal dysplasia: correction of deformity defined by new imaging modalities. *J Pediatr Orthop* 1997;17(2):247-254.

45. Ganz R, Parvizi J, Beck M, Leunig M, Nötzli H, Siebenrock KA: Femoroacetabular impingement: a cause for osteoarthritis of the hip. *Clin Orthop Relat Res* 2003; 417:112-120.

46. Clohisy JC, Carlisle JC, Beaulé PE, et al : A systematic approach to the plain radiographic evaluation of the young adult hip. *J Bone Joint Surg Am* 2008;90(suppl 4):47-66.

This review article describes the essential radiographic technique and assessment for hip deformity.

47. Dudda M, Albers C, Mamisch TC, Werlen S, Beck M: Do normal radiographs exclude asphericity of the femoral head-neck junction? *Clin Orthop Relat Res* 2009; 467(3):651-659.

Conventional radiographs can miss a subtle femoral head-neck junction abnormality. Radial MRI can detect these bony morphologic abnormalities, which can lead to FAI. Level of evidence: II.

48. Gosvig KK, Jacobsen S, Sonne-Holm S, Gebuhr P: The prevalence of cam-type deformity of the hip joint: A survey of 4151 subjects of the Copenhagen Osteoarthritis Study. *Acta Radiol* 2008;49(4):436-441.

A population-based radiographic survey using AP pelvic radiographs found cam-type deformity of the proximal femur to be present in approximately 17% of European men. Often these deformities are clinically silent.

49. Allen D, Beaulé PE, Ramadan O, Doucette S: Prevalence of associated deformities and hip pain in patients with cam-type femoroacetabular impingement. *J Bone Joint Surg Br* 2009;91(5):589-594.

Bilateral cam deformities were present in 78% of patients with symptomatic FAI. However, not all cam deformities are symptomatic; only 26% of the patients had bilateral hip pain. Hips with an α angle greater than 60° were 2.6 times more likely to have pain.

50. Bardakos NV, Villar RN: Predictors of progression of osteoarthritis in femoroacetabular impingement: A radiological study with a minimum of ten years follow-up. *J Bone Joint Surg Br* 2009;91(2):162-169.

A radiographic study looked at factors associated with the progression of osteoarthritis in hips with pistol-grip deformity. Not all hips had progression of arthritis. Varus angulation of the proximal femur and presence of a posterior wall sign were associated with arthritis progression.

51. Beaulé PE, Le Duff MJ, Zaragoza E: Quality of life following femoral head-neck osteochondroplasty for femoroacetabular impingement. *J Bone Joint Surg Am* 2007; 89(4):773-779.

A clinical outcome study using the Western Ontario and McMaster Universities Osteoarthritis Index and UCLA activity scores found significant improvement in quality of life after open surgical dislocation and osteochondroplasty for FAI. Level of evidence: IV.

52. Beck M, Leunig M, Parvizi J, Boutier V, Wyss D, Ganz R: Anterior femoroacetabular impingement: Part II. Midterm results of surgical treatment. *Clin Orthop Relat Res* 2004;418:67-73.

53. Byrd JW, Jones KS: Arthroscopic femoroplasty in the management of cam-type femoroacetabular impingement. *Clin Orthop Relat Res* 2009;467(3):739-746.

A noncontrolled cohort study of clinical outcome after arthroscopic osteoplasty for FAI found an average 20-point improvement in the Harris hip score, with clinical improvement in 83% of patients. No clear association was found between clinical outcome and articular cartilage damage. Level of evidence: IV.

54. Lincoln M, Johnston K, Muldoon M, Santore R: Combined arthroscopic and modified open approach for cam femoroacetabular impingement: A preliminary experience. *Arthroscopy* 2009;25(4):392-399.

A small clinical case study found clinical improvement and better range of motion after combined arthroscopic and limited open osteochondroplasty for FAI.

55. Philippon MJ, Yen YM, Briggs KK, Kuppersmith DA, Maxwell RB: Early outcomes after hip arthroscopy for femoroacetabular impingement in the athletic adolescent patient: A preliminary report. *J Pediatr Orthop* 2008;28(7):705-710.

A small clinical case study found a significant (average, 36 points) improvement in modified Harris hip scores in adolescents who underwent arthroscopic osteoplasty for FAI. Level of evidence: IV.

56. Wenger DE, Kendell KR, Miner MR, Trousdale RT: Acetabular labral tears rarely occur in the absence of bony abnormalities. *Clin Orthop Relat Res* 2004;426:145-150.

57. Bardakos NV, Vasconcelos JC, Villar RN: Early outcome of hip arthroscopy for femoroacetabular impingement: The role of femoral osteoplasty in symptomatic improvement. *J Bone Joint Surg Br* 2008;90(12):1570-1575.

In a consecutive comparison of the clinical outcomes of arthroscopic surgery in hips with FAI, with or without osteoplasty, both patient groups had significant improvement in outcomes. The proportion of good or excellent outcomes was higher in the patients who underwent osteoplasty.

58. Espinosa N, Rothenfluh DA, Beck M, Ganz R, Leunig M: Treatment of femoro-acetabular impingement: Preliminary results of labral refixation. *J Bone Joint Surg Am* 2006;88(5):925-935.

4: Lower Extremity

A consecutive clinical case study compared open surgical dislocation and osteochondroplasty, with or without labral repair. Patients who underwent labral repair after acetabular rim trimming had significantly better clinical results. Level of evidence: III.

59. Larson CM, Giveans MR: Arthroscopic debridement versus refixation of the acetabular labrum associated with femoroacetabular impingement. *Arthroscopy* 2009;25(4):369-376.

In a consecutive comparative clinical case study of arthroscopic osteochondroplasty with or without labral repair, patients in both groups had significant improvement in clinical outcome measures. The patients in the labral repair group had a slightly but significantly better clinical result. Level of evidence: III.

Chapter 19

Legg-Calvé-Perthes Disease

Travis Matheney, MD

Introduction

Legg-Calvé-Perthes (LCP) disease is a disorder of the hip in children. Its description is commonly credited to Arthur Legg, Jacques Calvé, and Georg Perthes, who in 1910 each independently reported on an apparently self-limiting condition of the hip in young children. However, Henning Waldenström also can be credited with much of the early insight into this condition through his pathohistologic evaluation and radiographic staging of hips in affected children. One hundred years later, the divergent theories on etiology are not yet reconciled, and a consensus on optimal treatment has not been reached.

Epidemiology and Pathogenesis

The true etiology of LCP disease is unknown. The age of onset typically is between 4 and 8 years, but the range is 2 to 12 years. The incidence is four times higher in boys than in girls, and the risk is relatively high in children with short stature and delayed bone age, a hyperactivity disorder, exposure to secondhand smoke, or a lower socioeconomic status. LCP disease is rare among children of African descent. LCP disease occurs bilaterally in approximately 10% to 15% of patients. [1-4]

An association with abnormal clotting factors has been described but not extensively supported by research. [5-7] Recently, the incidence of LCP disease was found to be increased in the presence of the factor V Leiden mutation, the prothrombin G20210A mutation, an elevated factor VIII level, or a protein S deficiency. [8] The underlying pathophysiology is believed to be related to osteonecrosis of the immature femoral head. The current belief is that during the child's early development, a vascular insult blocks epiphyseal blood flow within the tenuous arterial plexus on the femoral neck. Femoral head collapse occurs during the fragmentation phase of LCP disease because of presumed mechanical overload on a fragmenting epiphysis, and the collapse may become fixed during the healing phase. Biomechanical studies found significant increases in hip contact pressures in patients with normal hips during common activities such as walking or stair climbing (4 or 2.5 times body weight, respectively). [9] This finding historically has led clinicians to limit a child's activities during fragmentation. However, no correlation of specific activity limitations to outcomes of LCP disease has been published.

Clinical Evaluation

A child with LCP disease typically has a painless limp, with or without a Trendelenburg gait pattern. The child describes pain in the hip, thigh, or knee. The physical examination usually reveals a loss of abduction and internal rotation. The differential diagnosis during the early phase of LCP disease primarily includes toxic synovitis, osteomyelitis, and septic arthritis, and it also may include Meyer dysplasia (which has an appearance similar to that of bilateral LCP disease), an epiphyseal dysplasia, and sickle cell anemia.

The early phase of LCP disease is characterized by stiffness and contracture caused by joint synovitis. Activity restriction and nonsteroidal anti-inflammatory drugs can help relieve these symptoms. As the disease progresses and the femoral head heals, the synovitis resolves. If the femoral head is aspherical, however, the loss of motion may become permanent. Depending on the sphericity of the femoral head and its congruency with the acetabulum, premature osteoarthritis may develop in adulthood and lead to pain and disability.

Plain radiographs, including the AP pelvis and frog lateral views, and routine laboratory tests, including white blood cell count, erythrocyte sedimentation rate, and C-reactive protein level, can be useful in the diagnosis. The laboratory values typically are normal, although the erythrocyte sedimentation rate may be slightly elevated. Technetium-99m radionuclide scans can lead to diagnosis earlier in the disease process. MRI is useful for assessing early ischemia and can reveal changes in the femoral head months before they appear on plain radiographs. [10] MRI has not been shown to have prognostic value.

4: Lower Extremity

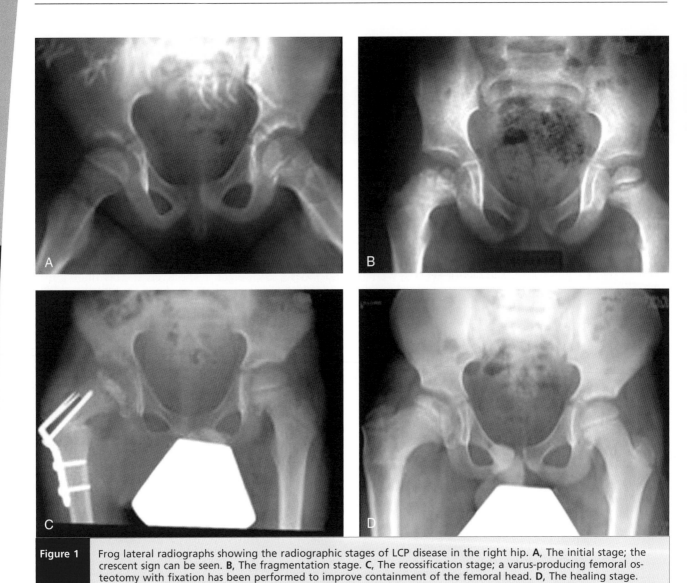

Figure 1 Frog lateral radiographs showing the radiographic stages of LCP disease in the right hip. **A,** The initial stage; the crescent sign can be seen. **B,** The fragmentation stage. **C,** The reossification stage; a varus-producing femoral osteotomy with fixation has been performed to improve containment of the femoral head. **D,** The healing stage.

Radiographic Stages

There may be no obvious abnormality during the initial radiographic stage of LCP disease[11] (**Figure 1**). Subtle signs may be present; these include an ossific nucleus that is smaller and/or more radiodense than on the asymptomatic side or a greater-than-normal space between the medial femoral head and the acetabulum. The initial stage is followed by fragmentation of the ossific nucleus and fracture of the subchondral plate. Normal-appearing bone density returns during the reossification stage, and the subchondral plate re-forms. Hip synovitis often resolves during this third stage, but the femoral head deformity may become fixed. During the healing stage, the femoral head assumes its permanent appearance, with residual deformity. This final stage lasts until skeletal maturity. If the femoral head shape is irregular, acetabular remodeling may continue during the healing stage.

Classification Systems

Multiple systems based on radiographic findings are used for classifying LCP disease. In the simple Salter-Thompson classification, femoral head involvement is determined to be less than or more than 50% (class A or B, respectively).[12] However, the crescent sign used to assess the extent of head involvement during the initial disease stage may be seen only in one third of patients, possibly because the timing of the initial radiographs varies. The Catterall classification similarly classifies epiphyseal involvement as less than 50% (groups I and II) or more than 50% (groups III and IV). The anterior head is involved in group I; the central and anterior head, in group II; most of the epiphysis, in group III; and the entire epiphysis, in group IV.[13] The Catterall classification was supplemented by a series of head-at-risk signs including the Gage sign, calcification of the lateral epiphysis, lateral subluxation of the femoral head, a horizontal growth plate, and metaphyseal cystic

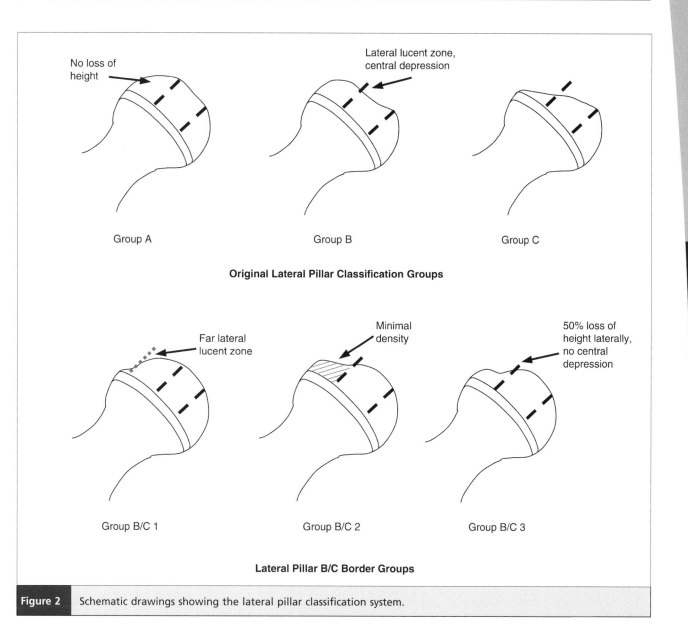

Original Lateral Pillar Classification Groups

Lateral Pillar B/C Border Groups

Figure 2 Schematic drawings showing the lateral pillar classification system.

lesions, but these signs were found to have poor intra-observer and interobserver reliability.[14,15]

The Herring lateral pillar system is the most commonly used classification system and has the best interrater reliability.[16] The lateral pillar is the lateralmost 30% of the femoral head, as seen on an AP hip radiograph. The classification initially included groups A, B, and C but has been modified to include the B/C border group (**Figure 2**). Hips classified into group A have no loss of height in the lateral pillar and no density changes. In group B, the hip has more than 50% of its original pillar height. In a group C hip, there is more lucency and a more-than-50% loss of height in the lateral pillar. In the B/C border group, the hip has more than 50% of its original height but is less than 2 to 3 mm wide (group B/C1); has more than 50% of its original height, but minimal ossification (group B/C2); or has exactly 50% of its original height but is depressed relative to the central pillar (group B/C3).[17]

After skeletal maturity, hips can be described using the Stulberg classification.[2] The Stulberg system describes radiographic features including congruency between the femoral head and the acetabulum. Class I hips are normal appearing, with spherical congruency. Class II hips have a spherical head in AP projections, with spherical congruency, but they have a larger than normal femoral head (coxa magna), a short femoral neck, and/or an abnormally steep acetabulum. Class III hips have an ovoid or mushroom-shaped (not flat) femoral head, a coxa magna, a short neck, and a steep acetabulum; they are now described as having aspherical congruency. Class IV hips are similar to class III hips except that there is flattening of the femoral head with continued aspherical congruency. Class V hips have a flat femoral head as well as a normally shaped femoral neck and acetabulum with aspherical congruency. Retrospective cohort studies determined the correlation between Stulberg class and risk of premature osteoarthritis; a hip classified as I, II, or III is at a relatively low risk of early osteoarthritis, but a hip classified as IV or V is at high risk.[18-24]

Treatment

Much of the treatment of LCP disease is based on the association between femoral head shape, the congruency of the femoral head with the acetabulum, and the development of osteoarthritis.[2] Aspherical, incongruent hips were found to develop osteoarthritis rapidly by the fifth decade of life; aspherical but congruent hips did not develop arthritis until the patient was well into midlife.[2,18-24] The treatment algorithm for early LCP disease is geared toward obtaining a spherical and congruent joint whenever possible. The choice of nonsurgical therapy or containment surgery primarily is based on multiple long-term studies that assessed outcomes in hips affected by LCP disease. Two of these, known as the Perthes Study Group and the Norwegian Perthes Study, were prospective, multicenter studies that assessed treatment outcomes by surgeon and hospital preference.

The Perthes Study Group found that outcome was correlated with both age at disease onset and lateral pillar classification. Patients who were younger than 8 years at onset and had a hip classified into lateral pillar group B did well regardless of whether they were treated with early containment surgery, observation, physical therapy, or bracing. Patients who were older than 8 years at onset with a hip classified into lateral pillar group B or B/C had a better outcome with surgical rather than nonsurgical treatment. Patients with a hip classified into lateral pillar group C (more than 50% involvement) had a poor outcome regardless of age at onset or treatment.[18,22-24]

The Norwegian Perthes Study had similar results. The strongest predictors of outcome were age at diagnosis (younger or older than 6 years), the percentage of the femoral head affected (less or more than 50%), and lateral pillar classification. Outcomes did not differ in hips with less than 50% necrosis, regardless of age at diagnosis or treatment; this finding differed from that of the Perthes Study Group in finding no age-dependent difference in outcomes among hips in lateral pillar group B. Femoral osteotomy yielded significantly better outcomes in children who were older than 6 years at diagnosis and had more than 50% necrosis of the femoral head. This finding also differed from that of the Perthes Study Group, which found that hips in lateral pillar group C had no improvement after femoral or pelvic osteotomy.[18,25] Regardless of the differences in their findings, these two studies indicate that no surgical intervention is warranted in children younger than 6 years.

Nonsurgical Treatment

Recommendations for the nonsurgical management of LCP disease are highly variable and often include initial bed rest accompanied by range-of-motion and adductor stretching, with or without the use of nonsteroidal anti-inflammatory drugs. Abduction casting has been used to assist with stretching, but full-time casting increases intra-articular pressures and is not commonly used. Physical therapy and bracing programs do not affect the natural history of the disease;[25] they no longer are a primary method of treatment but instead are used as an adjunct to observation or surgical treatment.

The use of bisphosphonates is an evolving area of research in LCP disease. Animal studies in which femoral head osteonecrosis was surgically induced found significant improvement in femoral head shape and structure when bisphosphonates were used.[26,27] The mechanism of action is a delay in necrotic bone resorption, without an apparent enhancement of bone anabolism. Clinical studies are at a very early stage, and the use of bisphosphonates therefore is not a standard of care for treating LCP disease.

Containment Surgery

Femoral and/or rotational pelvic osteotomy to keep the femoral head contained within the acetabulum is the most commonly recommended surgical method of treatment. Proponents consistently recommend that treatment should begin as early as possible during the fragmentation phase, when femoral head remodeling still may occur. A large study found that containment surgery during the osteonecrosis phase or early during the fragmentation phase caused the femoral head to bypass the fragmentation phase in 34% of hips, shorten the overall length of the disease, and minimize femoral head extrusion and metaphyseal changes.[28] It is believed that the younger the patient, the more time will be available for any needed acetabular remodeling. Both femoral and pelvic osteotomies require that the femoral head be mobile within the acetabulum, with no hinge abduction (**Figure 3**). A study of 38 hips found that the epiphyseal slip-in index is one of the best predictors of a good outcome after varus osteotomy. With the hip in 40° of abduction, this percentage measurement is obtained by dividing the distance from the bony acetabular edge to the apex of the epiphysis by the distance from the bony acetabular edge to the tip of the teardrop. The best outcomes were associated with an index greater than 20%.[29] The use of the slip-in index may help the surgeon decide whether a varus-producing proximal femoral osteotomy can achieve the most spherical femoral head possible.

No comparative study of femoral and pelvic osteotomies has been done in severity- and age-matched children with LCP disease. In a large uncontrolled study, proximal femoral osteotomy for LCP disease appeared to have the best results in children younger than 7 years with evident femoral head extrusion and in children age 7 years or older regardless of whether extrusion

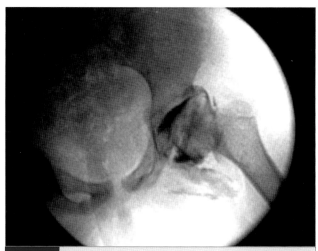

Figure 3 Arthrogram of the left hip, showing hinge abduction. With the hip abducted, the lateral edge of the epiphysis is hinging on the lateral acetabulum, with concomitant medial dye pooling.

was present.[28] The researchers added epiphysiodesis of the greater trochanter to prevent overgrowth and in the belief that it would minimize the risk of a later Trendelenburg gait pattern or extra-articular impingement. The extent to which epiphysiodesis of the greater trochanter limits these secondary problems remains unclear.[30]

Acetabular procedures have been recommended for improving femoral head containment. The Salter innominate osteotomy can be used in isolation or in combination with proximal femoral osteotomy. The Salter and varus-producing femoral osteotomies were found to have similar results.[31,32] If hinge abduction precludes a varus-producing femoral osteotomy, shelf acetabuloplasty can be used to improve femoral head containment and coverage, with good results.[33,34]

Better surgical outcomes appear to be obtainable when preoperative joint mobility is optimal. Traction, bracing, and physical therapy may be necessary to regain motion before surgery. If concentric motion cannot be achieved, acetabular augmentation procedures such as a shelf acetabuloplasty, with or without a valgus osteotomy, can be used for containment.

Salvage Osteotomy

Hips with poor sphericity and/or congruency may become symptomatic before the onset of end-stage osteoarthritis. The symptoms often result from impingement, instability, and poor range of motion caused by the misshapen femoral head. Flexion-valgus femoral osteotomy has been performed to reposition the limb in a more functional position and bring a relatively round portion of the femoral head into a weight-bearing position. The effect was found to be beneficial in selected skeletally immature and skeletally mature patients.[35,36]

In addition to its femoral head pathology, a hip with LCP disease may have acetabular dysplasia or retrover-

sion. Therefore, a combination of pelvic and femoral osteotomies may be required to achieve joint congruency and stability. Shelf acetabuloplasty (also called a labral support procedure), can further improve femoral head coverage and may improve acetabular depth and joint congruency in a skeletally immature patient, even in the presence of preoperative hinge abduction. These salvage procedures can improve the patient's symptoms, but their effect on long-term outcome is unclear.[35,36]

In a skeletally mature patient with severe residual deformity, pain and early arthrosis are significant concerns. The extent of deformity and the resulting instability or femoroacetabular impingement often dictate whether the hip will become symptomatic. It is important to recognize that instability in residual LCP disease can arise from a lack of anterolateral acetabular coverage over a large femoral head. Femoral and/or acetabular procedures (including labral support and periacetabular osteotomy) can provide good relief of symptoms and improve hip joint mechanics.[37] The presence of hip arthrosis and the radiographic appearance of the joint (classified using the Herring and Stulberg systems[16]) may dictate whether osteotomy and joint preservation are an option.

Summary

The exact etiology of LCP disease remains ill-defined, and the understanding of the progression of secondary deformity and treatment continues to evolve. Identifying a child at risk of LPC disease and applying corrective procedures that will predictably alter the natural history of the disease continue to be challenging. Most current treatment algorithms begin by minimizing excessive impact-loading activities and maintaining the hip's range of motion. Relatively few authors advocate nighttime bracing. The general principle of most nonsurgical and surgical interventions is to contain the diseased femoral head within the acetabulum, in an effort to attain the most congruent joint possible by the end of development. Current reports suggest that containment surgery has the best results when performed early in the disease process and in patients who have moderate disease and are older than 7 years. The use of bisphosphonates has had promising early results in minimizing changes in the shape and structure of the femoral head. If containment is not possible and the deformity is significant, the main treatment continues to be osteotomies of the femur and/or acetabulum, in an attempt to improve the congruency of the weight-bearing portion of the hip, increase the range of motion, and decrease femoroacetabular impingement. The long-term outcomes are variable, with the least-affected hips having the least progression of symptomatic hip arthrosis.

4: Lower Extremity

Annotated References

1. Herring JA, Lundeen MA, Wenger DR: Minimal Perthes' disease. *J Bone Joint Surg Br* 1980;62(1):25-30.

2. Stulberg SD, Cooperman DR, Wallensten R: The natural history of Legg-Calvé-Perthes disease. *J Bone Joint Surg Am* 1981;63(7):1095-1108.

3. Guille JT, Lipton GE, Szöke G, Bowen JR, Harcke HT, Glutting JJ: Legg-Calvé-Perthes disease in girls: A comparison of the results with those seen in boys. *J Bone Joint Surg Am* 1998;80(9):1256-1263.

4. Gordon JE, Schoenecker PL, Osland JD, Dobbs MB, Szymanski DA, Luhmann SJ: Smoking and socioeconomic status in the etiology and severity of Legg-Calvé-Perthes' disease. *J Pediatr Orthop B* 2004;13(6): 367-370.

5. Eldridge J, Dilley A, Austin H, et al: The role of protein C, protein S, and resistance to activated protein C in Legg-Perthes disease. *Pediatrics* 2001;107(6):1329-1334.

6. Hresko MT, McDougall PA, Gorlin JB, Vamvakas EC, Kasser JR, Neufeld EJ: Prospective reevaluation of the association between thrombotic diathesis and Legg-Perthes disease. *J Bone Joint Surg Am* 2002;84(9):1613-1618.

7. Mehta JS, Conybeare ME, Hinves BL, Winter JB: Protein C levels in patients with Legg-Calve-Perthes disease: Is it a true deficiency? *J Pediatr Orthop* 2006;26(2): 200-203.

   A possible link between a low protein C level (causing a hypercoagulable state) and LCP disease was investigated. A lower, but still normal, level of protein C was found in patients with LCP disease. The authors concluded there may be a link, despite other evidence to the contrary.

8. Vosmaer A, Pereira RR, Koenderman JS, Rosendaal FR, Cannegieter SC: Coagulation abnormalities in Legg-Calvé-Perthes disease. *J Bone Joint Surg Am* 2010; 92(1):121-128.

   A prospective, case-controlled study attempted to determine an association between some commonly studied clotting factors and LCP disease. After adjusting the odds ratios for sex and age, the authors found an increased incidence of LCP disease in the presence of factor V Leiden mutation (odds ratio, 3.3), prothrombin G20210A mutation (odds ratio, 2.6), elevated factor VIII level (odds ratio, 7.5), or protein S deficiency (odds ratio, 2.8). The effect was cumulative, with an increasing number of coincident abnormal clotting factors in boys but not in girls.

9. Bergmann G, Deuretzbacher G, Heller M, et al: Hip contact forces and gait patterns from routine activities. *J Biomech* 2001;34(7):859-871.

10. de Sanctis N, Rondinella F: Prognostic evaluation of Legg-Calvé-Perthes disease by MRI: Part II. Pathomorphogenesis and new classification. *J Pediatr Orthop* 2000;20(4):463-470.

11. Waldenström H: On necrosis of the joint cartilage by epiphysiolysis capitis femoris: 1930. *Clin Orthop Relat Res* 1996;322 :3-7.

12. Salter RB, Thompson GH: Legg-Calvé-Perthes disease: The prognostic significance of the subchondral fracture and a two-group classification of the femoral head involvement. *J Bone Joint Surg Am* 1984;66(4):479-489.

13. Catterall A: Natural history, classification, and x-ray signs in Legg-Calvé-Perthes' disease. *Acta Orthop Belg* 1980;46(4):346-351.

14. Smith SR, Ions GK, Gregg PJ: The radiological features of the metaphysis in Perthes disease. *J Pediatr Orthop* 1982;2(4):401-404.

15. Forster MC, Kumar S, Rajan RA, Atherton WG, Asirvatham R, Thava VR: Head-at-risk signs in Legg-Calvé-Perthes disease: Poor inter- and intra-observer reliability. *Acta Orthop Scand* 2006;77(3):413-417.

    The interobserver and intraobserver reliability of the Catterall head-at-risk signs was studied. Intraobserver reliability was found to be good for lateral subluxation and cystic metaphyseal changes, moderate for lateral calcification, and fair for the Gage sign and horizontal growth plate. Interobserver reliability was moderate for lateral subluxation, fair for lateral calcification and cystic metaphyseal changes, and slight for the Gage sign and horizontal growth plate. These results mean that the head-at-risk signs are difficult to use for predicting a poor prognosis in clinical practice.

16. Herring JA, Neustadt JB, Williams JJ, Early JS, Browne RH: The lateral pillar classification of Legg-Calvé-Perthes disease. *J Pediatr Orthop* 1992;12(2):143-150.

17. Herring JA, Kim HT, Browne R: Legg-Calve-Perthes disease: Part I. Classification of radiographs with use of the modified lateral pillar and Stulberg classifications. *J Bone Joint Surg Am* 2004;86(10):2103-2120.

    Intraobserver and interobserver reliability assessments are presented for modified versions of the lateral pillar and Stulberg classifications of LCP disease. Excellent reliability and generalizability were found for both classification systems.

18. Herring JA, Kim HT, Browne R: Legg-Calve-Perthes disease: Part II. Prospective multicenter study of the effect of treatment on outcome. *J Bone Joint Surg Am* 2004;86(10):2121-2134.

    A multicenter study evaluated multiple factors to assess outcome in LCP disease. Age at onset and lateral pillar classification were found to be strongly correlated with outcome.

19. Nathan Sambandam S, Gul A, Shankar R, Goni V: Reliability of radiological classifications used in Legg-

Calve-Perthes disease. *J Pediatr Orthop B* 2006;15(4): 267-270.

Radiologists evaluated the intraobserver and interrater reliability of the Salter-Thompson, lateral pillar, and Catterall classification systems. The lateral pillar classification was found to have the best intraobserver and interobserver reliability.

20. Meehan PL, Angel D, Nelson JM: The Scottish Rite abduction orthosis for the treatment of Legg-Perthes disease: A radiographic analysis. *J Bone Joint Surg Am* 1992;74(1):2-12.

21. Reinker KA: Early diagnosis and treatment of hinge abduction in Legg-Perthes disease. *J Pediatr Orthop* 1996; 16(1):3-9.

22. McAndrew MP, Weinstein SL: A long-term follow-up of Legg-Calvé-Perthes disease. *J Bone Joint Surg Am* 1984; 66(6):860-869.

23. Weinstein SL: Legg-Calvé-Perthes disease: Results of long-term follow-up. *Hip* 1985:28-37.

24. Kim WC, Hiroshima K, Imaeda T: Multicenter study for Legg-Calvé-Perthes disease in Japan. *J Orthop Sci* 2006;11(4):333-341.

A Japanese survey study examined factors that may affect outcome in LCP disease. Lateral pillar classification and age at diagnosis were found to be predictive of outcome. Surgically treated hips had a better outcome than nonsurgically treated hips, but the authors stated they could not determine the optimal treatment method.

25. Wiig O, Terjesen T, Svenningsen S: Prognostic factors and outcome of treatment of Perthes disease: A prospective study of 368 patients with five-year follow up. *J Bone Joint Surg Br* 2008;90(10):1364-1371.

The strongest predictors of outcome were found to be percentage of femoral head affected (less or more than 50%), lateral pillar classification, and patient age at diagnosis. There was no difference in outcome for hips with less than 50% necrosis, regardless of treatment and age at diagnosis. Conversely, femoral osteotomy yielded a significantly better outcome in children who were older than 6 years at diagnosis and had more than 50% necrosis of the femoral head.

26. Little DG, Peat RA, McEvoy A, Williams PR, Smith EJ, Baldock PA: Zoledronic acid treatment results in retention of femoral head structure after traumatic osteonecrosis in young Wistar rats. *J Bone Miner Res* 2003; 18(11):2016-2022.

27. Kim HK, Randall TS, Bian H, Jenkins J, Garces A, Bauss F: Ibandronate for prevention of femoral head deformity after ischemic necrosis of the capital femoral epiphysis in immature pigs. *J Bone Joint Surg Am* 2005; 87(3):550-557.

After an ischemic insult, the effect of ibandronate prophylaxis and postischemic treatment on the femoral head was compared with that of saline injection. Retention of femoral head shape was significantly improved

with both prophylactic and postinjury treatment. However, there was a significant decrease in the length of the nonischemic femur compared with that of noninjured femurs in saline-injected rats. The results were promising, but further work is needed to determine the optimal dose and duration of treatment.

28. Joseph B, Rao N, Mulpuri K, Varghese G, Nair S: How does a femoral varus osteotomy alter the natural evolution of Perthes' disease? *J Pediatr Orthop B* 2005;14(1): 10-15.

The outcomes of the 314 patients with LCP disease who underwent varus-producing femoral osteotomy were compared. The outcomes were better when the surgery was performed early in the fragmentation phase or in the osteonecrosis phase of disease. Of the hips that underwent femoral osteotomy in the osteonecrosis phase, 34% skipped the fragmentation phase altogether and had a shorter course of disease. A decrease in femoral head extrusion and metaphyseal changes also was noted.

29. Kamegaya M, Saisu T, Takazawa M, Nakamura J: Arthrographic indicators for decision making about femoral varus osteotomy in Legg-Calvé-Perthes disease. *J Child Orthop* 2008;2(4):261-267.

A new arthrographic assessment of how well the femoral head slips into the acetabulum appears to be a good predictor of outcome after varus femoral osteotomy for LCP disease. An epiphyseal slip-in index of 20% or more predicted an acceptable outcome with 80% sensitivity, 89% specificity, and a 7.2 likelihood ratio.

30. Shah H, Siddesh ND, Joseph B, Nair SN: Effect of prophylactic trochanteric epiphyseodesis in older children with Perthes' disease. *J Pediatr Orthop* 2009;29(8):889-895.

The effect of greater trochanteric epiphysiodesis on trochanteric overgrowth, range of motion, and development of Trendelenburg gait is noted. The authors were successful in creating a trochanteric arrest in only 60% of the patients, and 10% had overcorrection. No difference in range of motion was found, but the incidence of later Trendelenburg gait was believed to be decreased.

31. Kitakoji T, Hattori T, Kitoh H, Katoh M, Ishiguro N: Which is a better method for Perthes' disease: Femoral varus or Salter osteotomy? *Clin Orthop Relat Res* 2005; 430:163-170.

Femoral varus-producing osteotomy was performed in 46 patients, and Salter osteotomy was performed in 30 patients. There was no significant difference between baseline characteristics, but the sample was nonmatched. No significant difference was found in femoral head sphericity or hip joint congruency.

32. Ishida A, Kuwajima SS, Laredo Filho J, Milani C: Salter innominate osteotomy in the treatment of severe Legg-Calvé-Perthes disease: Clinical and radiographic results in 32 patients (37 hips) at skeletal maturity. *J Pediatr Orthop* 2004;24(3):257-264.

33. Domzalski ME, Glutting J, Bowen JR, Littleton AG: Lateral acetabular growth stimulation following a labral

support procedure in Legg-Calve-Perthes disease. *J Bone Joint Surg Am* 2006;88(7):1458-1466.

A review of 65 hips with unilateral LCP disease found an advantage to increased femoral head coverage and containment over a proximal femoral osteotomy alone. Coverage and depth were increased at 3-year follow-up when the authors' shelf acetabuloplasty procedure was used. Level of evidence: III.

34. Freeman RT, Wainwright AM, Theologis TN, Benson MK: The outcome of patients with hinge abduction in severe Perthes disease treated by shelf acetabuloplasty. *J Pediatr Orthop* 2008;28(6):619-625.

The outcome of shelf acetabuloplasty in unilateral LCP disease was prospectively assessed in 27 children with hinge abduction, more than 50% involvement, Catterall group III or IV classification, and lateral pillar group B or C classification. At an average 5-year follow-up, 24 of 27 hips had an overall good result.

35. Catterall A: The place of valgus extension femoral osteotomy in the late management of children with Perthes' disease. *Orthop Traumatol Rehabil* 2004;6(6):764-769.

36. Myers GJ, Mathur K, O'Hara J: Valgus osteotomy: A solution for late presentation of hinge abduction in Legg-Calvé-Perthes disease. *J Pediatr Orthop* 2008;28(2):169-172.

In this prospective study, 15 patients with unilateral LCP disease underwent femoral valgus osteotomy for hinge abduction. At an average 22-month follow-up, the mean Harris hip score had improved from 48 to 89 points. The score did not significantly improve thereafter (mean total follow-up, 6.5 years).

37. Clohisy JC, St John LC, Nunley RM, Schutz AL, Schoenecker PL: Combined periacetabular and femoral osteotomies for severe hip deformities. *Clin Orthop Relat Res* 2009;467(9):2221-2227.

The results of combined periacetabular osteotomy and proximal femoral osteotomy in hips with severe deformity were compared with the results of isolated periacetabular osteotomy in hips with less severe deformity. The average Harris hip score of patients who underwent the combined procedure had improved from 60.9 to 86.3 at a mean 44-month follow-up; 89% of patients had improvement of at least 10 points, and 75% had a Harris hip score higher than 80. Function was comparable to that of the patients with less severe deformity who underwent isolated periacetabular osteotomy.

Chapter 20

Slipped Capital Femoral Epiphysis

David A. Podeszwa, MD   Daniel J. Sucato, MD, MS

Introduction

Slipped capital femoral epiphysis (SCFE) is one of the most common adolescent hip disorders and one of the most challenging of all hip disorders to treat. The terminology is misleading because in SCFE the femoral epiphysis maintains its normal relationship to the acetabulum, and the femoral neck and shaft become displaced relative to the epiphysis. Most commonly, the metaphysis slips upward and anteriorly, inducing external rotation of the femur. Occasionally, the metaphysis displaces posteriorly or medially so that the femoral epiphysis is in a relatively anterior or lateral (valgus) position.

Epidemiology

The Kids' Inpatient Database, developed by the Healthcare Cost and Utilization Project, contains the inpatient records of the 6.7 million children discharged from US nonrehabilitation community hospitals during 1997 and the 7.3 million children discharged during 2000.[1] This database was used with US Census Bureau data to evaluate the epidemiology of SCFE in children age 9 to 16 years.[1] The overall incidence of SCFE in 1997 and 2000 was found to be 10.80 per 100,000 children. SCFE occurred significantly more frequently in boys than in girls (13.35 and 8.07 per 100,000 children, respectively; the ratio of boys to girls was 1.65). Boys were significantly older than girls at initial presentation (12.7 and 11.2 years, respectively). The average age for both genders was 12.2 years in 1997 and 12.1 years in 2000, 1.5 years younger than earlier reported. The incidence of SCFE was 3.94 times higher in African-American children and 2.53 times higher in Hispanic children than in white children.[1]

The incidence of SCFE in the northeastern United States (17.15 per 100,000 children) was significantly higher than the incidence in the West, South, or Mid-west (12.70, 8.12, or 7.69, respectively, per 100,000 children). Seasonal variations depended on latitude: north of 40° (the latitude of New York, NY), 57.4% of all SCFEs occurred during the summer; south of 40° latitude, 57.3% of all SCFEs occurred during the winter. These variations were independent of race and gender, suggesting an environmental component.[1]

Similar patterns of incidence and age at presentation were reported in Scotland, where an association was found between an increase in obesity and a significant increase in the incidence of SCFE.[2] Between 1981 and 2005, the percentage of overweight 13- to 15-year-olds doubled in Scotland, and the percentage of severely obese adolescents quadrupled. During the same period, the incidence of SCFE increased from 3.78 to 9.66 per 100,000 children, and the mean age at presentation decreased from 13.4 years to 12.6 years in boys and from 12.2 years to 11.6 years in girls.[2]

Etiology

The exact cause of SCFE usually is unknown but most likely is multifactorial. Mechanical, endocrine, and genetic factors may play a role in the development of SCFE. Several mechanical factors unique to the adolescent hip may predispose it to SCFE. The perichondral ring of the proximal femoral physis thins with maturation, thus altering the strength of the physis. The femoral neck of an adolescent with SCFE was found to have relative or absolute retroversion; the inclination of the proximal femoral physis is steeper in adolescents with SCFE, predisposing the hip to increased shear stress across the physis. Complex mathematical models with radiographic measurements of the contralateral hip were used to calculate shear stress and contact stress in 100 patients with a unilateral SCFE and 70 age-matched normal control subjects.[3] In the patients with SCFE, the contralateral hip had a significantly higher average shear stress than the hips of the control subjects, even when normalized for body weight. The inclination of the epiphysis was an average 8.9° more vertical in the contralateral hips of patients with SCFE than in the hips of the control subjects, thus confirming inclination and the associated shear stress as a risk factor.[3]

Common endocrine disorders associated with SCFE are hypothyroidism, conditions treated with growth hormone replacement, and chronic renal failure caused

Neither Dr. Podeszwa nor any immediate family member has received anything of value from or owns stock in a commercial company or institution related directly or indirectly to the subject of this chapter. Dr. Sucato or an immediate family member has received royalties and research or institutional support from Medtronic.

by uncontrolled secondary hyperparathyroidism. The genetic etiology of SCFE has yet to be identified. However, Amish children with SCFE were more likely to have a positive family history than non-Amish children with SCFE, and this finding lends credence to the theory that genetics or a combination of genetic and environmental factors has an influence.[4]

Assessment

A patient with SCFE most commonly is an adolescent boy who is obese; has had a few weeks or months of gradual-onset groin, thigh, or knee pain; and/or has a limp. Because pain referred to the knee may be the only symptom, any adolescent with knee pain must undergo a clinical and radiographic evaluation of the hips to rule out SCFE. The physical examination reveals ambulation with the affected foot externally rotated and a lower extremity resting position in external rotation. Flexion of the hip always is accompanied by obligate abduction and external rotation, with limited and painful internal rotation of the hip.

Stability or instability is the most clinically pertinent distinction in SCFE. The determination of physeal stability is based on the patient's ability to bear weight on the affected lower extremity during the initial emergency department or clinic visit. A patient with a stable SCFE is able to bear full or partial weight, with or without crutches, but a patient with unstable SCFE cannot bear any weight.[5] A patient with unstable SCFE may have had weeks or months of prodromal hip or knee pain that concluded with a sudden, fracturelike episode with severe pain and inability to bear weight, typically after relatively trivial trauma. Any attempt to assess the range of motion of the affected extremity elicits severe pain. The risk of osteonecrosis is as high as 47% in patients with unstable SCFE.[5] Classification of the SCFE as stable or unstable can influence the method of treatment; open reduction or fixation in situ using two screws may be necessary for an unstable SCFE.

AP and frog lateral plain radiographs of both hips are the primary imaging studies needed to diagnose SCFE. Widening and irregularity of the physis are the earliest radiographic signs; displacement may not be evident. In a normal hip, a line drawn on the AP radiograph tangential to the superior femoral neck (the Klein line) should intersect the lateral capital epiphysis. In a hip with the posterior displacement typical of SCFE, this line either intersects a smaller portion of the epiphysis or does not intersect it at all. The frog lateral radiograph usually is adequate for confirming SCFE because most slips are posterior. Ultrasonography, CT, and MRI generally are not needed for diagnosing SCFE. If radiographs are negative but the patient has symptoms, a body habitus, and a physical examination consistent with SCFE, MRI may be useful to detect physeal widening and irregularity, which are the earliest signs of SCFE.

Treatment

Stable SCFE

The goal of the initial treatment of any SCFE is to stabilize the epiphysis and prevent further displacement. The current standard treatment for a stable SCFE is in situ fixation under fluoroscopic guidance, using a single cannulated screw placed in the center of the epiphysis. This procedure can be successfully done on a fracture table or a radiolucent tabletop, with the affected lower extremity draped free.

A porcine model of SCFE was used to determine if a fully threaded cancellous screw provides greater stability than a partially threaded screw.[6] A 30° posterior slip was created, and a 7.3-mm–diameter screw (fully threaded or 16-mm partially threaded) was placed into the center-center position of the femoral head, with three threads crossing the physis and loaded in a posteroinferior direction to simulate slip progression. Increased loading was associated with increased epiphyseal displacement, but no significant biomechanical difference was identified between the use of a fully threaded or partially threaded screw. Nonetheless, the authors suggested that using a fully threaded screw is reasonable because bone healing around a fully threaded screw may provide greater stability, and implant removal may be easier.[6]

An adult cadaver model was used to evaluate screw head impingement on the acetabular rim during hip flexion after fixation of simulated moderate and severe SCFE.[7] A single, centrally placed screw was placed perpendicular to the simulated physis. In moderate SCFE (50° posterior, 10° inferior), the screw head caused a contour change in the acetabular labrum at 70° of hip flexion; 30° of external rotation of the femur was required to achieve 90° of hip flexion. In severe SCFE (80° posterior, 15° inferior), the screw head caused a labral contour change at 50° of hip flexion; 55° of external rotation was required to achieve 90° of hip flexion. Screw heads placed lateral to the intertrochanteric line, as seen on a fluoroscopic AP radiograph, were unlikely to impinge on the acetabular rim.[7] Therefore, avoiding placement of a screw perpendicular to the physis of a moderate or severe SCFE may decrease the risk of postoperative acetabular impingement and pain (Figure 1).

Unstable SCFE

The standard initial surgical treatment of an unstable SCFE is in situ pinning (with or without capsulotomy), or some form of open reduction. For in situ pinning of the unstable epiphysis, there has been debate over the use of single-screw or double-screw fixation. Single-screw fixation has been associated with postoperative slip progression, and double-screw fixation has been associated with an increased risk of complications such as pin penetration and chondrolysis. In a bovine shear model, double-screw fixation was found to be 33%

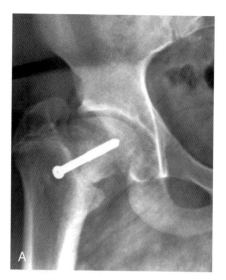

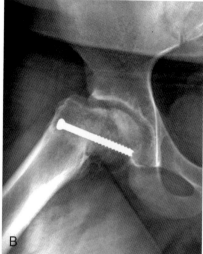

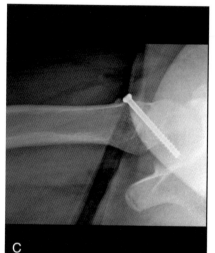

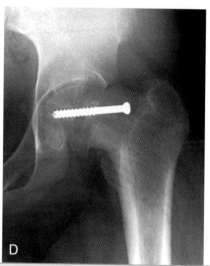

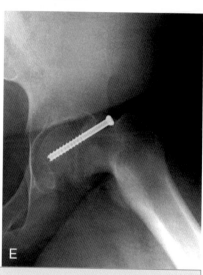

Figure 1   AP (**A**), frog lateral (**B**), and cross-table lateral (**C**) radiographs showing in situ screw fixation of a hip with a severe SCFE. The screw was not placed perpendicular to the physis, and the screw head is lateral to the intertrochanteric line; the patient is at risk of femoral acetabular impingement secondary to the deformity, but screw impingement is unlikely. AP (**D**) and frog lateral (**E**) radiographs showing screw impingement after in situ fixation of a hip with a severe SCFE. The screw is anterior in the neck, and the screw head is medial to the intertrochanteric line.

stiffer than single screw fixation.[8] However, when the same model was used under physiologic cyclical loading, there was no significant difference between single- and double-screw fixation.[9] The torsional stability of single- and double-screw fixation was not compared. Single-screw fixation was recommended because the risk of complications from using a second screw outweighed the biomechanical benefits.[8,9]

An immature bovine model with a reduced and a nonreduced slip was used in a torsional mode to test the stiffness of double-screw fixation. The goal was to reproduce the clinical conditions of in situ screw fixation of an unstable SCFE.[10] Short-threaded, 6.5-mm cannulated screws were placed perpendicular to the physis in a compression mode (with all threads placed across the physis). In the nonreduced model, double-screw fixation resulted in a 25% increase in axial stiff-

ness under shear and a 312% increase in torsional stiffness, in comparison with single-screw fixation. In the reduced model, double-screw fixation increased torsional stiffness by 137%. The authors concluded that the increased rotational stability of double-screw fixation justified its use in the stabilization of an unstable SCFE.[10]

An immature porcine model was used to determine whether the pattern of double-screw fixation affected the stability of the construct.[11] Mild-to-moderate unstable SCFEs were created and stabilized using one or two 7.3-mm stainless steel cannulated screws with a 16-mm thread length. A posteroinferior-directed physiologic load was applied because it was considered more relevant than a pure shear load. Compared with single-screw fixation, the double-screw constructs were 66% stiffer and 66% stronger. There was no significant dif-

4: Lower Extremity

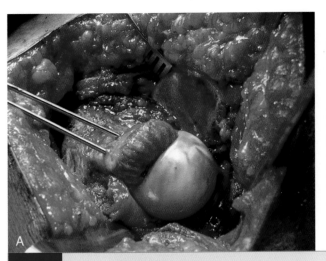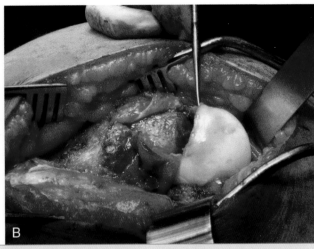

Figure 2   **A**, The typical appearance of an unstable SCFE at the time of surgical dislocation. The femoral epiphysis is severely displaced, and the metaphysis is prominent. **B**, A periosteal and retinacular sleeve created during open reduction of an unstable SCFE. The femoral neck has been shortened to allow reduction of the femoral epiphysis without tension on the retinacular periosteal sleeve.

ference between different double-screw configurations. The authors concluded that using a double-screw construct for an unstable SCFE is reasonable, but the biomechanical benefit must be weighed against the increased risk of screw-related complications.[11]

Double-screw in situ fixation for unstable SCFE has had very good clinical outcomes, according to recent reports. Twenty-eight patients with 30 unstable SCFEs underwent urgent reduction and fixation, usually 12 to 24 hours after the onset of acute symptoms. Two 6.5-mm cannulated screws were used, with two exceptions.[12] Positional reduction was accepted in 25 hips; an open arthrotomy was necessary in 5, with reduction to the preacute position under direct visualization and without femoral neck shortening. A percutaneous arthrotomy was done in an additional 16 hips.[12] At an average 5.5-year follow-up (range, 2 to 11.2 years), 4 hips (13%) had radiographic findings consistent with osteonecrosis, and 3 of these hips required at least one additional surgery. None of the hips with osteonecrosis underwent open capsulotomy. Two additional patients (7%) had mild pain with prolonged sitting, 6 (20%) had a mild limp, and 2 (7%) had a moderate limp. There was no statistical association between the development of osteonecrosis and age, duration of prodromal symptoms, time to reduction, severity of slip, presence of an arthrotomy, or noncompliance with weight-bearing restrictions.[12]

Open reduction has been studied as a means of improving the extent of epiphyseal reduction and, more importantly, lessening the risk of osteonecrosis. A recent study found that urgent open reduction of an unstable SCFE is safe and that it results in a near-anatomic alignment of the femoral epiphysis, almost eliminating the need for secondary procedures to correct residual deformity.[13] Sixty-four consecutive incidences of unstable SCFE were studied in patients who

had experienced a relatively low-energy fall followed by acute hip pain, with radiographic evidence of SCFE and ultrasonographic evidence of a joint effusion. All patients were treated with an anterior arthrotomy, evacuation of the intra-articular effusion or hematoma, controlled gentle reduction (with no attempt to reduce a preexisting chronic SCFE), and fixation with smooth Kirschner wires. For gentle reduction, the surgeon's finger palpates the gap between the metaphysis and epiphysis, taking care to avoid any abrupt motions, while the hip is carefully flexed, abducted, and internally rotated. Only the unstable portion of the slip is reduced, leaving deformity secondary to any preexisting slip.[13] Only three patients (5%) developed partial osteonecrosis after surgery, and there was no relationship to the severity of slip. All incidences of osteonecrosis were recognized within 6 months after the reduction, and all required an additional surgical intervention. At an average 4.9-year follow-up (range, 1.5 to 8.67 years), the average Iowa Hip Score was 94.5 on a 100-point scale.[13]

A modified Dunn procedure is used as a more aggressive means of reducing an unstable slip.[14,15] The advantage of this procedure is that an extensive subperiosteal exposure and an extended retinacular soft-tissue flap can be created to allow circumferential femoral neck visualization, removal of the callus, and shortening of the femoral neck, thus relieving tension on the retinacular vessels and allowing a safe anatomic reduction of the femoral head (**Figure 2**). In the short term, there was no osteonecrosis after capital realignment with the modified Dunn procedure in 12 moderately or severely unstable SCFEs at two institutions.[16] A normal or near-normal α angle or slip angle was restored in every hip, with a near-normal hip range of motion (**Figure 3**).

If in situ percutaneous pinning is chosen, an additional capsulotomy may lessen the risk of osteonecro-

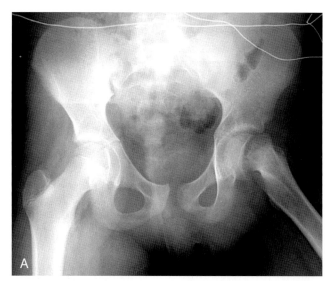

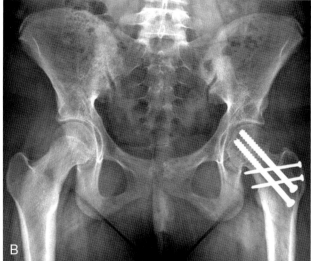

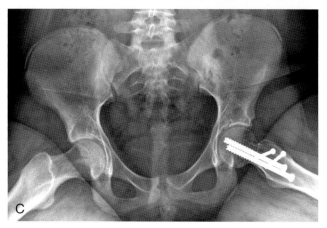

Figure 3 | **A,** AP pelvic radiograph showing a severe, unstable left SCFE. AP (**B**) and frog lateral (**C**) pelvic radiographs showing the left hip 2 years after capital realignment using the modified Dunn procedure. There is near-anatomic alignment of the proximal femur, with no evidence of osteonecrosis.

sis. A study that measured the intracapsular pressure of hips with unstable SCFE found that the pressure increased to a mean 75 mm Hg with reduction and was significantly greater than the mean pressure of 23 mm Hg in the contralateral hip. The authors concluded that the increased pressure would have a tamponade effect on the retinacular vessels and recommended opening the capsule with pinning.[17]

Reconstruction of Residual Deformity

All SCFE deformities distort the proximal femoral anatomy. The offset of the femoral head and neck is decreased as a result of femoral head retroversion and the presence of a metaphyseal prominence. This metaphyseal deformity has been recognized as a source of femoral acetabular impingement (FAI) and hip pain. Significant intra-articular pathology can result, including labral and articular cartilage damage, leading to premature osteoarthritis in the hip.[18]

Deformity correction can be challenging because often the patient is obese and the deformity is severe. The Southwick or Imhauser intertrochanteric osteotomy has been the procedure of choice for correcting deformity

associated with a moderate or severe slip angle. These procedures are successful in correcting the deformity and improving hip mechanics, thereby decreasing pain and improving function, with a low risk of osteonecrosis.[19,20]

CT-based simulation of intertrochanteric corrective osteotomy for SCFE with a moderate or severe slip angle found that a uniplanar proximal femoral flexion osteotomy and a multiplanar proximal femoral osteotomy led to similar improvement in hip range of motion.[21] However, the improvement in hip flexion, unlike the improvement in abduction and internal rotation, was unsatisfactory for the requirements of daily activities. This study finding highlights the need for preoperative planning to consider all factors that can affect postoperative range of motion, including metaphyseal prominence, proximal femoral varus, and femoral retroversion, as well as the slip angle.[21]

In an alternative osteotomy and fixation technique, a transverse percutaneous subtrochanteric osteotomy is used with external fixation.[22] This technique was used to correct severe residual deformity associated with pain, limp, and limited function in 13 patients. At a minimum 32-month follow-up, 12 patients had good or excellent function, and 11 patients had good or excellent pain relief. The rate of pin tract infection was higher than rates reported in the literature and was believed to be related to the body habitus of the typical patient. The significant advantage of this procedure may be the flexibility it offers for changing the correction or adding a lengthening procedure.[22]

The development of the Ganz surgical technique for hip dislocation greatly expanded the appreciation of and ability to treat intra-articular pathology secondary to changes in proximal femoral and acetabular anatomy.[15] The association between FAI and significant articular cartilage and labral injury, particularly the prominent femoral metaphysis, has been well documented through the use of this technique.[18] An early report of the surgical dislocation technique, with or without concomitant intertrochanteric osteotomy to treat FAI associated with SCFE, found no observed osteonecrosis, trochanteric nonunion, or other major complications at an average 12-month follow-up.[23] This technique allows an osteoplasty of the metaphyseal prominence to be done in addition to the intertrochanteric osteotomy, possibly improving the impingement at the site of deformity. Identifying the ideal patients and indications for this procedure will require more study, with longer follow-up.

A disadvantage of a proximal femoral osteotomy is that the surgical correction is distant from the site of deformity. Techniques for subcapital reorientation have been associated with rates of osteonecrosis as high as 100%. A modified Dunn procedure has been used through a surgical dislocation approach to achieve capital realignment of moderate or severe residual deformity of stable SCFE.[16] This technically demanding procedure allows full exposure of the proximal femur and subperiosteal dissection of the entire femoral neck, thus protecting the femoral head blood supply. At a minimum 1-year follow-up, patients had excellent correction of the capital alignment, with no osteonecrosis or chondrolysis and the restoration of near-normal hip range of motion. The procedure also allows labral and articular cartilage damage to be assessed and treated. Twenty-five of 26 stable SCFEs were found to have articular cartilage damage, and longer symptom duration was associated with the presence of cartilage damage.[16]

Prophylactic Pinning

Between 20% and 40% of all patients with SCFE have bilateral involvement, and approximately 50% of these patients have bilateral SCFE at their initial clinical visit. Patients who initially have unilateral involvement typically develop a contralateral SCFE within 18 months. The arguments for prophylactic pinning include the high risk of an asymptomatic contralateral slip, which is associated with osteoarthritic changes at long-term follow-up, and the prevention of an unstable contralateral slip, which is associated with osteonecrosis. These advantages must be weighed against the risks and cost of an additional procedure.

Of 227 patients with a unilateral SCFE, 82 (36%) developed a contralateral slip, 18 (22%) of which were moderate or severe; 5 patients (6%) developed osteonecrosis or chondrolysis of the hip.[24] Moderate or severe residual deformity and the development of osteonecrosis or chondrolysis are associated with early osteoarthrosis. Because of the great likelihood of a contralateral slip, the risk of early osteoarthrosis, and the established complications associated with a contralateral slip, prophylactic pinning was recommended as preferable to observation and symptomatic treatment.[24]

Although there are no widely accepted guidelines for determining when a contralateral slip should be pinned, the procedure should be strongly considered for some patients. A patient with chronic renal failure or an endocrinopathy-related SCFE is at the highest risk for bilateral involvement. Clinical and radiographic assessment every 4 to 6 months is mandatory if prophylactic pinning is not done. Prophylactic pinning should be strongly considered for all patients younger than 12 years. A score of 16 points or lower on the modified Oxford bone age assessment or the presence of an open triradiate cartilage is an excellent predictor of a subsequent contralateral slip.[25] A recent review of 90 patients with SCFE, 70 of whom had unilateral SCFE, reported each patient's age at presentation, sex, race, modified Oxford bone age score, and open or closed triradiate cartilage status. Sixteen patients with unilateral SCFE (23%) developed a contralateral SCFE after an average of 11 months. Chronologic age was the only significant predictor of a contralateral slip. All girls younger than 10 years and all boys younger than 12 years who initially had a unilateral SCFE developed a contralateral SCFE.[26]

Summary

SCFE is a relatively common condition among adolescents. The patient typically is obese; has hip, thigh, or knee pain; and has an external foot progression angle. The keys to diagnosis are a low index of suspicion, a physical examination that reveals obligate external rotation with hip flexion, and confirmation by AP and frog lateral pelvic radiographs. Stable SCFE usually is successfully treated with in situ pinning using one screw. Unstable SCFE often requires two screws to prevent delayed slip progression. Some methods of open treatment with a safe or partial reduction and/or opening of the capsule appear to lessen the risk of osteonecrosis. The high incidence of osteonecrosis in unstable SCFE and improved recognition of FAI with residual deformity have led to the increased use of more aggressive surgical approaches that include open reduction and stable fixation, with early successful results. A young patient with a low modified Oxford bone age score and open triradiate cartilage should be considered for prophylactic pinning of the contralateral hip.

Annotated References

1. Lehmann CL, Arons RR, Loder RT, Vitale MG: The epidemiology of slipped capital femoral epiphysis: An update. *J Pediatr Orthop* 2006;26(3):286-290.

    This study reports geographic, racial, and seasonal variations in the incidence of SCFE using the Kids' Inpatient Database, coupled with US Census Bureau data for 1997 and 2000.

2. Murray AW, Wilson NI: Changing incidence of slipped capital femoral epiphysis: A relationship with obesity? *J Bone Joint Surg Br* 2008;90(1):92-94.

    The incidence of SCFE increased 2.5 times over two decades and was strongly correlated with a similar increase in adolescent obesity. The mean age at diagnosis fell significantly for both boys and girls.

3. Zupanc O, Krizancic M, Daniel M, et al: Shear stress in epiphyseal growth plate is a risk factor for slipped capital femoral epiphysis. *J Pediatr Orthop* 2008;28(4):444-451.

    Mathematical models compared shear stress and contact hip stress of the contralateral hip in patients with SCFE to age- and gender-matched patients with normal hips. Hips in the patients with SCFE had significantly higher average shear stress and more vertically inclined physeal angles.

4. Loder RT, Nechleba J, Sanders JO, Doyle P: Idiopathic slipped capital femoral epiphysis in Amish children. *J Bone Joint Surg Am* 2005;87(3):543-549.

    Amish children with SCFE were not obese and had a significantly higher rate of familial involvement compared with non-Amish children. This finding may reflect a genetic or environmental component in SCFE or an interaction between them. Level of evidence: II.

5. Loder RT, Richards BS, Shapiro PS, Reznick LR, Aronson DD: Acute slipped capital femoral epiphysis: The importance of physeal stability. *J Bone Joint Surg Am* 1993;75(8):1134-1140.

6. Miyanji F, Mahar A, Oka R, Pring M, Wenger D: Biomechanical comparison of fully and partially threaded screws for fixation of slipped capital femoral epiphysis. *J Pediatr Orthop* 2008;28(1):49-52.

    Although no biomechanical difference was identified between fully and partially threaded screws for stabilization of the femoral head, there may be an unproved clinical benefit to using a fully threaded screw.

7. Goodwin RC, Mahar AT, Oswald TS, Wenger DR: Screw head impingement after in situ fixation in moderate and severe slipped capital femoral epiphysis. *J Pediatr Orthop* 2007;27(3):319-325.

    A biomechanical study evaluating screw head impingement after in situ fixation perpendicular to the physis of a simulated moderate or severe SCFE found that screw heads placed lateral to the intertrochanteric line were unlikely to impinge on the acetabulum.

8. Karol LA, Doane RM, Cornicelli SF, Zak PA, Haut RC, Manoli A II: Single versus double screw fixation for treatment of slipped capital femoral epiphysis: A biomechanical analysis. *J Pediatr Orthop* 1992;12(6):741-745.

9. Kibiloski LJ, Doane RM, Karol LA, Haut RC, Loder RT: Biomechanical analysis of single- versus double-screw fixation in slipped capital femoral epiphysis at physiological load levels. *J Pediatr Orthop* 1994;14(5):627-630.

10. Segal LS, Jacobson JA, Saunders MM: Biomechanical analysis of in situ single versus double screw fixation in a nonreduced slipped capital femoral epiphysis model. *J Pediatr Orthop* 2006;26(4):479-485.

    In a bovine model, double-screw fixation was 312% stiffer under torsional loading than single-screw fixation in a nonreduced SCFE and 137% stiffer in a reduced SCFE. The increased stability may warrant double-screw use in unstable SCFE.

11. Kishan S, Upasani V, Mahar A, et al: Biomechanical stability of single-screw versus two-screw fixation of an unstable slipped capital femoral epiphysis model: Effect of screw position in the femoral neck. *J Pediatr Orthop* 2006;26(5):601-605.

    A biomechanical evaluation of one- and two-screw fixation of unstable SCFEs using physiologic loading found that stabilization with a two-screw construct was stiffer and stronger than stabilization with a one-screw construct.

12. Chen RC, Schoenecker PL, Dobbs MB, Luhmann SJ, Szymanski DA, Gordon JE: Urgent reduction, fixation, and arthrotomy for unstable slipped capital femoral epiphysis. *J Pediatr Orthop* 2009;29(7):687-694.

    This review of 30 unstable SCFEs found that urgent positional reduction with an arthrotomy (percutaneous or open) and fixation with two cannulated screws resulted in a low rate of slip progression (3%) and osteonecrosis (13%). Level of evidence: IV.

13. Parsch K, Weller S, Parsch D: Open reduction and smooth Kirschner wire fixation for unstable slipped capital femoral epiphysis. *J Pediatr Orthop* 2009;29(1):1-8.

    Hip capsulotomy with evacuation of hemarthrosis and gentle reduction of an unstable SCFE followed by smooth wire fixation can be done safely (osteonecrosis, 4.7%), with an excellent functional outcome. Level of evidence: IV.

14. Leunig M, Slongo T, Kleinschmidt M, Ganz R: Subcapital correction osteotomy in slipped capital femoral epiphysis by means of surgical hip dislocation. *Oper Orthop Traumatol* 2007;19(4):389-410.

    The surgical technique for subcapital correction of SCFE using hip dislocation is described, with a report of the early Bernese experience.

15. Ganz R, Gill TJ, Gautier E, Ganz K, Krügel N, Berlemann U: Surgical dislocation of the adult hip a technique with full access to the femoral head and

acetabulum without the risk of avascular necrosis. *J Bone Joint Surg Br* 2001;83(8):1119-1124.

16. Ziebarth K, Zilkens C, Spencer S, Leunig M, Ganz R, Kim YJ: Capital realignment for moderate and severe SCFE using a modified Dunn procedure. *Clin Orthop Relat Res* 2009;467(3):704-716.

    Short-term follow-up of 40 patients treated with a modified capital reorientation procedure through a surgical dislocation approach found that the technique is safe, has an acceptable complication rate, and allows full correction of moderate and severe slips.

17. Herrera-Soto JA, Duffy MF, Birnbaum MA, Vander Have KL: Increased intracapsular pressures after unstable slipped capital femoral epiphysis. *J Pediatr Orthop* 2008;28(7):723-728.

    Compared with uninvolved hips, hips with an unstable SCFE had a significantly increased intracapsular pressure, which could be reduced by a percutaneous arthrotomy. Manipulation of an unstable SCFE causes a significant increase in the intracapsular pressure.

18. Leunig M, Casillas MM, Hamlet M, et al: Slipped capital femoral epiphysis: Early mechanical damage to the acetabular cartilage by a prominent femoral metaphysis. *Acta Orthop Scand* 2000;71(4):370-375.

19. Southwick WO: Osteotomy through the lesser trochanter for slipped capital femoral epiphysis. *J Bone Joint Surg Am* 1967;49(5):807-835.

20. Imhauser G: Zur Pathogenese and Therapie der jugendlichen Hüftkopflösung. *Z Orthop Ihre Grenzgeb* 1957; 88:3.

21. Mamisch TC, Kim YJ, Richolt J, et al: Range of motion after computed tomography-based simulation of intertrochanteric corrective osteotomy in cases of slipped capital femoral epiphysis: Comparison of uniplanar flexion osteotomy and multiplanar flexion, valgisation, and rotational osteotomies. *J Pediatr Orthop* 2009; 29(4):336-340.

    A computer-model comparison of different intertrochanteric osteotomy techniques found an increased hip range of motion with each procedure, but the resultant hip flexion is not acceptable for daily activities.

22. Tjoumakaris FP, Wallach DM, Davidson RS: Subtrochanteric osteotomy effectively treats femoroacetabular impingement after slipped capital femoral epiphysis. *Clin Orthop Relat Res* 2007;464:230-237.

    The clinical and radiographic outcomes of 13 patients are presented, at an average 43-month follow-up after treatment for residual deformity of severe SCFE with a percutaneous subtrochanteric osteotomy using external fixation.

23. Spencer S, Millis MB, Kim YJ: Early results of treatment of hip impingement syndrome in slipped capital femoral epiphysis and pistol grip deformity of the femoral head-neck junction using the surgical dislocation technique. *J Pediatr Orthop* 2006;26(3):281-285.

    At an average 12-month follow-up of 19 patients who underwent a surgical dislocation for residual deformity of SCFE or a pistol grip deformity, patients with preexisting cartilage damage had a worse outcome. The procedure was found to be safe.

24. Yildirim Y, Bautista S, Davidson RS: Chondrolysis, osteonecrosis, and slip severity in patients with subsequent contralateral slipped capital femoral epiphysis. *J Bone Joint Surg Am* 2008;90(3):485-492.

    A high prevalence of contralateral slip (36%) was found; 6% of contralateral slips developed chondrolysis or osteonecrosis, and 21% of contralateral hips with moderate or severe SCFE had a potential for poor outcome because of the risk of osteoarthritis.

25. Stasikelis PJ, Sullivan CM, Phillips WA, Polard JA: Slipped capital femoral epiphysis: Prediction of contralateral involvement. *J Bone Joint Surg Am* 1996;78(8): 1149-1155.

26. Riad J, Bajelidze G, Gabos PG: Bilateral slipped capital femoral epiphysis: Predictive factors for contralateral slip. *J Pediatr Orthop* 2007;27(4):411-414.

    Of 70 patients with a unilateral SCFE, 16 (23%) developed a contralateral SCFE. Chronologic age (younger than 10 years in girls and 12 years in boys) was the only significant predictor of a contralateral slip. Modified Oxford bone age score and the presence of triradiate cartilage were not predictive.

4: Lower Extremity

Chapter 21

Congenital Deformities of the Knee

John D. Polousky, MD

Introduction

Congenital deformities about the knee are unusual. Diagnosing and treating these deformities in infants is challenging for several reasons: most children are not ambulatory until approximately age 12 months, so there is no noticeable disability at birth; most of the skeleton surrounding the knee is unossified, so that a diagnosis from plain radiographs is difficult; and subtle differences in length and alignment may not be readily apparent in a newborn. This chapter outlines the clinical features and treatment of the more common congenital deformities occurring around the knee.

Congenital Knee Dislocation

Congenital dislocation of the knee ranges from a simple hyperextension deformity to a complete dislocation of the tibiofemoral joint. The etiology of congenital knee dislocation is not well understood. The anatomic findings include a shortened and fibrotic quadriceps mechanism, anterior displacement of the hamstring tendons and iliotibial band, contracted anterior capsule, loss of the suprapatellar pouch, and absence or abnormality of the cruciate ligaments. Congenital knee dislocation has been most frequently associated with female sex, premature birth, or a breech delivery presentation. Several other abnormalities are associated with congenital dislocation of the knee, including congenital dislocation of the hip, myelodysplasia, arthrogryposis, Larsen syndrome, and achondroplasia.[1-3]

Congenital knee dislocations are classified based on severity. Recurvatum is defined as hyperextension greater than 15° with full flexion and normal radiographic findings. Subluxation is hyperextension greater than 15° without full flexion or with a component of instability. Dislocation is instability with 100% radiographic anterior displacement of the tibia with respect to the femur (Figure 1).

The mainstay of treatment is serial manipulation and splinting in flexion, beginning within 6 weeks of the patient's birth. Nonsurgical treatment leads to a good or excellent long-term result if begun early. Surgical treatment, including quadriceps lengthening, capsular release, and reduction, is reserved for an older patient or a patient with an unsuccessful closed reduction.[1-3] The use of a minimally invasive technique combined with casting recently was described for treating patients with Larsen syndrome.[4]

Congenital Patellar Dislocation

Congenital patellar dislocation is an irreducible lateral dislocation that is present but often undiagnosed in a newborn. Congenital patellar dislocation sometimes is defined to include a similar condition in which the patella is located in the trochlear groove at birth and subsequently develops lateral subluxation, which becomes a fixed dislocation during childhood. Congential patellar dislocation is a rare condition that must be differentiated from the more common obligatory subluxation, which develops later in childhood and adolescence. Although congenital patellar dislocation can occur in isolation, commonly it is associated with Larson syndrome, arthrogryposis, diastrophic dysplasia, nail-patella syndrome, Down syndrome, or Ellis–van Creveld syndrome.[5]

The pathoanatomy of congenital patellar dislocation is characterized by thickened, tight lateral soft-tissue structures, including the iliotibial band and lateral retinaculum. In contrast, the medial soft tissues are atrophic. The quadriceps is shortened, and the patella is situated proximally. The osseous abnormalities include a dysplastic trochlea and a small patella, which is delayed in its ossification and lateral tibial torsion. Often, subluxation of the quadriceps posterior to the center of rotation of the knee joint causes the quadriceps to act as a flexor.[6] With continued growth, genu valgum may develop as a result of the lateral soft-tissue tether.

Congenital patellar dislocation can be difficult to diagnose but should be suspected in children with knee flexion contractures, delayed walking, genu valgum, external tibial torsion, or an associated condition or syndrome. Physical examination reveals that the femoral condyles are abnormally prominent to palpation. The patella is small and difficult to palpate laterally. Patients generally have a flexion contracture and very limited active flexion. Functionally, congenital patellar dislocation can mimic a neuromuscular disorder such as cerebral palsy.[5] In a child younger than 3 years, plain

Dr. Polousky or an immediate family member serves as a paid consultant to or is an employee of Orthopediatrics.

4: Lower Extremity

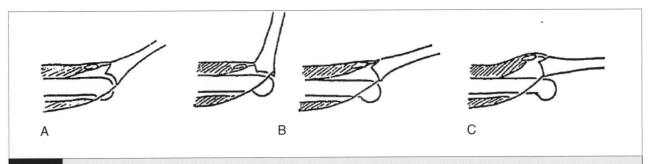

Figure 1 Schematic drawings showing the classification of congenital knee dislocation. **A,** Hyperextension (greater than 15°, with full flexion). **B,** Subluxation (hyperextension greater than 15°, with a relatively severe hyperextension deformity [*left*] or instability [*right*]). **C,** Dislocation (instability, with variable extension and flexion). (Adapted with permission from Laurence M: Genu recurvatum congenitum. *J Bone Joint Surg Br* 1967;49B:121.)

radiographs are not diagnostic because the patella has not yet ossified. Ultrasonography or MRI can reveal the position of the patella.

Nonsurgical measures cannot correct congenital patellar dislocation. Some authors consider this condition to be benign and recommend observation, but most recommend early surgical correction (**Figure 2**). Multiple procedures have been described, most of which involve extensive release of the contracted lateral structures, extensor mechanism realignment, tightening of the lax medial structures, and repositioning of the tibial attachment of the patellar tendon.[7-9] More limited procedures to reposition the patella and augment the medial structures tend to be inadequate, having high rates of recurrence. Remodeling of the trochlea can occur when the surgical reduction is done in a young child. In the recommended Andrish technique,[7] the lateral retinaculum is divided between the oblique and transverse layers so that it can be lengthened and repaired. The vastus lateralis is dissected sharply from the intermuscular septum and advanced proximally on the quadriceps tendon. Distally, patellomeniscal ligaments are released. Patella alta is corrected by lengthening the quadriceps tendon and shortening the patellar tendon. Finally, the attenuated medial structures are augmented by a medial patellofemoral ligament reconstruction in which the semitendinosus tendon is rerouted through a slip in the proximal medial collateral ligament and attached to the patella. With adequate release, distal realignment usually is not necessary. Avoiding distal realignment is advantageous in children because the surgical options are limited by the tibial apophysis. However, the Roux-Goldthwait procedure is a viable option.

Congenital Pseudarthrosis of the Tibia

Congenital pseudarthrosis of the tibia (CPT) is a relatively rare condition that appears in infancy or early childhood and is characterized by anterolateral bowing and variable shortening of the tibia. CPT may be present with a true pseudarthrosis at birth. A fracture frequently occurs during childhood, and achieving and maintaining a union can be challenging. CPT is associated with neurofibromatosis type I; approximately 6% of children with neurofibromatosis type I have CPT, and approximately 55% of children with CPT have neurofibromatosis type I. Anterolateral bowing is often the first recognized manifestation of neurofibromatosis type I. Although multiple classification systems for CPT have been proposed, they are based on radiographic appearance, and no correlation with outcomes has been found.[10]

The etiology of CPT is unclear. Histologically, the pseudarthrosis site consists of thick, abnormal periosteum and fibrovascular tissue. Neurofibromas have not been found to be part of the lesion. Some authors have suggested that CPT is primarily a disorder of the periosteum. The initial assessment of a child with suspected CPT should include gross and radiographic examination of the lower limbs. The skin should be inspected for café au lait spots. A diagnosis of CPT should be followed by a diagnostic workup for neurofibromatosis.

The treatment of CPT is one of the most challenging undertakings in pediatric orthopaedics. The goals are to prevent fracture until skeletal maturity (if it has not been reached), achieve and maintain union, and minimize the angular deformity and length discrepancy. The patient's family should be cautioned from the beginning of treatment that the condition may require multiple surgical procedures and, ultimately, amputation.

In children with anterolateral bowing alone, full-time bracing with a custom orthosis during weight-bearing activities is indicated to prevent fracture. Bracing is continued until the child reaches skeletal maturity. Unfortunately, compliance with bracing is difficult to quantify and often is a therapeutic obstacle.

Many surgical procedures have been described to correct fracture in CPT. The principles of surgical correction consider both mechanical stability and biology. In general, the area of pseudarthrosis is resected to a more normal-appearing section of bone, the defect is shortened and grafted with bone, and the segments are stabilized. A variety of means can be used, including intramedullary nailing, vascularized fibular grafting, and Ilizarov lengthening and transport techniques.

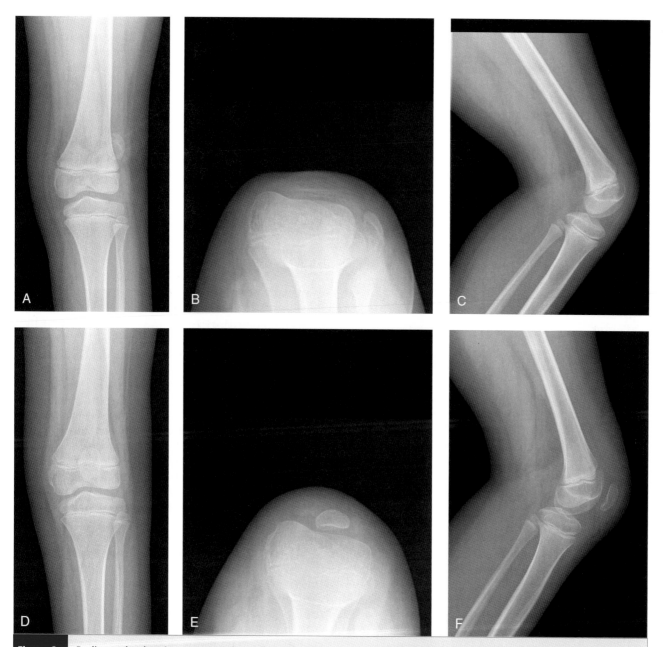

Figure 2 Radiographs showing congenital patellar dislocation in a 9-year-old girl before and after surgical reduction and stabilization. AP (**A**), sunrise (**B**), and lateral (**C**) radiographs showing the laterally dislocated patella. AP (**D**), sunrise (**E**), and lateral (**F**) radiographs showing the patellar position after stabilization.

Long-term results of resection of the pseudarthrosis, autologous bone grafting, and intramedullary fixation have been reported.[11] Union was initially achieved in 18 of 21 patients, but 12 of the 18 patients had a fracture after the initial union, requiring further treatment. Refracture was associated with earlier removal of the intramedullary nail after initial union. Limb-length discrepancy and valgus deformity were frequently found at follow-up. Five patients ultimately underwent amputation, two because of persistent pseudarthrosis and three because of marked deformity and/or limb-length

discrepancy. A comparison study of intramedullary nailing and bone grafting found that better results and union rates were achieved when the procedure was combined with resection of the pseudarthrosis and appropriate shortening of both the tibia and fibula to facilitate apposition of more normal bone than when the procedure was done without resection.[12]

A refracture-free survival rate of 47% was found 5 years after Ilizarov osteosynthesis, with no subsequent change.[13] In 12 of 23 patients, two or more surgical procedures were required after the initial osteosynthesis operation. Risk of refracture was associated with age younger than 4 years, small tibia diameter, and persistence of the fibula pseudarthrosis.

There has been recent interest in using recombinant human bone morphogenetic protein (rhBMP) to increase union rates in CPT. When rhBMP-2 was used in conjunction with resection of the pseudarthrosis, autogenous bone grafting, and intramedullary nailing, five of seven patients had initial union. Union was maintained in four patients at a mean 5.4-year follow-up.[14] No adverse effects of the rhBMP were noted. However, the use of rhBMP for this purpose has not been approved by the US Food and Drug Administration.

Although rates of union are high after the initial procedure, subsequent refracture and progressive deformity are not infrequent. Long-term intramedullary stabilization of the tibia and treatment of the fibular pseudarthrosis are recommended for maintaining union. Stabilization of the ankle joint with intramedullary fixation is controversial.

Posterior Medial Bow of the Tibia

Posterior medial bow of the tibia is a congenital malformation associated with calcaneovalgus foot deformity. Although the child's deformity at birth is distressing to families and health care providers, the condition tends to diminish greatly during the first 12 months of life. Posterior medial bow is not associated with neurofibromatosis and does not carry the risk of fracture characteristic of anterolateral bowing. Treatment generally is reserved for residual valgus deformity and limblength discrepancy.

The etiology of posterior medial bowing is not well understood. The possible causes include a genetically mediated error in limb development or in utero mechanical forcing of the foot into dorsiflexion against the tibia. The assessment of posterior medial bowing begins at birth. It is important to differentiate between a simple calcaneovalgus foot deformity and a calcaneovalgus foot associated with a posterior medial bow. A calcaneovalgus foot deformity is not associated with a residual limb-length discrepancy, and the family should be made aware of this distinction during counseling on the prognosis. Radiographs are helpful in quantifying the extent of the deformity. The hips should be carefully examined because the calcaneovalgus foot deformity is associated with congenital dislocation of the hip and acetabular dysplasia.[15]

Residual limb-length discrepancy is directly related to the initial severity of the tibial bow. The affected tibia grows proportionately to the unaffected side, and therefore, the discrepancy at maturity can be predicted using accepted methods of growth prediction. During childhood, serial limb-length radiographs are required to assess both limb length and residual deformity.[15-17]

The treatment generally is aimed at addressing the residual limb-length discrepancy and the deformity. For a milder discrepancy, appropriately timed epiphysiodesis of the proximal tibia is an attractive option that carries a relatively low complication rate and low morbidity. The drawback to this procedure is that the patient's adult stature will be diminished. Hemiepiphysiodesis is a good option for correction of a valgus deformity, if present. The Ilizarov lengthening method is an option for a larger discrepancy, with the advantage of allowing both the length and the angular deformity to be corrected using one device. Lengthening is usually done through a proximal, metaphyseal osteotomy; the angular deformity can be better treated through a more distal osteotomy. The complications of external fixation and lengthening are well documented, and the entire treatment process requires a significant commitment by the patient, caregivers, and surgeon.

Congenital Tibial Deficiency

Congenital deficiency of the tibia (CDT) is rare; the reported incidence is one per one million live births. In CDT, in contrast to congenital fibular deficiency, the medial aspect of the limb is dysplastic. The tibia is commonly absent or markedly dysplastic. Knee and quadriceps function may be severely limited, and the foot and ankle are supinated and in varus. The first ray is shortened. Unlike fibular deficiency, CDT can occur in families. CDT usually is associated with other malformations of the ipsilateral limb or another area, including cleft lip and palate, cleft hand, polydactyly, and congenital femoral deficiency. CDT has no known cause.[18]

Assessment of a newborn with suspected CDT begins with a comprehensive physical examination to identify any associated anomalies and assess the affected extremity. Particular attention should be paid to the integrity of the hip, knee, and ankle joints. The classification of CDT is based on plain radiographic findings[19] (Figure 3). Type IA is characterized by an absent tibia with a hypoplastic distal femoral epiphysis, and type IB by an absent tibia with a normal distal femoral epiphysis. In type II, the distal tibia is absent; in type III, the proximal tibia is absent; and in type IV, there is diastasis of the syndesmosis with proximal migration of the talus.

The goal of treating CDT is to maximize the patient's functioning. Although the family may prefer immediate surgical reconstruction, it is important to realize that the growth rate of the affected limb will be significantly slower than that of the normal side, necessitating multiple lengthening procedures. An early amputation with prosthetic fitting generally yields the most functional and predictable results. Types IA and IB generally are associated with poor knee function as well as very poor or absent quadriceps function, and knee disarticulation is recommended. Patients with type II CDT often have good knee and quadriceps function, and below-knee amputation is more desirable. A synostosis between the dysplastic tibia and fibula can be cre-

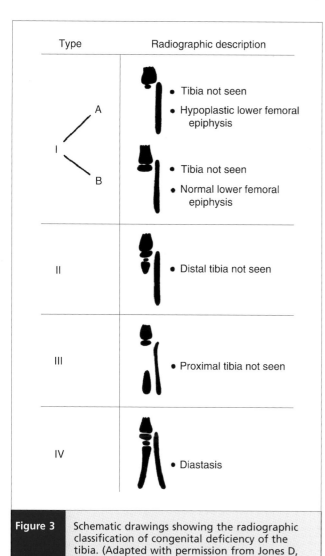

Type	Radiographic description
I A	• Tibia not seen • Hypoplastic lower femoral epiphysis
I B	• Tibia not seen • Normal lower femoral epiphysis
II	• Distal tibia not seen
III	• Proximal tibia not seen
IV	• Diastasis

Figure 3 Schematic drawings showing the radiographic classification of congenital deficiency of the tibia. (Adapted with permission from Jones D, Barnes J, Lloyd-Roberts GC: Congenital aplasia of the tibia with intact fibula: Classification and management. *J Bone Joint Surg Br* 1978;60: 31-39.)

ated for these patients, followed by a Syme or Boyd amputation. Type III CDT can be treated with a Boyd or Syme amputation with a calcaneofibular arthrodesis. The management of type IV is more controversial. The traditional treatment is talectomy, closure of the diastasis, and a Syme amputation; however, centralization of the talus, closure of the distal diastasis, and lengthening have been described.[20,21]

Infantile Tibia Vara (Blount Disease)

Infantile tibia vara, also called Blount disease, has an age of onset between approximately 1 year (when the child begins to walk) and 3 years; it is first seen as worsening genu varum. The less common adolescent form appears when the child is older than 6 to 8 years. Both the infantile and adolescent forms are character-

ized by disordered endochondral ossification. Although the two forms of tibia vara have similar risk factors and pathology, they should be considered separate pathologic processes.[22]

Infantile tibia vara is not a congenital deformity but instead is a developmental deformity of the proximal medial tibial physis. Clinically, it is important to distinguish pathologic tibia vara from physiologic genu varum, which represents the normal progression from overall varus alignment at birth, to a maximal valgus alignment at approximately age 3 years, and, finally, to normal adult alignment at age 7 to 8 years. The other differential diagnoses include metaphyseal chondrodysplasia, hypophosphatemic rickets, and focal fibrocartilaginous dysplasia.[22]

The exact cause of infantile tibia vara is not known and probably is multifactorial. The disease is most common in children who are obese, female, or of African descent, as well as children who began walking before age 1 year. (In general, children who are male or have another racial identity begin walking later.) Many of the associated factors suggest that the condition at least partly results from a mechanical overload of the medioproximal tibial physis. According to the Hueter-Volkmann principle, the growth of a physis can be slowed by increasing the transphyseal pressure and can be stimulated by decreasing the transphyseal pressure.

The evaluation of a child with suspected pathologic tibia vara begins with a thorough history. A complete birth and developmental history should include the age at which the child began walking. The medical history should identify any renal disease, endocrinopathies, or known skeletal dysplasias. Parents should be asked whether there is a family history of rickets or skeletal dysplasia. The physical examination should include the child's height and weight; height below the 25th percentile should arouse suspicion of rickets or skeletal dysplasia. The physical examination also should include the child's overall lower extremity alignment and symmetry, hip and knee motion, ligamentous stability, and tibial torsion.

A radiographic evaluation is the most accurate means of quantifying the deformity and measuring progression or resolution. Standing radiographs, with the beam centered at the knees and including both the hips and ankles, provide the most reliable measure of overall alignment. Bilateral radiographs can be useful for differentiating between physiologic genu varum and infantile tibia vara. The metaphyseal-diaphyseal angle has been proposed for use as a tool to predict the progression of infantile tibia vara (**Figure 4**). A metaphyseal-diaphyseal angle greater than 11° was found to be predictive of pathologic progression.[23,24] It is believed that treatment should not be undertaken until the metaphyseal-diaphyseal angle reaches 14° to 16°, especially if the child is younger than 3 years.

The Langenskiöld radiographic classification describes metaphyseal changes progressing from a mild, beaked appearance to a marked slope with bony bar

4: Lower Extremity

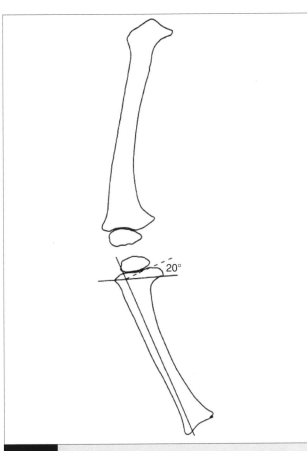

Figure 4 Schematic drawing showing the metaphyseal-diaphyseal angle, as used in predicting the progression of infantile tibia vara. Lines are drawn parallel to the lateral tibial cortex (the diaphyseal line) and the tibial metaphysis (the metaphyseal line). At their intersection, a third line (*shown by dashes*) is drawn perpendicular to the diaphyseal line; the metaphyseal-diaphyseal angle is between this line and the metaphyseal line. (Adapted with permission from Levine AM, Drennan JC: Physiologic bowing and tibia vara: The metaphyseal-diaphyseal angle in the measurement of bowleg deformities. *J Bone Joint Surg Am* 1982;64:1158-1163.)

formation[25] (**Figure 5**). This system is useful for describing the proximal tibia but is unreliable for predicting disease progression or deformity recurrence after treatment.

The lack of understanding of the natural history of infantile tibia vara creates difficulty in differentiating this condition from physiologic genu varum. In general, tibia vara should be suspected in children whose condition fails to improve or progress after they reach age 3 years and in children who have a unilateral deformity.

Bracing is the traditional first-line treatment for infantile tibia vara. The proposed mechanism of action of the brace is believed to be a mechanical unloading of the medial physis that takes advantage of the Hueter-Volkmann effect. Compliance with bracing is difficult to measure, and studies of bracing efficacy have lacked control subjects. A natural history study found no advantage to bracing over simple observation, even in patients with Langenskiöld stage II or III changes.[26] Therefore, observation is recommended until the child reaches age 4 years, with consideration of corrective osteotomy for children who do not have spontaneous correction.

Surgery should be considered for children whose correction does not continue beyond age 3 or 4 years. Early studies reported low rates of recurrence in children with changes at Langenskiöld stage IV or lower, but later studies found less favorable long-term results. The use of multiple surgical techniques has been reported, ranging from osteotomies with acute correction to gradual correction with external fixation devices, but the studies generally have been small and retrospective. To prevent recurrence, the most important factor is detection of a physeal bar, preferably with MRI. If a physeal bar is present and not addressed, there is a high risk of recurrence after realignment osteotomy. The presence of a physeal bar should be suspected in any child with changes at Langenskiöld stage IV or higher. MRI is also useful in determining joint orientation. On plain radiographs, the medial plateau may appear severely depressed, leading to an overestimation of the

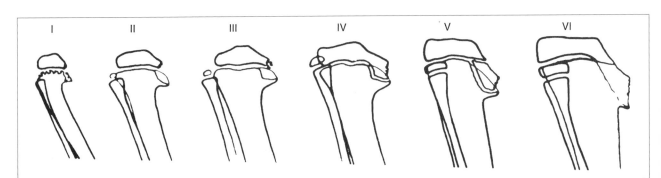

Figure 5 Schematic drawings showing the Langenskiöld radiographic classification of infantile tibia vara, by stage. I: Mild beaking of the tibial metaphysis. II: Beaking with slight depression. III: Depression with early fragmentation. IV: More severe depression with early bar formation. V: Severely disrupted physis with abnormal growth. VI: Definite bar formation with severe disruption of the articular surface. (Reproduced with permission from Langenskiöld A: Tibia vara: A critical review. *Clin Orthop Rel Res* 1989;246:195-207.)

need for a medial plateau elevation osteotomy. MRI can reveal a relative absence of ossification in the medial epiphysis and a hypertrophic medial meniscus. Because patient weight is associated with an increased risk of recurrence, slight overcorrection can be considered if the patient is obese.

Corrective osteotomies can be done acutely with internal fixation or with gradual correction and external fixation. A recent systematic literature review found no advantage to using one method over the other.[27] Various osteotomy techniques have been described. In general, the osteotomy should be performed distal to the tibial tuberosity to prevent damage to the apophysis and a subsequent recurvatum deformity. The osteotomy should correct both the varus and internal rotation deformities.

Physeal bar resection can be both difficult and unpredictable. For a patient with less than 50% physeal involvement (and preferably less than 30%), resection and interposition with fat or polymethylmethacrylate combined with realignment osteotomy should be considered.[28] If there is more than 50% involvement, realignment combined with lateral epiphysiodesis and later lengthening is a viable option. For children with severe medial plateau depression, a hemiplateau elevation osteotomy combined with a distal osteotomy can be considered, although MRI often shows this to be unnecessary.

Summary

Congenital deformities about the knee represent a broad spectrum of pathology. The physician must keep in mind that congenital musculoskeletal anomalies often are associated with anomalies of other organ systems. During infancy, the diagnosis may be obvious, but often the deformity is very subtle. In general, prompt diagnosis and treatment during the first few years of life lead to the most functional outcome.

Annotated References

1. Ferris B, Aichroth P: The treatment of congenital knee dislocation: A review of nineteen knees. *Clin Orthop Relat Res* 1987;216:135-140.

2. Nogi J, MacEwen GD: Congenital dislocation of the knee. *J Pediatr Orthop* 1982;2(5):509-513.

3. Laurence M: Genu recurvatum congenitum. *J Bone Joint Surg Br* 1967;49(1):121-134.

4. Dobbs MB, Boehm S, Grange DK, Gurnett CA: Case report: Congenital knee dislocation in a patient with larsen syndrome and a novel filamin B mutation. *Clin Orthop Relat Res* 2008;466(6):1503-1509.

   A novel point mutation was found in a patient with Lar-

sen syndrome. The authors describe their clinical algorithm for treatment of congenital knee dislocation, in which serial casting is recommended for 6 to 7 weeks, followed by a minimally invasive quadriceps tenotomy and anterior capsular release if casting does not achieve 90° of flexion. The casting and surgical techniques are described.

5. Eilert RE: Congenital dislocation of the patella. *Clin Orthop Relat Res* 2001;389 :22-29.

6. Ghanem I, Wattincourt L, Seringe R: Congenital dislocation of the patella: Part I. Pathologic anatomy. *J Pediatr Orthop* 2000;20(6):812-816.

7. Andrish J: Surgical options for patellar stabilization in the skeletally immature patient. *Sports Med Arthrosc* 2007;15(2):82-88.

   The different features of patellar instability in children are outlined. Surgical approaches based on the underlying pathoanatomy are discussed in detail.

8. Ghanem I, Wattincourt L, Seringe R: Congenital dislocation of the patella: Part II. Orthopaedic management. *J Pediatr Orthop* 2000;20(6):817-822.

9. Langenskiöld A, Ritsilä V: Congenital dislocation of the patella and its operative treatment. *J Pediatr Orthop* 1992;12(3):315-323.

10. Vander Have KL, Hensinger RN, Caird M, Johnston C, Farley FA: Congenital pseudarthrosis of the tibia. *J Am Acad Orthop Surg* 2008;16(4):228-236.

    The literature on the etiology, evaluation, and treatment of congenital pseudarthrosis of the tibia is reviewed.

11. Dobbs MB, Rich MM, Gordon JE, Szymanski DA, Schoenecker PL: Use of an intramedullary rod for treatment of congenital pseudarthrosis of the tibia: A long-term follow-up study. *J Bone Joint Surg Am* 2004;86-A(6):1186-1197.

12. Johnston CE II: Congenital pseudarthrosis of the tibia: Results of technical variations in the Charnley-Williams procedure. *J Bone Joint Surg Am* 2002;84-A(10):1799-1810.

13. Cho TJ, Choi IH, Lee SM, et al: Refracture after Ilizarov osteosynthesis in atrophic-type congenital pseudarthrosis of the tibia. *J Bone Joint Surg Br* 2008; 90(4):488-493.

    A refracture-free survival rate of 47% at 5 years did not decrease after the 5-year mark. Increased risk of refracture was associated with age younger than 4 years and a small tibial cross-section area.

14. Richards BS, Oetgen ME, Johnston CE: The use of rhBMP-2 for the treatment of congenital pseudarthrosis of the tibia: A case series. *J Bone Joint Surg Am* 2010; 92(1):177-185.

    The use of rhBMP-2 is described as an addition to resection, autogenous bone grafting, and intramedullary rod-

4: Lower Extremity

ding. Five of seven patients achieved union, with only one refracture at a mean 5.4-year follow-up.

15. Hofmann A, Wenger DR: Posteromedial bowing of the tibia: Progression of discrepancy in leg lengths. *J Bone Joint Surg Am* 1981;63(3):384-388.

16. Pappas AM: Congenital posteromedial bowing of the tibia and fibula. *J Pediatr Orthop* 1984;4(5):525-531.

17. Shah HH, Doddabasappa SN, Joseph B: Congenital posteromedial bowing of the tibia: A retrospective analysis of growth abnormalities in the leg. *J Pediatr Orthop B* 2009;18(3):120-128.

    In a retrospective review of 20 patients, most of the angular deformity was found to resolve during the first year of life, and limb-length discrepancy was found to be proportional to the degree of initial bowing.

18. Kalamchi A, Dawe RV: Congenital deficiency of the tibia. *J Bone Joint Surg Br* 1985;67(4):581-584.

19. Jones D, Barnes J, Lloyd-Roberts GC: Congenital aplasia and dysplasia of the tibia with intact fibula: Classification and management. *J Bone Joint Surg Br* 1978;60(1):31-39.

20. Schoenecker PL, Capelli AM, Millar EA, et al: Congenital longitudinal deficiency of the tibia. *J Bone Joint Surg Am* 1989;71(2):278-287.

21. Tokmakova K, Riddle EC, Kumar SJ: Type IV congenital deficiency of the tibia. *J Pediatr Orthop* 2003;23(5):649-653.

22. Greene WB: Infantile tibia vara. *J Bone Joint Surg Am* 1993;75(1):130-143.

23. Levine AM, Drennan JC: Physiological bowing and tibia vara: The metaphyseal-diaphyseal angle in the measurement of bowleg deformities. *J Bone Joint Surg Am* 1982;64(8):1158-1163.

24. Lavelle WF, Shovlin J, Drvaric DM: Reliability of the metaphyseal-diaphyseal angle in tibia vara as measured on digital images by pediatric orthopaedic surgeons. *J Pediatr Orthop* 2008;28(6):695-698.

    The interobserver and intraobserver reliability of the measurement of the metaphyseal-diaphyseal angle using either the lateral cortex of the tibia or the center of the tibial shaft as the long axis of the tibia is examined. Excellent intraobserver and interobserver reliability was found for both methods among pediatric orthopedic surgeons. There was no significant difference between the two methods of measurement.

25. Langenskiöld A: Tibia vara: A critical review. *Clin Orthop Relat Res* 1989;246(246):195-207.

26. Shinohara Y, Kamegaya M, Kuniyoshi K, Moriya H: Natural history of infantile tibia vara. *J Bone Joint Surg Br* 2002;84(2):263-268.

27. Gilbody J, Thomas G, Ho K: Acute versus gradual correction of idiopathic tibia vara in children: A systematic review. *J Pediatr Orthop* 2009;29(2):110-114.

    The authors systematically reviewed the published literature assessing the radiographic restoration of alignment produced by gradual correction and acute correction. Radiographic alignment was the primary outcome measure. Only one study found a small advantage to gradual correction with external fixation. The remaining 17 articles found no differences, although they were of lower quality design.

28. Andrade N, Johnston CE: Medial epiphysiolysis in severe infantile tibia vara. *J Pediatr Orthop* 2006;26(5):652-658.

    In 27 tibiae treated with epiphysiolysis (24 patients; average age at surgery, 7 years), recurrent varus deformity was prevented and growth was restored in 16 tibiae. Mild recurrence of deformity and significant growth was seen in 6 tibia. In the 11 unsuccessful procedures, failure was associated with age older than 7 years, undercorrection of the mechanical axis, and an earlier unsuccessful epiphysiolysis.

Chapter 22
Congenital Disorders of the Foot

David M. Scher, MD   Gaia Georgopoulos, MD

Introduction

Pediatric foot conditions are common and range from normal variants to severe deformities. The response correspondingly ranges from parental reassurance to prompt and intensive treatment during the perinatal period. The literature, diagnoses, and treatment protocols pertaining to some of the most significant foot conditions are discussed here.

Clubfoot

Clubfoot is a heterogeneous congenital foot deformity. Several abnormalities are universally present, although they vary in severity. The major osseous deformities include hindfoot equinus, heel varus, medial displacement of the navicular with lateral uncovering of the talar head, abduction of the midfoot, cavus with plantar flexion of the first ray, and relative pronation of the forefoot in relation to the position of the hindfoot.[1] Deformities of the tarsal bones themselves also are present to a varying extent, including plantar flexion, medial deviation of the talar neck, and wedging of the navicular. The major soft-tissue abnormalities are contractures and, often, thickening of the posterior, medial, and plantar soft tissues including the Achilles tendon, the posterior tibial and medial flexor tendons, and, to a varying extent, the medial and plantar ligaments (the superficial deltoid ligament, the spring ligament, and the plantar fascia).[1]

The most effective and most commonly used treatment for clubfoot is the Ponseti method, in which the deformities are gradually and simultaneously corrected by manipulation and serial long leg casting of the foot (Figure 1). The first cast is applied with the forefoot in supination to bring it in line with the hindfoot, which is in varus, and with the first ray in dorsiflexion. This cast typically corrects the cavus deformity. Subsequent casts are applied to abduct the foot around the head of the talus. When the foot is maximally abducted, the talar head is covered and the heel is in valgus. The final cast is applied with the foot in at least 15° of dorsiflexion. Achieving this degree of dorsiflexion requires a percutaneous Achilles tenotomy in approximately 90% of patients. The final cast remains in place for 3 weeks and is followed by a strict regimen of bracing. Full-time bracing is used for several months, followed by several years of part-time bracing during sleep. The brace consists of a bar with attached shoes that maintain the feet in a position of wide abduction, with approximately 70° of external rotation and 15° of dorsiflexion at the end of the bar.[1]

Several recent studies found poor long-term results after surgical treatment and better results when the Ponseti method was used. Patients treated with extensive soft-tissue releases had poor long-term outcomes on measures of foot function and quality of life (the physical function domain).[2] Patients treated with the Ponseti method also were compared with patients treated using another method of manipulation, followed by posteromedial surgical release of the clubfoot. Follow-up studies were done at a mean age of 25 years for those treated with the Ponseti method and 19 years for those treated with surgery.[3] A good or excellent result was achieved in 78% of those treated with the Ponseti method and 43% of those treated with surgery. A short-term comparison of the Ponseti method with posteromedial release also found superior results for the Ponseti method, based on range of motion and a functional rating system.[4] There have been many early reports of good outcomes from multiple centers using the Ponseti method, and medium-term reports continue to find good results.[5]

A comparison of the Ponseti method with the French functional physical therapy method found the two to be equally effective.[6] Both methods are nonsurgical and include regular manipulation. In the French method, the manipulations are performed daily by physical therapists; temporary, between-session immobilization with taping is used instead of casting. Initial correction was achieved in 95% of patients in both groups and was maintained at 4 years in 84% of patients. Gait analysis found that more children in the physical therapy group had normal sagittal plane ankle motion (kinematics) than in the Ponseti group.[7] However, there were dis-

Dr. Scher or an immediate family member serves as a board member, owner, officer, or committee member of the American Academy for Cerebral Palsy and Developmental Medicine and the Pediatric Orthopaedic Club of New York. Neither Dr. Georgopoulos nor any immediate family member has received anything of value from or owns stock in a commercial company or institution related directly or indirectly to the subject of this chapter.

4: Lower Extremity

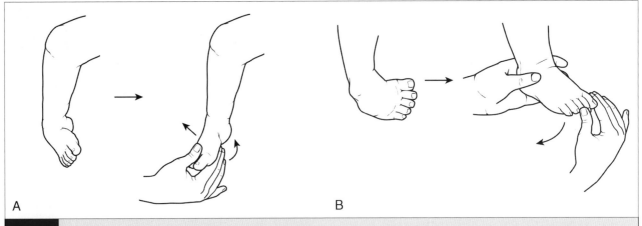

Figure 1 Schematic drawings showing the foot position for the Ponseti method of correcting clubfoot. **A,** An uncorrected clubfoot, showing the medial crease and cavus deformity *(left)*. The hindfoot is supinated to bring it in line with the forefoot, and the first ray is dorsiflexed; the medial crease dissipates as the foot is manipulated *(right)*. The first cast is applied with the foot in this position. **B,** Subsequent casts are applied with the foot abducted around the talar head *(left)*. To abduct the foot and reduce the talar head beneath the navicular, the examiner's left thumb is positioned on the talar head just anterior to the lateral malleolus, and the right hand is used to abduct the foot *(right)*.

tinct differences in the nature of the gait deviations. The children in the physical therapy group had an equinus gait and footdrop, whereas the children in the Ponseti group had mildly increased dorsiflexion in the stance phase. These differences may be attributable to the Achilles tenotomy used in the Ponseti method but not in the physical therapy method. Two centers found that physical therapists can effectively administer the Ponseti casting method, with results comparable to those achieved by orthopaedic surgeons.[8,9]

Traditionally, long leg plaster casts have been used in the Ponseti method; almost all of the studies on the effectiveness of this method have adhered to this protocol. The use of below-knee, semirigid fiberglass casts was found to be successful in a group of 51 patients at 2-year follow-up.[10] However, a randomized, prospective comparison study of plaster casts and semirigid fiberglass casts found better correction with the plaster casts.[11]

Physical, rather than radiographic, examination of the foot typically is used in the Ponseti method to assess both the initial deformity and the success of correction. Radiographs can be effectively used after the Achilles tenotomy to confirm correction of ankle equinus, as shown by the lateral tibiocalcaneal angle. Radiographs also can be useful to ensure that the equinus is being corrected by movement at the ankle joint rather than by a break in the midfoot.[12]

The Ponseti method originally was described for treating idiopathic clubfoot, but recent studies have documented its success in treating clubfoot associated with arthrogryposis or myelomeningocele. Only short-term studies involving a small number of patients are available to evaluate the Ponseti method in arthrogryposis. These results suggest that initial correction can be obtained in all patients but that more casts are required than for patients with idiopathic clubfoot.[13,14]

The risk of recurrence persists and may be related to brace intolerance; however, few patients require extensive soft-tissue releases.[13] In a small group of patients with clubfoot related to myelomeningocele, the success rate was equivalent to that of patients with idiopathic clubfeet, but the rate of recurrence was significantly higher.[15] Most recurrences were managed using repeat casting or casting with repeat tenotomy; there was no significant difference from idiopathic clubfoot in the need for extensive soft-tissue releases. Brace intolerance was associated with some of the recurrences. Some recurrences occurred despite adequate bracing, however, suggesting that muscle imbalance has a role in recurrence. In a larger study comparing idiopathic clubfoot with nonidiopathic clubfoot related to arthrogryposis, myelomeningocele, and other conditions, more casts were required and both recurrences and failures were more common in the patients with nonidiopathic clubfoot; however, initial correction was achieved in 90% of these patients.[16]

There is no evidence to suggest that the risk of recurrence is related to the severity of the initial deformity. Bracing is crucial for preventing a recurrence of the deformity. Brace intolerance and relatively low parent educational level (less than high school) were found to be associated with recurrence.[17-19] Cultural factors appear to have a role in brace intolerance and recurrence. Early brace discontinuation was associated with recurrence in a rural Native American population and may have been the result of deficient communication and education provided to the patient and family by the physician.[20]

The so-called complex clubfoot is particularly resistant to treatment.[21] The complex clubfoot is short and wide and in severe equinus, with plantar flexion of all of the metatarsals, a short and hyperextended first toe, and often a deep transverse plantar crease accompanied by a deep posterior crease. These characteristics often are not initially recognizable and become apparent only after the first several casts slip. A different method of manipulation is required, with less emphasis on abduction and more on gradual dorsiflexion of the entire foot. The objective is to achieve final abduction of no more than approximately 40°, unlike the 60° to 70° achieved in the typical clubfoot. To help prevent slippage, the cast is applied in approximately 110° of flexion at the knee, rather than the typical 90°.

If supination recurs after either the Ponseti method or a posteromedial release is used, the preferred treatment is a complete tibialis anterior tendon transfer to the lateral cuneiform. For recurrent equinus, the transfer can be combined with an Achilles tendon lengthening.[21-23] Treatments for more severe recurrent or residual deformity after surgical correction have been less extensively studied. The reported results of using the Ilizarov method for soft-tissue correction are conflicting. More than 50% of children age 2 to 10 years had a poor outcome and limited radiographic correction after Ilizarov soft-tissue correction.[24] However, a similar method was used in children age 5 to 10 years with mostly good or excellent results.[25] A talonavicular arthrodesis can effectively correct symptomatic dorsal subluxation of the navicular and relieve symptoms.[26] Talectomy can be used as a salvage procedure for severe recurrent clubfoot deformity in patients with arthrogryposis or myelomeningocele. At 20-year follow-up, all patients treated with talectomy were pain free, and 75% had a good or fair result.[27] However, 25% had pain with walking, some developed tibiocalcaneal arthritis or spontaneous tibiocalcaneal fusion, and many required additional surgery to correct residual deformities.

Flatfoot

Flexible Flatfoot

Flatfoot, or pes planus, can be characterized as flexible or rigid. In a flexible flatfoot, the arch is reconstituted on toe rise or when not bearing weight. The hindfoot is flexible on examination. There is supple and unrestricted subtalar motion with passive inversion and eversion of the foot, and the heel rolls into varus during active toe rise. Flexible flatfoot in children is considered a normal anatomic variant that occurs with ligamentous laxity. Prevalence studies have found flexible flatfoot to be present in 28% to 59% of children in different populations.[28-30] Flexible flatfoot is associated with younger age, male sex, and obesity.[27-30] Treatment is not warranted for painless flexible flatfoot because the condition has no effect on arch development. Athletic performance, as measured by the ability to perform a series of physical function tests, does not differ between children with flatfoot and those with a normal arch height.[31]

A flexible flatfoot can become painful, although there are no data indicating the frequency or incidence

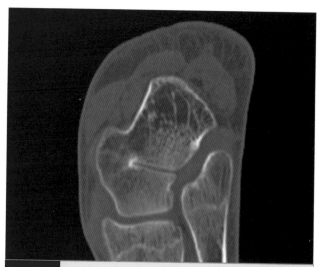

Figure 2 Coronal CT section of a talocalcaneal tarsal coalition, showing approximately 40% involvement of the posterior facet.

of pain. Painful flatfoot may be associated with contractures of the gastrocnemius or Achilles tendon, but there are no substantiating studies.[32] The described surgical treatments for painful flatfoot include gastrocnemius recession in the setting of gastrocnemius equinus, subtalar arthroereisis (placement of a cylindrical implant within the sinus tarsi), lateral column-lengthening osteotomy, and combined osteotomies of the hindfoot and midfoot.[32-35] No controlled or comparative studies have been done to support the use of one treatment over another.

Rigid Flatfoot

Rigid flatfoot, in which the arch does not reconstitute itself with toe rise or when not bearing weight, usually indicates an abnormality in the joints of the hindfoot. These abnormalities can include subtalar arthritis, infection, and tumor. Talocalcaneal and calcaneonavicular tarsal coalitions are among the most common causes. The initial diagnostic studies should include AP, lateral, and internal oblique radiographs of the foot. An axial view of the heel occasionally reveals a talocalcaneal coalition. If plain radiographs are normal, CT is warranted to investigate for a talocalcaneal coalition. In the presence of a calcaneonavicular coalition, an axial radiograph or CT is advisable to rule out a concomitant talocalcaneal coalition. MRI can be useful if a cartilaginous or fibrous coalition is suspected. In the absence of a coalition on multiplanar imaging studies of a painful rigid flatfoot, laboratory studies are warranted as part of a complete rheumatologic and infectious disease investigation.

A talocalcaneal coalition usually involves the middle facet of the subtalar joint. Resection of the coalition is indicated if nonsurgical treatment fails to relieve the symptoms. Surgical resection has good results if the coalition measured less than 50% of the width of the en-

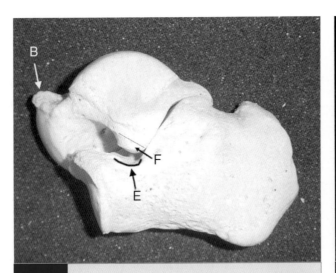

Figure 3 Photograph showing a lateral view of the talus and calcaneus, with beaking of the dorsal part of the talar neck (B), a calcaneal neck anterior extension facet (E), and an accessory anterolateral talar facet (F). (Reproduced with permission from Martus JE, Femino JE, Caird MS, Hughes RE, Browne RH, Farley FA: Accessory anterolateral facet of the pediatric talus: An anatomic study. *J Bone Joint Surg Am* 2008;90[11]: 2452-2459.)

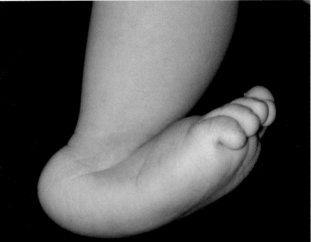

Figure 4 Photograph of a rocker-bottom deformity in a child with congenital vertical talus. Hindfoot equinus and dorsiflexion of the forefoot are shown. (Reproduced with permission from Georgopoulos G: Myelomeningocele, in Drennan JC, ed: *The Child's Foot and Ankle*, ed 2. Philadelphia, PA, Lippincott, Williams & Wilkins, 2009, pp 209-217.)

tire posterior facet and the hindfoot valgus measured less than 16° to 21° on a coronal CT section (**Figure 2**). Fat or tendon is placed in the area of the resection to prevent recurrence.[36,37] Resection of the coalition along with complete excision of the sustentaculum tali also was found to be effective in relieving symptoms, with no recurrences or complications.[38]

A study of human skeletons found that the anatomy of calcaneonavicular coalitions is quite variable. The presence of multiple, extensive osseous abnormalities and connections between the navicular and calcaneus was notable. There was a tendency for the anterior facet of the calcaneus to be deficient or absent and partially or completely replaced by a projection of bone from the navicular, forming part of the coalition. This abnormality has implications for the manner in which the bone is resected, and it may lead to instability at the talonavicular joint after resection.[39] Resection of calcaneonavicular coalitions with the interposition of fat autograft leads to good symptom improvement and restoration of both subtalar motion and plantar flexion.[40] A cadaver study found that interposed extensor digitorum brevis muscle fills an average of 64% of the tunnel created by resection of the calcaneonavicular coalition; in comparison, 100% of the tunnel is filled when fat autograft is used. This finding suggests that the risk of recurrence may be lower if fat autograft is used.[40] Gait analysis of subtalar kinematics after resection of talocalcaneal and calcaneonavicular coalitions revealed no improvement in eversion and inversion during walking, despite improvements in passive range of motion and sagittal plane foot motion.[41] The gait remains abnormal despite clinical improvement after surgical resection of a tarsal coalition.

Another cause of hindfoot stiffness and pain is arthrofibrosis of the middle facet of the subtalar joint without a coalition, consisting of hypervascular synovium with thickened joint capsule. Surgical exploration of the middle facet with excision of the abnormal tissue was performed in 19 patients, with 17 having a good result.[42] The accessory anterolateral facet of the talus, consisting of a projection from the lateral process of the talus, is another anatomic variant implicated in painful flatfoot in children[43,44] (**Figure 3**). In a study of pediatric skeletal specimens, the presence of this facet was associated with male sex, dorsal talar beaking, and a decreased angle of Gissane.[43]

Congenital Vertical Talus

Congenital vertical talus is an uncommon foot deformity characterized by hindfoot equinus and an irreducible dorsolateral dislocation of the navicular on the talar head and neck. The foot has a rocker-bottom appearance, and the talar head is visible and palpable on the plantar medial aspect of the foot (**Figure 4**). The etiology is unknown; the proposed possibilities include intrauterine growth compression, arrested development during the second month of gestation, a central nervous system abnormality, and a neuromuscular disorder. Vascular abnormalities exist in both congenital vertical talus and clubfoot. Examination using arteriography or magnetic resonance angiography showed that the posterior tibial artery was deficient or absent in the lower extremities of patients with congenital vertical talus.[45]

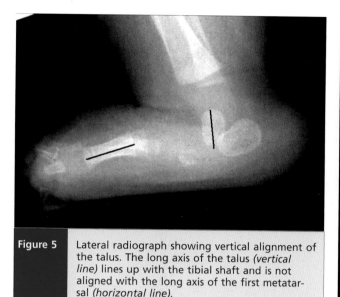

Figure 5 Lateral radiograph showing vertical alignment of the talus. The long axis of the talus *(vertical line)* lines up with the tibial shaft and is not aligned with the long axis of the first metatarsal *(horizontal line)*.

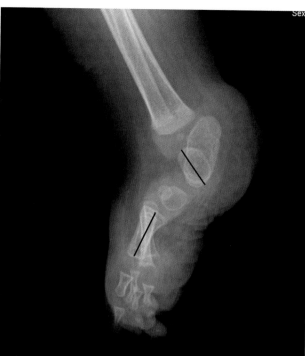

Figure 6 Plantar flexion lateral radiograph in which the lines show that the talus and first metatarsal are not aligned. This hallmark of a true vertical talus suggests that the navicular remains dorsally dislocated on the talar head and neck.

There may be a genetic component to the etiology.[46] A positive family history was found in 12% to 20% of patients with congenital vertical talus, suggesting an autosomal dominant inheritance pattern with incomplete penetrance.[47] A mutation was identified in the homeobox D10 *(Hoxd-10)* gene in several families with congenital vertical talus, and a mutation in the cartilage-derived morphogenetic protein–1 *(CDMP-1)* gene was identified in a family with hand and foot abnormalities including congenital vertical talus.[47]

Approximately 50% of congenital vertical tali are classified as idiopathic. In the other 50%, the patient has an associated condition; these include myelomeningocele, a contractural syndrome such as arthrogryposis, a chromosomal abnormality, a spinal cord abnormality, and myopathy.[48] Because of the high incidence of an associated condition, it is important to evaluate patients with congenital vertical talus for other general or skeletal abnormalities. The deformity is bilateral in 50% to 70% of patients, and it accounts for 10% of all foot deformities associated with myelomeningocele.

The pathoanatomy of congenital vertical talus consists of a navicular that is dorsally and laterally displaced on the neck of the talus.[49] The talar neck is elongated and deviated medially and plantarly, along with the talar head. There is a contracture of the dorsal tendons, tibialis anterior, extensor hallucis longus, and extensor digitorum, as well as a contracture of the dorsal talonavicular, posterior ankle, and subtalar joint capsules. The tibialis posterior and the peroneal tendons are displaced anterior to the axis of the ankle, and therefore they act as dorsiflexors of the midfoot.

The diagnosis is confirmed with AP, lateral, and plantar flexion lateral radiographs to determine the AP and lateral talocalcaneal and talus–first metatarsal angles. On the lateral radiograph, the talus is in a vertical position, lining up with the long axis of the tibial shaft, and the calcaneus is in equinus (**Figure 5**). On the AP radiograph, there is an increased talocalcaneal angle, and the talus is directed medially. The diagnosis is confirmed on a plantar flexion lateral radiograph. In true congenital vertical talus, the navicular does not reduce with plantar flexion. Because the navicular is not ossified in the newborn, the talus does not line up with the first metatarsal (**Figure 6**).

An untreated foot with congenital vertical talus has a stiff rocker bottom, develops calluses, is painful, and is difficult to fit with shoes. Because of the hindfoot equinus, the heel never touches the ground, and push-off strength is poor. Treatment should be initiated after the diagnosis is made. As with clubfoot deformity, the initial treatment is serial manipulation and casting. Serial casting does not correct the dorsal dislocation of the navicular, but it stretches the dorsal soft tissues and thereby allows less invasive surgery. Several surgical procedures have been described for treating congenital vertical talus. The method used depends on the age of the child, the severity of the deformity, and the surgeon's preference.

Historically, surgical correction was performed in two stages: reduction of the talonavicular joint with lengthening of the tibialis anterior and the extensor tendons, followed by Achilles tendon lengthening, peroneal tendon lengthening, and posterior ankle and subtalar release. This method led to several complications, the most significant of which was osteonecrosis of the talus. Most surgeons now prefer a single-stage proce-

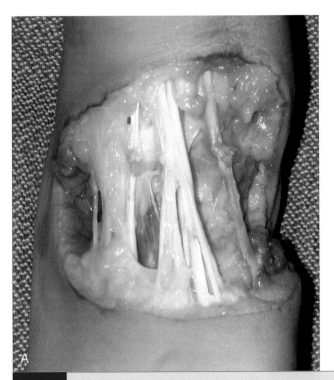
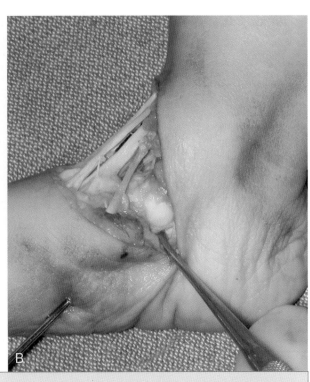

Figure 7 The correction of congential vertical talus through a dorsal approach. **A,** The dorsal tendons have undergone Z lengthening. **B,** The talonavicular joint has been reduced and pinned. The Achilles tenotomy has not yet been performed. (Reproduced with permission from Georgopoulos G: Myelomeningocele, in Drennan JC, ed: *The Child's Foot and Ankle,* ed 2. Philadelphia, PA, Lippincott, Williams & Wilkins, 2009, pp 209-217.)

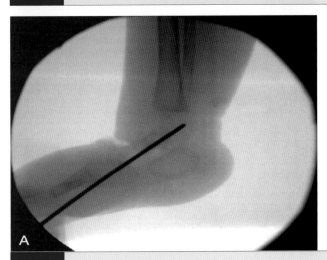
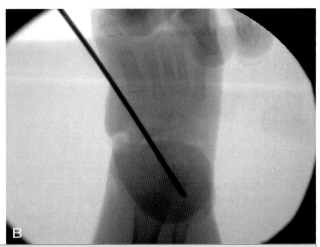

Figure 8 Intraoperative C-arm **(A)** and lateral **(B)** radiographs showing reduction and pinning of the talonavicular joint. Note that the long axis of the talus is now aligned with the first metatarsal in both views.

dure that can be performed through a posterior or a dorsal approach. The posterior approach uses a Cincinnati incision, and an extensive ankle and subtalar release is done with the reduction of the talonavicular joint. The peroneal tendons can be lengthened, and the calcaneocuboid joint can be reduced, if needed. Lengthening of the dorsal tendons can be done through a separate incision.[50,51] In the dorsal approach, the incision runs from just inferior to the medial malleolus across the dorsum of the foot to the tip of the fibula. This in-

cision allows direct access to the dorsally dislocated navicular and the contracted tibialis anterior and extensor tendons, as well as the peroneal tendons and the calcaneocuboid joint (**Figure 7**). After the talonavicular joint is pinned, a percutaneous Achilles tenotomy is done to correct the equinus (**Figure 8**). A formal posterior release occasionally is required.[52] The short-term results of both procedures have been good, but the dorsal approach requires less time and leads to fewer complications.[53]

In a recently described minimally invasive technique adapted from the Ponseti method for clubfeet, serial casting of a congenital vertical talus is followed by a limited surgical release. Serial casts are applied in the opposite direction from the position used for casts to correct clubfoot. After the first several casts are applied, a lateral radiograph is used to assess the reduction of the talonavicular joint. If the talus lines up with the first metatarsal, the talonavicular joint is surgically pinned, and a percutaneous Achilles tenotomy is done. If the talonavicular joint cannot be reduced, a limited open reduction of the joint is done. Occasionally, the dorsal tendons also require lengthening. Although this surgery may involve an open capsule and tendon lengthening, it is much less extensive than the surgical alternatives.[54] Regardless of the surgical procedure, the tibialis anterior can be lengthened or transferred to the neck of the talus. No studies are available to determine whether a lengthening or transfer is preferable, although transfer may be more beneficial in a deformity secondary to myelomeningocele.

Corrective procedures are more successful in younger children. Although the upper age limit for success is unknown, more extensive surgery is usually required in children older than 3 years. In addition to soft-tissue procedures, it may be necessary to perform a Grice-Green extra-articular subtalar arthrodesis or a naviculectomy to shorten the medial column, combined with a lateral column lengthening. A triple arthrodesis may be considered as a salvage procedure.

Juvenile Hallux Valgus

Juvenile hallux valgus is a deformity of the foot in which the first metatarsal is medially deviated and the great toe is laterally deviated. The true incidence and etiology of juvenile hallux valgus are unknown. Several conditions are associated with hallux valgus, including flatfoot (pes planus), metatarsus adductus, a long first metatarsal, deformity of the medial cuneiform, a hypermobile first ray, and a lateral-sloping distal metatarsal articular surface. Shoe wear has been implicated as a cause of hallux valgus, as the condition is rare in populations that do not wear shoes. Approximately 80% of patients with hallux valgus are female. A high percentage of female patients have a mother with hallux valgus, and therefore a sex-linked dominant trait is suggested.[55]

Examination of a patient with hallux valgus should include a gait evaluation. The foot should be examined with the patient sitting and bearing weight, with particular attention to the arch, position of the hindfoot, and severity of the deformity. The range of motion of the ankle, subtalar, metatarsal medial cuneiform, and metatarsophalangeal joints should be assessed. Ankle dorsiflexion should be checked with the knee flexed and extended to look for gastrocnemius and/or soleus contracture. Hypermobility of the medial cuneiform–

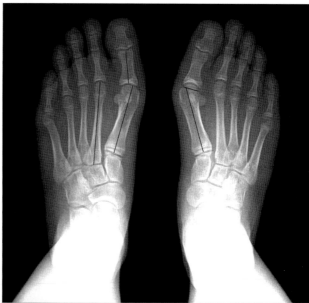

Figure 9   AP standing radiograph showing the measurement of the intermetatarsal angle and the hallux valgus angle (*left*) and the measurement of the distal metatarsal articular angle (*right*). In this patient, the metatarsal articular surface is laterally deviated, with a distal metatarsal articular angle greater than 6°.

first metatarsal joint should be assessed. On standing AP and lateral radiographs, the hallux valgus angle, first and second intermetatarsal angle, and distal metatarsal articular angle are determined (**Figure 9**). A normal hallux valgus angle is 10° or less, a normal intermetatarsal angle is less than 9°, and a normal distal metatarsal articular angle is less than 6°.[56] The congruency of the first metatarsophalangeal joint also should be assessed, as it is particularly important in determining the appropriate surgical procedure.

The condition is asymptomatic in some patients, who primarily are concerned with the cosmetic deformity. A symptomatic patient reports pain over the medial prominence with shoe wear, pain with activities, and difficulty in fitting shoes (especially shoes with a narrow toe box). The initial treatment of all patients should be nonsurgical. Shoes should have a wide toe box and be constructed of soft materials. Orthotics and some splints may be of benefit.[55,57]

Surgery can be considered when nonsurgical methods have failed to relieve the symptoms. Several surgical procedures have been described, in five major categories: distal soft-tissue realignment procedures, distal osteotomies, proximal osteotomies, first metatarsal–medial cuneiform fusions, and combination procedures. Obtaining a good result and avoiding a recurrence requires that the chosen procedure correct all aspects of the deformity. Distal soft-tissue realignment procedures performed alone have fallen out of favor because they have a high recurrence rate.

The most appropriate procedure is chosen based on

the location of the specific deformities, the size of the distal metatarsal articular angle or the intermetatarsal angle, and the congruity of the metatarsophalangeal joint. In general, a distal soft-tissue procedure with a proximal realignment osteotomy is indicated if the metatarsophalangeal joint is incongruent and the intermetatarsal angle is greater than normal. Both proximal and distal realignment procedures are required if the joint is congruent, with greater than normal distal metatarsal articular and intermetatarsal angles.

A high percentage of juvenile hallux valgus deformities have a large distal metatarsal articular angle, indicating a laterally deviated articular surface. The larger the distal metatarsal articular angle is, the more severe the hallux valgus angle. Juvenile hallux valgus deformities also are often associated with a congruent metatarsophalangeal joint.[55] Soft-tissue procedures alone would create an incongruent metatarsophalangeal joint, leading to stiffness and recurrence. The addition of distal realignment osteotomies, such as the Mitchell procedure, is indicated to correct moderate or severe hallux valgus deformities with an incongruent metatarsophalangeal joint. Distal realignment osteotomies also can be successful if the distal metatarsal articular angle is only moderately elevated. The distal chevron osteotomy cannot correct an increased distal metatarsal articular angle but is indicated if the hallux valgus angle is less than 30° and the intermetatarsal angle is normal.

The scarf osteotomy can be successful if the intermetatarsal angle is increased and the distal metatarsal articular angle is normal. This osteotomy has been popular in Europe for many years and recently has been used in the United States. A longitudinal Z osteotomy of the first metatarsal is performed, in which the distal dorsal fragment is shifted laterally then internally fixed. The scarf osteotomy should be used with care in skeletally immature patients, as good initial correction of the intermetatarsal and hallux valgus angles was found to be followed by gradual loss of correction by final follow-up.[58] A lateral epiphysiodesis of the first metatarsal gradually corrects the metatarsus primus varus in skeletally immature patients and may be an alternative in patients with symptomatic hallux valgus who are younger than 10 years.[59] The first metatarsal double osteotomy can be successful if the joint was congruent, with increased distal metatarsal articular and intermetatarsal angles. The Lapidus procedure is indicated for moderate or severe hallux valgus with an increased intermetatarsal angle and associated hypermobility of the medial cuneiform–first metatarsal joint. The difficult diagnosis of this hypermobility is made both radiographically and clinically.[60] Hypermobility of the medial cuneiform–first metatarsal joint may be secondary to the deformity, and correction of the deformity with a distal soft-tissue procedure and a proximal crescentic osteotomy could result in less hypermobility.[61]

The complications of surgical treatment include recurrence of the deformity, osteonecrosis of the metatarsal head, hallux varus, and stiffness of the metatarsophalangeal joint. Surgery should not be undertaken for cosmetic reasons only. Because of the high recurrence rate, it has been stated that surgical correction should be delayed until the patient reaches skeletal maturity. The recurrence rate was not found to be greater in pediatric patients.[55] Care should be taken to avoid damaging the physis, however, because damage to the physis shortens the first metatarsal and could cause recurrence. A shortened first metatarsal can lead to transfer lesions in the rest of the foot and a poor result.[62]

Cavus Deformities

Cavus deformities of the foot are characterized by an elevated arch in stance (Figure 10). The position of the hindfoot most often is in varus but also can be in valgus, calcaneus, or equinus. Although the condition can be idiopathic, often it is the result of an underlying central neurologic condition such as cerebral palsy or Friedreich ataxia. The associated spine abnormalities include tethered cord syndrome, diastematomyelia, syringomyelia, and myelodysplasia. Peripheral neuropathies are a common cause of cavovarus foot deformities, with Charcot-Marie-Tooth disease the most common of the hereditary sensory motor neuropathies. An extensive evaluation is indicated to detect any underlying neuromuscular diagnosis. The patient should be referred to a neurologist or physiatrist for serologic testing. Electromyography and nerve conduction studies also should be considered. MRI of the spinal cord should be obtained, especially with a unilateral deformity, to rule out any intraspinal abnormality.

The pathoanatomy and pathomechanics of cavus deformities have been well described.[63,64] In Charcot-Marie-Tooth disease, the first metatarsal becomes plantar flexed because of weak intrinsic muscles and unopposed long extensors; the peroneus longus maintains its strength compared with the peroneus brevis, accentuating the plantar flexion of the first ray and leading to shortening of the plantar fascia. As the deformity progresses from flexibility to rigidity, the hindfoot must assume a varus position to maintain the tripod of the foot.

The clinical evaluation should include a thorough neurologic examination. The position of the hindfoot and the forefoot must be evaluated. Flexibility of the deformity is determined using the Coleman block test or the kneeling method[65] (Figure 10). Standing AP and lateral radiographs of the feet should be obtained. The radiographic hallmarks of a cavus foot include increased calcaneal pitch, Meary angle, navicular height, and Hibbs angle[63] (Figure 11).

Nonsurgical treatment has a small role for most patients. If the deformity is flexible, an orthotic device may provide support for an unstable ankle.

Surgery usually is needed to correct the condition. Several surgical treatments are available, and the choice of treatment is primarily based on the flexibility of the foot. The surgery should be performed before the de-

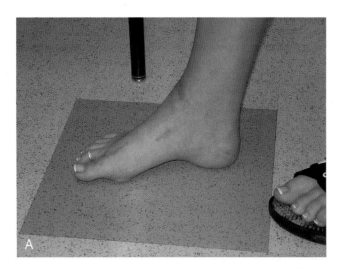

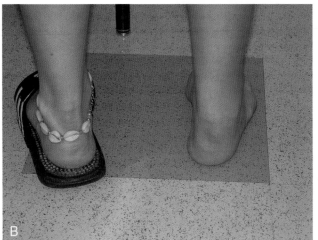

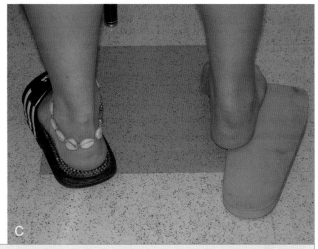

Figure 10	Clinical photographs of a cavus foot deformity. **A,** Elevation of the arch with weight bearing. **B,** The hindfoot is in varus when the patient is standing. **C,** In the Coleman block test, the block under the lateral aspect of the foot allows the first metatarsal to drop to the floor; if the hindfoot is flexible, the heel is now in valgus. This patient has only a partial correction of the hindfoot varus.

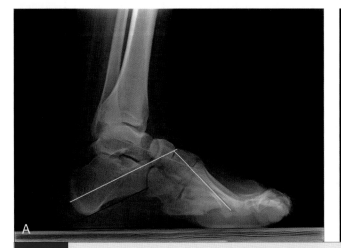

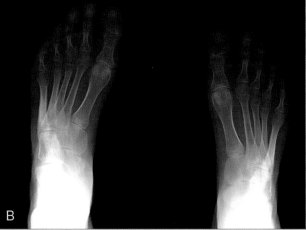

Figure 11	A cavovarus foot deformity. **A,** Lateral radiograph showing an increased calcaneal pitch *(black line)*, increased Meary angle *(red lines)*, and increased Hibbs angle *(yellow lines)*. **B,** AP standing radiograph showing hindfoot varus with a decreased talocalcaneal angle and a supinated foot.

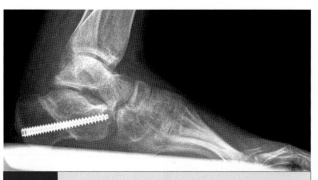

Figure 12   Postoperative lateral radiograph of a cavus foot treated with a soft-tissue release and a calcaneal slide osteotomy.

formity becomes fixed to release the soft-tissue contractures of the planter fascia and abductor hallucis, with bony surgery as indicated. The goal is to obtain a plantigrade foot with muscle balance adequate to prevent recurrence of the deformity.

In a patient with Charcot-Marie-Tooth disease, soft-tissue procedures performed alone have been successful in correcting flexible deformity.[66] A study of the long-term results of releasing the plantar fascia, transferring the peroneus longus to the peroneus brevis, performing a dorsal closing-wedge osteotomy of the first metatarsal, and transferring the anterior tibial tendon to the lateral cuneiform found that the patients maintained a flattened arch, although some had recurrent hindfoot varus.[66] None of the patients required triple arthrodesis. A combination of soft-tissue and bony procedures is needed to correct a rigid deformity; a stepwise approach to the deformity correction allows all of the components to be treated. Because the primary pathology is in the forefoot, one author recommends first treating the forefoot with a dorsal closing-wedge osteotomy of the first metatarsal and a plantar opening-wedge osteotomy of the medial cuneiform.[65] A closing-wedge osteotomy of the cuboid can then be done for residual adductus, followed by a calcaneal slide osteotomy for hindfoot varus. A plantar fasciotomy can be added if necessary. If the deformity is secondary to Charcot-Marie-Tooth disease, a peroneus longus to peroneus brevis transfer is added. In contrast, a soft-tissue release, followed by bony procedures in a staged fashion, also has been recommended[67] (Figure 12). Triple arthrodesis always should be avoided; several studies found severe degenerative changes of the mobile joints in patients who underwent triple arthrodesis.[67,68] Several dorsal midfoot osteotomies have been described, and they may be considered primarily as salvage procedures.[69,70] Dorsal midfoot osteotomies have the benefit of correcting the deformity where it occurs, but they do not treat the hindfoot and forefoot deformities and may be better suited to cavus deformities associated with clubfoot.

Patients with an underlying neurologic condition, especially a progressive disorder such as Charcot-Marie-

Tooth disease, should be warned that further surgery may be required. Tethered cord syndrome also can lead to recurrent deformity.

Summary

Intervention is required for many common foot deformities in children. It is important to remember that an extensive evaluation is necessary to rule out other underlying pathology in a number of pediatric foot deformities. The treatment of clubfoot has significantly changed during the past 10 years. A resurgence in the use of the Ponseti technique has led to a decrease in the use of extensive surgical procedures to correct this common foot deformity.

Annotated References

1. Ponseti IV: *Congenital Clubfoot.* New York, NY, Oxford University Press, 1996, p 140.

2. Dobbs MB, Nunley R, Schoenecker PL: Long-term follow-up of patients with clubfeet treated with extensive soft-tissue release. *J Bone Joint Surg Am* 2006; 88(5):986-996.

   At a mean 31-year follow-up, patients treated with soft-tissue releases for idiopathic clubfoot had impaired function as measured using three outcomes instruments. Functional scores were worse than those reported at a 30-year follow-up of patients treated with the Ponseti method. Level of evidence: III.

3. Ippolito E, Farsetti P, Caterini R, Tudisco C: Long-term comparative results in patients with congenital clubfoot treated with two different protocols. *J Bone Joint Surg Am* 2003;85(7):1286-1294.

4. Zwick EB, Kraus T, Maizen C, Steinwender G, Linhart WE: Comparison of Ponseti versus surgical treatment for idiopathic clubfoot: A short-term preliminary report. *Clin Orthop Relat Res* 2009;467(10):2668-2676.

   The Ponseti method was compared with the use of another casting technique followed by posteromedial release. At 3-year follow-up, range of motion and functional scores were better in patients treated with the Ponseti method. Level of evidence: III.

5. Bor N, Coplan JA, Herzenberg JE: Ponseti treatment for idiopathic clubfoot: Minimum 5-year followup. *Clin Orthop Relat Res* 2009;467(5):1263-1270.

   At 5-year follow-up, 89% of patients with clubfoot had a good outcome after treatment with the Ponseti method. An additional surgical procedure was required in 32% and was associated with poor brace use. Level of evidence: IV.

6. Richards BS, Faulks S, Rathjen KE, Karol LA, Johnston CE, Jones SA: A comparison of two nonoperative methods of idiopathic clubfoot correction: The Ponseti

method and the French functional (physiotherapy) method. *J Bone Joint Surg Am* 2008;90(11):2313-2321.

The Ponseti and French physical therapy methods were found to achieve equivalent results. Initial correction was achieved in 94.4% and 95% of patients, respectively. At 2-year follow-up, a good outcome was achieved in 72% and 67%, respectively. Parents were more likely to choose the Ponseti method. Level of evidence: II.

7. El-Hawary R, Karol LA, Jeans KA, Richards BS: Gait analysis of children treated for clubfoot with physical therapy or the Ponseti cast technique. *J Bone Joint Surg Am* 2008;90(7):1508-1516.

Gait analysis was performed for 105 patients treated with physical therapy or the Ponseti method. Children treated with physical therapy had more knee hyperextension, equinus, and foot drop, with increased internal foot progression. Stance-phase dorsiflexion was more common in the children treated with the Ponseti method. Level of evidence: II.

8. Shack N, Eastwood DM: Early results of a physiotherapist-delivered Ponseti service for the management of idiopathic congenital talipes equinovarus foot deformity. *J Bone Joint Surg Br* 2006;88(8):1085-1089.

The success of the Ponseti method administered by a physical therapist is reported.

9. Janicki JA, Narayanan UG, Harvey BJ, Roy A, Weir S, Wright JG: Comparison of surgeon and physiotherapist-directed Ponseti treatment of idiopathic clubfoot. *J Bone Joint Surg Am* 2009;91(5):1101-1108.

The results of the Ponseti method administered by a surgeon and a physical therapist are compared. Patients treated by a physical therapist had fewer recurrences or additional surgical procedures. Level of evidence: III.

10. Brewster MB, Gupta M, Pattison GT, Dunn-van der Ploeg ID: Ponseti casting: A new soft option. *J Bone Joint Surg Br* 2008;90(11):1512-1515.

The authors' modification of the Ponseti method to use short leg casts with semirigid fiberglass casting tape was found to be successful.

11. Pittner DE, Klingele KE, Beebe AC: Treatment of clubfoot with the Ponseti method: A comparison of casting materials. *J Pediatr Orthop* 2008;28(2):250-253.

A randomized, prospective study compared the use of plaster casts to semirigid fiberglass in the Ponseti method. Better results were achieved with plaster. Level of evidence: II.

12. Radler C, Manner HM, Suda R, et al: Radiographic evaluation of idiopathic clubfeet undergoing Ponseti treatment. *J Bone Joint Surg Am* 2007;89(6):1177-1183.

The lateral tibiocalcaneal angle was found to be increased, with no change in the talocalcaneal angle, after Achilles tenotomy. This change reflects a true increase in ankle dorsiflexion rather than a midfoot break. Level of evidence: IV.

13. Boehm S, Limpaphayom N, Alaee F, Sinclair MF, Dobbs MB: Early results of the Ponseti method for the treatment of clubfoot in distal arthrogryposis. *J Bone Joint Surg Am* 2008;90(7):1501-1507.

The Ponseti method was as successful in correcting clubfoot in patients with distal arthrogryposis as in patients with idiopathic clubfoot, although more casts were necessary. The risk of recurrence and the long-term results are unknown. Level of evidence: IV.

14. van Bosse HJ, Marangoz S, Lehman WB, Sala DA: Correction of arthrogrypotic clubfoot with a modified Ponseti technique. *Clin Orthop Relat Res* 2009;467(5):1283-1293.

The Ponseti method was found to be successful in patients with arthrogryposis. A modification is described in which tenotomy is performed before the first casting and again, if necessary, before the last casting.

15. Gerlach DJ, Gurnett CA, Limpaphayom N, et al: Early results of the Ponseti method for the treatment of clubfoot associated with myelomeningocele. *J Bone Joint Surg Am* 2009;91(6):1350-1359.

The Ponseti method initially was successful in 96% of children with myelomeningocele-associated clubfoot and 100% of children with idiopathic clubfoot. Relapses occurred in 68% and 26%, respectively. Most children were treated without the need for extensive soft-tissue release.

16. Janicki JA, Narayanan UG, Harvey B, Roy A, Ramseier LE, Wright JG: Treatment of neuromuscular and syndrome-associated (nonidiopathic) clubfeet using the Ponseti method. *J Pediatr Orthop* 2009;29(4):393-397.

The Ponseti method was used to treat nonidiopathic and idiopathic clubfeet. The nonidiopathic feet required more casts and had more recurrences and failures, but correction was obtained in more patients. Level of evidence: II.

17. Dobbs MB, Rudzki JR, Purcell DB, Walton T, Porter KR, Gurnett CA: Factors predictive of outcome after use of the Ponseti method for the treatment of idiopathic clubfeet. *J Bone Joint Surg Am* 2004;86(1):22-27.

18. Thacker MM, Scher DM, Sala DA, van Bosse HJ, Feldman DS, Lehman WB: Use of the foot abduction orthosis following Ponseti casts: Is it essential? *J Pediatr Orthop* 2005;25(2):225-228.

After successful casting, patients who used the foot abduction brace had better results at early follow-up than those who did not.

19. Haft GF, Walker CG, Crawford HA: Early clubfoot recurrence after use of the Ponseti method in a New Zealand population. *J Bone Joint Surg Am* 2007;89(3):487-493.

Patients who did not comply with the bracing protocol had more major and minor recurrences than those who did comply. Level of evidence: II.

20. Avilucea FR, Szalay EA, Bosch PP, Sweet KR, Schwend RM: Effect of cultural factors on outcome of Ponseti

treatment of clubfeet in rural America. *J Bone Joint Surg Am* 2009;91(3):530-540.

Communication failures resulting from cultural differences may be to blame for poor compliance with bracing in a rural Native American population. Level of evidence: I.

21. Ponseti IV, Zhivkov M, Davis N, Sinclair M, Dobbs MB, Morcuende JA: Treatment of the complex idiopathic clubfoot. *Clin Orthop Relat Res* 2006;451:171-176.

    The modified technique for treating the complex clubfoot (a severe variant of idiopathic clubfoot) is described. Level of evidence: IV.

22. Farsetti P, Caterini R, Mancini F, Potenza V, Ippolito E: Anterior tibial tendon transfer in relapsing congenital clubfoot: Long-term follow-up study of two series treated with a different protocol. *J Pediatr Orthop* 2006;26(1):83-90.

    A complete transfer of the tibialis anterior to the lateral cuneiform was successful in stabilizing a recurrence in clubfeet initially treated with posteromedial release or the Ponseti method. Although patients in both groups had radiographic abnormalities, those treated with the Ponseti method had better functional scores.

23. Dietz FR: Treatment of a recurrent clubfoot deformity after initial correction with the Ponseti technique. *Instr Course Lect* 2006;55:625-629.

    The protocol for managing recurrences after treatment with the Ponseti method is described.

24. Freedman JA, Watts H, Otsuka NY: The Ilizarov method for the treatment of resistant clubfoot: Is it an effective solution? *J Pediatr Orthop* 2006;26(4):432-437.

    The Ilizarov method led to poor outcomes when used for older children with recurrent clubfoot after surgical treatment.

25. Prem H, Zenios M, Farrell R, Day JB: Soft tissue Ilizarov correction of congenital talipes equinovarus: 5 to 10 years postsurgery. *J Pediatr Orthop* 2007;27(2):220-224.

    Soft-tissue distraction using the Ilizarov method for clubfeet in older children had good short-term results that were maintained in all but one patient at 5-year follow-up.

26. Swaroop VT, Wenger DR, Mubarak SJ: Talonavicular fusion for dorsal subluxation of the navicular in resistant clubfoot. *Clin Orthop Relat Res* 2009;467(5):1314-1318.

    Talonavicular arthrodesis was used for symptomatic dorsal subluxation of the navicular in recurrent clubfeet, with good outcomes and few complications. Level of evidence: IV.

27. Legaspi J, Li YH, Chow W, Leong JC: Talectomy in patients with recurrent deformity in club foot: A long-term follow-up study. *J Bone Joint Surg Br* 2001;83(3):384-387.

28. Pfeiffer M, Kotz R, Ledl T, Hauser G, Sluga M: Prevalence of flat foot in preschool-aged children. *Pediatrics* 2006;118(2):634-639.

    The prevalence of flatfoot was found to be 44% in 3- to 6-year-old children; it decreased with increasing age. Flatfoot was more prevalent among boys and children who were overweight.

29. Chang JH, Wang SH, Kuo CL, Shen HC, Hong YW, Lin LC: Prevalence of flexible flatfoot in Taiwanese school-aged children in relation to obesity, gender, and age. *Eur J Pediatr* 2010;169(4):447-452.

    Boys and children who were overweight were more likely to have a flexible flatfoot. The prevalence was greatest among boys who were overweight.

30. Chen JP, Chung MJ, Wang MJ: Flatfoot prevalence and foot dimensions of 5- to 13-year-old children in Taiwan. *Foot Ankle Int* 2009;30(4):326-332.

    Children who were obese had a higher incidence of flatfoot than children of normal weight.

31. Tudor A, Ruzic L, Sestan B, Sirola L, Prpic T: Flatfootedness is not a disadvantage for athletic performance in children aged 11 to 15 years. *Pediatrics* 2009;123(3):e386-e392.

    There was no difference in motor skills and athletic performance on several physical tests between children with flexible flatfoot and those with normal arch height.

32. Hansen ST: *Functional Reconstruction of the Foot and Ankle*. Philadelphia, PA, Lippincott Williams & Wilkins, 2000, p 196.

33. Giannini BS, Ceccarelli F, Benedetti MG, Catani F, Faldini C: Surgical treatment of flexible flatfoot in children: A four-year follow-up study. *J Bone Joint Surg Am* 2001;83(suppl 2, pt 2):73-79.

34. Mosca VS: Calcaneal lengthening for valgus deformity of the hindfoot: Results in children who had severe, symptomatic flatfoot and skewfoot. *J Bone Joint Surg Am* 1995;77(4):500-512.

35. Rathjen KE, Mubarak SJ: Calcaneal-cuboid-cuneiform osteotomy for the correction of valgus foot deformities in children. *J Pediatr Orthop* 1998;18(6):775-782.

36. Olney BW, Asher MA: Excision of symptomatic coalition of the middle facet of the talocalcaneal joint. *J Bone Joint Surg Am* 1987;69(4):539-544.

37. Raikin S, Cooperman DR, Thompson GH: Interposition of the split flexor hallucis longus tendon after resection of a coalition of the middle facet of the talocalcaneal joint. *J Bone Joint Surg Am* 1999;81(1):11-19.

38. Westberry DE, Davids JR, Oros W: Surgical management of symptomatic talocalcaneal coalitions by resection of the sustentaculum tali. *J Pediatr Orthop* 2003;23(4):493-497.

39. Cooperman DR, Janke BE, Gilmore A, Latimer BM, Brinker MR, Thompson GH: A three-dimensional study of calcaneonavicular tarsal coalitions. *J Pediatr Orthop* 2001;21(5):648-651.

40. Mubarak SJ, Patel PN, Upasani VV, Moor MA, Wenger DR: Calcaneonavicular coalition: Treatment by excision and fat graft. *J Pediatr Orthop* 2009;29(5):418-426.

    Resection of a calcaneonavicular coalition with interposition of fat graft yielded better results than reported in most studies of extensor digitorum brevis interposition. Plantar flexion and subtalar motion improved in 82% and 74% of patients, respectively. A cadaver study found better filling of the gap when fat graft was used.

41. Hetsroni I, Nyska M, Mann G, Rozenfeld G, Ayalon M: Subtalar kinematics following resection of tarsal coalition. *Foot Ankle Int* 2008;29(11):1088-1094.

    There were no significant differences in subtalar motion during walking between patients who had tarsal coalitions and those who had undergone resection of tarsal coalitions. Sagittal kinematics were better in those who had undergone resection. Level of evidence: III.

42. El Rassi G, Riddle EC, Kumar SJ: Arthrofibrosis involving the middle facet of the talocalcaneal joint in children and adolescents. *J Bone Joint Surg Am* 2005;87(10):2227-2231.

    A previously undescribed condition of inflammatory arthrofibrosis of the subtalar joint was found in patients with painful rigid flatfeet. The results of treatment are reported. Level of evidence: IV.

43. Martus JE, Femino JE, Caird MS, Hughes RE, Browne RH, Farley FA: Accessory anterolateral facet of the pediatric talus: An anatomic study. *J Bone Joint Surg Am* 2008;90(11):2452-2459.

    A survey of a pediatric osteologic collection found that 34% of the specimens had accessory anterolateral talar facets, which were associated with dorsal talar beaking in 29%. The authors suggest an association with painful talocalcaneal impingement.

44. Martus JE, Femino JE, Caird MS, Kuhns LR, Craig CL, Farley FA: Accessory anterolateral talar facet as an etiology of painful talocalcaneal impingement in the rigid flatfoot: A new diagnosis. *Iowa Orthop J* 2008;28:1-8.

    An association between an accessory facet on the anterolateral aspect of the talus was found in six children with painful flatfeet and is believed to be a source of pain. Early results of treatment are reported.

45. Kruse L, Gurnett CA, Hootnick D, Dobbs MB: Magnetic resonance angiography in clubfoot and vertical talus: A feasibility study. *Clin Orthop Relat Res* 2009; 467(5):1250-1255.

    Magnetic resonance angiography was used to diagnose vascular anomalies associated with clubfoot and congenital vertical talus. This is a noninvasive means of detecting absent or deficient posterior tibial arteries in association with congenital vertical talus.

46. Alaee F, Boehm S, Dobbs MB: A new approach to the treatment of congenital vertical talus. *J Child Orthop* 2007;1(3):165-174.

    Congenital vertical talus is reviewed in terms of diagnosis, pathogenesis, pathoanatomy, and genetics. The incidence of a positive family history in congenital vertical talus is 12% to 20%. The condition may have an autosomal dominant inheritance pattern with incomplete penetrance. A new *Hoxd-10* gene has been identified in several families with congenital vertical talus. A treatment using serial stretching casts and minimal surgery is similar to the Ponseti method for clubfoot.

47. Dobbs MB, Schoenecker PL, Gordo JE: Autosomal dominant transmission of isolated congenital vertical talus. *Iowa Orthop J* 2002;22:25-27.

48. Aroojis AJ, King MM, Donohoe M, Riddle EC, Kumar SJ: Congenital vertical talus in arthrogryposis and other contractural syndromes. *Clin Orthop Relat Res* 2005; 434:26-32.

    The treatment of congenital vertical talus associated with arthrogryposis and other contractural syndromes is described. The five contractural syndromes are classic amyoplasia, distal arthrogryposis, limb contractures associated with a specific syndrome, musculoskeletal contracture with organ system involvement, and extremity contracture not otherwise classified. None of the patients with classic amyoplasia had congenital vertical talus. The children in the second and fifth groups had good results from surgery, but those in the third and fourth groups had poor results or did not undergo surgery because they had severe health issues or were not ambulatory.

49. Drennan JC: Congenital vertical talus. *Instr Course Lect* 1996;45:315-322.

50. Duncan RD, Fixsen JA: Congenital convex pes valgus. *J Bone Joint Surg Br* 1999;81(2):250-254.

51. Kodros SA, Dias LS: Single-stage surgical correction of congenital vertical talus. *J Pediatr Orthop* 1999;19(1):42-48.

52. Saini R, Gill SS, Dhillon MS, Goyal T, Wardak E, Prasad P: Results of dorsal approach in surgical correction of congenital vertical talus: An Indian experience. *J Pediatr Orthop B* 2009;18(2):63-68.

    The results of correcting vertical talus using both a dorsal and a posterior incision are retrospectively reviewed. The dorsal incision allowed a direct approach to the contracted structures and the dorsally dislocated navicular. Talonavicular reduction was achieved and maintained in all 20 patients at an average 4-year follow-up. The average patient age was 16 months.

53. Mazzocca AD, Thomson JD, Deluca PA, Romness MJ: Comparison of the posterior approach versus the dorsal approach in the treatment of congenital vertical talus. *J Pediatr Orthop* 2001;21(2):212-217.

54. Dobbs MB, Purcell DB, Nunley R, Morcuende JA: Early results of a new method of treatment for idiopathic con-

4: Lower Extremity

genital vertical talus: Surgical technique. *J Bone Joint Surg Am* 2007;89(suppl 2, pt 1):111-121.

Serial manipulation and casting for congenital vertical talus, followed by minimal surgery, is described. The surgical procedures included percutaneous Achilles tenotomy and occasional fractional lengthening of the tibialis anterior and peroneus brevis, with pinning at the talonavicular joint. Three patients had recurrent dorsal subluxation of the talonavicular joint, but the remaining 16 maintained the correction at 2-year follow-up. The recommendation is to proceed with an open talonavicular joint reduction if closed reduction does not achieve complete talonavicular reduction.

55. Coughlin MJ: Juvenile hallux valgus: Etiology and treatment. *Foot Ankle Int* 1995;16(11):682-697.

56. Scott G, Wilson DW, Bentley G: Roentgenographic assessment in hallux valgus. *Clin Orthop Relat Res* 1991;267:143-147.

57. Robinson AH, Limbers JP: Modern concepts in the treatment of hallux valgus. *J Bone Joint Surg Br* 2005;87(8):1038-1045.

This comprehensive review of hallux valgus includes etiology, clinical and radiographic assessment, and nonsurgical and surgical treatments. A successful surgical outcome depends on correct procedure selection and technical performance.

58. George HL, Casaletto J, Unnikrishnan PN, et al: Outcome of the scarf osteotomy in adolescent hallux valgus. *J Child Orthop* 2009;3(3):185-190.

Scarf osteotomy was performed in 13 patients (19 feet). There was significant improvement in the mean postoperative intermetatarsal angle, which was maintained at follow-up. Despite initial improvement in both the hallux valgus and distal metatarsal articular angles, this correction was lost at the last follow-up. Scarf osteotomy should be used with caution in symptomatic adolescent hallux valgus, as the rate of recurrence is high.

59. Davids JR, McBrayer D, Blackhurst DW: Juvenile hallux valgus deformity: Surgical management by lateral hemiepiphyseodesis of the great toe metatarsal. *J Pediatr Orthop* 2007;27(7):826-830.

The results of proximal lateral hemiepiphysiodesis of the first metatarsal for the treatment of juvenile hallux valgus are reviewed. The procedure was effective in halting the progression of deformity in all feet, and it achieved significant correction of the intermetatarsal angle and hallux valgus angle in more than 50%. There was no significant decrease in first metatarsal length.

60. Coughlin MJ, Jones CP: Hallux valgus and first ray mobility: A prospective study. *J Bone Joint Surg Am* 2007;89(9):1887-1898.

The clinical and radiographic diagnosis of medial cuneiform–first metatarsal hypermobility is described in adults. Although several patients had hallux valgus associated with the hypermobility, they did well after a distal soft-tissue realignment and proximal crescentic osteotomy.

61. Coughlin MJ, Smith BW: Hallux valgus and first ray mobility: Surgical technique. *J Bone Joint Surg Am* 2008;90(suppl 2, pt 2):153-170.

After a distal soft-tissue realignment with a proximal crescentic osteotomy to treat moderate to severe subluxated hallux valgus, first-ray hypermobility was reduced to a normal level without fusing the cuneiform metatarsal joint.

62. Stephens MM: Does shortening of the first ray in the treatment of adolescent hallux valgus prejudice the outcome? *J Bone Joint Surg Br* 2006;88(7):858-859.

As hallux valgus deformity increases, the first ray becomes dysfunctional. Ground reaction force is then transferred to the more lateral rays, particularly the second ray, and they become much less mobile than the first metatarsal. Any corrective osteotomy that shortens the first ray results in a further transfer of load and leads to symptomatic transfer lesions. Shortening of the first ray should be avoided with corrective osteotomy.

63. Aminian A, Sangeorzan BJ: The anatomy of the cavus foot. *Foot Ankle Clin* 2008;13(2):191-198.

A comprehensive description of the cavus foot is presented, with its biomechanics, associated gait abnormalities, and radiographic abnormalities.

64. Schwend RM, Drennan JC: Cavus foot deformity in children. *J Am Acad Orthop Surg* 2003;11(3):201-211.

65. Mubarak SJ, Van Valin SE: Osteotomies of the foot for cavus deformities in children. *J Pediatr Orthop* 2009;29(3):294-299.

In a retrospective review of multiple osteotomies done in a stepwise fashion to treat 20 rigid cavus feet, almost all feet were found to have a good or excellent result. Undercorrection of the hindfoot varus led to a poor result. Progression of the deformity was secondary to symptomatic tethered cord.

66. Ward CM, Dolan LA, Bennett DL, Morcuende JA, Cooper RR: Long-term results of reconstruction for treatment of a flexible cavovarus foot in Charcot-Marie-Tooth disease. *J Bone Joint Surg Am* 2008;90(12):2631-2642.

Long-term results are presented for a soft-tissue procedure to treat flexible cavovarus foot deformities associated with Charcot-Marie-Tooth disease. The procedure included a plantar release, peroneus longus–peroneus brevis transfer, first metatarsal dorsal closing-wedge osteotomy, Jones transfer, and tibialis anterior tendon transfer to the lateral cuneiform. At follow-up, no patient had recurrent cavus, although some had recurrent hindfoot varus. None of the patients required triple arthrodesis. Level of evidence: IV.

67. Mosca VS: The cavus foot. *J Pediatr Orthop* 2001;21(4):423-424.

68. Wetmore RS, Drennan JC: Long-term results of triple arthrodesis in Charcot-Marie-Tooth disease. *J Bone Joint Surg Am* 1989;71(3):417-422.

69. Wicart P, Seringe R: Plantar opening-wedge osteotomy of cuneiform bones combined with selective plantar release and dwyer osteotomy for pes cavovarus in children. *J Pediatr Orthop* 2006;26(1):100-108.

In a retrospective review of surgical results, all deformities were found to have a neurologic etiology. Good results were found in 64% of patients, and poor results in 36%. Most of the poor results were from progression of the deformity, and they required further surgical correction.

70. Weiner DS, Morscher M, Junko JT, Jacoby J, Weiner B: The Akron dome midfoot osteotomy as a salvage procedure for the treatment of rigid pes cavus: A retrospective review. *J Pediatr Orthop* 2008;28(1):68-80.

Residual clubfoot deformity was the etiology in most of the 139 patients who underwent an Akron dome midfoot osteotomy, although a few feet had a neuromuscular etiology. At long-term follow-up, the procedure was found to correct only the midfoot cavus and did not treat hindfoot or forefoot deformities. The percentage of satisfactory results decreased with the length of follow-up. Younger age at the time of surgery was a significant risk factor for a poor result. The procedure was initially successful in correcting midfoot cavus and probably should be considered an intermediate procedure to delay the need for triple arthrodesis until adulthood. Level of evidence: III.

4: Lower Extremity

Chapter 23

Limb-Length Discrepancy and Limb Lengthening

Samantha A. Spencer, MD   Roger F. Widmann, MD

4: Lower Extremity

Introduction

Lower limb-length discrepancy is common. More than half of military recruits were found to have a limb-length discrepancy, most of which were 1 cm or less.[1] Gait studies have had equivocal findings as to whether gait patterns may be altered if a lower extremity discrepancy exceeds 2 cm.[2,3] The treatment of a limb-length discrepancy depends on both its etiology and its severity. Thus, observation is the recommended treatment of a discrepancy smaller than 2 cm. The treatment of a larger discrepancy ranges from orthotic management to guided growth procedures such as epiphysiodesis. Limb lengthening usually is done if the discrepancy at skeletal maturity is likely to exceed 5 cm. A very large discrepancy (more than 20 cm) or a discrepancy in a limb that is unsuitable for lengthening or reconstruction may be best treated with amputation and fitting of a prosthesis.

The limb-length discrepancy must be carefully analyzed before any treatment decision is made. The etiology of the discrepancy needs to be understood for the purpose of predicting the total amount of discrepancy and deformity at skeletal maturity. The analysis can be completed when the etiology is understood, and a treatment plan can then be implemented.

Etiology

The etiology of limb-length discrepancy can be classified as interference in length, interference in growth, or stimulation of growth.[4] An interference in length results from an acute change such as a fracture, surgical procedure, or unreduced dislocation. An interference in growth can be caused by a congenital difference, an infection or inflammation, paralysis, a tumor, or a trau-

matic injury. Many of these factors also lead to stimulation of growth. In some patients, such as those with a congenital short femur, a constant rate of growth inhibition is expected throughout childhood. In other patients, such as those with osteomyelitis, a temporary stimulus or inhibition to physeal growth may later resolve. In patients with a pediatric femur fracture, stimulation of growth is expected for a finite time after fracture healing.

A limb-length discrepancy also can be categorized as congenital-syndromic or acquired. Within these two groups, the specific cause may be an inhibition or a stimulation of growth. The congenital causes include an isolated limb deficiency such as a congenital short femur, proximal femoral focal deficiency (PFFD), tibial hemimelia, or fibular hemimelia; an overgrowth syndrome such as Beckwith-Wiedemann hemihypertrophy; and a vascular malformation syndrome such as Sturge-Weber or Klippel-Trénaunay syndrome. The acquired causes include physeal trauma leading to growth disturbance, an inflammatory condition such as juvenile inflammatory arthritis, Legg-Calvé-Perthes disease, slipped capital femoral epiphysis, tumor, a diaphyseal fracture that healed with shortening or caused overgrowth, and hemiplegic cerebral palsy (which causes undergrowth). Additional causes are listed in **Table 1**.

Assessment

Clinical Evaluation

The review of the patient's history should include an understanding of any congenital syndrome, past trauma, tumor, infection, or joint inflammation that could create a predisposition for limb-length discrepancy. The patient should be examined with the arms, pelvis, back, and legs bare; the inspection is facilitated if the patient is wearing shorts rather than a back-tied gown. The Tanner stage of pubertal maturity should be noted.[5] The symmetry of the back, arms, and legs should be observed, as well as any skin markings. Significant side-to-side differences in girth and length may indicate hemihypertrophy or hemiplegia. A patient with a vascular malformation often has characteristic skin

Neither Dr. Spencer nor any immediate family member has received anything of value from or owns stock in a commercial company or institution related directly or indirectly to the subject of this chapter. Dr. Widmann or an immediate family member has received research or institutional support from Medtronic Sofamor Danek.

Table 1

Etiologies of Lower Limb Deformity and Length Discrepancy

Congenital	Acquired
Beckwith-Wiedemann syndrome	Acute bone loss
Congenital short femur	Acute brain injury
Fibrous dysplasia	Burns
Fibula deficiency	Cerebral palsy
Hemiatrophy	Enchondromatosis
Hemihypertrophy	Fracture healing process
Hypoplasia syndromes	Hemangioma
Idiopathic etiology	Hemophilia
Klippel-Trénaunay syndrome	Iatrogenic etiology
Multiple hereditary exostoses	Infection
	Inflammation
Neurofibromatosis	Irradiation
Ollier disease	Juvenile rheumatoid arthritis
Proteus syndrome	Myelomeningocele
Proximal femoral focal deficiency	Neurologic etiology
	Osteomyelitis
Skeletal dysplasia	Peripheral nerve injury
Sturge-Weber syndrome	Physeal injury
Tibial deficiency	Pigmented villonodular synovitis
	Poliomyelitis
	Purpura fulminans
	Septic arthritis
	Spinal cord injury
	Trauma
	Tumor
	Tumor treatment

(Adapted with permission from Finch GD, Dawe CJ: Hemiatrophy. *J Pediatr Orthop* 2003;23[1]:99-101; and Stanitski DF: Limb-length inequality: Assessment and treatment options. *J Am Acad Orthop Surg* 1999;7[3]:143-153.)

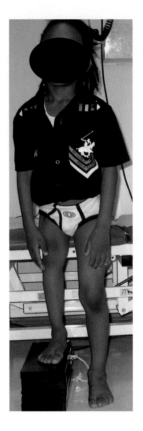

Figure 1 Photograph of a 6-year-old boy with proximal femoral focal deficiency. The characteristic short, broad thigh can be seen.

markings, such as a pinkish lacy discoloration of capillary malformation associated with overgrowth. Patients with neurofibromatosis have multiple café-au-lait spots as well as axillary and inguinal freckling. Some congenital limb differences have a characteristic appearance that may include skin dimpling, foot deformity, a short and broad thigh, genu valgum with a lax anterior drawer or absent anterior cruciate ligament, a midtibial dimple, or a valgus foot with missing lateral rays (in fibular hemimelia with associated PFFD) (**Figure 1**).

Several methods are used to measure limb-length discrepancy. A standing pelvic obliquity can be measured by leveling it with blocks placed under the foot on the shorter side. The Galeazzi test, which is performed with the patient supine and both hips flexed to 90°, provides an estimate of femur length equality as long as the hips are not dislocated (**Figure 2**). The total limb lengths of the two sides can be compared by measuring from the anterosuperior iliac spine to the medial malleolus on each side, although these landmarks are imprecise. Measuring from the umbilicus to the medial malleolus yields the apparent leg length. Prone heel heights can be

compared with the patient prone and both knees flexed to 90°. All joints should be examined because the presence of a contracture or angular deformity can disrupt the accuracy of the measurements. In particular, a hip flexion-adduction contracture can cause the limb to appear much shorter than its actual length. The standing block test was found to yield more accurate and reliable measurements than the other clinical methods.[6]

Radiographic Evaluation

Femur length is radiographically measured from the top of the femoral head to the medial femoral condyle, and tibia length is measured from the medial femoral condyle to the middle of the ankle mortise. A supine scanogram consists of three separate radiographs of the hips, knees, and ankles, with a tape measure placed beside one or both legs (**Figure 3**). A standing AP hips-to-ankles radiograph from a 6-ft distance can be used to assess limb-length discrepancy as well as angular deformity (**Figure 4**). A CT scanogram also can be used to calculate the radiographic distance between points on the long bones (**Figure 5**). A CT scanogram eliminates the need for multiple images and is comparable to other methods in radiation exposure and cost. The accuracy of all radiographic methods can be affected by the presence of a joint contracture. A lateral-position CT scanogram may be helpful if hip and knee contractures are present.

Ultrasonography or MRI may be helpful if the radiographic landmarks are not easily discernible. For example, skeletal dysplasias and limb differences often are

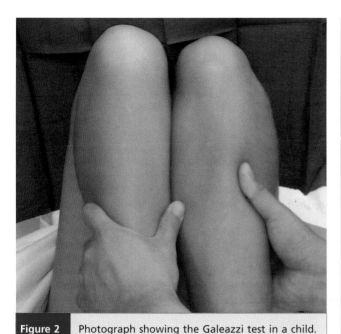

Figure 2 | Photograph showing the Galeazzi test in a child. A difference in knee heights is caused by differing femur lengths.

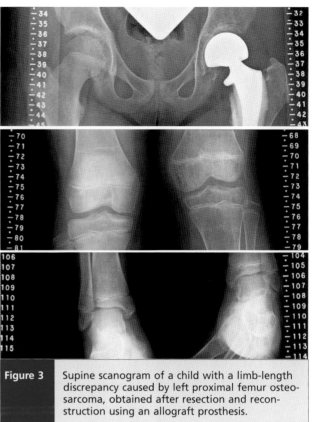

Figure 3 | Supine scanogram of a child with a limb-length discrepancy caused by left proximal femur osteosarcoma, obtained after resection and reconstruction using an allograft prosthesis.

diagnosed from measurements taken during fetal ultrasonographs. MRI can help in assessing the true extent of discrepancy and deformity in a young child with PFFD, whose proximal femur and hip may be slow to ossify.[7,8]

Children reach skeletal maturity at different ages, and therefore an assessment of skeletal or bone age is important in the radiographic assessment of deformity. The Greulich and Pyle atlas of normal standards contains AP radiographs showing the left hands of boys and girls at different ages.[9] The patient's AP left hand and wrist radiograph can be compared with radiographs in the Greulich and Pyle atlas to determine the patient's bone age, which may differ from the chronologic age. This method has diminished accuracy in children who are younger than 10 years, are at peak height velocity, or have a congenital hand anomaly. Skeletal age also can be measured by radiographically comparing growth centers around the elbow.[10,11]

Data Analysis

Several analysis methods accurately calculate the best timing of epiphysiodesis (premature physeal arrest) to achieve a limb-length discrepancy of no more than 2 cm at skeletal maturity. However, all of the analysis methods assume a constant rate of growth inhibition, which is not the pattern in all conditions.[4,12,13]

The Arithmetic Method

The arithmetic method uses the Green and Anderson growth charts to predict the best timing of epiphysiodesis. The use of this method requires the assumption that skeletal maturity occurs at age 14 years in girls and at age 16 years in boys. The assumed growth rate per

year is 0.375 inch (10 mm) in the distal femoral physis and 0.25 inch (6 mm) in the proximal tibial physis. This method is simple and remains useful. For children who do not mature at the assumed ages or who do not have a constant rate of growth inhibition, the use of this method may yield an inaccurate result.[4]

The Growth-Remaining Method

The Green and Anderson growth charts are used to calculate future limb-length discrepancies based on skeletal age. The past rate of growth is used to calculate an inhibition rate for the shorter leg. Growth data for the longer leg are plotted on a Green and Anderson leg-length chart, and the length of the longer leg at maturity is determined from the graph. The future limb-length discrepancy is calculated by multiplying the inhibition rate by the length of the longer leg at maturity and adding the result to the existing limb-length discrepancy. The appropriate timing for epiphysiodesis of the longer leg can be selected based on the amount of correction needed.[14,15]

The Moseley Straight-Line Graph Method

In the Moseley straight-line graph method, the growth of the legs is represented graphically by straight lines, and a nomogram is used to determine the growth percentile from the skeletal age and leg length[4] (Figure 6). The lengths of both legs and the skeletal age are plotted at several patient visits over a minimum of 1 year, and a

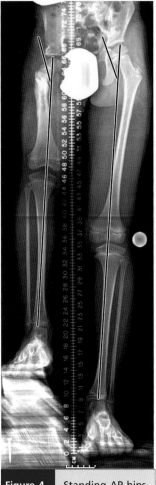

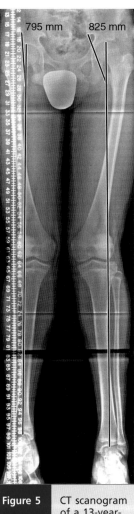

| Figure 4 | Standing AP hips-to-ankles radiograph of the child shown in Figure 1. The congenital short right femur is balanced with blocks. |

| Figure 5 | CT scanogram of a 13-year-old boy with hemihypertrophy affecting the left lower extremity. |

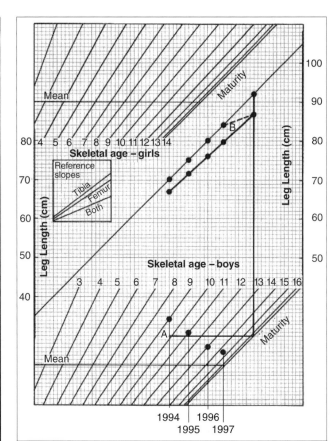

| Figure 6 | Sample graph showing the use of the Moseley straight-line method of predicting limb-length discrepancy at skeletal maturity. Measurements over 4 consecutive years are shown for a boy with idiopathic hemiatrophy. In the first year (1994) the longer leg was 70 cm, the shorter leg was 67 cm, and the radiographically determined skeletal age was 9 years. The findings of annual scanograms and bone-age radiographs also were plotted for each of the subsequent 3 years. Horizontal line *A* is the best-fit horizontal bone-age line, which intersects the maturity line at the end of skeletal growth. At skeletal maturity, the length of the longer leg is projected to be 92 cm, and that of the shorter leg is projected to be 87 cm. Dashed line *B* projects the effect of epiphysiodeses of the distal femur and proximal tibia performed when the length of the longer leg is 84 cm; the projected result is limb equalization by skeletal maturity. (Reproduced with permission from Beaty JH: Congenital anomalies of lower extremity, in Canale ST, ed: *Campbell's Operative Orthopaedics*, ed 9. St. Louis, MO, Mosby, 1998, p 988.) |

horizontal line is drawn to best fit the skeletal ages. The length of both legs at skeletal maturity is plotted by drawing a vertical line from the intersection of the horizontal line and the skeletal maturity line. A sloped line corresponding to a possible date for epiphysiodesis (distal femur, proximal tibia, or combined) is inserted to show the resulting growth-rate modification. The predicted limb-length discrepancy at skeletal maturity can by seen by extrapolating the new slope out to the skeletal maturity line.[16]

The Paley Multiplier Method
The Paley multiplier method is based on a finding that rates of growth and growth inhibition are constant across different ethnic populations.[17] Thus, the amount of future growth can be calculated based on the patient's chronologic age and its assigned multiplier, as taken from a chart. For example, the multiplier for a

4-year-old boy is 2; if a 4-year-old boy has a 2-cm discrepancy, a 4-cm discrepancy can be expected at skeletal maturity. Several mathematical formulas are presented to calculate the timing of epiphysiodesis. The advantages of the multiplier method are that it considers the question of differences in growth rates among different ethnic populations and does not require multiple data points or rely on accurate skeletal age[17] (Table 2).

Morbidity

Several studies examined the morbidity of limb-length discrepancy in children and its possible association with gait abnormality, joint pain, and premature osteoarthritis. A gait analysis study of 35 children with limb-length discrepancy ranging from 0.8% to 15.8% of the length of the long extremity (0.6 to 11.1 cm) found that when the discrepancy was 5.5% or more, more mechanical work was performed by the long extremity and there was a greater vertical displacement of the center of body mass.[18] It can be inferred from this finding that a limb with a discrepancy of 5.5% or more is less energy efficient. A force plate study concluded that in adults with a limb-length discrepancy of 1 to 3 cm, the shorter limb sustains a greater proportion of the load and loading rate.[19] Limb lengthening was found to lead to significant improvement in the quantifiable stance phase parameters of gait and limp.[20]

Treatment

Goals

The goals of treatment include a limb-length discrepancy of less than 2 cm at skeletal maturity; a level pelvis; a vertical lumbar spine; relatively equal knee heights; and a symmetric, efficient gait pattern that minimizes the work of ambulation.[4,18] The empiric treatment guidelines found in standard orthopaedic textbooks predate the development of modern limb equalization techniques.[4]

There is general consensus that a limb-length discrepancy of less than 2 cm at skeletal maturity does not require surgical intervention. If the child or parent perceives symptoms, a shoe lift can be used; the appropriate size of the lift generally is 50% of the measured discrepancy. A tapered lift can be used inside the shoe for a discrepancy as large as 1 cm, but a larger lift usually must be placed outside the shoe to maintain the foot inside the heel counter.

If the child has a predicted limb-length discrepancy of 2 to 6 cm at skeletal maturity, the decision-making process should compare the risks and benefits of a relatively simple surgical epiphysiodesis with the risks and benefits of limb lengthening. Lengthening of the lower limb historically has had a higher rate of complications. The recommended treatment for a 2- to 6-cm discrepancy has been the use of shoe lifts, epiphysiodesis, or a shortening procedure. As experience with limb lengthening has grown and outcomes have improved, the role of limb lengthening for a 3- to 6-cm discrepancy has been debated, especially in skeletally mature individuals who may have missed the opportunity for epiphysiodesis. If a 6- to 20-cm discrepancy is predicted, it is recommended that as many as three lengthening procedures be performed, possibly accompanied by epiphysiodesis. A discrepancy of more than 20 cm is treated with amputation, fitting of a prosthesis, or,

Table 2

Lower Limb Multipliers for Boys and Girls

Age, in Years + Months	Multiplier	
	Boys	Girls
0 + 0 (at birth)	5.080	4.630
0 + 3	4.550	4.155
0 + 6	4.050	3.725
0 + 9	3.600	3.300
1 + 0	3.240	2.970
1 + 3	2.975	2.750
1 + 6	2.825	2.600
1 + 9	2.700	2.490
2 + 0	2.590	2.390
2 + 3	2.480	2.295
2 + 6	2.385	2.200
2 + 9	2.300	2.125
3 + 0	2.230	2.050
3 + 6	2.110	1.925
4 + 0	2.000	1.830
4 + 6	1.890	1.740
5 + 0	1.820	1.660
5 + 6	1.740	1.580
6 + 0	1.670	1.510
6 + 6	1.620	1.460
7 + 0	1.570	1.430
7 + 6	1.520	1.370
8 + 0	1.470	1.330
8 + 6	1.420	1.290
9 + 0	1.380	1.260
9 + 6	1.340	1.220
10 + 0	1.310	1.190
10 + 6	1.280	1.160
11 + 0	1.240	1.130
11 + 6	1.220	1.100
12 + 0	1.180	1.070
12 + 6	1.160	1.050
13 + 0	1.130	1.030
13 + 6	1.100	1.010
14 + 0	1.080	1.000
14 + 6	1.060	NA
15 + 0	1.040	NA
15 + 6	1.020	NA
16 + 0	1.010	NA
16 + 6	1.010	NA
17 + 0	1.000	NA

NA = not applicable.

4: Lower Extremity

Table 3

Treatment Guidelines for Limb-Length Equalization

Predicted Discrepancy at Skeletal Maturity	Preferred Treatment
< 2 cm	None Optional shoe lift
2 to 6 cm	Epiphysiodesis, shortening, or shoe lift
3 to 20 cm	Lengthening, with or without epiphysiodesis
> 20 cm	Prosthesis use, with or without amputation

rarely, so-called heroic lengthening procedures (Table 3). No functional outcome data have established superior results from the use of one method over another or supported the use of a particular treatment algorithm.

The treatment must be individualized based on the patient's underlying diagnosis, the family's expectations, and the skills and experience of the treating orthopaedic surgeon. The factors that should be considered include the expected height of the child at skeletal maturity as well as the complication profile of each treatment being considered, its predicted morbidity, the timing of treatment and recovery, and the growth potential of the shorter limb. In general, epiphysiodesis is the preferred option for managing hemiatrophy or hemihypertrophy, idiopathic limb-length discrepancy, or limb-length discrepancy resulting from traumatic growth arrest in adolescence. Lengthening may be a better option for traumatic or infectious growth arrest about the knee with onset before age 10 years or for a congenital limb-length discrepancy predicted to be greater than 5 cm at skeletal maturity.

Shortening Procedures

Epiphysiodesis

Epiphysiodesis is a fairly predictable procedure with low morbidity. This method is used to achieve limb-length equalization at maturity in children with predictable growth inhibition and a limb-length discrepancy of 2 to 6 cm. Notwithstanding the proven accuracy of all four methods of predicting limb-length discrepancy at skeletal maturity, it is reasonable to expect that a limb-length discrepancy of less than 1.5 cm at maturity will be achieved in 70% of patients.[21,22] The techniques for achieving a predictable epiphysiodesis have evolved rapidly from the traditional open bone-block Phemister technique to percutaneous drill-curettage techniques and percutaneous epiphysiodesis using transphyseal screws.[23-25] Although all three techniques have been successfully used, the latter two techniques have the advantage of requiring minimal incisions and allowing full weight bearing shortly after the procedure. Percuta-

neous epiphysiodesis using transphyseal screws has the further advantage of achieving an immediate cessation of longitudinal growth because of the placement of large, fully threaded cannulated screws across the physis. The patient is able to almost immediately return to full activities, including sports (Figure 7). The complications associated with the percutaneous drill-curettage technique include an occasional delayed physeal closure, knee effusion, knee stiffness, intra-articular drill or curet penetration, and a delayed return to athletic participation. In a patient with more than 3 years of remaining growth, a concomitant open anterior proximal fibula growth arrest procedure should be considered whenever proximal tibia epiphysiodesis is performed to prevent proximal fibular overgrowth.[26]

Femur Shortening

A femur-shortening procedure can be considered to treat a limb-length discrepancy of as much as approximately 5 cm, if the patient has reached skeletal maturity and has missed the opportunity for a minimally invasive, predictable epiphysiodesis.[27] Tibia shortening has been associated with high rates of compartment syndrome, limb edema, and muscle weakness, and this procedure is not generally performed to treat limb-length discrepancy. Closed femur shortening over an intramedullary nail is a good option if the patient will be unable to comply with the close follow-up and intensive physical therapy required after a lengthening procedure or if the patient is obese (lengthening may lead to soft-tissue complications in such patients). The shortening procedure generally is performed proximally; this location is believed to minimize the effect on quadriceps function, and the muscle coverage is adequate for using the split intercalary femur segment as local bone graft at the shortening site (Figure 8).

The disadvantages of femur shortening include a loss of mature skeletal height and a predictable weakening of the quadriceps musculature, which may persist even at 2-year postoperative assessment.[28] Closed femur shortening over an intramedullary nail also may be associated with fat embolism syndrome, which is believed to be caused by increased intramedullary pressure from reaming and nail placement.[29] This factor has led to the recommendation that the distal femur be vented before reaming and nail placement. Femur shortening also can be performed as a proximal or distal open procedure, with removal of the intercalary segment and stabilization using a blade plate.

Lengthening Procedures

Distraction osteogenesis has rapidly become the accepted method of limb lengthening.[30] The alternative methods, including acute lengthening with the transiliac method and acute femur lengthening, are limited by the high rate of sciatic nerve injury if the lengthening is greater than 2.5 cm.[31] The key elements in successful distraction osteogenesis are a low-energy, minimally invasive corticotomy and gradual rhythmic distraction at

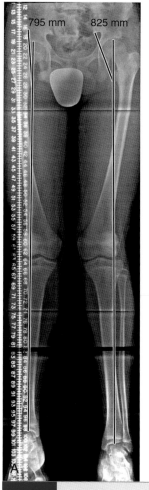

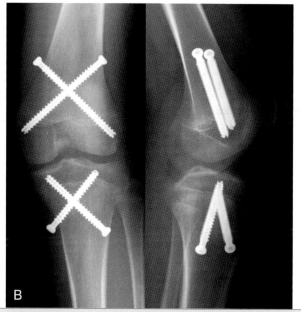

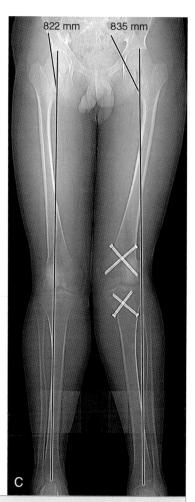

Figure 7   **A**, Preoperative scanogram showing a lower limb-length discrepancy of 3.0 cm in a 13-year-old boy with hemihypertrophy and left leg overgrowth. **B**, AP *(left)* and lateral *(right)* radiographs showing percutaneous epiphysiodesis using transphyseal screws. **C**, CT scanogram showing the final lower limb deficiency of 1.3 cm at skeletal maturity.

the corticotomy site, beginning 5 to 7 days after the corticotomy. The Ilizarov technique for limb lengthening with external fixation using circular frames and tensioned fine wires has been successfully modified by using segmental half-pins rather than wires for fixation.[32] Optimal regenerate bone formation is associated with daily fixator lengthening of up to 1 mm, done at three or more widely spaced intervals throughout the day. Fewer complications occur if the goal is limited to 3 to 6 cm of lengthening or a 20% to 30% lengthening of an individual bone during one treatment period.[33] Predictable lengthening can be achieved with monolateral external fixators, circular Ilizarov fixators and variants, hybrid fixation systems (external fixators with lengthening over an intramedullary nail), and fully implantable intramedullary lengthening devices. The complication profiles of the external fixation systems are similar. The risk of intramedullary infection is higher with lengthening over an intramedullary nail, however, especially if the patient had an earlier open fracture or other trauma. Intramedullary lengthening devices hold great promise as their motorized systems become in-

creasingly predictable and reliable. These devices are especially promising for use in skeletally mature patients, in whom the physis is already closed.

Monolateral Frame

The monolateral external fixator frame with a lengthening rail system offers a technically simple application, compared with Ilizarov's early circular–fine wire systems. This technique uses two different pin blocks with segmental fixation and tapered half-pins. A wrench and a lengthening device attached to the mobile block on the rail system are used to adjust the length 0.25 mm as many as four times per day. After desired length is achieved, the lengthening device is removed and the pin blocks are locked to the rail system until adequate bone healing and regenerate strength are achieved. The disadvantages of the monolateral rail system include the limited ability to correct deformities associated with limb lengthening. Varus and valgus correction devices have been developed; the Multi-Axial Correction device (Biomet, Parsippany, NJ) allows for six-degree correction using a monolateral frame system.[34]

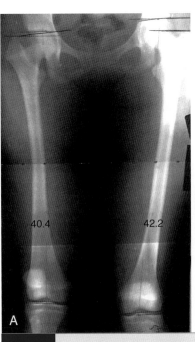
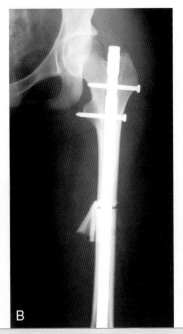
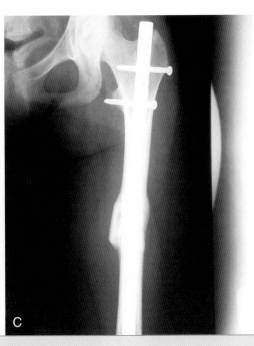

Figure 8 **A,** Preoperative AP radiograph showing a femoral difference at skeletal maturity of 3.8 cm in a 17-year-old girl. **B,** AP radiograph 1 month after closed femur shortening over an intramedullary nail. **C,** AP radiograph showing union with remodeling of the split intercalary fragment 4 months after the shortening.

Circular External Fixation Systems

A circular external fixation system, as originally developed by Ilizarov, is extremely versatile, adaptable with the use of 90° and 120° arches, and usable across joints, especially in situations such as lengthening for congenital short femur, in which knee subluxation and dislocation is a predictable complication. To simplify frame application and decrease the risk of soft-tissue complications, the use of fine wires has been modified to include half-pins whenever possible. The greatest advantage of the circular fixation system is its ability to correct the predictable deformities associated with limb lengthening, such as procurvatum of the femur, without the need for a return trip to the operating room or significant frame modification.

The Taylor Spatial Frame (Smith & Nephew, Memphis, TN) is a computer-assisted system for limb lengthening and deformity correction. Limb length, bony translation, and bone segment rotation can be simultaneously controlled (**Figure 9**). Any deformity occurring during limb lengthening can be easily treated as a secondary residual correction without modifying the frame. As greater length is achieved, the struts are simply and easily exchanged in the office with no need for anesthesia or sedation. Controversy exists regarding the advantages and disadvantages of the Taylor Spatial Frame in children, however. A recent study of 15 pediatric patients who underwent lengthening with the Taylor system concluded that the time required for lengthening was significantly greater than for 6 patients who were treated using the traditional Ilizarov frame with clickers.[35] This result is believed to be related to increased bone travel with concomitant deformity correc-

tion as well as the greater stiffness of the Taylor Spatial Frame. A larger study of 20 tibia lengthenings using the Taylor Spatial Frame found no difference in the time required for lengthening compared with 27 tibia lengthenings using the Ilizarov frame.[36] The advantages of the Taylor Spatial Frame for treating limb-length discrepancy with deformity include the ability to simultaneously correct length, angulation, rotation, and translation without the use of hinge constructs as well as the ability to fine-tune the deformity correction with residual adjustments.

Lengthening Over a Nail

Lengthening over an intramedullary nail was developed as a means of decreasing the patient's time in the external fixator frame. To avoid bony impingement during lengthening, this technique requires accurate application of the external fixator colinear with the mechanical axis of the bone. The risk of pin site infection leading to intramedullary osteomyelitis is greatly increased if the patient had an earlier infection or open fracture.[37] The significant advantage of this technique is that the external fixator is removed after lengthening has been achieved but before regenerate maturation occurs.

Closed Intramedullary Distraction

Several fully implantable internal-lengthening devices are under development for use in limb lengthening. The Intramedullary Skeletal Kinetic Distractor (Orthofix, McKinney, TX) is the only such device currently approved by the US Food and Drug Administration.[38] These devices offer several potential advantages over external fixators, including the elimination of soft-

4: Lower Extremity

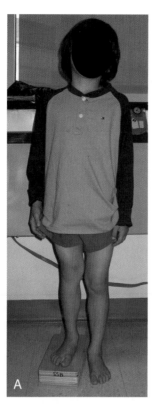
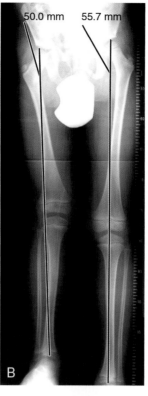
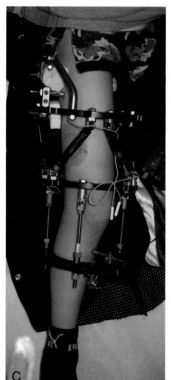
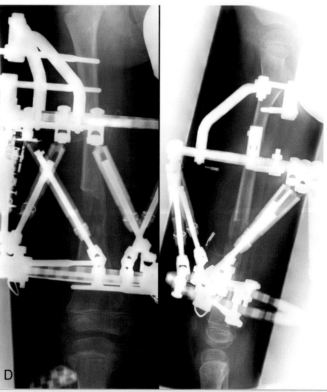
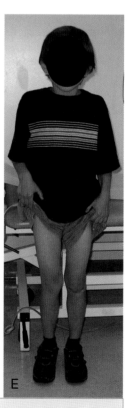

Figure 9   **A**, Photograph showing the preoperative appearance of a 7-year-old boy with congenital short femur. **B**, Presurgical AP radiograph showing a femoral difference of 5.7 cm. **C**, Photograph showing a femur-lengthening frame with the device extended across the knee to prevent subluxation or contracture during lengthening. **D**, AP *(left)* and lateral *(right)* radiographs of the right femur showing regenerate bone formation during lengthening. **E**, Photograph showing the child's posttreatment clinical appearance, with the pelvis and knees well balanced.

4: Lower Extremity

tissue transfixation with wires and half-pins and the associated risk of pin tract infection and osteomyelitis. However, the device can be used only in a large-diameter bone, and it must not cross the growth plate in children with significant remaining growth. These factors may limit the use of the technique to patients with relatively large bones who are at or near skeletal maturity.

Amputation and Prosthesis Fitting

Amputation and the fitting of a prosthesis may be an option if the patient is predicted to have an extreme limb-length discrepancy (more than 20 cm) or has a limb-length condition associated with a nonfunctional foot and ankle. These patients generally have a congenital limb deficiency syndrome such as a PFFD, a congenital short femur, or tibia or fibula hemimelia. The status of the foot often is the primary consideration before limb lengthening. At a minimum the patient must have a three-ray foot that is or can be made plantigrade.[39] The stability and development of the hip and knee also must be considered. If a stable, plantigrade, weight-bearing foot or a stable, functional hip cannot be achieved, a prosthesis fitting must be considered, with possible amputation. The currently available dynamic, energy-conserving prostheses allow the patient to have an extremely active lifestyle. If limb-length equalization will require more than three or four surgical procedures during childhood, many families consider amputation and prosthesis fitting as an alternative. Limited studies found that patients with a condition such as fibula hemimelia have an excellent, similar quality of life after serial lengthening or amputation with a fitted prosthesis.[40]

Complications of Limb-Lengthening Surgery

Limb-lengthening surgery is associated with a broad range of complications. The specific complications and their frequency vary with the diagnosis, the device, the affected limb segment, and the extent of the lengthening. For example, the risk of knee subluxation or dislocation is specifically associated with lengthening of a congenital short femur, and the risk is increased if a monolateral frame is used rather than a circular frame extending across the knee. The complications associated with limb lengthening may involve pins or wires, joint contracture, joint subluxation or dislocation, neurologic injury, vascular injury, axial deviation (malunion), regenerate bone delay or failure (delayed union or nonunion, late refracture), device failure, or growth inhibition.

The complications associated with limb lengthening have been classified into several systems. In the Paley classification, a difficulty during limb lengthening is called a problem, an obstacle, or a complication.[41] A problem, such as a pin tract infection, does not require surgery to resolve. An obstacle, such as joint sublux-

ation, requires surgery. A complication is any intraoperative injury or other issue encountered during limb lengthening that is not resolved by the end of treatment. The Velazquez definition of a complication is any untoward occurrence to a patient during the course of treatment or after removal of the fixator.[42] A major complication necessitates an additional surgical procedure, causes lasting sequelae, or prolongs the treatment; a minor complication responds to nonsurgical treatment and does not lead to lasting sequelae. The Dahl scheme classifies complications as minor, serious, or severe.[33] A minor complication does not affect the outcome or require extensive intervention. The focus of the Dahl system is on serious and severe complications that are either major and temporary or minor and permanent. In general, complications are more common if the limb lengthening exceeds 15% to 25% of the bone length.[43]

Pin and wire site complications may be iatrogenic, such as those associated with pin or wire insertion, soft-tissue and bony infection around an implant, or pin or wire loosening or breakage. Soft-tissue infection is common. A minor infection is treated with local care and oral antibiotics, and it rarely leads to permanent sequelae. The incidence of half-pin loosening and pin tract infection has been greatly reduced with the implantation of hydroxyapatite-coated external fixation pins.[44]

Limb lengthening frequently is associated with limitations in joint range of motion. Postoperative positioning, splinting, and physical therapy are widely used to avoid loss of motion and contractures. Sometimes the goals of lengthening are modified to prevent a loss of motion. Joint subluxation or dislocation is most frequently associated with lengthening of a congenital short femur and may be associated with hip dysplasia or an absent cruciate ligament with anteroposterior knee instability (**Figure 10**). A stable hip is a prerequisite for successful lower limb lengthening. The recommendations for the knee range from extending the frame across the knee (with a hinge at the knee's center of rotation) to no extension across the knee and aggressive physical therapy. Most published research supports extending the frame across the knee to avoid subluxation, rather than dealing with the complication after it develops.[45] Lengthening of the Achilles tendon before or after surgery occasionally must be considered to treat or prevent equinus contractures.

Acute nerve or vascular injury is a rarely encountered iatrogenic complication that can be avoided by becoming familiar with the local anatomy and using an axial cross-sectional imaging atlas before wire or half-pin insertion.[46] The typical lengthening of 1 mm per day rarely leads to neurovascular complications, but uncorrected nerve compression by the wire or half-pin can lead to neurapraxia or permanent neurologic damage. A retrospective study of 814 limb-lengthening procedures found a 9.3% incidence of nerve lesions, 86% of which occurred during the lengthening process.[47]

Nerve lesions can be managed by slowing or stopping the distraction process and/or decompressing the involved nerve. Patients undergoing double-level tibia lengthening or lengthening associated with skeletal dysplasia had an increased risk of developing a nerve lesion. Angular deviations, premature consolidation, and delayed union or nonunion have been reported during or after limb lengthening.[41,42] A variety of techniques for fixation, osteotomy, and dynamization of frames have been used.

Evidence-based criteria for frame removal are lacking. Fracture occurred after frame removal in as many as 30% of patients who underwent lengthening of a congenital short femur.[45] This risk of refracture can be decreased by modifying the technique to include lengthening over a rod or intramedullary rod fixation after lengthening is completed.[48] Device failure is rare when current monolateral and circular fixator frames are used.

Because the risk of complications increases with the percentage of the bone being lengthened, the use of conservative lengthening procedures or a combination of lengthening and epiphysiodesis has been suggested.[49] Repeated lengthening of a limb segment has not led to significantly increased complication rates.[50] Techniques have been developed to decrease or eliminate the patient's time in the external fixator but have been used primarily for adults or skeletally mature adolescents. These techniques include lengthening over a nail with an external fixator, lengthening followed by nailing, and using an intramedullary lengthening device with or without an internal motor.[51] Limb lengthening with a submuscular locking plate has been proposed to allow early removal of the fixator.[35]

Lengthening for Short Stature

Proponents of limb lengthening to correct short stature argue that society is oriented toward people who are taller than 5 ft and that shorter people face many barriers (such as limited access to public toilets, sinks, and telephones) as well as psychosocial problems because of discrimination or poor self-image. So-called symmetric extended limb lengthening (ELL) may require two episodes of femur-tibia lengthening and one episode of humerus lengthening.

Opponents argue that ELL has a high risk of complications including permanent nerve injury, failure to achieve normal height, scarring leading to a poor cosmetic appearance of the limbs, and permanent limb weakness and stiffness. An adolescent's psychosocial development may be more impaired by the loss of social time during ELL than by short stature. The cause of short stature is not removed by ELL; for example, a patient with achondroplasia may have spinal stenosis after ELL and will still have the characteristic facial morphology.[52,53] The position of the Little People of America is that there are no established medical indica-

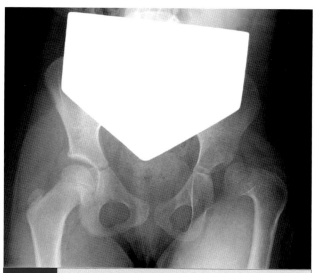

Figure 10 AP supine radiograph showing postoperative hip subluxation in a patient with congenital short femur. After femur lengthening with a monolateral frame, the patient developed hip and knee subluxation that led to 90° contractures of both joints. The hip subluxation was caused by a dysplastic acetabulum that was not treated before lengthening.

tions for ELL but that cosmetic, adaptive, and psychosocial indications do exist.[52] An extensive preoperative workup should be done, along with psychological assessment and counseling.

Some individuals who were extensively interviewed after undergoing ELL had achieved a short-average stature with no permanent disabilities and were quite happy with the outcome, but others had disastrous complications or were not satisfied with the outcome.[53] The topic remains controversial. ELL is a complex undertaking that has high complication rates, requires lengthy and costly care, and is not medically necessary. The use of adaptive devices can compensate for the practical disadvantages of short stature. However, ELL can have a successful functional outcome in carefully selected, well-managed patients.[54,55]

Annotated References

1. Rush WA, Steiner HA: A study of lower extremity length inequality. *Am J Roentgenol Radium Ther* 1946; 56(5):616-623.

2. Murrell P, Cornwall MW, Doucet SK: Leg-length discrepancy: Effect on the amplitude of postural sway. *Arch Phys Med Rehabil* 1991;72(9):646-648.

3. Soukka A, Alaranta H, Tallroth K, Heliövaara M: Leg-length inequality in people of working age: The association between mild inequality and low-back pain is questionable. *Spine (Phila Pa 1976)* 1991;16(4):429-431.

4. Moseley CF: Leg length discrepancy, in Morrisy RT, Weinstein SL, eds: *Lovell and Winter's Pediatric Orthopaedics.* New York, NY, Lippincott Williams & Wilkins, 2006, pp 1213-1256.

   This is a comprehensive chapter in a major pediatric orthopaedic textbook on the etiology, assessment, and treatment of leg-length discrepancy.

5. Tanner J, Whitehouse RH, Cameron N, et al: *Assessment of Skeletal Maturity and Prediction of Adult Height (TW2 Method).* London, England, Academic Press, 1975.

6. Terry MA, Winell JJ, Green DW, et al: Measurement variance in limb length discrepancy: Clinical and radiographic assessment of interobserver and intraobserver variability. *J Pediatr Orthop* 2005;25(2):197-201.

   This study prospectively followed 16 patients with limb-length discrepancy and compared intraobserver and interobserver reliability of clinical measurements and standing slit scanograms. Direct measurement of slit scanograms was found most reliable (0.1 cm mean difference, intraclass correlation coefficient 0.99, confidence interval 0.4 cm). Level of evidence: I.

7. Leitzes AH, Potter HG, Amaral T, Marx RG, Lyman S, Widmann RF: Reliability and accuracy of MRI scanogram in the evaluation of limb length discrepancy. *J Pediatr Orthop* 2005;25(6):747-749.

   Twelve cadaver femurs were measured with conventional AP scanograms, CT scanograms, and MRI scanograms, and they were compared to the gold standard of electronic calipers. AP scanogram was the most accurate, but all methods were accurate and reliable. Level of evidence: I.

8. Sabharwal S, Kumar A: Methods for assessing leg length discrepancy. *Clin Orthop Relat Res* 2008;466(12):2910-2922.

   This review of limb-length discrepancy measurement publications from 1950 to 2008 concludes that the best initial imaging study usually is a standing full-length computed radiograph of both legs, with the pelvis leveled. Level of evidence: IV.

9. Greulich W, Pyle S: *Radiographic Atlas of the Skeletal Development of the Hand and Wrist.* Stanford, CA, Stanford University Press, 1959.

10. Charles YP, Diméglio A, Canavese F, Daures JP: Skeletal age assessment from the olecranon for idiopathic scoliosis at Risser grade 0. *J Bone Joint Surg Am* 2007;89(12):2737-2744.

    During peak height velocity, the skeletal age is determined at 6-month intervals based on olecranon radiographs using a simplified radiographic classification modified from the Sauvegrain method. There was excellent interobserver reliability (0.987). Level of evidence: II.

11. Diméglio A, Charles YP, Daures JP, de Rosa V, Kaboré B: Accuracy of the Sauvegrain method in determining skeletal age during puberty. *J Bone Joint Surg Am* 2005;87(8):1689-1696.

    The Sauvegrain method of determining skeletal age based on elbow radiographs was assessed and compared with Greulich and Pyle bone ages of the hand and wrist. The correlation was 0.85. Level of evidence: II.

12. Aguilar JA, Paley D, Paley J, et al: Clinical validation of the multiplier method for predicting limb length at maturity, part I. *J Pediatr Orthop* 2005;25(2):186-191.

    This study retrospectively applied the multiplier method to 60 patients previously treated for limb-length discrepancy. The multiplier method using chronologic age was slightly better than the Moseley and Anderson methods at predicting leg length at maturity. Level of evidence: III.

13. Aguilar JA, Paley D, Paley J, et al: Clinical validation of the multiplier method for predicting limb length discrepancy and outcome of epiphysiodesis: Part II. *J Pediatr Orthop* 2005;25(2):192-196.

    This study retrospectively applied the multiplier method to 60 patients treated for limb-length discrepancy. Residual leg-length discrepancy after epiphysiodesis was more accurately predicted by the multiplier method than the Moseley method. Level of evidence: III.

14. Anderson M, Green WT, Messner MB: Growth and predictions of growth in the lower extremities. *J Bone Joint Surg Am* 1963;45:1-14.

15. Anderson M, Green WT: Lengths of the femur and the tibia; norms derived from orthoroentgenograms of children from 5 years of age until epiphysial closure. *Am J Dis Child* 1948;75(3):279-290.

16. Moseley CF: A straight-line graph for leg-length discrepancies. *J Bone Joint Surg Am* 1977;59(2):174-179.

17. Paley D, Bhave A, Herzenberg JE, Bowen JR: Multiplier method for predicting limb-length discrepancy. *J Bone Joint Surg Am* 2000;82(10):1432-1446.

18. Song KM, Halliday SE, Little DG: The effect of limb-length discrepancy on gait. *J Bone Joint Surg Am* 1997;79(11):1690-1698.

19. White SC, Gilchrist LA, Wilk BE: Asymmetric limb loading with true or simulated leg-length differences. *Clin Orthop Relat Res* 2004;421:287-292.

20. Bhave A, Paley D, Herzenberg JE: Improvement in gait parameters after lengthening for the treatment of limb-length discrepancy. *J Bone Joint Surg Am* 1999;81(4):529-534.

21. Moseley CF: Assessment and prediction in leg-length discrepancy. *Instr Course Lect* 1989;38:325-330.

22. Kemnitz S, Moens P, Fabry G: Percutaneous epiphysiodesis for leg length discrepancy. *J Pediatr Orthop B* 2003;12(1):69-71.

23. Phemister DB: Epiphysiodesis for equalizing the length of the lower extremities and for correcting other defor-

mities of the skeleton. *Mem Acad Chir (Paris)* 1950; 76(26-27):758-763.

24. Canale ST, Russell TA, Holcomb RL: Percutaneous epiphysiodesis: Experimental study and preliminary clinical results. *J Pediatr Orthop* 1986;6(2):150-156.

25. Métaizeau JP, Wong-Chung J, Bertrand H, Pasquier P: Percutaneous epiphysiodesis using transphyseal screws (PETS). *J Pediatr Orthop* 1998;18(3):363-369.

26. McCarthy JJ, Burke T, McCarthy MC: Need for concomitant proximal fibular epiphysiodesis when performing a proximal tibial epiphysiodesis. *J Pediatr Orthop* 2003;23(1):52-54.

27. Sasso RC, Urquhart BA, Cain TE: Closed femoral shortening. *J Pediatr Orthop* 1993;13(1):51-56.

28. Barker KL, Simpson AH: Recovery of function after closed femoral shortening. *J Bone Joint Surg Br* 2004; 86(8):1182-1186.

29. Edwards KJ, Cummings RJ: Fat embolism as a complication of closed femoral shortening. *J Pediatr Orthop* 1992;12(4):542-543.

30. Ilizarov GA: Clinical application of the tension-stress effect for limb lengthening. *Clin Orthop Relat Res* 1990; 250:8-26.

31. Millis MB, Hall JE: Transiliac lengthening of the lower extremity: A modified innominate osteotomy for the treatment of postural imbalance. *J Bone Joint Surg Am* 1979;61(8):1182-1194.

32. De Bastiani G, Aldegheri R, Renzi-Brivio L, Trivella G: Limb lengthening by callus distraction (callotasis). *J Pediatr Orthop* 1987;7(2):129-134.

33. Dahl MT, Gulli B, Berg T: Complications of limb lengthening: A learning curve. *Clin Orthop Relat Res* 1994;301:10-18.

34. McCarthy JJ, Ranade A, Davidson RS: Pediatric deformity correction using a multiaxial correction fixator. *Clin Orthop Relat Res* 2008;466(12):3011-3017.

Twenty-five limb deformities treated with a multiaxial monolateral fixator had satisfactory results, with few major complications. This type of fixator is an alternative to a circular fixator. Level of evidence: IV.

35. Iobst CA, Dahl MT: Limb lengthening with submuscular plate stabilization: A case series and description of the technique. *J Pediatr Orthop* 2007;27(5):504-509.

Six patients were treated with limb lengthening over a submuscular plate. The technique, complications, and results are described. Mean external fixator duration was 45 days. There were three serious and two severe complications. Level of evidence: IV.

36. Kristiansen LP, Steen H, Reikerås O: No difference in tibial lengthening index by use of Taylor spatial frame or Ilizarov external fixator. *Acta Orthop* 2006;77(5): 772-777.

The results of 20 tibia lengthenings with the Taylor Spatial Frame were compared with the results of 27 tibia lengthenings with the Ilizarov external fixator. The time required for lengthening was equivalent. Residual deformities were more easily corrected with the Taylor Spatial Frame. Level of evidence: III.

37. Herzenberg JE, Paley D: Tibial lengthening over nails (LON). *Tech Orthop* 1997;12:250-259.

38. Simpson AH, Shalaby H, Keenan G: Femoral lengthening with the Intramedullary Skeletal Kinetic Distractor. *J Bone Joint Surg Br* 2009;91(7):955-961.

Of 33 femurs treated with an Intramedullary Skeletal Kinetic Distractor, 32 achieved the desired length. Difficulty with lengthening was observed in 24%, and uncontrolled lengthening was observed in 21%. Level of evidence: IV.

39. Birch JG, Lincoln TL, Mack PW: Functional classification of fibular hemimelia, in Herring JA, Birch JG: *The Child With a Limb Deficiency*. Rosemont, IL, American Academy of Orthopaedic Surgeons, 1998, pp 161-170.

40. Walker JL, Knapp D, Minter C, et al: Adult outcomes following amputation or lengthening for fibular deficiency. *J Bone Joint Surg Am* 2009;91(4):797-804.

Sixty-two patients with fibular deficiency were identified; 36 had amputation and 26 had lengthening. Quality-of-life questionnaire results were compared with those of 28 control subjects. The patients with amputation and lengthening both had high function and an average to above-average quality of life. Level of evidence: III.

41. Paley D: Problems, obstacles, and complications of limb lengthening by the Ilizarov technique. *Clin Orthop Relat Res* 1990;250:81-104.

42. Velazquez RJ, Bell DF, Armstrong PF, Babyn P, Tibshirani R: Complications of use of the Ilizarov technique in the correction of limb deformities in children. *J Bone Joint Surg Am* 1993;75(8):1148-1156.

43. Karger C, Guille JT, Bowen JR: Lengthening of congenital lower limb deficiencies. *Clin Orthop Relat Res* 1993;291:236-245.

44. Pommer A, Muhr G, Dávid A: Hydroxyapatite-coated Schanz pins in external fixators used for distraction osteogenesis: A randomized, controlled trial. *J Bone Joint Surg Am* 2002;84(7):1162-1166.

45. Aston WJ, Calder PR, Baker D, Hartley J, Hill RA: Lengthening of the congenital short femur using the Ilizarov technique: A single-surgeon series. *J Bone Joint Surg Br* 2009;91(7):962-967.

46. Maiocchi AB, ed: *Atlas for the Insertion of Transosseous Wires and Half-Pins*. Milan, Italy, Smith & Nephew, 2003.

The safe insertion of wires and half-pins in an external frame was reviewed, with clinical photographs and cross-sectional anatomy diagrams.

47. Nogueira MP, Paley D, Bhave A, Herbert A, Nocente C, Herzenberg JE: Nerve lesions associated with limb-lengthening. *J Bone Joint Surg Am* 2003;85(8):1502-1510.

48. Herzenberg JE, Branfoot T, Paley D, Violante FH: Femoral nailing to treat fractures after lengthening for congenital femoral deficiency in young children. *J Pediatr Orthop B* 2010;19(2):150-154.

    Nine patients had femur fractures after lengthening for congenital short femur. Fractures were successfully treated with Rush rod nailing. The surgical technique is detailed, and prophylactic nailing after removal of fixators is discussed. Level of evidence: IV.

49. Antoci V, Ono CM, Antoci V Jr, Raney EM: Bone lengthening in children: How to predict the complications rate and complexity? *J Pediatr Orthop* 2006;26(5):634-640.

    This review of 116 lower extremity–lengthening complications established a linear correlation between lengthening percentage and complications such as neurologic compromise and joint contracture. At a 40% lengthening index, neurologic and joint contracture complications were 60%. Level of evidence: IV.

50. Griffith SI, McCarthy JJ, Davidson RS: Comparison of the complication rates between first and second (repeated) lengthening in the same limb segment. *J Pediatr Orthop* 2006;26(4):534-536.

    Twelve limbs (seven femurs and five tibias) underwent two lengthenings. The complication rates were similar after the second lengthening, but the patients' time in an external fixator was longer, and amount of length achieved was less. Level of evidence: IV.

51. Rozbruch SR, Kleinman D, Fragomen AT, Ilizarov S: Limb lengthening and then insertion of an intramedullary nail: A case-matched comparison. *Clin Orthop Relat Res* 2008;466(12):2923-2932.

    A group of patients who underwent lengthening in a frame followed by frame removal and nailing were compared with patients treated only in a frame. Nailing allowed earlier frame removal (12 versus 29 weeks), earlier healing, and prevention of refracture. Level of evidence: III.

52. Little People of America Medical Advisory Board: Extended Limb Lengthening: Position Summary. Tustin, CA, Little People of America, 2006. http://www.lpaonline.org/mc/page.do?sitePageId=56366&orgId=lpa. Accessed September 10, 2010.

    The Little People of America Medical Advisory Board has issued a position statement on limb lengthening. Level of evidence: V.

53. Adelson BA: *Dwarfism: Medical and Psychosocial Aspects of Profound Short Stature.* Baltimore, MD, The Johns Hopkins University Press, 2005.

    This book reviews the medical and social aspects of short stature and includes many interviews with patients, some of whom have undergone extended limb lengthening.

54. Aldegheri R, Dall'Oca C: Limb lengthening in short stature patients. *J Pediatr Orthop B* 2001;10(3):238-247.

55. Vaidya SV, Song HR, Lee SH, Suh SW, Keny SM, Telang SS: Bifocal tibial corrective osteotomy with lengthening in achondroplasia: An analysis of results and complications. *J Pediatr Orthop* 2006;26(6):788-793.

    Forty-seven bifocal tibia lengthenings for achondroplasia are reviewed. A lengthening index of more than 40% total and 15% in the distal segment resulted in a 100% incidence of equinus. Distal segment lengthening of more than 15% is not recommended. Level of evidence: IV.

Chapter 24

Lower Limb Prosthetics

John A. Herring, MD   Donald R. Cummings, CP(LP)

4: Lower Extremity

Introduction

Clinicians have developed strategies for prescribing and fitting prostheses to meet the dynamic needs of growing children with an amputation or limb deficiency. Research and development in limb prosthetics initially emphasized the needs of the much larger adult population. However, materials, components, and techniques specifically for children are gradually being introduced and implemented.

Children and Prosthesis Use

In orthopaedic clinics that routinely treat pediatric patients with an amputation or limb deficiency, approximately 30% of the children younger than 16 years have undergone amputation because of traumatic injury (often involving a motor vehicle crash, lawn mower or power tool accident, or electrical or thermal burns) or disease (such as cancer or meningococcemia). The remaining 70% have a congenital limb deficiency that either is treated as or requires an amputation.[1] These amputations can be the result of amniotic band constriction (Streeter dysplasia), longitudinal deficiency of the tibia or fibula, proximal femoral focal deficiency, or transverse limb deficiencies that are homologues of different amputation levels. Children with a congenital limb deficiency often have unstable proximal joints, inadequate proximal musculature, malrotation, and leg-length inequality.[2] As many as 40% of children with a congenital limb anomaly have multiple limb involvement.[3]

A child born with a lower limb absence generally is considered ready for prosthesis use and early gait training when she or he starts pulling up to stand; even a child with a high or bilateral deficiency usually reaches this developmental milestone by age 9 to 16 months.[4,5] A first transfemoral or knee disarticulation prosthesis,

for use until the child has learned to walk safely, commonly incorporates a locked knee or excludes the knee joint altogether (**Figure 1**). However, the resulting need for the toddler to circumduct often creates difficulty in crawling, playing on the floor, and even sitting. In recent years, the availability of smaller knee components, some of which have increased stance-phase stability, has allowed many first prostheses to include an articulating knee (**Figure 2**). The ability of the toddler to adapt to such a prosthesis has not been well documented; the important factors probably are individual development, limb length, access to prosthetic care, physical therapy, and consistent caregiver involvement.

A child's prosthesis needs growth adjustments several times per year until skeletal maturity, and a new prosthesis is required an average of every 15 months. Therefore, the clinic team has relatively frequent opportunities to work with the child and caregiver. Consecutive prostheses are chosen based on the child's history of successful or problematic prosthesis use, the child's current needs and interests, and the availability of appropriate new technology. The child's physical, intellectual, or emotional readiness for particular devices, interventions, or surgeries may require decision making to be accelerated or delayed.

Recent Advances in Pediatric Prosthetics

Underlying knowledge as well as materials, components, and techniques related to the construction and fitting of pediatric prostheses has advanced incrementally during the past 5 years. In particular, there have been advances in component development for adult patients with an amputation. The microprocessor-controlled knee prosthesis is a relatively recent innovation backed by years of development, and multiple versions of this prosthesis are now available from at least five competing manufacturers in the United States and Europe. However, all are designed and sized to fit an adult or possibly a moderately active adolescent,[6] and published results are lacking to clarify selection criteria and clinical outcomes.

The barriers to the introduction of microprocessor-controlled knees for preadolescent children are related to patent protection, cost, technology, and prosthesis size. Nonetheless, there have been some advances in pediatric prostheses. Several polycentric and other

Dr. Herring or an immediate family member has received royalties from Medtronic Sofamor Danek and has received research or institutional support from Saunders/Mosby-Elsevier. Neither Mr. Cummings nor any immediate family member has received anything of value from or owns stock in a commercial company or institution related directly or indirectly to the subject of this chapter.

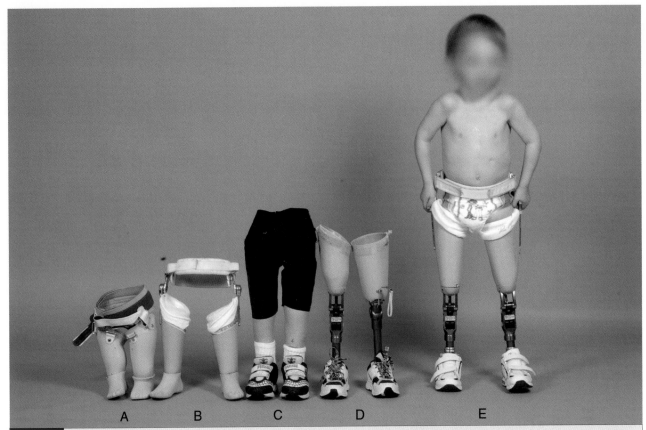

Figure 1   This child was born with multiple lower limb deficiencies, including a dislocated right hip that was much weaker than the left hip. He underwent bilateral knee disarticulations at age 15 months. Over 3 years, he was fitted with a progression of prostheses: nonarticulated "stubbies" with solid ankle, cushion heel feet (**A**); stubbies with metal hip joints, a pelvic band, and waist belt suspension (**B**); taller, nonarticulated prosthetic legs with elastic-fiber waist belt suspension (**C**); a right polycentric knee and a left manually locking knee (**D**); and bilateral polycentric knees with thrust-bearing hip joints (**E**). By age 4 the metal hip joints were no longer being used, and the child was walking with free knees. By age 6 years, he was running in a second pair of prostheses.

non–microprocessor-controlled knee prostheses now are available in most pediatric sizes. Pediatric modular components provide interchangeability and ease of growth adjustment. Prosthetic feet designed to meet the high functional demands of children also are available. Children's activity levels generally are high, and their interests are diverse. A single type of prosthesis often does not allow a child to fully participate in a diverse range of activities (for example, soccer, swimming, skateboarding, marching in a band, cheerleading, golf, rock climbing, dancing [**Figure 3**]). Therefore, children and adolescents often benefit from using a sports prosthesis customized to specific activities, such as a running prosthesis with a J- or C-shaped carbon-composite foot (**Figure 4**). Carbon-composite feet designed for adult sprinters became available during the early 1990s, and they were gradually resized or redesigned for children. Several manufacturers now offer pediatric running feet based on a child's foot size, weight, and activity level. Such components and well-fitted, safely suspended sockets have made running an increasingly more achievable goal for many children, even those with bilateral lower limb involvement (**Figure 5**).

Although research still is not available to allow the practice of adult or pediatric prosthetics to become evidence based,[7] an awareness of the growing array of prosthetic options can help the patient, family, surgeon, and rehabilitation team make informed choices about strategies for amputation and prosthesis use.

General Considerations in Pediatric Prosthetics

The unique aspects of fitting a growing child with a limb prosthesis have been well described.[8] Gradual movement from simple to more complex components, design and alignment based on the child's level of development, and methods of accommodating growth changes must be considered. In comparison with adults, children are more likely to require a fitting after a Syme amputation (ankle disarticulation) or knee disarticulation, a distal pad adjustment for overgrowth after a transdiaphyseal amputation, and refitting after relatively frequent surgical revisions. For example, the prosthesis may require refitting to accommodate angular changes resulting from growth modulation surgery.

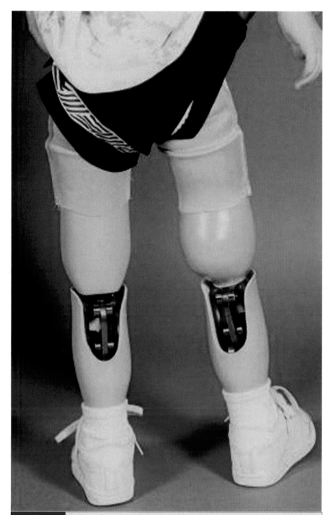

Figure 2 A typical fitting for a child with bilateral knee disarticulations who is transitioning to articulated knees. These polycentric knees lock at heel contact and remain locked until toe-off, when the ground reaction force generates a hyperextension force that disengages the knee lock and allows the limb to flex and extend freely through the swing phase.

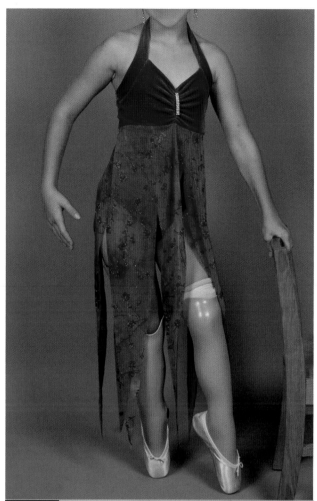

Figure 3 A pair of prostheses designed specifically to allow the child to dance and pivot on her toes in ballet.

Prosthesis replacement often is necessary after surgical removal of terminal bone overgrowth.[9] Although these common considerations have not changed, the prosthetist increasingly has available an array of components and techniques that will influence the treatment of children with an amputation.

Evolving Treatment Strategies

Changing surgical strategies often influence the development of prosthetic components or techniques. For example, the prosthetist must use adapted techniques and components to treat a child who has undergone rotationplasty required for a proximal femoral focal deficiency or a malignant tumor of the proximal tibia or

distal femur (**Figure 6**). The metal joint used to protect the child's rotated ankle and enable it to assume the function of the amputated knee generally is load bearing and otherwise intended for a patient with transtibial or through-knee amputation. The leather thigh lacer traditionally used for anchoring such a prosthetic joint now is frequently replaced by a custom thermoplastic thigh cuff using Velcro closures. The patient's rotated foot must absorb considerable axial load, shear, and rotational force. A socket for the rotated foot is modified to distribute pressures as evenly as possible over the foot; although strategies and materials vary, a soft protective liner usually is incorporated.[10] Most patients who have undergone rotationplasty are capable of high activity levels, and some form of energy-storage-and-return (ESAR) prosthetic foot is indicated.[11] The specific foot is chosen based on the patient's shoe size, weight, and activity level, as well as the space available below the patient's toes. Modular components and lightweight, durable materials with carbon fiber reinforcement are used whenever possible.

4: Lower Extremity

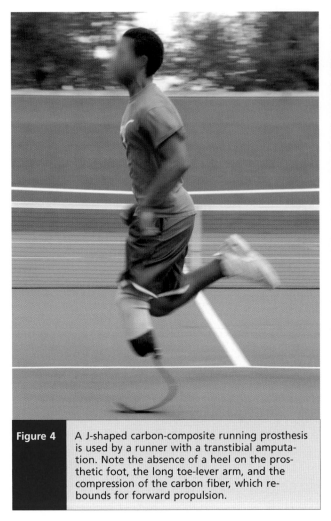

Figure 4 A J-shaped carbon-composite running prosthesis is used by a runner with a transtibial amputation. Note the absence of a heel on the prosthetic foot, the long toe-lever arm, and the compression of the carbon fiber, which rebounds for forward propulsion.

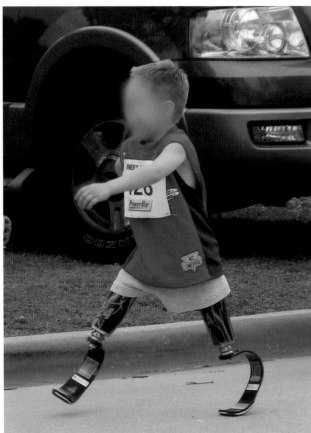

Figure 5 This 6-year-old child with bilateral knee disarticulations is able to run with C-shaped carbon-composite running feet from which prosthetic knees have been excluded. The child can run efficiently and more safely without the need to control the knees. This strategy is often used for patients with a bilateral or unilateral transfemoral amputation.

Surgical decision making often must take into account recent advances in prosthetics. For example, the use of the ESAR foot, which is designed for a transtibial or higher level of amputation, should be considered in the decision to perform an epiphysiodesis for a child with a Syme or Boyd amputation. The currently available pediatric prosthetic feet offer increased ESAR capability, multiaxial ankle function, or both. At least six manufacturers supply such prosthetic feet for children. Most of these are available in lengths as short as 14 cm, allowing them to be used in children as young as 2 to 3 years. There is almost no evidence to indicate the best age for fitting a child with a first dynamic response foot. It is recommended that the child should have a heel-to-toe gait and be actively attempting to run. Most of the available prostheses allow selection of foot stiffness, skin tone, a foot shell with cosmetic toes, attachment hardware, and spacers in varying widths so the device can easily be lengthened as the child grows. Foot components specifically designed for sprinting and running are available for young children. These prosthetic feet are popular with children and adolescents, but their specific functional benefit for children is the subject of debate and ongoing research.[12-15] Studies in

adults found a strong patient preference for the ESAR prosthetic foot, which has better performance than a conventional prosthetic foot, especially in activities of daily living other than walking on a level surface.[16]

Advances in the function of prosthetic feet have led to a reevaluation of amputation strategies. A child with a long amputation, such as the Syme or Boyd amputation, cannot usually be fit with an ESAR foot. Instead, a very low profile Syme foot or an even lower profile carbon deflection plate often is required (**Figure 7**). The choice is limited because very few such prosthetic feet have been designed for these amputation levels. For a child with a unilateral amputation, the presence of at least 7 cm beneath the distal end of the amputation allows the use of many ESAR prosthetic feet, and a 14-cm difference also allows the use of a foot designed for running or other sports (**Figure 8**). Some clinics recently have emphasized the possible need for ipsilateral tibiofibular epiphyseodeses at the time of a Syme or Boyd amputation or soon thereafter to enable the patient to benefit from these components at skeletal ma-

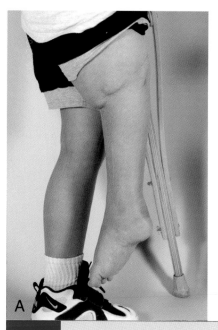
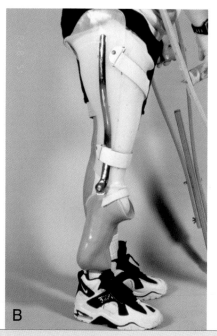
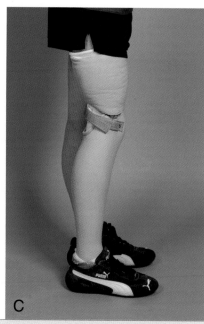

Figure 6 **A,** A recent rotationplasty in an adolescent boy. **B,** The prosthesis includes a socket with a soft interface to support the rotated foot and a supracalcaneal strap for suspension. The rotated ankle is now functioning in place of the ablated knee; it is protected from trauma by two external metal joints that attach to a plastic thigh cuff. The thigh section uses anterior and posterior plastic shells to contain and protect the hardware and surgical site. When the bone has completely healed, the thigh section can be lowered and the anterior shell removed for comfort. **C,** A rotationplasty prosthesis with a cosmetic cover.

turity.[17] Because of the frequency with which new components become commercially available, a knowledgeable prosthetist should be consulted before a decision is made concerning any residual limb-length alteration.

Sports of all kinds have been an important consideration in the development of pediatric components and techniques during the past 20 years. Children and adolescents with an amputation now have many opportunities to participate in regional, national, and international competitions for athletes with a limb deficiency. Sports events and clinics are sponsored by the Paralympic Games, Challenged Athletes Foundation, Amputee Coalition of America, and other organizations. More patients are becoming involved at an increasingly young age in sports such as track and field, snow skiing, skateboarding, surfing, bicycle riding, basketball, football, and tennis. In response, prosthetists, researchers, and component developers are creating innovative studies and products. Many of their efforts focus on the needs of young adults, which are pertinent to adolescents and children. Published research on sports participation by patients with an amputation has focused on methodologies to measure running biomechanics, high-jump techniques, human turning gait analysis in the development of transverse rotation (torque) leg adapters, the biomechanics of cycling with a transtibial prosthesis, and a unique below-knee prosthesis designed for snowboarding.[18-22] Many of these reports are based on a single patient or a small group of patients, however,

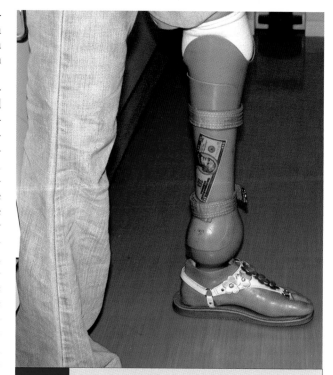

Figure 7 A Syme amputation generally allows excellent distal loading, rotational control, and prosthesis suspension. The selection of prosthetic feet is limited by the relatively small space available for components below the end of the amputation.

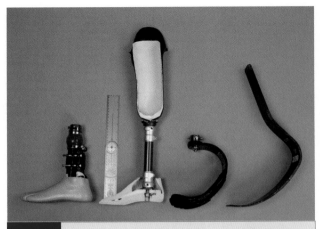

Figure 8 Four variations on the ESAR foot for an adolescent or small adult, including a transected transtibial prosthesis. The lowest profile foot depicted is approximately 7 cm high. Additional space usually is required for liners, distal pads, the plastic socket, and attachment hardware.

and do not reflect emerging techniques or project development.

Children who have an active lifestyle that includes sports are more likely to continue to be active into adulthood. Both elite and recreational athletes with an amputation challenge prosthetists to address their needs by developing specialized knowledge and collaborating with other health care professionals. This trend will continue to push the development of better techniques and components for active children with an amputation.[23]

Socket Designs and Interfaces

Providing a comfortable, biomechanically appropriate socket always has been the prosthetist's first priority, regardless of the patient's age. The particular challenge in providing a well-fitted socket for a child is that the child will outgrow the socket. A new socket is required approximately every 15 months until skeletal maturity and every 3 to 4 years thereafter.[24] These growth changes commonly are handled with frequent follow-up, varying prosthetic sock thicknesses, flexible thermoplastic inner sockets, and gel or foam liners. Gel liners now are routinely used for adult patients as a means of protecting the residual limb. For children, the prosthetist often can adjust for growth by switching to a thinner gel liner or reducing the thickness or number of socks worn over the liner. The socket surrounding the liner is suspended using a distal pin-and-shuttle lock mechanism, lanyard, or vacuum. For adults and some adolescents, gel liners can be combined with an elevated vacuum generated through a valve and a mechanical or battery-powered pump. Reports on the use of an elevated vacuum system in children are anecdotal, and the efficacy of such systems remains to be seen. Ther-

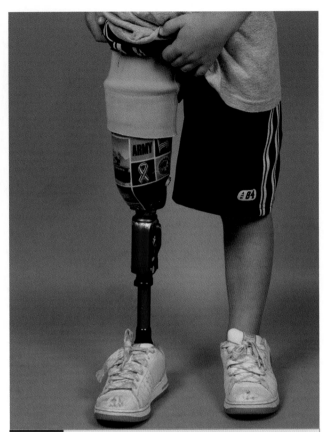

Figure 9 A child with a knee disarticulation has been fitted with a gel liner and a suction socket. A pediatric hydraulic knee is used. Because the child can tolerate full distal loading through his femoral condyles, the socket does not extend beyond the upper third of the thigh. A gel suspension sleeve can be worn to provide additional security.

moplastic gel liners based on silicon, urethane, or mineral oil are being used for children as manufacturers increasingly offer them in appropriate sizes, along with pins, locks, suction valves, and other suspension adaptors. These systems appear to work well for many children as a means of suspending transtibial, knee disarticulation, and some transfemoral prostheses (**Figure 9**).

In general, the prosthetist first selects and orders the liner; a cast is then taken of the child's residual limb over the liner. A limb that has burn or other scars, an angular deformity, an unusually sharp bony prominence, or another challenging feature sometimes can be most successfully fitted using a custom-made gel liner created by a fabrication service using a cast or scanned shape. The process is more expensive and time consuming than the use of a ready-made liner, but it enables the prosthetist to specify the thickness of the material in each region of the socket as well as the gel durometer (hardness) and the overall liner shape. The advantages of a gel liner for a child or an adult may be outweighed by a commonly reported skin condition such as an allergic reaction, ingrown hair, heat rash, odor, or excessive sweating.[25] The treatment can involve a dermatologic consultation, more frequent cleaning of the residual limb, the use of another type of liner, or the substitution of prosthetic socks.

Summary

Most major advances in prosthetic technology during the past several years have been geared toward relatively active adults or older patients with diabetes. These advances include the development of vacuum pumps and valves, gel liners, microprocessor-controlled knees, and ESAR feet. The techniques used to successfully fit such products are continually changing. Most manufacturers who develop prosthetic products now offer pediatric components, and usually it is only a matter of time before products are targeted to the challenges presented by the growing child. Prosthetists who work with children are likely to continue seeing a rapid expansion in techniques and component options.

Annotated References

1. Challenor YB: Limb deficiencies and amputation surgery in children, in Molnary GE, ed: *Pediatric Rehabilitation*. Baltimore, MD, Williams & Wilkins, 1985.

2. Aitken GT, Pellicore RJ: Introduction to the child amputee, in American Academy of Orthopaedic Surgeons, ed: *Atlas of Limb Prosthetics*. St Louis, MO, CV Mosby, 1981, pp 493-500.

3. Gibson D: Child and juvenile amputee, in Banjerjee S, Khan N, eds: *Rehabilitation Management of Amputees*. Baltimore, MD, Williams & Wilkins, 1982, pp 394-414.

4. Bochmann D: Prosthetic devices for the management of proximal femoral focal deficiency. *Orthot Prosthet* 1980;12(1):4-19.

5. Kruger LM: Congenital limb deficiencies: Lower limb deficiencies, in American Academy of Orthopaedic Surgeons, ed: *Atlas of Limb Prosthetics*. St Louis, MO, CV Mosby, 1981, pp 522-552.

6. Berry D, Olson M, Larntz K: Perceived stability, function, and satisfaction among transfemoral amputees using microprocessor and nonmicroprocessor controlled prosthetic knees: A multicenter survey. *J Prosthet Orthot* 2009;21(1):32-41.

   Self-reports from 368 adults with unilateral transfemoral amputation indicated that their C-leg microprocessor-controlled hydraulic knee provided significantly better comfort, security, maneuverability, cosmetic appearance, and safety than their non-microprocessor-controlled knee, with fewer adverse effects.

7. Ramstrand N, Brodtkorb TH: Considerations for developing an evidenced-based practice in orthotics and prosthetics. *Prosthet Orthot Int* 2008;32(1):93-102.

   The need for research in prosthetics to become more relevant to clinical practice and for prosthetists to lead future research is emphasized.

8. Cummings DR: Pediatric prosthetics: An update. *Phys Med Rehabil Clin N Am* 2006;17(1):15-21.

   Clinical experience and recent literature are summarized, with an emphasis on the need for clinicians to match prosthetic components, socket designs, and fitting techniques to the individual child and his or her state of development.

9. Herring J: Limb deficiencies, in *Tachdjian's Pediatric Orthopedics*, ed 3. Philadelphia, PA, WB Saunders Co, 2002, pp 1745-1810.

10. Wessling M, Aach M, Hardes J, et al: Improvement of the soft socket after rotationplasty: A single case study. *Prosthet Orthot Int* 2009;33(1):10-16.

    A rotationplasty socket with a soft interface was used in a very active 28-year-old patient, with related efforts to reduce blistering and callusing by emphasizing broader pressure distribution on the rotated foot.

11. Gebert C, Hardes J, Vieth V, Hillmann A, Winkelmann W, Gosheger G: The effect of rotationplasty on the ankle joint: Long-term results. *Prosthet Orthot Int* 2006;30(3):316-323.

    Radiographs and MRI were used to evaluate the affected ankle joints of 21 patients treated with rotationplasty for bone tumor or proximal femoral focal deficiency; the patients also wore an exoprosthesis. Most ankles had minimal changes at a mean 13.5-year follow-up. Rotationplasty was found not to result in inevitable arthrosis.

12. Hafner BJ, Sanders JE, Czerniecki J, Fergason J: Energy storage and return prostheses: Does patient perception correlate with biomechanical analysis? *Clin Biomech (Bristol, Avon)* 2002;17(5):325-344.

13. McMulkin M, Osebold W, Mildes R, Rosenquist R: Comparison of three pediatric prosthetic feet during functional activities. *J Prosthet Orthot* 2004;16(3):78-84.

14. Menard MR, McBride ME, Sanderson DJ, Murray DD: Comparative biomechanical analysis of energy-storing prosthetic feet. *Arch Phys Med Rehabil* 1992;73(5):451-458.

15. Perry J: Amputee gait, in Smith DG, Michael JW, and Bowker JH, eds: *Atlas of Amputations and Limb Deficiencies: Surgical, Prosthetic and Rehabilitation Principles*, ed 3. Rosemont, IL, American Academy of Orthopaedic Surgeons, 2004, pp 367-384.

16. Hafner B: Perceptive evaluation of prosthetic foot and ankle systems. *J Prosthet Orthot* 2005;17(4):S42-S46.

4: Lower Extremity

No strong correlation was evident between perceptive and objective outcomes measures used to evaluate prosthetic feet and/or patient preference. Both types of studies suggest that amputees prefer ESAR feet and have better function than with conventional prosthetic feet.

17. Osebold WR, Lester EL, Christenson DM: Problems with excessive residual lower leg length in pediatric amputees. *Iowa Orthop J* 2001;21(21):58-67.

18. Childers WL, Kistenberg RS, Gregor RJ: The biomechanics of cycling with a transtibial amputation: Recommendations for prosthetic design and direction for future research. *Prosthet Orthot Int* 2009;33(3):256-271.

   The biomechanical challenges for a cyclist with an amputation include a fixed ankle position without power generation. Adaptations include modifying the pedal, adjusting the cycling cleat placement, and adjusting the functional length of the prosthesis.

19. Flick KC, Orendurff MS, Berge JS, Segal AD, Klute GK: Comparison of human turning gait with the mechanical performance of lower limb prosthetic transverse rotation adapters. *Prosthet Orthot Int* 2005;29(1):73-81.

20. Minnoye SL, Plettenburg DH: Design, fabrication, and preliminary results of a novel below-knee prosthesis for snowboarding: A case report. *Prosthet Orthot Int* 2009;33(3):272-283.

   A prototype prosthesis with a multiaxial ankle was developed for a competitive snowboarder with a transtibial amputation. The purpose was to simulate the ankle motion of nonamputee snowboarders. The prototype was well accepted.

21. Nolan L, Patritti BL: The take-off phase in transtibial amputee high jump. *Prosthet Orthot Int* 2008;32(2):160-171.

   Motion analysis was used to study the sound-side take-off technique used by two Paralympic high jumpers with a unilateral transtibial amputation. Differences in body position and vertical velocity may be related to the preceding step arising on the prosthetic side.

22. Wilson JR, Asfour S, Abdelrahman KZ, Gailey R: A new methodology to measure the running biomechanics of amputees. *Prosthet Orthot Int* 2009;33(3):218-229.

   Spring-mass model and symmetry index were used to evaluate the effect of prosthesis changes on the running biomechanics of individuals with a transtibial amputation. The measures were sufficiently sensitive to detect biomechanical differences caused by small changes in prosthetic height and stiffness, and they hold promise for future studies.

23. Gailey RS, Cooper RA: Sports-medicine for the disabled: The time for specialization in prosthetics and orthotics is now. *Prosthet Orthot Int* 2009;33(3):187-191.

   The development of techniques and technology benefiting athletes with an amputation has accelerated since the 1988 Paralympic Games in Seoul. Specialization in sports prosthetics is considered advantageous.

24. Lambert CN: Amputation surgery in the child. *Orthop Clin North Am* 1972;3(2):473-482.

25. Hall M, Shurr D, VanBeek M, Zimmerman M: The prevalence of dermatological problems for transtibial amputees using a roll-on liner. *J Prosthet Orthot* 2008;20(4):134-139.

   In 110 adults with a transtibial amputation, a survey by questionnaire (with dermatologic examination in 26) found that 91% had experienced manageable skin irritation with the use of roll-on gel liners. Ulceration, dermatitis, and folliculitis were most commonly reported.

Section 5

Spine

SECTION EDITOR:
PETER O. NEWTON, MD

Chapter 25
Early-Onset Scoliosis

Sumeet Garg, MD   Charles E. Johnston, MD

Introduction

Scoliosis usually is classified by its etiology. The possible etiologies include congenital anomalies of the spine and thorax, genetic syndromes, and neuromuscular disorders. Scoliosis with no known cause (idiopathic scoliosis) traditionally has been classified by patient age at recognition: infantile idiopathic scoliosis appears before age 4 years, juvenile idiopathic scoliosis between ages 4 and 10 years, and adolescent idiopathic scoliosis after age 10 years.

Recent progress in understanding the relationship of pulmonary development to spine growth and chest wall deformity has led to classification based on age of scoliosis onset. Early-onset scoliosis (EOS) is deformity occurring while the spine undergoes its most rapid growth before age 5 to 6 years. EOS encompasses both idiopathic and nonidiopathic etiologies. The focus in treating children with EOS is to promote the growth of the thoracic cage. Late-onset scoliosis occurs after age 6 years. The primary focus in treating children with late-onset scoliosis is on managing the spinal column deformity.

Growth and Development of the Thorax

The growth of the spinal column is not steady throughout childhood and adolescence. There are periods of rapid growth during early childhood and adolescence, with slower growth during late childhood. An investigation of normal growth rates found increases in thoracic height of 1.4 cm per year from birth to age 5 years, 0.6 cm per year between ages 5 and 10 years, and 1.2 cm per year between age 10 years and skeletal maturity.[1] This varied pattern of longitudinal thoracic

spine growth is not matched by the volumetric growth of the thorax. In children with no spine deformity, chest volume at age 4 years is only 33% of adult chest volume, and at age 10 years it is 55%. The overall volume triples between ages 4 and 16 years and doubles between ages 10 and 16 years[2] (**Figure 1**).

The volumetric growth of the thorax is critical to pulmonary development. In early childhood, pulmonary development primarily results from a multiplication in the number of alveoli (hyperplasia).[3] This phase is at its peak from birth to age 2 years, and it ends by age 8 years.[4] The 20 to 50 million alveoli present at birth are estimated to increase eightfold by age 8 years. The subsequent increase in pulmonary volume results

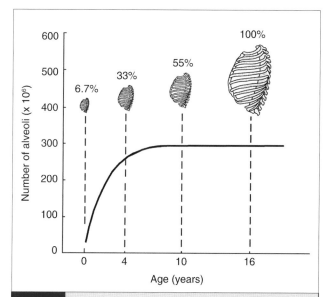

Figure 1 Graph showing normal alveolar hyperplasia (*curved line*) and thoracic volume (*rib cage drawings*) as a function of age. By age 5 to 6 years, alveolar multiplication is essentially complete, but thoracic volume is only about one third of the normal adult volume (*Adapted with permission from Campbell RM Jr, Smith MD: Thoracic insufficiency syndrome and exotic scoliosis. J Bone Joint Surg Am 2007;89[suppl 1]: 108-122; and Charles YP, Diméglio A, Marcoul M, Bourgin JF, Marcoul A, Bozonnat MC: Influence of idiopathic scoliosis on three-dimensional thoracic growth. Spine [Phila Pa 1976] 2008;33[11]: 1209-1218.*)

Dr. Johnston or an immediate family member serves as a board member, owner, officer, or committee member of the Scoliosis Research Society and the Texas Scottish Rite Hospital for Children; has received royalties from Medtronic; is a member of a speakers' bureau or has made paid presentations on behalf of Medtronic; serves as an unpaid consultant to Medtronic; and has received research or institutional support from Medtronic. Neither Dr. Garg nor any immediate family member has received anything of value from or owns stock in a commercial company or institution related directly or indirectly to the subject of this chapter.

5: Spine

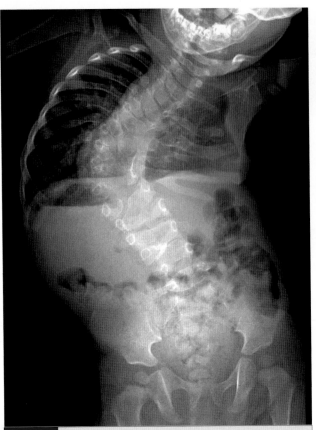

Figure 2 AP radiograph showing absence of the upper ribs and fusion of the lower ribs in the left thorax, producing an incompetent chest wall in a 2-year-old child with VATER association (vertebral, anal, tracheoesophageal, and renal defects) and complex unclassifiable congenital scoliosis. There are no normal vertebral elements between T1 and L5.

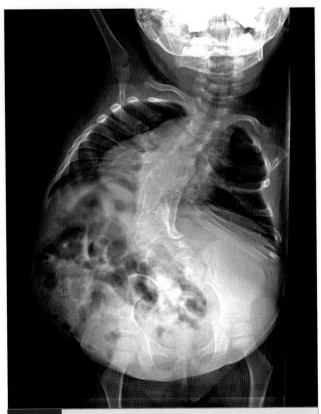

Figure 3 AP radiograph showing the characteristic multiple bilateral vertebral body and rib fusions in a child with the spondylothoracic dysplasia variant of Jarcho-Levin syndrome.

from the growth of the alveoli (hypertrophy).[3] The differentiation between early- and late-onset scoliosis is based on the timing of alveolar multiplication, which largely occurs during the so-called golden period before age 6 years. Alveolar multiplication is crucial for achieving normal lung volume through later hypertrophy.

Normal lung development is impaired by EOS and the associated chest wall deformity. Children with untreated, progressive EOS have a greater incidence of respiratory failure and mortality than unaffected children. In contrast, the mortality rate for patients with untreated adolescent idiopathic scoliosis is no greater than that of the general population.[5] Respiratory failure in patients with EOS results from both intrinsic alveolar hypoplasia (a smaller-than-normal number of alveoli) and extrinsic disturbance of chest wall function. The inability of the thorax to support normal respiration and lung growth is called thoracic insufficiency syndrome.[6]

Extrinsic disturbance of chest wall function occurs because of impaired chest wall compliance associated with progressive scoliosis, congenital scoliosis with fused ribs, or chest wall incompetence associated with absent ribs (**Figure 2**). The most dramatically impaired compliance is found in patients with extensive bilateral rib fusions and spine shortening (Jarcho-Levin syndrome; **Figure 3**), and those with extreme bilateral narrowing of the thorax (Jeune syndrome). Even if the patient does not have rib fusions or a syndromic etiology, the concavity of thoracic scoliosis narrows the intercostal spaces and impairs expansion during inspiration (**Figure 4**). Axial plane deformity in progressive EOS further impairs chest wall function. The resulting rib hump deformity produces a less compliant, narrowed convex hemithorax (**Figure 5**). In severe EOS, the thoracic deformity compresses the pulmonary parenchyma, leading to pulmonary hypertension and right heart failure.

With increasing recognition of the consequences of thoracic insufficiency syndrome, the focus of EOS treatment has shifted toward promoting thoracic growth while controlling spine deformity. In the past, early fusion was recommended because a short, straight spine was believed to be preferable to a longer, curved spine. Recent studies have found that pulmonary func-

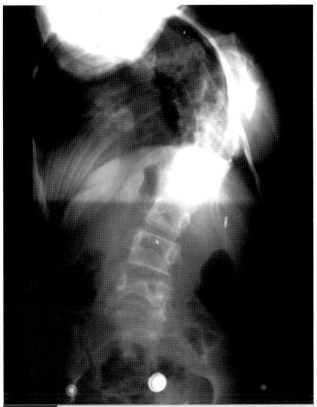

Figure 4 | AP radiograph showing severely narrowed intercostal spaces on the concavity of a severe scoliosis and marked narrowing of the convex hemithorax caused by axial plane deformity. The patient died of respiratory failure at age 20 years.

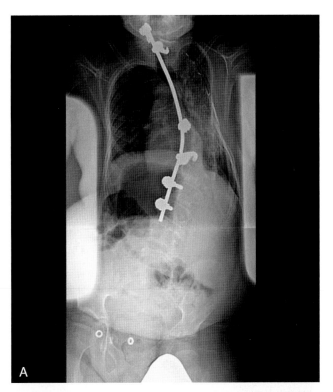

A

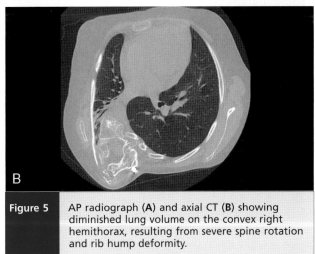

B

Figure 5 | AP radiograph (A) and axial CT (B) showing diminished lung volume on the convex right hemithorax, resulting from severe spine rotation and rib hump deformity.

tion can be severely reduced after early spine fusion. It is debatable, however, whether the decrease is caused by the effect of the fusion on thoracic growth or by the deformity itself. Children with infantile idiopathic scoliosis who were treated with fusion at an average age of 4 years had an average forced vital capacity (FVC) at follow-up of 41% of predicted value; those treated after age 10 years had an average FVC of 70% of predicted value.[7] In another study, 28 children with non-neuromuscular scoliosis who had spine fusion before age 9 years had an average FVC of 57.8% of predicted value. All 12 patients with an FVC lower than 50% of predicted value had a thoracic spine length (T1-T12) less than 18 cm. The worst pulmonary function was noted in those who had the greatest number of fused thoracic segments as well as a proximal thoracic fusion extending to T1 or T2.[8] Quality of life, as measured using functional scales, also was found to be decreased in children treated with early spine fusion.[9] Thus, growth-sparing methods designed to manage EOS without resorting to spine fusion during the golden period before age 6 years have become popular. These methods include casting, the use of growing rods, and chest wall expansion.

Natural History

The natural history of EOS varies based on the etiology. Idiopathic EOS, often called infantile idiopathic scoliosis, has an onset before age 4 years and occurs with slightly greater frequency in boys than in girls. EOS often presents as a left thoracic curve. Spontaneous resolution occurs in as many as 90% of patients.[10] Certain radiologic characteristics have prognostic significance.[11] Patients with a rib-vertebral angle difference less than 20° had a more than 80% likelihood of a nonprogressive deformity; patients with a rib-vertebral angle difference exceeding 20° had a more than 80% likelihood of a progressive deformity. Patients with severe rotation causing overlap of the rib head and the

5: Spine

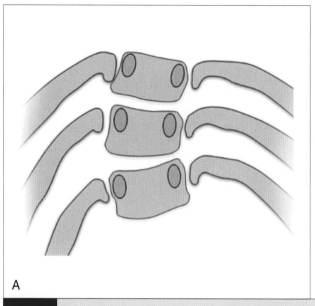 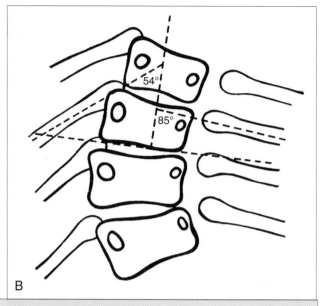

Figure 6 Schematic drawings showing the rib-vertebral angle difference. **A**, Phase I rotation in which the ribs do not overlie the adjacent pedicle. **B**, Phase II rotation with the ribs overlying the adjacent pedicle. The rib-vertebral angle difference is measured at the apical vertebra of the deformity, as shown.

vertebral body in the frontal plane (a so-called phase II rib) had near-certain progression of deformity (**Figure 6**). Observation is recommended for patients who are at low risk for progression. Patients who have progression are treated with a variety of nonsurgical and surgical methods.

Congenital scoliosis, described as deformity associated with a congenital vertebral anomaly, is characterized as a failure of formation, a failure of segmentation, or both. Hemivertebrae and wedged vertebrae result from a failure of formation, and block vertebrae and unilateral bars result from a failure of segmentation. A fully segmented hemivertebra anatomically includes half of a vertebral body, both inferior and superior end plates, a single pedicle, and a single lamina, and it has a corresponding extra unilateral rib. A semisegmented hemivertebra has only one identifiable end plate, with the other end plate fused to the adjacent vertebral body. A nonsegmented hemivertebra has no identifiable end plates. The greatest risk of progressive deformity is found with a fully segmented hemivertebra and a unilateral bar opposite the hemivertebra.[12] If not treated during childhood, the spine deformity may progress 14° per year during adolescence. The lowest risk of progression is in children with block vertebrae and a nonsegmented or fully incarcerated hemivertebra.

The most severe congenital scoliosis may involve failures of both segmentation and formation in a complex combination defying classification. In this so-called jumbled spine, rib fusions and other chest wall malformations lead to thoracic insufficiency syndrome (**Figure 2**). Precisely describing the vertebral anatomy often is difficult from plain radiographs. CT and three-dimensional CT surface reconstruction are invaluable

for defining the anatomy, determining the likelihood of progression, and planning surgery[13] (**Figure 7**).

Jarcho-Levin syndrome is one of the more dramatic syndromic conditions that can lead to EOS. The two variations of Jarcho-Levin syndrome are spondylothoracic dysplasia and the less severe spondylocostal dysostosis (**Figure 3**), both of which involve markedly decreased thoracic height. In spondylothoracic dysplasia, the ribs fuse posteriorly near the spinal column, and extensive vertebral fusions may cause the spinal column to appear as a single block vertebra. The mortality rate approaches 100% during the first year of life; a child who survives the first year may require mechanical ventilatory support. Spondylocostal dysostosis has a different radiographic appearance in which a jumbled-spine pattern of congenital defects is accompanied by hypoplasia as well as both rib fusion and absence. Patients with either form of Jarcho-Levin syndrome may have severe restrictive lung disease. Nonetheless, some patients with spondylocostal dysostosis survive well into the sixth decade of life.[14,15] Jeune, Larsen, and cerebrocostomandibular syndromes also commonly lead to EOS.[16,17]

A neural axis abnormality such as Chiari malformation, syrinx, or tethered spinal cord may be associated with progressive deformity in EOS. Ten of 46 children with infantile idiopathic scoliosis (22%) were found to have a neural axis abnormality, and 8 of these children required neurosurgical intervention.[18] A study of 54 patients with idiopathic infantile scoliosis found that 7 (13%) had a neural axis anomaly, and 3 of them required neurosurgical intervention.[19] Children with progressive, nonsyndromic EOS should routinely undergo MRI of the spine to detect a possible neural axis deformity.

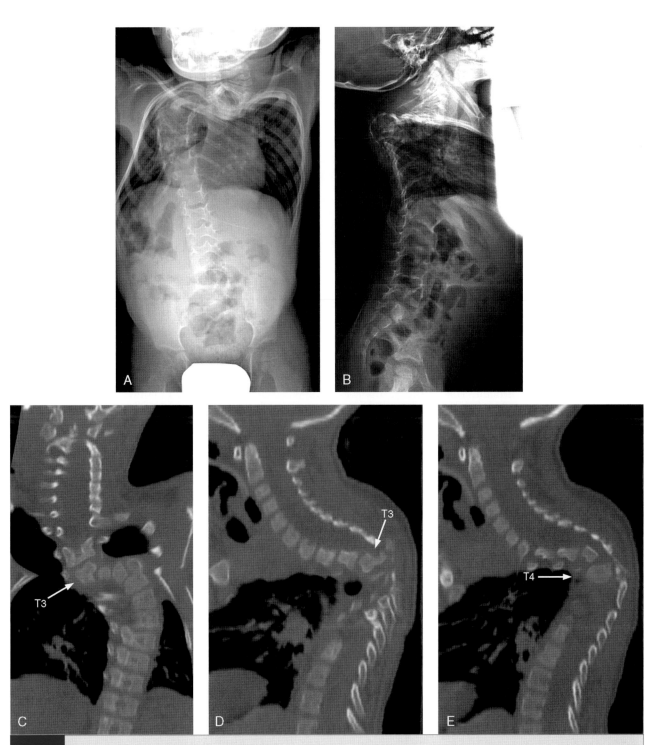

Figure 7 AP (**A**) and lateral (**B**) radiographs showing severe kyphoscoliosis in a 3-year-old child. Plain radiographs were insufficient for classifying the deformity. Coronal CT showing hemivertebrae at T3 and T6 (**C**) and severe canal stenosis at T3 (**D**) and T4 (**E**) at the apex of the kyphosis.

Nonsurgical Treatment

Spine fusion in a child younger than 6 years is suspected to limit thoracic growth and impair respiratory function.[7,8] The goal of nonsurgical treatment is to delay the need for spine fusion as long as possible to maximize thoracic growth. The typical nonsurgical treatment includes bracing or casting. Bracing generally is reserved for patients with modest idiopathic EOS deformity. Bracing can be detrimental in a child with EOS because of pressure on the rib cage; the Milwaukee brace may be generally preferable to the Boston-style

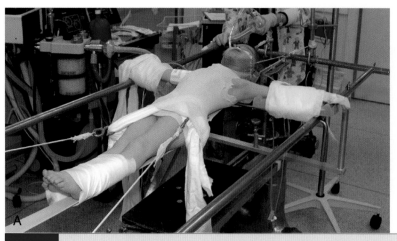
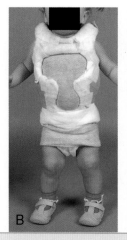
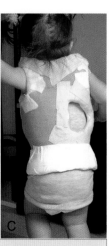

Figure 8   Photographs of casting. **A**, Application of a cast under general anesthesia, using an open-frame table with traction. Anterior (**B**) and posterior (**C**) views of a 1-year-old child in a cast. A cast window allows for abdominal and pulmonary expansion and settling of concave ribs.

thoracolumbosacral orthosis because constriction of the chest wall is less rigid. Patients with congenital scoliosis or a thoracic cage anomaly may have inflexibility that renders brace use difficult. This consideration is especially important for a patient with a larger curve because of the poor fit on a distorted thorax. Casting under general anesthesia, with longitudinal and rotational corrective forces, is useful to decrease the magnitude of deformity and perhaps permit orthotic management.

Casting has been used for decades to treat scoliosis and recently has increased in popularity.[20,21] The largest study reported results for 136 children with idiopathic deformity. The goal of treatment was to reach less than 10° of deformity. If casting failed to achieve the needed correction, an orthosis was used. At long-term follow-up, 96 of 136 children had resolution to less than 10° of deformity.[21]

Casting should be performed under general anesthesia on an open-frame table, with head and pelvic traction (**Figure 8, *A***). A traditional Risser table or the Mehta modified casting table is used for a technique involving a rotational force directed posterior to anterior on the rib hump, with counterforce on the pelvis and/or shoulders. A generous anterior window should be cut into the cast to allow abdominal and chest expansion, and a posterior window on the concave side of the cast allows space for the concave ribs to translate (**Figure 8, *B* and *C***). The cast is changed every 2 to 4 months, depending on the patient's age and cast hygiene. Complications are minimized with careful cast application and appropriately placed windows.

Traction also is used as a delaying tactic and a means of loosening the spine before fusion or fusionless surgical treatment. Traction is especially useful if the patient has a rigid curve that cannot be improved by bracing or casting. Longitudinally directed traction force is biomechanically more efficient than laterally directed force for correcting a severe curve.[22] Halo-femoral traction is useful intraoperatively to help correct a stiff curve. Halo-gravity traction is advantageous because it allows the child to be mobile with a walker or wheelchair (**Figure 9**); in contrast, a child undergoing halo-femoral traction is confined to bed. Halo-gravity traction was found to be safe and effective;[23,24] in 33 children treated with halo-gravity traction for a mean of 13 weeks before surgery, the average improvement was 65% in trunk shift, 35% in the coronal plane, and 30% in kyphosis. Trunk height increased as much as 11.5 cm (average, 5.3 cm).[24] In another study, halo-gravity traction did not improve the ultimate correction in children with severe congenital scoliosis, but it significantly decreased the need for vertebral column resection to achieve correction.[25] The benefit of preoperative traction correction thus lies in allowing a more complex and risky procedure to be avoided.

The halo is applied under general anesthesia using multiple pins. Individual pin torque is approximately the same as the child's age in years; for example, pins should be tightened to 2 in-lb in a 2-year-old child. Six to 8 pins are used for most children and adolescents, but as many as 12 pins may be used for toddlers. Adequate clearance of the halo ring around the entire skull is important, and forehead pins should not tether the eyebrows or eyelids. Traction weight is added gradually, with frequent neurologic surveillance. Patients can tolerate traction of 50% or more of their body weight. A cranial nerve deficit or motor weakness requires prompt reduction or removal of traction. Pulmonary function usually is assessed while the patient is in traction. The traction is continued until deformity correction or pulmonary improvement has reached a plateau.

Complications are uncommon in halo-gravity traction.[23,26] Nystagmus or other signs of cranial nerve traction generally resolve quickly after the traction weight is decreased. The use of multiple pins lessens the incidence of individual pin loosening and infection. If a pin

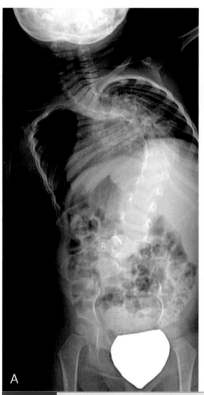
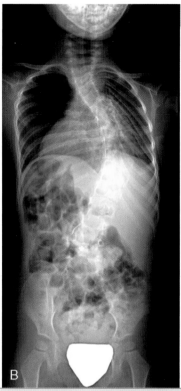
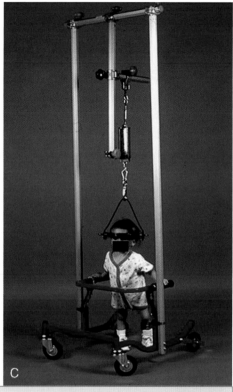

Figure 9 AP radiographs obtained before (**A**) and after (**B**) halo-gravity traction was used to treat a child with EOS. **C**, Photograph of the child using a halo-walker for mobility during treatment.

site infection does not respond to oral antibiotics, the pin should be removed and possibly relocated to a clean site on the ring. Halo-gravity traction is contraindicated for an infant with open cranial sutures, if the patient is unable to tolerate prolonged traction because of a severe cognitive defect, or if the patient has a sharp kyphosis, a cervical anomaly of uncertain stability, an intraspinal neoplasm, or a skull defect.

Surgical Treatment

Spine fusion traditionally has been considered the definitive treatment for EOS, but the apparent detrimental effects of early fusion on pulmonary function have stimulated a shift toward growth-sparing treatments during the period of rapid thoracic growth. These treatments may involve growth modulation, an extendable growing-rod construct, or the vertical expandable prosthetic titanium rib (VEPTR). Unlike other fusionless spine implants, the VEPTR has been approved by the US Food and Drug Administration (FDA) for use in skeletally immature patients with thoracic insufficiency syndrome.

Short-segment fusion remains an important treatment for some types of congenital scoliosis, despite the general goal of delaying definitive spine fusion to allow thoracic and pulmonary growth. Hemivertebra excision with short-segment fusion is an excellent procedure for a congenital deformity involving as many as four vertebrae. Earlier treatments focused on fusion in situ or convex hemiepiphysiodesis, which attempts to guide correction by producing asymmetric growth. Hemiepiphysiodesis does not often achieve actual curve correction, but fusion in situ and convex hemiepiphysiodesis generally can achieve long-term stabilization of a short-segment deformity.[27-32]

Hemivertebra excision with short-segment fusion through anterior and posterior approaches was found to be efficacious in 60 patients. Correction was safely achieved in nearly 50% of patients, with neurologic improvement in 10 patients (17%) who had a kyphotic deformity.[33] Several other studies have confirmed the efficacy of hemivertebra resection using anterior and posterior approaches in patients with congenital scoliosis[34-36] (**Figure 10**). Congenital scoliosis can also be safely and effectively corrected using the technically challenging posterior-only approach.[37,38] The procedure involves hemivertebra excision and osteotomy of a bar, if present, with transpedicular instrumentation used for short-segment spine fusion. Forty-one patients age 1 to 6 years achieved stable correction at an average 6-year follow-up, with spine growth maintained outside the fusion mass.[37-39] A posterolateral approach to hemivertebra excision was used in 24 patients; correction was adequate at intermediate follow-up, and there were no

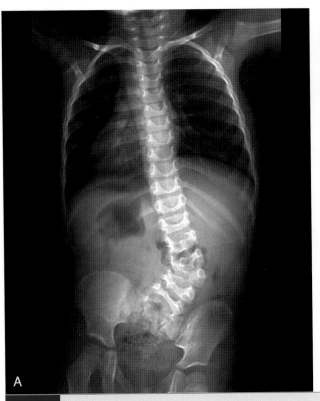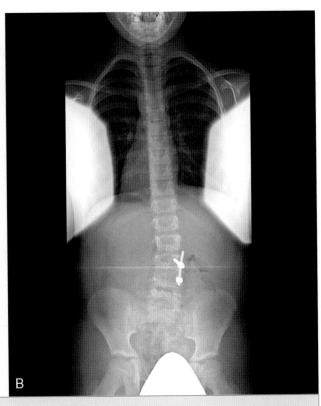

Figure 10   AP radiographs obtained before (**A**) and 6 years after (**B**) hemivertebra excision and short-segment fusion at L3 in a 4-year-old child.

major neurologic complications.[40] No study has reported the effect of convex hemiepiphysiodesis or hemivertebra excision on pulmonary function.

Spine growth modulation using vertebral body staples was developed for treating juvenile idiopathic scoliosis.[41,42] All disks involved in the Cobb angle are stapled using nitinol staples, which have shape memory; as the tines of the staple warm to body temperature, they close to compress across a disk space. At early follow-up, only 2 of 21 patients (10%) had required definitive spine fusion, and 87% had deformity progression of less than 10°.[41,42] No results have been reported for four patients with idiopathic EOS who were younger than 8 years at the time of treatment.[41,42]

The current growth-sparing treatments primarily use serially lengthened distraction instrumentation that combines spine, rib, and pelvic fixation points. The first reported fusionless instrumentation (the Moe procedure) used a single subcutaneous Harrington rod and hook, with optional end-vertebrae fusion.[43] Subperiosteal exposure of the spine was avoided, except at the end levels, to discourage spontaneous fusion. Although this procedure prevented progressive deformity until the time of definitive fusion, spine elongation averaged only 2 to 3 cm, despite multiple lengthening procedures.[44,45] Disappointing amounts of growth and the occurrence of severe crankshaft phenomenon have stimulated the search for a better method of treatment.[28,46]

In response to limited growth and frequent rod failure with the Moe procedure, the use of two subcutaneous rods with end-vertebrae fusion was introduced by Akbarnia.[47] Tandem or transverse connectors are used to link proximal and distal rods anchored to end-vertebrae (**Figure 11**). The construct is lengthened every 6 months until complications occur or no further gains in length are achieved.[47] Increasing the strength of fixation with a second rod is believed to improve the stability of the construct as it is lengthened, improve the maintenance of the gained correction, and decrease the risk of implant failure. In 13 children with noncongenital EOS who underwent this procedure and were followed to definitive fusion, the average increase in T1-S1 length was more than 10 cm. The average growth rate of 1.46 cm per year is in line with normal growth.[48] Growth was even greater when a regular schedule of lengthening at 6-month intervals was maintained. The final deformity correction was 64%, with most of the correction resulting from the initial procedure. Six of 13 patients had a complication, including 4 who had more than one complication.[47]

The Akbarnia technique uses hook anchors proximally and a mixture of hooks and screws distally (**Figure 11, C and D**). The recent trend has been to use only screws both proximally and distally. It is believed that increased stability of fixation will reduce the incidence of implant complications and particularly the incidence of fixation pullout, which has been problematic in de-

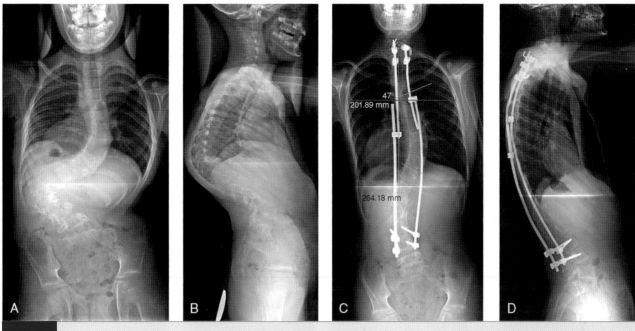

Figure 11 Preoperative AP (**A**) and lateral (**B**) radiographs of a 4-year-old boy with congenital muscular dystrophy and collapsing scoliosis. AP (**C**) and lateral (**D**) radiographs after eight procedures over the next 5 years to implant and lengthen growing-rod instrumentation. The T1-12 and T1-S1 spine length measurements were normal.

formities with a significant kyphosis component. Biomechanical studies found that growing-rod constructs had greater stability if two-level screw fixation was used at each end, rather than hook fixation.[49] However, anecdotal reports of gradual thoracic pedicle screw migration into the spinal canal reinforces the need for great caution if this type of proximal anchor is selected for a nonfusion procedure (**Figure 12**). Pedicle screw fixation has not been approved by the FDA for use in the pediatric population and, therefore, is an off-label use.

Growing-rod fixation also has been used to treat congenital scoliosis.[44,50] The largest available study involved 19 patients treated at several centers; growth rates averaged 1.2 cm per year, with improvement in the space available for the lungs.[50] Growing-rod fixation can be considered for treating congenital scoliosis in two groups of patients: those who have a long flexible-motion segment containing a short anomalous segment and those who have a jumbled spine with multiple anomalies not amenable to excision and short-segment fusion. Provided that short-segment fusion, with or without hemivertebra and/or bar excision, can restore spine balance, it remains an attractive choice for patients with congenital scoliosis.

The so-called guided growth method involves a limited fusion at the apex of the deformity, with bilateral pedicle screw instrumentation.[51] Pedicle screws also are placed extraperiosteally at more cephalad and caudal segments. Bilateral rods are placed, but set screws are not tightened at the end anchors so that the spine can grow in a guided manner, with the rods sliding through

the nonfixed pedicle screws cephalad and caudal to the apical fusion. The obvious advantage of this method over the use of growing rods is that repeated surgical procedures are not required for lengthening. Ten children, age 2 to 10 years and having different diagnoses, had a correction from a mean of 71° (range, 40° to 86°) before surgery to a mean of 27° (range, 7° to 52°) at 6-week-follow-up. The correction was maintained at 2-year follow-up. The average increase in trunk height was 12%. Additional surgery was required in five children (three procedures because of implant difficulties and two because of infection).[51]

In children with a primary chest wall deformity such as a rib fusion or rib absence, primary spinal column fixation may not promote growth of the pulmonary system or chest wall. The VEPTR was developed to allow thoracic cage expansion after an opening-wedge thoracoplasty in children with congenital scoliosis involving fused ribs and thoracic insufficiency syndrome.[17] The VEPTR is FDA approved under a humanitarian-use exemption for skeletally immature patients with thoracic insufficiency syndrome. The device can be secured to the ribs, spine, or pelvis to provide distraction across the chest concavity, stabilize flail segments of the chest, and expand thoracic volume (**Figure 13**). Spine deformity correction or stabilization is obtained by means of chest wall distraction resulting from the increased corrective moment provided by the lateral placement of the device in relation to the spine. As with growing rods, periodic lengthening is required to maintain thoracic expansion. In 27 children with thoracic insufficiency syndrome, the use of VEPTR led

5: Spine

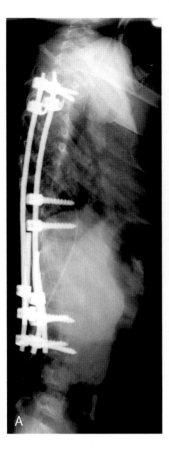
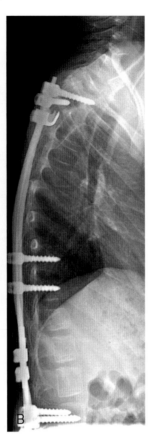
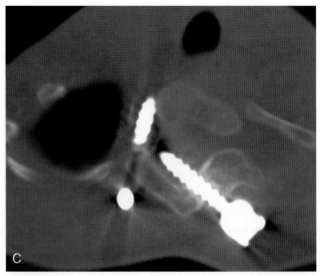

Figure 12   **A,** Immediate postoperative lateral radiograph showing the insertion of pedicle screws at the proximal end of a growing-rod construct. **B,** Lateral radiograph obtained 2 years later showing a change in position of one of the screws. **C,** Five months after the final, uneventful lengthening procedure, the patient had gradual paraparesis. CT showed migration of the left pedicle screw into and through the spinal canal.

to thoracic growth of 0.7 cm per year, a mean 33% scoliosis correction, and most importantly, stabilization of pulmonary function. Absolute FVC was significantly increased in the children who began treatment before age 2 years and who had not had previous spine surgery, although the percentage predicted vital capacity did not change. Complications occurred in 22 children. The most common complication was proximal migration of the implant through the ribs, which usually was managed by repositioning the fixation device during a scheduled lengthening procedure.[52] Other studies have reported similar results.[53-55] The increase in thoracic volume was found to be maintained into adulthood; chest CT revealed an average 147% increase in total lung volume, with a 217% increase on the concave side.[56] The increases in absolute FVC did not lead to an increase in percentage predicted vital capacity for age, which remained steady.[56]

The pulmonary findings were similar in a study of 24 children treated with VEPTR, but there was a notable new finding related to chest wall compliance.[53] Respiratory compliance, as measured by a passive deflation technique, declined 56% after VEPTR treatment. This suspected iatrogenic decrease in chest compliance may help explain why the percentage predicted vital capacity for age does not appear to improve in patients treated with VEPTR, despite increases in overall vital capacity. This finding indicates that routine use of VEPTR may not be appropriate for children who do not have rib fusions or flail chest.

The use of VEPTR can lead to a unique complication: upper extremity neurologic injury secondary to brachial plexus stretch or compression, directly or by scapular traction during wound closure. Proximal VEPTR anchors should not be placed higher than the second rib to avoid direct compression on the plexus. A recent review of neurologic injuries in VEPTR treatment confirmed that upper extremity injuries were the most commonly identified adverse events after VEPTR surgery (in 0.5% of 1,736 procedures).[57] Mortality rates remain high, despite improvement in pulmonary function and spine deformity, because of the severity of preoperative disease in some patients. Of 43 children treated with VEPTR for Jeune or Jarcho-Levin syndrome, 4 (9%) died within 1 year of the index surgery.[58] Two of the deaths resulted from respiratory failure, one from renal failure, and one from liver failure. An additional 4 children (9%) had a life-threatening event.

Although eventual spine fusion is anticipated with growth-sparing techniques after maximum pulmonary gain has been achieved, a recent study found that many patients with hypoplastic or flail chest are being treated without the need for definitive fusion at the end of growth.[59] Similar reports have not emerged for patients treated with growing-rod or apical fusion techniques, and definitive fusion still must be anticipated for almost all children treated with those techniques.

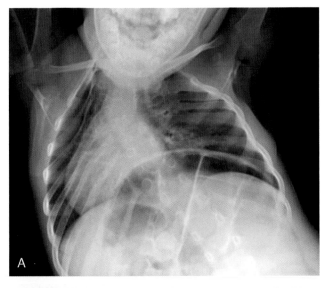

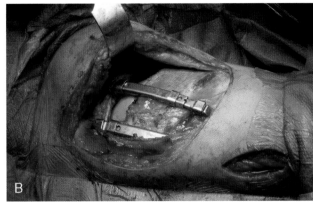

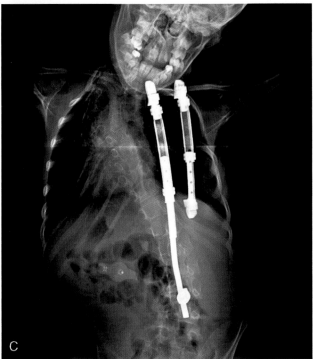

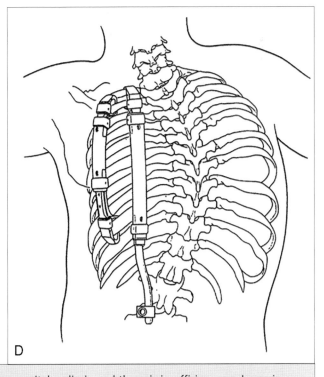

Figure 13 A, Preoperative AP radiograph showing fused ribs, congenital scoliosis, and thoracic insufficiency syndrome in a 4-year-old child. B, Intraoperative photograph showing medial rib-to-spine and lateral rib-to-rib VEPTR implantation. C, AP radiograph 3 years after serial VEPTR lengthening, showing increased thoracic height, hemithoracic volume, and control of the spine deformity. D, Schematic drawing showing VEPTR implantation with rib-to-rib and rib-to-spine anchoring.

Summary and Future Directions

The resurgent use of nonsurgical treatments for EOS has benefitted patients by allowing improvement in spine and chest deformity without the morbidity associated with surgical treatment. Effective casting can completely correct the spine deformity and improve pulmonary development in many patients with mild to moderate deformity.

When surgery is indicated, the options include both conventional spine fusion and growth-sparing methods such as growing-rod and VEPTR fixation. Each method has particular indications and challenges. The results of growth modulation techniques such as spine stapling have not been reported for patients with EOS. Growth guidance is promising, but only short-term follow-up results are available. The future directions include flexible spine tethering and modulation of vertebral growth centers, which are being studied in animal models but have not yet been applied to the challenging treatment of EOS.

Annotated References

1. Diméglio A: Growth of the spine before age 5 years. *J Pediatr Orthop B* 1992;1:102-107.

2. Charles YP, Diméglio A, Marcoul M, Bourgin JF, Marcoul A, Bozonnat MC: Influence of idiopathic scoliosis on three-dimensional thoracic growth. *Spine (Phila Pa 1976)* 2008;33(11):1209-1218.

   This landmark study calculated thoracic volume, circumference, and other parameters from optical surface scanning data and related them to age, weight, and height in 130 children with scoliosis and 126 without deformity.

3. Emery JL, Mithal A: The number of alveoli in the terminal respiratory unit of man during late intrauterine life and childhood. *Arch Dis Child* 1960;35:544-547.

4. Reid L: Lung growth, in Zorab PA, ed: *Scoliosis and Growth*. Edinburgh, Scotland, Churchill Livingstone, 1971, pp 117-121.

5. Pehrsson K, Nachemson A, Olofson J, Ström K, Larsson S: Respiratory failure in scoliosis and other thoracic deformities: A survey of patients with home oxygen or ventilator therapy in Sweden. *Spine (Phila Pa 1976)* 1992;17(6):714-718.

6. Campbell RM Jr, Smith MD, Mayes TC, et al: The characteristics of thoracic insufficiency syndrome associated with fused ribs and congenital scoliosis. *J Bone Joint Surg Am* 2003;85A(3):399-408.

7. Goldberg CJ, Gillic I, Connaughton O, et al: Respiratory function and cosmesis at maturity in infantile-onset scoliosis. *Spine (Phila Pa 1976)* 2003;28(20):2397-2406.

8. Karol LA, Johnston C, Mladenov K, Schochet P, Walters P, Browne RH: Pulmonary function following early thoracic fusion in non-neuromuscular scoliosis. *J Bone Joint Surg Am* 2008;90(6):1272-1281.

   Of 28 patients with spine fusion at a mean age of 3.3 years, 12 had FVC of less than 50% of predicted volume at 11-year follow-up. Diminished pulmonary function correlated with the extent of thoracic segment fusion, a proximal extension of fusion to T1-T2, and a T1-T12 length of less than 18 cm. Level of evidence: IV.

9. Vitale MG, Matsumoto H, Bye MR, et al: A retrospective cohort study of pulmonary function, radiographic measures, and quality of life in children with congenital scoliosis: An evaluation of patient outcomes after early spinal fusion. *Spine (Phila Pa 1976)* 2008;33(11):1242-1249.

   Children with congenital scoliosis who were treated with early spine fusion had worse pulmonary function tests and quality-of-life outcomes at follow-up than healthy peers. Early thoracic fusion led to shorter spine length, lower FVC and forced expiratory volume in 1 second, and more pain.

10. Lloyd-Roberts GC, Pilcher MF: Structural idiopathic scoliosis in infancy: A study of the natural history of 100 patients. *J Bone Joint Surg Br* 1965;47:520-523.

11. Mehta MH: The rib-vertebra angle in the early diagnosis between resolving and progressive infantile scoliosis. *J Bone Joint Surg Br* 1972;54(2):230-243.

12. McMaster MJ, Ohtsuka K: The natural history of congenital scoliosis: A study of two hundred and fifty-one patients. *J Bone Joint Surg Am* 1982;64(8):1128-1147.

13. Newton PO, Hahn GW, Fricka KB, Wenger DR: Utility of three-dimensional and multiplanar reformatted computed tomography for evaluation of pediatric congenital spine abnormalities. *Spine (Phila Pa 1976)* 2002;27(8):844-850.

14. Ramírez N, Cornier AS, Campbell RM Jr, Carlo S, Arroyo S, Romeu J: Natural history of thoracic insufficiency syndrome: A spondylothoracic dysplasia perspective. *J Bone Joint Surg Am* 2007;89(12):2663-2675.

    In a long-term outcome and survival study of 28 patients with thoracic insufficiency syndrome secondary to spondylothoracic dysplasia, 20 of 28 patients survived despite severe restrictive respiratory disease and enjoyed a reasonable quality of life.

15. Cornier AS, Ramírez N, Arroyo S, et al: Phenotype characterization and natural history of spondylothoracic dysplasia syndrome: A series of 27 new cases. *Am J Med Genet* 2004;128A(2):120-126.

16. Campbell RM Jr: Spine deformities in rare congenital syndromes: Clinical issues. *Spine (Phila Pa 1976)* 2009;34(17):1815-1827.

    This is a focused review of medical and surgical treatment considerations in six exotic syndromes associated with thoracic insufficiency syndrome, including arthrogryposis and Marfan, Jeune, Jarcho-Levin, cerebrocostomandibular, and Larsen syndromes.

17. Campbell RM Jr, Hell-Vocke AK: Growth of the thoracic spine in congenital scoliosis after expansion thoracoplasty. *J Bone Joint Surg Am* 2003;85(3):409-420.

18. Dobbs MB, Lenke LG, Szymanski DA, et al: Prevalence of neural axis abnormalities in patients with infantile idiopathic scoliosis. *J Bone Joint Surg Am* 2002;84(12):2230-2234.

19. Pahys JM, Samdani AF, Betz RR: Intraspinal anomalies in infantile idiopathic scoliosis: Prevalence and role of MRI. *44th Annual Meeting Final Program*. Milwaukee, WI, Scoliosis Research Society, 2009, paper 37. http://www.srs.org.meetings/am09/am09-final-program.pdf. Accessed September 17, 2010.

Of 54 patients with idiopathic scoliosis greater than 20° that was diagnosed before age 36 months, 7 (13%) had neural axis abnormality and 5 required neurosurgical intervention.

20. D'Astous JL, Sanders JO: Casting and traction treatment methods for scoliosis. *Orthop Clin North Am* 2007;38(4):477-484, v.

    The methods, rationale, and results of casting (with the Cotrel-Mehta technique) and halo-gravity traction are described, with an emphasis on equipment and principles.

21. Mehta MH: Growth as a corrective force in the early treatment of progressive infantile scoliosis. *J Bone Joint Surg Br* 2005;87(9):1237-1247.

    This is the largest published study (136 patients) of casting for growth guidance treatment of infantile scoliosis. Unique phenotype patterns (sturdy, slender, known syndromic, unknown syndromic) are presented with their prognostic implication. Full correction was achieved in 94 patients and partial correction in 42, with treatment more successful before age 2 years.

22. White AA III, Panjabi MM: The clinical biomechanics of scoliosis. *Clin Orthop Relat Res* 1976;118:100-112.

23. Rinella A, Lenke L, Whitaker C, et al: Perioperative halo-gravity traction in the treatment of severe scoliosis and kyphosis. *Spine (Phila Pa 1976)* 2005;30(4):475-482.

    Thirty-three patients (mean age, 13.8 years) underwent halo-gravity traction as a preoperative and intraoperative method of maximizing curve reduction. The mean preoperative curve was 84°. There were no permanent neurologic sequelae, and surgical correction was achieved in 46%.

24. Sink EL, Karol LA, Sanders J, Birch JG, Johnston CE, Herring JA: Efficacy of perioperative halo-gravity traction in the treatment of severe scoliosis in children. *J Pediatr Orthop* 2001;21(4):519-524.

25. Sponseller PD, Takenaga RK, Newton P, et al: The use of traction in the treatment of severe spinal deformity. *Spine (Phila Pa 1976)* 2008;33(21):2305-2309.

    Thirty patients treated with halo-gravity traction were compared with 23 patients treated without traction. No differences in curve correction, surgical time, or blood loss were noted. The complication rate was 27% with traction and 52% without traction. Those not treated with traction were treated with vertebral column resection more frequently (39% versus 3%).

26. Walick K, McClung A, Sucato DJ, Johnston CE: Halo-gravity traction in severe pediatric spinal deformity. *43rd Annual Meeting Scientific Program Abstracts*. Milwaukee, WI, Scoliosis Research Society, 2008, paper 80. http://www.srs.org.meetings/am08/doc/oral_abstracts.pdf. Accessed September 17, 2010.

    Fifty patients undergoing halo-gravity traction were divided into three groups: patients younger than 8 years with no previous treatment, patients older than 8 years with no previous treatment, and patients with previous treatment. Patients in all groups had equal benefit in percentage deformity correction, T1-T12 height increase, and trunk shift. Patients with earlier fusion equally benefitted from traction.

27. Cil A, Yazici M, Alanay A, Acaroglu RE, Uzumcugil A, Surat A: The course of sagittal plane abnormality in the patients with congenital scoliosis managed with convex growth arrest. *Spine (Phila Pa 1976)* 2004;29(5):547-553.

28. Terek RM, Wehner J, Lubicky JP: Crankshaft phenomenon in congenital scoliosis: A preliminary report. *J Pediatr Orthop* 1991;11(4):527-532.

29. Thompson AG, Marks DS, Sayampanathan SR, Piggott H: Long-term results of combined anterior and posterior convex epiphysiodesis for congenital scoliosis due to hemivertebrae. *Spine (Phila Pa 1976)* 1995;20(12):1380-1385.

30. Winter RB, Lonstein JE, Denis F, Sta-Ana de la Rosa H: Convex growth arrest for progressive congenital scoliosis due to hemivertebrae. *J Pediatr Orthop* 1988;8(6):633-638.

31. Winter RB, Moe JH: The results of spinal arthrodesis for congenital spinal deformity in patients younger than five years old. *J Bone Joint Surg Am* 1982;64(3):419-432.

32. Winter RB, Moe JH, Lonstein JE: Posterior spinal arthrodesis for congenital scoliosis: An analysis of the cases of two hundred and ninety patients, five to nineteen years old. *J Bone Joint Surg Am* 1984;66(8):1188-1197.

33. Leatherman KD, Dickson RA: Two-stage corrective surgery for congenital deformities of the spine. *J Bone Joint Surg Br* 1979;61(3):324-328.

34. Deviren V, Berven S, Smith JA, Emami A, Hu SS, Bradford DS: Excision of hemivertebrae in the management of congenital scoliosis involving the thoracic and thoracolumbar spine. *J Bone Joint Surg Br* 2001;83(4):496-500.

35. Hedequist DJ, Hall JE, Emans JB: Hemivertebra excision in children via simultaneous anterior and posterior exposures. *J Pediatr Orthop* 2005;25(1):60-63.

    Eighteen children (mean age, 3.2 years) underwent simultaneous anterior and posterior hemivertebra excision using unilateral compression implants. An average correction of 71% was achieved, with no pseudarthroses or neurologic complications.

36. Klemme WR, Polly DW Jr, Orchowski JR: Hemivertebral excision for congenital scoliosis in very young children. *J Pediatr Orthop* 2001;21(6):761-764.

37. Ruf M, Harms J: Hemivertebra resection by a posterior approach: Innovative operative technique and first results. *Spine (Phila Pa 1976)* 2002;27(10):1116-1123.

5: Spine

38. Ruf M, Harms J: Posterior hemivertebra resection with transpedicular instrumentation: Early correction in children aged 1 to 6 years. *Spine (Phila Pa 1976)* 2003; 28(18):2132-2138.

39. Ruf M, Jensen R, Letko L, Harms J: Hemivertebra resection and osteotomies in congenital spine deformity. *Spine (Phila Pa 1976)* 2009;34(17):1791-1799.

    At a mean 6.17-year follow-up of 41 patients (mean age, 3 years 5 months) after hemivertebra resection through a posterior-only approach, those without a unilateral bar had curve correction from 36° to 7°, with spontaneous correction of compensatory curves. Patients with a bar had curve correction from 69° to 23°, also with good compensatory curve correction.

40. Li X, Luo Z, Li X, Tao H, Du J, Wang Z: Hemivertebra resection for the treatment of congenital lumbarspinal scoliosis with lateral-posterior approach. *Spine (Phila Pa 1976)* 2008;33(18):2001-2006.

    Twenty-four patients (mean age, 9.4 years) underwent posterolateral resection of lumbar hemivertebrae. The main curve was corrected in 61%, with normal lordosis. No major complications or neurologic deficit occurred.

41. Betz RR, D'Andrea LP, Mulcahey MJ, Chafetz RS: Vertebral body stapling procedure for the treatment of scoliosis in the growing child. *Clin Orthop Relat Res* 2005; 434:55-60.

    In patients older than 8 years with a curve of less than 50°, thoracoscopic vertebral body stapling achieved 87% stability with less than 10° progression at 1-year follow-up.

42. Betz RR, Kim J, D'Andrea LP, Mulcahey MJ, Balsara RK, Clements DH: An innovative technique of vertebral body stapling for the treatment of patients with adolescent idiopathic scoliosis: A feasibility, safety, and utility study. *Spine (Phila Pa 1976)* 2003;28(20):S255-S265.

43. Moe JH, Kharrat K, Winter RB, Cummine JL: Harrington instrumentation without fusion plus external orthotic support for the treatment of difficult curvature problems in young children. *Clin Orthop Relat Res* 1984;185:35-45.

44. Klemme WR, Denis F, Winter RB, Lonstein JW, Koop SE: Spinal instrumentation without fusion for progressive scoliosis in young children. *J Pediatr Orthop* 1997; 17(6):734-742.

45. Mineiro J, Weinstein SL: Subcutaneous rodding for progressive spinal curvatures: Early results. *J Pediatr Orthop* 2002;22(3):290-295.

46. Acaroglu E, Yazici M, Alanay A, Surat A: Three-dimensional evolution of scoliotic curve during instrumentation without fusion in young children. *J Pediatr Orthop* 2002;22(4):492-496.

47. Akbarnia BA, Breakwell LM, Marks DS, et al: Dual growing rod technique followed for three to eleven years until final fusion: The effect of frequency of lengthening. *Spine (Phila Pa 1976)* 2008;33(9):984-990.

    Thirteen patients with noncongenital EOS had a mean curve correction from 81° to 36° during lengthening and 28° after fusion. An average of five lengthenings every 9 months produced a mean growth rate of 1.5 cm per year, with more frequent lengthening (less than 6 months) producing a growth rate of 1.8 cm per year. Six of 13 patients experienced complications, and 13 complications (5 after final fusion) required treatment.

48. Diméglio A, Bonnel F: *Le Rachis en Croissance*. Paris, France, Springer, 1990.

49. Mahar AT, Bagheri R, Oka R, Kostial P, Akbarnia BA: Biomechanical comparison of different anchors (foundations) for the pediatric dual growing rod technique. *Spine J* 2008;8(6):933-939.

    Four pedicle screws over adjacent segments provide the strongest resistance to pullout testing, compared with foundations with hooks. Cross-linking does not add to pullout strength. Hook constructs resist pullout better in the lumbar vertebrae than in the thoracic vertebrae.

50. Elsebaie HB, Yazici M, Thompson GH, et al: Safety and efficacy of growing rod technique for pediatric congenital spinal deformities. *First International Congress of Early Onset Scoliosis and Growing Spine*. Wheaton, IL, International Congress of Early Onset Scoliosis and Growing Spine, 2007, paper 10. http://www.growingspine.org/files/abstracts_and_journal.doc. Accessed September 17, 2010.

    Nineteen patients with congenital scoliosis underwent growing-rod treatment. An average of 4.3 lengthenings over 2.5 to 6 years produced curve correction from 65° to 47°, with 5 cm of T1-S1 growth (1.2 cm per year) achieved. There were 15 complications in eight patients, after 11 procedures.

51. McCarthy RE, McCullough FL, Luhmann SJ, Lenke LG: Shilla growth enhancing system for the treatment of scoliosis in children: Greater than two year follow-up. *43rd Annual Meeting Scientific Program Abstracts*. Milwaukee, WI, Scoliosis Research Society, 2008, p 53. http://www.srs.org.meetings/am08/doc/oral_abstracts.pdf. Accessed September 17, 2010.

    Ten patients (mean age, 7 years 6 months) underwent growth guidance surgery using apical pedicle screws and fusion to achieve curve correction and nonconstrained guidance screws at the end vertebrae. At 2-year follow-up, correction to 34° was obtained, from an initial 70.5°. Five unplanned surgeries were necessary for complications, compared to an estimated 49 surgeries for a standard periodic-lengthening protocol.

52. Campbell RM Jr, Smith MD, Mayes TC, et al: The effect of opening wedge thoracostomy on thoracic insufficiency syndrome associated with fused ribs and congenital scoliosis. *J Bone Joint Surg Am* 2004;86(8):1659-1674.

53. Motoyama EK, Yang CI, Deeney VF: Thoracic malformation with early-onset scoliosis: Effect of serial VEPTR expansion thoracoplasty on lung growth and function in children. *Paediatr Respir Rev* 2009;10(1):12-17.

Absolute FVC (measured under anesthesia) increased by 11% per year in 24 children undergoing VEPTR treatment. Children younger than 6 years had a greater FVC increase than older children (14.5% versus 6.5%). Percentage predicted FVC did not keep up with body growth. Respiratory system compliance decreased 56% despite clinically successful thoracic expansion.

54. Ramirez N, Flynn JM, Serrano JA, Carlo S, Cornier AS: The Vertical Expandable Prosthetic Titanium Rib in the treatment of spinal deformity due to progressive early onset scoliosis. *J Pediatr Orthop B* 2009;18(4):197-203.

In 17 patients, primarily with congenital scoliosis, who underwent VEPTR treatment, curve correction of 59% was achieved, with a 13% complication rate, at 25-month follow-up.

55. Samdani AF, Ranade A, Dolch HJ, et al: Bilateral use of the vertical expandable prosthetic titanium rib attached to the pelvis: A novel treatment for scoliosis in the growing spine. *J Neurosurg Spine* 2009;10(4):287-292.

At 25-month follow-up, 11 patients with bilateral rib-to-pelvis VEPTR had improvement in Cobb angle (81.7° to 58°), T2-T12 kyphosis (43° to 37°), and T1-S1 length (23.1 cm to 29.4 cm), with a 36% complication rate after a mean of 3.7 lengthenings.

56. Emans JB, Caubet JF, Ordonez CL, Lee EY, Ciarlo M: The treatment of spine and chest wall deformities with fused ribs by expansion thoracostomy and insertion of vertical expandable prosthetic titanium rib: Growth of thoracic spine and improvement of lung volumes. *Spine (Phila Pa 1976)* 2005;30(17, suppl):S58-S68.

In 31 patients with congenital scoliosis and fused ribs, thoracic spine length increased a mean of 4.3 cm through device expansion. Scoliosis was corrected from 55° to 43° after a mean of 3.5 lengthenings. CT lung volume increased from a mean of 369 cc to 736 cc at last follow-up, and lung volume on the treated hemithorax increased 219%.

57. Skaggs DL, Choi PD, Rice C, et al: Efficacy of intraoperative neurologic monitoring in surgery involving a vertical expandable prosthetic titanium rib for early-onset spinal deformity. *J Bone Joint Surg Am* 2009;91(7):1657-1663.

Eight neurologic injuries, including six in the upper extremity, occurred in 1,736 VEPTR-related surgeries in six centers. There were two incidences of false-negative somatosensory-evoked potential monitoring and one false-negative somatosensory-evoked or motor-evoked potential monitoring. Neurologic monitoring is indicated in primary implantation and exchange of VEPTR devices.

58. Betz RR, Mulcahey MJ, Ramirez N, et al: Mortality and life-threatening events after vertical expandable prosthetic titanium rib surgery in children with hypoplastic chest wall deformity. *J Pediatr Orthop* 2008;28(8):850-853.

Four of 43 patients with Jeune syndrome (9%) died during the first year after VEPTR treatment. Four additional patients with Jeune or Jarcho-Levin syndrome had a life-threatening event. Respiratory, cardiac, renal, and bowel necrosis events were the main causes of mortality and morbidity in these patients with hyoplastic thorax. Level of evidence: IV.

59. Flynn JM, St. Hilaire T, Emans JB, et al: Is definitive spinal fusion, or VEPTR removal, needed after VEPTR expansions are over? An analysis of 39 "VEPTR graduates." *43rd Annual Meeting Scientific Program Abstracts*. Milwaukee, WI, Scoliosis Research Society, 2008, p 17. http://www.srs.org.meetings/am08/doc/oral_abstracts.pdf. Accessed September 17, 2010.

The final surgical procedures for 39 VEPTR patients approaching skeletal maturity included 18 spine fusions, 11 VEPTR-only treatments, and 10 indeterminate treatments. Sixty-eight percent of patients with congenital scoliosis and fused ribs had a final fusion, but only 16% of patients with a hypoplastic thorax required final fusion.

5: Spine

Chapter 26

The Treatment of Neuromuscular Spine Deformities

Paul D. Sponseller, MD

Introduction

Any disorder affecting axial strength and balance during growth carries a high risk for spine deformity. The likelihood of severe deformity at an early age, limited response to nonsurgical treatment, osteopenia, and complications must be considered in treatment decision making for a child with such a disorder. It is important to understand the general principles of neuromuscular deformity as well as the commonly seen upper motor neuron, lower motor neuron, and myopathic conditions.

Patient Assessment

A patient with a neuromuscular spine deformity may be functionally assessed as a sitter (dependent or independent) or an ambulator (therapeutic, household, or community).[1] The examiner should document the presence of voluntary motor activity, especially in the lower extremities, for future comparison. The patient should be screened for neuromuscular scoliosis at least once yearly. It also is necessary to screen for hip contractures affecting the spine. A hip that does not flex to 90° requires increased spinal kyphosis to allow sitting; at the other extreme, increased lumbar lordosis often compensates for a flexion contracture.

A pelvic radiograph is necessary for treatment decision making about the spine. Pelvic obliquity is measured as the angle between the top of the iliac crests and a T1-S1 line in the upright position. Spine flexibility can be determined with forced supine bending for moderate curves or traction for larger curves.

Dr. Sponseller or an immediate family member serves as a board member, owner, officer, or committee member of the Pediatric Orthopaedic Society of North America; has received royalties from Globus Medical and DePuy, a Johnson & Johnson company; is a member of a speakers' bureau or has made paid presentations on behalf of DePuy, a Johnson & Johnson company; serves as a paid consultant to or is an employee of DePuy, a Johnson & Johnson company; and has received research or institutional support from DePuy, a Johnson & Johnson company.

Orthotic Treatment

Orthosis use generally is not successful for halting the progression of a neuromuscular spine deformity. A retrospective study found that patients with cerebral palsy and scoliosis reached a need for surgery at the same age regardless of whether they had been treated with a brace.[2] However, an orthosis may improve sitting balance for a patient with a long, flexible, unbalanced C-shaped curve.[3] These findings are consistent with those for virtually every other neuromuscular disease characterized by progressive scoliosis. A rational approach has been to offer orthosis use to a child with a developing neuromuscular deformity who meets several conditions: the child is still growing, the curve is still small (less than 40°), and the curve is flexible. If the orthosis is well tolerated, it can be continued as long as it proves useful. Generally, there is no reason to delay surgery after a curve reaches 75° to 90°.[4]

Wheelchair modification may allow some patients to avoid surgery. Custom supports for the trunk and head are incorporated to increase the patient's comfort level. A custom-contoured wheelchair back may be best for a patient with a relatively well-balanced double curve who nonetheless has substantial posterior rib prominences.

Surgical Treatment

Decision Making

The decision to correct a neuromuscular curve should be made jointly by the patient's family, the physical therapist (if applicable), the primary pediatric care team, and the surgeon. The scoliosis may be causing sitting intolerance, pain, pulmonary impairment, and physical deformity.[5,6] There is no clear evidence that spine surgery can prolong the life of a patient with any of the neuromuscular disorders.[7-9] However, surgery can improve the quality of life of some patients and enhance caregiver satisfaction. Patients and their families reported relatively low satisfaction if the patient had a residual spine deformity or developed hyperlordosis or a complication after surgery.[10]

5: Spine

Patient Preparation

Adequate nutrition may lower the risk of surgical complications. The patient's weight should be at the 10th percentile or higher as related to height or armspan.[11-13] A change in the feeding regimen, gastrostomy or jejunostomy tube feeding, or supplemental nighttime tube feeding all have been proposed to prepare the patient for surgery.

The patient's pulmonary status should be optimized. Many patients have reactive airway disease and can benefit from several days of pretreatment with steroids. Children with spinal muscular atrophy or Duchenne muscular dystrophy were found to have a high incidence of sleep apnea and hypopnea, and preoperative noninvasive positive-pressure ventilation was found to be beneficial during the perioperative period.[14] Awareness that the patient has sleep apnea allows for adequate monitoring after extubation. Patients with scoliosis caused by Duchenne muscular dystrophy should have surgery before their forced vital capacity declines below 30% of the predicted value. An echocardiogram may be used to assess right heart function in patients with severe restrictive lung disease because primary or secondary cardiomyopathy may be present.

Surgical Approach

Early clinical reports have shown the value of combined anterior-posterior spine fusion for many types of neuromuscular scoliosis. However, improvements in technique allow an isolated posterior procedure or even an isolated anterior procedure to accomplish the surgical goals.[15] There may still be a role for anterior release and fusion followed by an instrumented posterior fusion if the patient is younger than 11 years and has a large or rigid curve that cannot be corrected to less than approximately 40° with traction.[16] Deficient posterior elements, rigid hyperkyphosis, and hyperlordosis represent other relative indications for anterior fusion. The goal is to correct not only the curve but also any associated pelvic obliquity.[15,16]

Anterior and posterior fusion may be done on the same day or on separate days. Same-day, single-stage surgery is associated with lower overall blood loss, lower total surgical time, and a shorter hospital stay.[17,18] However, a single-stage procedure is not feasible for all patients; some patients may develop a coagulopathy or cardiopulmonary difficulty during prolonged surgery. The relative indications for performing the surgery in two stages include a preexisting cardiac or pulmonary condition or a complication during the first stage of the procedure (such as loss of more than half of blood volume or increasing difficulty with ventilation).[19,20] Patients with extreme pelvic obliquity because of a large curve may benefit from traction before surgery, between surgical stages, or intraoperatively.[21]

Routine posterior fusion to the pelvis is controversial. It is generally believed that a frontal-plane sitting balance with weight distribution balanced between the thighs and ischium and coccyx is desirable and that lumbar lordosis should be preserved for this purpose. A shorter fusion may better preserve some flexibility, lower surgical time, and reduce blood loss.[22] Fusion short of the pelvis may be valuable for a patient with a neuromuscular spine deformity who is ambulatory or has reasonably active trunk balance; such patients are rare, however. A negative consequence of a too-short fusion may be the development of increased pelvic obliquity below the curve. The preference of most surgeons is to treat most patients with fusion to the pelvis. Strong indications for fusion to the pelvis are a curve apex below L2, a rigid curve, and a pelvic obliquity greater than 15°.[23]

Many patients develop a large curve at a young age. Distraction-based guided growth using instrumentation without fusion may be appropriate to optimize pulmonary and abdominal growth and function in these patients. Growing rods and the vertically expandable prosthetic titanium rib (VEPTR) can be used for this purpose, but they require serial surgical procedures. The fixation may dislodge because of poor bone density and spine kyphosis. In addition, the child's comorbidities may make the treatment too risky. The optimal construct, the application criteria, and the benefits of this form of treatment in comparison with early fusion have not been established.[24]

Surgical Technique

Uncontrolled studies suggest that patients with Duchenne muscular dystrophy may have less blood loss during spine surgery if controlled hypotension and transexamic acid are used.[25] Spinal cord monitoring is challenging and controversial in patients with a neuromuscular deformity because of the underlying neurologic disorder. Neurologic injury can have a devastating effect even on a patient who cannot stand or walk. Monitoring can be done using spinal cord as well as cortical stimulation and recording.[26] Seizure activity is a relative contraindication to the use of transcranial motor-evoked potentials. It is important to discuss the possibility of neurologic injury with the family before surgery and to decide what will be done if spinal cord monitoring abnormalities develop.

Vertebral column resection (as an alternative to a separate anterior procedure), Ponte osteotomies, or pedicle subtraction osteotomies can be used intraoperatively to increase the correction of rigid focal segments.[5] The available internal fixation constructs greatly vary. The unit rod still is widely used because of its versatility, leverage, and reliable achievement of pelvic balance; however, the smooth iliac segments may pull out if the patient has lumbar kyphosis. Modular systems with a combination of pedicle screws, hooks, and wires increasingly are being used to correct neuromuscular curves.[27,28] The benefits of these systems have yet to be established.

Pelvic fixation often is critical to provide the desired correction of extreme pelvic obliquity or sagittal deformity in a neuromuscular curve. The many successfully

5: Spine

used pelvic fixation devices are either rod based or screw based (Table 1). They are anchored into the ilia, sacrum, or both. In the Galveston rod, a modification of the Luque rod, a long portion of the rod is anchored into the tables of the ilium.[29] The unit rod is a modification of the Galveston rod in which the right and left rods are joined together. The S rod is a different configuration of the Luque rod in which the distal limb of the rod is bent into a modified S shape to fit over the sacral ala.[13] Another variation includes a bend that allows the rod to be inserted into the first sacral foramen to correct severe myelomeningocele kyphosis.[13] Some techniques also use sacral or iliac screws. Iliac fixation with long (60- to 100-mm) screws generally can be accommodated in the column of bone between the posterior sacroiliac spine and the anteroinferior iliac spine. Alternatively, iliac screws can be inserted through the sacral ala, across the sacroiliac joint, and into the ilium. This insertion leaves the head of the iliac screws in line with the other spine anchors.[30]

Adequate autograft bone may not be available in a patient with neuromuscular scoliosis, and allograft, osteoconductive material, or osteobiologic agents may be needed. No comparative studies of autograft and allograft have been published. The efficacy, safety, and need for osteoconductive and osteobiologic materials in children also have yet to be established.

Complications and Postoperative Care

Complications are more frequent after surgery for neuromuscular scoliosis than for idiopathic spine deformities. A recent study found a 28% overall rate of major complications,[31] and another study reported a 22% rate after anterior surgery for neuromuscular scoliosis, with pulmonary complications the most common.[20] Severity of neurologic involvement was found to predict the risk of complications in patients with cerebral palsy.[32] A curve magnitude of more than 60° or 100° also was found to be a risk factor for complications.[5,31,32]

Infection is a common postoperative complication for children with neuromuscular scoliosis. A 1998 meta-analysis of the literature found an overall infection rate of 8%;[6] the risk factors for infection included severe mental retardation and the surgical use of allograft.[6,12] However, a subsequent study did not bear out the use of allograft as a risk factor.[33] Infections in patients with neuromuscular spine deformity generally are polymicrobial; this factor suggests contamination through the wound itself rather than through hematogenous seeding. The most common pathogens were coagulase-negative *Staphylococcus, Enterobacter, Enterococcus,* and *Escherichia coli.*[34] Prevention is the most important strategy. Perioperative antibiotic coverage is recommended by the Joint Commission for prevention of infection in all major surgical procedures. The generally recommended broad-spectrum antibiotic prophylaxis covers gram-negative organisms as well as *Staphylococcus.* A retrospective study of children with

Table 1

Methods of Pelvic Fixation

Rod Based

Galveston rod
S rod
Unit rod
Warner-Fackler

Screw Based

Iliac
Iliosacral
M/W iliosacral-iliac
S1-S2
Transsacral rod
Spinopelvic transiliac

myelodysplasia highlighted the value of urine cultures and preoperative treatment of bacterial colonization or urinary tract infection.[35]

Any sign of infection after surgery should be promptly evaluated. The involved pathogens should be determined, as well as whether the infection is superficial or deep. Wound aspiration can be performed through intact skin using sterile technique. Irrigation and débridement of the wound usually should be performed if deep infection is suspected.[34] Suppressive antibiotic coverage may be necessary. The instrumentation almost always can be preserved, at least until the fusion is complete. The use of frequent dressing changes or vacuum-assisted closure increasingly is being reported.[36] The risk of pseudarthrosis is increased after any deep wound infection.

Intensive or intermediate-level nursing care usually is required for at least 1 to 2 days after surgery. Pulmonary complications are anticipated, and upright positioning, frequent suctioning, and the use of a positive-pressure mask or chest physical therapy should be instituted.[14] The most common cause of pulmonary decline during the first 3 days after surgery is mucous plugging of the airways.

Nutritional supplementation is begun as soon as possible after surgery, with intravenous hyperalimentation if a delay in feeding is anticipated. Postoperative bracing is rarely needed. A neck brace may be helpful in a patient with poor head control to prevent cervicothoracic kyphosis from developing during the early postoperative period of weakness. Wheelchair adjustments may be indicated because of the patient's changed body shape.

Functional Results

The functional results of neuromuscular spine surgery are complex to assess. Alterations in trunk height and pelvic obliquity can affect the ability of children to perform independent transfers and self-care using their upper extremities. Few medical benefits were found in small level IV studies. A study of institution-dwelling patients with cerebral palsy found no difference in the rate of medical complications between those who had or had not undergone spine surgery.[7] There was no difference in pulmonary medication, occurrence of decubitus ulcers, or care burden between patients with neuromuscular scoliosis based on whether the patient had undergone spine fusion.[8] Nonetheless, caregivers had a high satisfaction rate after surgery.[10] Prospective testing and retesting at 1-year follow-up revealed significant improvement not only in caregiver satisfaction but also in perceived patient comfort and happiness.[37]

Upper Motor Neuron Disorders

Cerebral Palsy

More than two thirds of nonambulatory patients with severe cerebral palsy (Gross Motor Function Classification System level IV or V) develop scoliosis, whereas very few patients with less severe cerebral palsy (level I, II, or III) develop scoliosis. A recent evidence-based review challenges the validity of the long-held assumption that the risk of progression is related to the severity of involvement.[38] The risk of scoliosis appears to be best predicted by the presence or absence of independent sitting balance. Only a small proportion of children will develop a predominant kyphosis, which may be functionally disabling. The mean age of curve development is 7 years, but a few patients develop a curve much earlier. Some of these patients develop a curve after undergoing rhizotomy. Concern has been raised about an association between the performance of a selective dorsal rhizotomy and the development of scoliosis and spondylolisthesis,[39] but no cause-and-effect relationship has been established. No increase in the risk of scoliosis progression was found when intrathecal baclofen was used.[40]

Brace treatment does not appear to decrease the risk or the rate of curve progression in patients with cerebral palsy, although it may facilitate sitting in some patients.[2] Progression is likely even after skeletal maturity if the curve exceeds 40°.[41,42] The indications for surgery are variable and poorly established. One study found that a greater curve magnitude is a strong predictor of complications,[31] but a threshold deformity for recommending surgery was not established. No studies have compared the widely used unit rod and segmental wire type of instrumentation with the increasingly popular but more expensive modular screw-and-hook systems in patients with cerebral palsy (**Figure 1**).[27,28,43,44]

The routine use of intraoperative spinal cord monitoring is controversial in patients with cerebral palsy. Because of these patients' cortical impairment, spinal cord monitoring is more difficult to obtain than in patients with another type of neuromuscular deformity. Proponents of spinal cord monitoring argue that although patients with cerebral palsy have relatively little function to lose, a spinal cord deficit after surgery may alter respiratory function and protective sensation. Neuromonitoring was found to be possible in 91% of patients with cerebral palsy, usually by relying on brainstem potentials.[45] Signal changes occurred in one third of the patients, mostly related to the insertion of hooks or wires or to the amount of correction. There was one false-positive signal change, and there was one undetected neurologic injury in a patient who could not be monitored. The clinical significance of the observed changes was not described.[45]

As posterior techniques improve, anterior release and fusion is less commonly performed in relatively young patients or in patients with a relatively large curve. Using modern techniques, it should be possible to correct a balanced curve that is greater than 60° and has pelvic obliquity of less than 10°.[16,21,27,28,43]

Rett Syndrome

Rett syndrome is an X-linked dominant neurodegenerative disorder. The cause is a defect in the gene encoding methyl-CgP-binding protein (*MeCP2*),[46] which causes a defect in DNA methylation. The condition almost always occurs in girls. Patients lack language development and display stereotypic hand movements. Seizures, spasticity, ataxia, and contractures may develop. Approximately 60% of patients develop scoliosis and/or kyphosis, often at a young age.[47,48] Bracing does not seem to control curve progression. Patients have reduced bone density. Spine fusion is indicated in approximately 10% of patients. The surgical techniques follow the standard rules for the management of neuromuscular scoliosis. Fusion to the pelvis may be necessary if the curve is large and the patient is nonambulatory.[49]

Friedreich Ataxia

Friedreich ataxia is an autosomal recessive disorder with spinocerebellar degeneration. The physical findings include ataxia, dysarthria, and cavus feet. Cardiomyopathy is common and often leads to death during the third or fourth decade of life. Many patients with Friedreich ataxia develop scoliosis. A double major curve is the most common pattern,[50] but any curve pattern can occur. Approximately 15% of patients have significant pelvic obliquity.[50] Most patients also have increased kyphosis. Bracing is poorly tolerated because of the movement disorder. The likelihood of curve progression seems to be related to age at curve development; most patients who develop curves before puberty will have significant progression.[51] Because not all curves progress, surgery is recommended for a curve greater than 60° or a curve greater than 40° that began at a young age.[50] A cardiac evaluation should be performed before surgery.[52]

Charcot-Marie-Tooth Disease

Charcot-Marie-Tooth disease is a peripheral neuropathy that usually is of autosomal dominant inheritance.

5: Spine

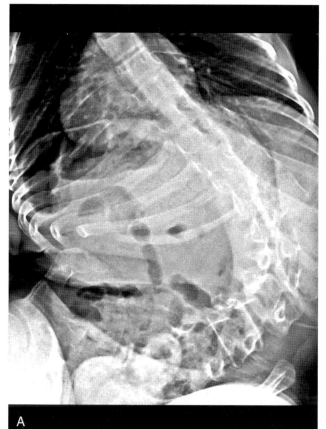

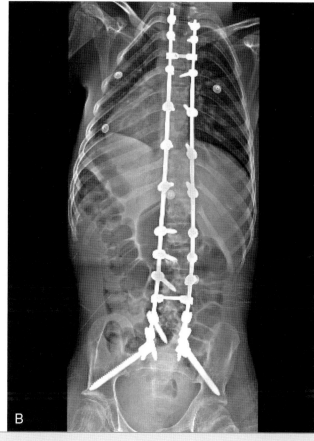

Figure 1 AP radiographs showing a 95° scoliosis curve in a 14-year-old child with cerebral palsy before (**A**) and after (**B**) surgery. Segmental fixation was used, with screws in the pedicles and sacroilium.

It is classified by electrodiagnostic criteria as a type I or II hereditary motor and sensory neuropathy. Kyphosis and scoliosis occur in 10% to 50% of patients.[53,54] Spine deformity is more common in girls and patients with type I neuropathy than in boys or patients with type II neuropathy. A patient with a thoracic scoliosis curve is more likely to have an apex convex to the left than other patients with scoliosis. It is not known whether bracing changes the natural history of Charcot-Marie-Tooth disease. The natural history of curves into adulthood has not been studied. Fewer than 5% of patients with Charcot-Marie-Tooth disease develop curves that are considered for surgical treatment.[54]

Spinal Cord Injury

Spinal cord injury to a child younger than 10 years almost always results in scoliosis if there is a significant residual neurologic deficit. Early, full-time bracing of a relatively small curve may slow, but not prevent, deformity progression.[55] No consistent indications for surgery have been developed. The child may develop pressure sores if there is too little or too much lordosis.

Myelomeningocele

Patients with myelomeningocele may present the greatest challenge to a pediatric spine surgeon because of the combination of severe deformity, poor skin coverage, lack of viable muscular covering of the lower spine, and concomitant neurologic and medical conditions. The spine deformity can occur through at least three potential mechanisms: trunk muscle weakness; neurogenic factors including tethering, syrinx, and Chiari malformation; and congenital malformation (at least 20% of patients have hemivertebrae and/or bars). Children with myelomeningocele have a high incidence of latex allergy, often are small for their age, have early skeletal and physical maturity, and often have a neurogenic bladder with a propensity for chronic urinary tract infection or bacterial colonization.[35,56]

Scoliosis occurs with greater frequency in patients with a higher level spinal dysraphism. More than half of patients who lack function below the thoracic level develop scoliosis. No published study has found bracing to be efficacious in these children. In view of the significant challenges of surgical fusion and its aftereffects, bracing may be used for a deformity between 20° and 40°. Progression is possible if the patient has an increasing curve with a low-level lesion or other clinical

5: Spine

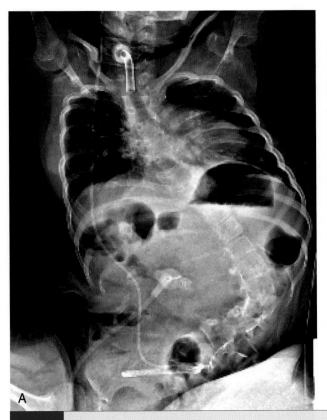 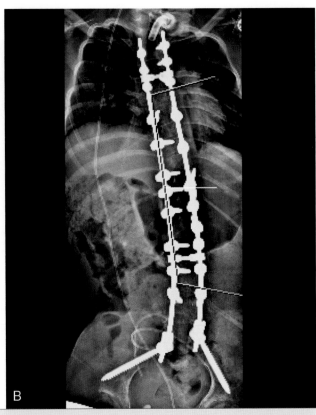

Figure 2   AP radiographs showing severe scoliosis that impaired sitting balance in an 11-year-old girl with an L3 myelomeningocele and a Chiari malformation requiring tracheostomy. **A**, The curve was 90° before surgery. **B**, The posterior-only procedure included a vertebral column resection at T12 to shorten the spine. Segmental fixation was used, with screws in the pedicles and the sacroilium.

signs of tethering. Tether release has been recommended for progressive curves, but 60% of patients with scoliosis and a cord diagnosed as tethered have progression despite untethering.[57] In a skeletally immature patient, a curve greater than 40° will progress after untethering.[57,58] Tether release carries some neurologic risk, and not all patients have return of function.[59]

Many patients have a curve greater than 45° that is likely to progress. The scoliosis may produce few adverse effects if the curve is purely lumbar and is distal or balanced; the patient's relatively short trunk height produces little sitting imbalance. However, a patient with a long, unbalanced curve may have difficulty sitting without using the hands, braces, or an adapted chair.

When a patient is being considered for surgery, it is useful for a multidisciplinary team to be involved, including a neurosurgeon, a plastic surgeon, an orthopaedic surgeon, and experienced anesthesia and operating room personnel. Historically, the combination of posterior instrumented fusion with an anterior fusion (with or without instrumentation) generally has been recommended.[18,60-63] This approach evolved because frequent infections and dysraphic posterior spine elements led to a risk of pseudarthrosis when posterior fu-

sion was used alone. Indications for using anterior instrumentation with the anterior fusion, in combination with posterior fusion and instrumentation, have not been defined. Decreasing the use of anterior surgery has been recommended with the use of currently used segmental fixation systems (**Figure 2**). No comparative studies have been published, however. Whether to fuse to the sacrum also is a matter of debate. Some surgeons have described a rigid corrective fixation (usually anteroposterior), stopping at L4 or L5, for a curve with a high apex, to preserve some distal mobility and prevent ischial pressure sores.[64] An anterior fusion with instrumentation alone may suffice for selected patients with a single nonkyphotic curve of moderate size.[65]

Spinal cord monitoring can be used for patients with a lower lumbar level myelomeningocele and should include quadriceps monitoring (the quadriceps usually are the best innervated and most functionally significant muscles).

Thoracolumbar and lumbar kyphosis occurs in approximately 10% of patients with myelomeningocele and usually affects patients with higher level paralysis. The etiology appears to be a deficiency in the posterior elements and a lack of posterior muscle and ligamentous support. Three types of kyphosis have been defined: paralytic (in 44% of patients), which usually is a

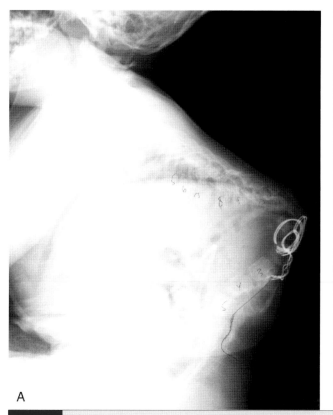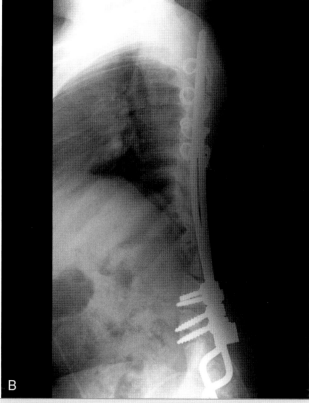

| **Figure 3** | Lateral radiographs showing myelokyphosis in a 6-year-old girl. **A,** Pressure sores over the bony apex before surgery. After kyphectomy, the child grew 6 cm in the instrumented thoracic region, and the wires moved up the rod. **B,** Revision surgery was necessitated by growth. |

smooth curve; sharply angled (in 38%); and congenital (in 14%), which results from an anterior bar or hemivertebra.[66] Virtually all of these deformities progress. Kyphosis can lead to skin breakdown, difficulty in sitting, increased abdominal and intrathoracic pressure, and altered body image.

The indications and ideal age for surgery are a matter of debate. A patient younger than approximately 10 years has a less pronounced gibbus and a less fixed compensatory thoracic lordosis. However, the vertebrae are smaller and more difficult to use for fixation, and growth maximization is a concern. Most experts believe that surgery at age 5 to 8 years probably is ideal, but the procedure may be done at an earlier or later age as clinically indicated.

Correction of a gradual (paralytic) kyphosis uses multiple decancellation osteotomies and sometimes can be done without resecting the cord. In a recent study, bilateral VEPTR with anchorage into the ilia was used as a means of supporting the trunk during growth.[67] A sharp gibbus requires that the cord be mobilized and usually transected at the apex of the gibbus. Gradual-onset shunt malfunction has been reported after transection of the spinal cord and should be watched for.[68] The deformed apical vertebra must be resected, as well as the proximal (horizontal) vertebrae leading into

the lordotic segment. Enough bone must be resected to fit within the soft-tissue envelope of the body. Kyphectomy may be performed in a newborn if the gibbus is prominent and skin closure is difficult. A variety of techniques have been reported, but fixation is difficult and residual kyphosis and translation often remain at the resection site.

Multiple techniques exist for fixation of the spine during a kyphectomy.[69] The most widely accepted techniques involve rods to stabilize a long segment of the spine to the pelvis. The instrumentation should be carried sufficiently proximally to counteract any thoracic lordosis and/or scoliosis (**Figure 3**). In a child younger than 10 years, the spine can be fused only at the level of the resection to allow spine growth along the rods using sublaminar wires. In an older child, in whom remaining growth is not a consideration, the use of proximal hooks and screws may provide rigid fixation for fusion.

Congenital scoliosis occurs in approximately 20% of patients with spina bifida. It is best to obtain a full spine radiograph of a patient with spina bifida. Congenital scoliosis is treated according to standard principles.

The complications of spine fusion in patients with myelomeningocele include deep wound infection in 8% to 19%.[62] Shunt malfunction and cerebrospinal fluid

5: Spine

leakage may occur during the postoperative period. The rate of pseudarthrosis is reported to be as high as 15%.[61-63]

Lower Motor Neuron Disorder: Spinal Muscular Atrophy

Spinal muscular atrophy is an autosomal recessive disorder that appears in early childhood as a degeneration of anterior horn cells. Most patients have a stable clinical course. The disorder has been classified based on age at presentation: type I, younger than 6 months; type II, 6 to 18 months; and type III, older than 18 months. Patients with a type I disorder are unlikely to survive past early childhood. Spine specialists most often see patients with a type II disorder, many of whom survive into adulthood. The development of a severe, collapsing curve at a very young age poses unique challenges. The criteria for bracing have not been established. Prophylactic bracing has not prevented curve development and progression, but it may assist sitting balance and delay spine fusion.[70] The reported mean age at surgery is 10 to 11 years.[71-73] In patients younger than 9 to 10 years, spine instrumentation without fusion may be appropriate to maintain growth. Loss of function in the upper and lower extremities has been reported after surgery, but risk can be minimized with rigid fixation to the pelvis and early mobilization.[72]

Myopathic Disorders

Duchenne Muscular Dystrophy

Duchenne muscular dystrophy causes scoliosis before puberty in almost all patients because of a defect in dystrophin. Most of these curves become severely collapsed and impair sitting balance. The patient's life expectancy typically is into the third decade. However, the advent of corticosteroid treatment is extending the lifespan of affected children. It has been reported that scoliosis development was delayed or possibly prevented by the long-term use of corticosteroids.[74,75] Progression is less likely if the curve developed after age 14 years and pulmonary vital capacity remains above 1,900 mL.[76,77] Pulmonary function declines not only because of the scoliosis but also as part of the natural history of the dystrophy; each year of age and each 10° curve increase leads to a 4% decrease in forced vital capacity.[78] Bracing has not been shown to prevent curve progression, but it may slow progression in the early juvenile period. To minimize pulmonary complications, most patients should undergo surgical treatment before forced vital capacity drops below 30%. In addition to pulmonary function tests, the preoperative assessment should include electrocardiography and echocardiography. (Cardiomyopathy is associated with the disease, and pulmonary impairment leads to right heart strain.)

Patients with Duchenne muscular dystrophy have an increased risk of malignant hyperthermia, and surgical blood loss is high.[79] The collapsing nature of the curve means that the fusion should include most of the spine, usually from T2 to the pelvis.[80] Because the patient has diminished bone density, the surgeon should maximize the number of fixation points.[81] The reported postoperative complication rate is as high as 27%, including a 5% to 10% incidence of wound infection.[82,83] However, the surgery improves patients' quality of life, and its results are enthusiastically received by most parents and neurologists who care for these patients.[82-84]

Arthrogryposis

The term arthrogryposis refers to a group of conditions characterized by stiffness and contracture in multiple joints. The classic form is idiopathic and is called amyoplasia or arthrogryposis multiplex congenita; it includes extension contractures of the elbows, knees, and fingers, with variable positioning of the hips, which often are dislocated. Other disorders that fall into the spectrum of arthrogryposis include multiple pterygium (Escobar syndrome), congenital contractual arachnodactyly (Beals syndrome), Freeman-Sheldon syndrome, and more than 100 less common conditions. Spine deformities occur in approximately 10% to 25% of patients with arthrogryposis and tend to be stiff. Bracing has not been proved to slow curve progression. Surgery may be indicated if the deformity is large and progressive, with a risk of pulmonary function or sitting impairment. The young age at which the curve can begin suggests that the use of a growing system occasionally can be attempted. The role of hip contractures should be analyzed in assessing balance. For instance, a hip extension contracture often necessitates a compensatory lumbar kyphosis. In the coronal plane, a hip with limited abduction often is accommodated by an elevation of the entire pelvis on that side.

Summary

The challenges posed by neuromuscular spine deformities include the early age of onset, the large size of curves, an increased risk of infection, comorbidities caused by cardiac and pulmonary dysfunction, osteopenia, and varied functional impairments that may be affected by progressive spine deformity and surgical treatment. The complication rates after surgical management are higher than those reported for idiopathic scoliosis and generally are related to preexisting comorbidities. Awareness of all of these factors is needed for optimal care of the patient.

Annotated References

1. Lonstein JE, Akbarnia A: Operative treatment of spinal deformities in patients with cerebral palsy or mental

retardation: An analysis of one hundred and seven cases. *J Bone Joint Surg Am* 1983;65(1):43-55.

2. Miller A, Temple T, Miller F: Impact of orthoses on the rate of scoliosis progression in children with cerebral palsy. *J Pediatr Orthop* 1996;16(3):332-335.

3. Leopando MT, Moussavi Z, Holbrow J, Chernick V, Pasterkamp H, Rempel G: Effect of a Soft Boston Orthosis on pulmonary mechanics in severe cerebral palsy. *Pediatr Pulmonol* 1999;28(1):53-58.

4. Olafsson Y, Saraste H, Al-Dabbagh Z: Brace treatment in neuromuscular spine deformity. *J Pediatr Orthop* 1999;19(3):376-379.

5. Yazici M, Asher MA, Hardacker JW: The safety and efficacy of Isola-Galveston instrumentation and arthrodesis in the treatment of neuromuscular spinal deformities. *J Bone Joint Surg Am* 2000;82(4):524-543.

6. Benson ER, Thomson JD, Smith BG, Banta JV: Results and morbidity in a consecutive series of patients undergoing spinal fusion for neuromuscular scoliosis. *Spine (Phila Pa 1976)* 1998;23(21):2308-2318.

7. Kalen V, Conklin MM, Sherman FC: Untreated scoliosis in severe cerebral palsy. *J Pediatr Orthop* 1992;12(3):337-340.

8. Cassidy C, Craig CL, Perry A, Karlin LI, Goldberg MJ: A reassessment of spinal stabilization in severe cerebral palsy. *J Pediatr Orthop* 1994;14(6):731-739.

9. Thomson JD, Banta JV: Scoliosis in cerebral palsy: An overview and recent results. *J Pediatr Orthop B* 2001;10(1):6-9.

10. Watanabe K, Lenke LG, Daubs MD, et al: Is spine deformity surgery in patients with spastic cerebral palsy truly beneficial? A patient/parent evaluation. *Spine (Phila Pa 1976)* 2009;34(20):2222-2232.

    Eighty-four patients and families of patients with cerebral palsy completed a questionnaire an average 6 years after spine fusion. High satisfaction was reported for sitting balance (93%), cosmesis (94%), and patient quality of life (71%). Lower satisfaction was correlated with late complications, less correction of deformity, and hyperlordosis of the lumbar spine. Level of evidence: IV.

11. Jevsevar DS, Karlin LI: The relationship between preoperative nutritional status and complications after an operation for scoliosis in patients who have cerebral palsy. *J Bone Joint Surg Am* 1993;75(6):880-884.

12. Tolo VT: Surgical treatment of adolescent idiopathic scoliosis. *Instr Course Lect* 1989;38:143-156.

13. McCarthy RE, Bruffett WL, McCullough FL: S rod fixation to the sacrum in patients with neuromuscular spinal deformities. *Clin Orthop Relat Res* 1999;364:26-31.

14. Bach JR, Sabharwal S: High pulmonary risk scoliosis surgery: Role of noninvasive ventilation and related techniques. *J Spinal Disord Tech* 2005;18(6):527-530.

    A small group of children with neuromuscular scoliosis who were at high risk for pulmonary compromise had intermittent positive-pressure ventilation or mechanical vest treatment after spine fusion. All had rapid weaning from the ventilator, and none had perioperative pulmonary complications. Level of evidence: IV.

15. Boachie-Adjei O, Lonstein JE, Winter RB, Koop S, vanden Brink K, Denis F: Management of neuromuscular spinal deformities with Luque segmental instrumentation. *J Bone Joint Surg Am* 1989;71(4):548-562.

16. Auerbach JD, Spiegel DA, Zgonis MH, et al: The correction of pelvic obliquity in patients with cerebral palsy and neuromuscular scoliosis: Is there a benefit of anterior release prior to posterior spinal arthrodesis? *Spine (Phila Pa 1976)* 2009;34(21):E766-E774.

    Sixty-one patients with neuromuscular scoliosis had either anterior-posterior or posterior-only fusion with a unit rod. The final results were comparable for curve correction and pelvic obliquity. The children with anteroposterior fusion had a larger, stiffer curve. The criteria for performing anterior-posterior fusion were not tested. Level of evidence: IV.

17. Shufflebarger HL, Grimm JO, Bui V, Thomson JD: Anterior and posterior spinal fusion: Staged versus same-day surgery. *Spine (Phila Pa 1976)* 1991;16(8):930-933.

18. Banta JV: Combined anterior and posterior fusion for spinal deformity in myelomeningocele. *Spine (Phila Pa 1976)* 1990;15(9):946-952.

19. O'Brien T, Akmakjian J, Ogin G, Eilert R: Comparison of one-stage versus two-stage anterior/posterior spinal fusion for neuromuscular scoliosis. *J Pediatr Orthop* 1992;12(5):610-615.

20. Sarwahi V, Sarwark JF, Schafer MF, et al: Standards in anterior spine surgery in pediatric patients with neuromuscular scoliosis. *J Pediatr Orthop* 2001;21(6):756-760.

21. Takeshita K, Lenke LG, Bridwell KH, Kim YJ, Sides B, Hensley M: Analysis of patients with nonambulatory neuromuscular scoliosis surgically treated to the pelvis with intraoperative halo-femoral traction. *Spine (Phila Pa 1976)* 2006;31(20):2381-2385.

    In a retrospective review, 20 of 40 patients with neuromuscular scoliosis and pelvic obliquity had intraoperative halo-femoral traction. The selection criteria were not controlled. A larger correction of the lumbar curve and a greater correction of the pelvic obliquity were found in the patients with halo-femoral traction. Level of evidence: IV.

22. Huang MJ, Lenke LG: Scoliosis and severe pelvic obliquity in a patient with cerebral palsy: Surgical treatment utilizing halo-femoral traction. *Spine (Phila Pa 1976)* 2001;26(19):2168-2170.

5: Spine

23. Whitaker C, Burton DC, Asher M: Treatment of selected neuromuscular patients with posterior instrumentation and arthrodesis ending with lumbar pedicle screw anchorage. *Spine (Phila Pa 1976)* 2000;25(18):2312-2318.

24. Vitale MG, Gomez JA, Matsumoto H, Roye DP Jr; Members of Chest Wall and Spine Deformity Study Group: Variability of expert opinion in treatment of early-onset scoliosis. *Clin Orthop Relat Res*; published online September 2010.

   Eight of 12 patients with early-onset scoliosis were believed by all 13 reviewing surgeons to require surgery. Poor agreement was found as to the type of surgery, extent of surgery, and method of stabilization.

25. Shapiro F, Zurakowski D, Sethna NF: Tranexamic acid diminishes intraoperative blood loss and transfusion in spinal fusions for Duchenne muscular dystrophy scoliosis. *Spine (Phila Pa 1976)* 2007;32(20):2278-2283.

   Fifty-six patients with Duchenne muscular dystrophy were evaluated for blood loss during spine fusion. Thirty-six patients did not receive tranexamic acid, and 20 did. The mean blood loss for the patients receiving tranexamic acid was 1,944 mL; mean blood loss for the other patients was 3,382 mL. The criteria for transfusion were not defined. The data were corrected for patient weight, blood volume, and surgical time. Level of evidence: IV.

26. Owen JH, Sponseller PD, Szymanski J, Hurdle M: Efficacy of multimodality spinal cord monitoring during surgery for neuromuscular scoliosis. *Spine (Phila Pa 1976)* 1995;20(13):1480-1488.

27. Teli MG, Cinnella P, Vincitorio F, Lovi A, Grava G, Brayda-Bruno M: Spinal fusion with Cotrel-Dubousset instrumentation for neuropathic scoliosis in patients with cerebral palsy. *Spine (Phila Pa 1976)* 2006;31(14):E441-E447.

   In patients with cerebral palsy, the average curve correction was 60%, and the pelvic obliquity correction was 40%. There were major complications in 13.5% of patients and minor complications in an additional 10%. Level of evidence: IV.

28. Modi HN, Hong JY, Mehta SS, et al: Surgical correction and fusion using posterior-only pedicle screw construct for neuropathic scoliosis in patients with cerebral palsy: A three-year follow-up study. *Spine (Phila Pa 1976)* 2009;34(11):1167-1175.

   The average curve correction was 56% and the average pelvic obliquity was 43% in patients with cerebral palsy. The overall rate of complications was 32%, of which most were pulmonary. Level of evidence: IV.

29. Allen BL Jr, Ferguson RL: L-rod instrumentation for scoliosis in cerebral palsy. *J Pediatr Orthop* 1982;2(1):87-96.

30. Chang TL, Sponseller PD, Kebaish KM, Fishman EK: Low profile pelvic fixation: Anatomic parameters for sacral alar-iliac fixation versus traditional iliac fixation. *Spine (Phila Pa 1976)* 2009;34(5):436-440.

   A method is described for inserting long iliac screws through a sacral starting point that is deep under a midline muscle flap and in line with other spinal anchors. Level of evidence: I.

31. Master DL, Son-Hing JP, Poe-Kochert C, Armstrong DG, Thompson GH: Risk factors for major complications after surgery for neuromuscular scoliosis. *Spine (Phila Pa 1976)*; published online July 2010.

   In 131 patients with neuromuscular scoliosis, there were 46 major complications in 37 patients (28%) after different types of surgery. Nonambulatory status and a curve greater than 60° were associated with a higher risk of complications. Level of evidence: IV.

32. Lipton GE, Miller F, Dabney KW, Altiok H, Bachrach SJ: Factors predicting postoperative complications following spinal fusions in children with cerebral palsy. *J Spinal Disord* 1999;12(3):197-205.

33. Yazici M, Asher MA: Freeze-dried allograft for posterior spinal fusion in patients with neuromuscular spinal deformities. *Spine (Phila Pa 1976)* 1997;22(13):1467-1471.

34. Sponseller PD, LaPorte DM, Hungerford MW, Eck K, Bridwell KH, Lenke LG: Deep wound infections after neuromuscular scoliosis surgery: A multicenter study of risk factors and treatment outcomes. *Spine (Phila Pa 1976)* 2000;25(19):2461-2466.

35. Hatlen T, Song K, Shurtleff D, Duguay S: Contributory factors to postoperative spinal fusion complications for children with myelomeningocele. *Spine (Phila Pa 1976)* 2010;35(13):1294-1299.

   In a retrospective review of children with myelomeningocele who underwent spine fusion, there were lower infection rates when preoperative urine cultures were obtained, with prophylactic treatment for urinary tract infection and/or colonization. Level of evidence: IV.

36. Sponseller PD, Shah SA, Abel MF, Newton PO, Letko L, Marks M: Infection rate after spine surgery in cerebral palsy is high and impairs results: Multicenter analysis of risk factors and treatment. *Clin Orthop Relat Res* 2010;468(3):711-716.

   A review of spine fusion in 157 patients with cerebral palsy performed at eight centers found a 10% infection rate. Fourteen of 16 patients had débridement, and hardware was removed in 2 patients. Level of evidence: IV.

37. Jones KB, Sponseller PD, Shindle MK, McCarthy ML: Longitudinal parental perceptions of spinal fusion for neuromuscular spine deformity in patients with totally involved cerebral palsy. *J Pediatr Orthop* 2003;23(2):143-149.

38. Loeters MJ, Maathuis CG, Hadders-Algra M: Risk factors for emergence and progression of scoliosis in children with severe cerebral palsy: A systematic review. *Dev Med Child Neurol* 2010;52(7):605-611.

   A review of the literature from 1966 to 2009 found 10 papers with sufficient information for ascertaining the risk factors for scoliosis emergence and progression in children with Gross Motor Function Classification System level IV or V cerebral palsy. There was weak evidence for an association between the severity of cerebral palsy, hip dislocation, and pelvic obliquity and scoliosis.

39. Golan JD, Hall JA, O'Gorman G, et al: Spinal deformities following selective dorsal rhizotomy. *J Neurosurg* 2007;106(6, suppl):441-449.

   In 98 patients with cerebral palsy who had selective dorsal rhizotomy, the mean age at surgery was 5 years and the mean follow-up was 6 years. Mild scoliosis was found in 45% on standing radiographs, and 19% had spondylolisthesis. Cerebral palsy severity and ambulatory status were predictors of these findings. Level of evidence: IV.

40. Shilt JS, Lai LP, Cabrera MN, Frino J, Smith BP: The impact of intrathecal baclofen on the natural history of scoliosis in cerebral palsy. *J Pediatr Orthop* 2008;28(6): 684-687.

   Fifty patients with an intrathecal baclofen pump were matched to 50 patients with similarly severe cerebral palsy and a similar Cobb angle. The average per-year rate of scoliosis progression was not significantly different between the two groups (6.6° versus 5°). Level of evidence: IV.

41. Thometz JG, Simon SR: Progression of scoliosis after skeletal maturity in institutionalized adults who have cerebral palsy. *J Bone Joint Surg Am* 1988;70(9):1290-1296.

42. Saito N, Ebara S, Ohotsuka K, Kumeta H, Takaoka K: Natural history of scoliosis in spastic cerebral palsy. *Lancet* 1998;351(9117):1687-1692.

43. Tsirikos AI, Lipton G, Chang WN, Dabney KW, Miller F: Surgical correction of scoliosis in pediatric patients with cerebral palsy using the unit rod instrumentation. *Spine (Phila Pa 1976)* 2008;33(10):1133-1140.

   In 287 children treated for neuromuscular scoliosis with a unit rod and a variety of fusion methods, the overall infection rate was 6.7%. The average curve correction was 68%, and the average pelvic obliquity correction was 71%. Level of evidence: IV.

44. Sponseller PD, Shah SA, Abel MF, et al: Scoliosis surgery in cerebral palsy: Differences between unit rod and custom rods. *Spine (Phila Pa 1976)* 2009;34(8):840-844.

   Unit rods provided more consistent correction of pelvic obliquity than custom rods but required more blood replacement and had more prominence at the cranial end. Level of evidence: III.

45. DiCindio S, Theroux M, Shah S, et al: Multimodality monitoring of transcranial electric motor and somatosensory-evoked potentials during surgical correction of spinal deformity in patients with cerebral palsy and other neuromuscular disorders. *Spine (Phila Pa 1976)* 2003;28(16):1851-1856.

46. Van den Veyver IB, Zoghbi HY: Mutations in the gene encoding methyl-CpG-binding protein 2 cause Rett syndrome. *Brain Dev* 2001;23(suppl 1):S147-S151.

47. Bassett GS, Tolo VT: The incidence and natural history of scoliosis in Rett syndrome. *Dev Med Child Neurol* 1990;32(11):963-966.

48. Loder RT, Lee CL, Richards BS: Orthopedic aspects of Rett syndrome: A multicenter review. *J Pediatr Orthop* 1989;9(5):557-562.

49. Holm VA, King HA: Scoliosis in the Rett syndrome. *Brain Dev* 1990;12(1):151-153.

50. Labelle H, Tohmé S, Duhaime M, Allard P: Natural history of scoliosis in Friedreich's ataxia. *J Bone Joint Surg Am* 1986;68(4):564-572.

51. Daher YH, Lonstein JE, Winter RB, Bradford DS: Spinal deformities in patients with Friedreich ataxia: A review of 19 patients. *J Pediatr Orthop* 1985;5(5):553-557.

52. Cady RB, Bobechko WP: Incidence, natural history, and treatment of scoliosis in Friedreich's ataxia. *J Pediatr Orthop* 1984;4(6):673-676.

53. Hensinger RN, MacEwen GD: Spinal deformity associated with heritable neurological conditions: Spinal muscular atrophy, Friedreich's ataxia, familial dysautonomia, and Charcot-Marie-Tooth disease. *J Bone Joint Surg Am* 1976;58(1):13-24.

54. Walker JL, Nelson KR, Stevens DB, Lubicky JP, Ogden JA, VandenBrink KD: Spinal deformity in Charcot-Marie-Tooth disease. *Spine (Phila Pa 1976)* 1994;19(9): 1044-1047.

55. Mehta S, Betz RR, Mulcahey MJ, McDonald C, Vogel LC, Anderson C: Effect of bracing on paralytic scoliosis secondary to spinal cord injury. *J Spinal Cord Med* 2004;27(suppl 1):S88-S92.

56. Zerin JM, McLaughlin K, Kerchner S: Latex allergy in patients with myelomeningocele presenting for imaging studies of the urinary tract. *Pediatr Radiol* 1996;26(7): 450-454.

57. Pierz K, Banta J, Thomson J, Gahm N, Hartford J: The effect of tethered cord release on scoliosis in myelomeningocele. *J Pediatr Orthop* 2000;20(3):362-365.

58. McGirt MJ, Mehta V, Garces-Ambrossi G, et al: Pediatric tethered cord syndrome: Response of scoliosis to untethering procedures. Clinical article. *J Neurosurg Pediatr* 2009;4(3):270-274.

   In children who had a tethered cord with scoliosis and were skeletally immature (as determined by the Risser sign), a curve greater than 40° carried a high risk of progression after cord untethering. Level of evidence: IV.

59. Al-Holou WN, Muraszko KM, Garton HJ, Buchman SR, Maher CO: The outcome of tethered cord release in secondary and multiple repeat tethered cord syndrome. *J Neurosurg Pediatr* 2009;4(1):28-36.

60. Osebold WR: Stability of myelomeningocele spines treated with the Mayfield two-stage anterior and posterior fusion technique. *Spine (Phila Pa 1976)* 2000; 25(11):1344-1351.

61. Banit DM, Iwinski HJ Jr, Talwalkar V, Johnson M: Posterior spinal fusion in paralytic scoliosis and myelomeningocele. *J Pediatr Orthop* 2001;21(1):117-125.

62. Geiger F, Parsch D, Carstens C: Complications of scoliosis surgery in children with myelomeningocele. *Eur Spine J* 1999;8(1):22-26.

63. Parsch D, Geiger F, Brocai DR, Lang RD, Carstens C: Surgical management of paralytic scoliosis in myelomeningocele. *J Pediatr Orthop B* 2001;10(1):10-17.

64. Wild A, Haak H, Kumar M, Krauspe R: Is sacral instrumentation mandatory to address pelvic obliquity in neuromuscular thoracolumbar scoliosis due to myelomeningocele? *Spine (Phila Pa 1976)* 2001;26(14):E325-E329.

65. Sponseller PD, Young AT, Sarwark JF, Lim R: Anterior only fusion for scoliosis in patients with myelomeningocele. *Clin Orthop Relat Res* 1999;364(364):117-124.

66. Carstens C, Koch H, Brocai DR, Niethard FU: Development of pathological lumbar kyphosis in myelomeningocele. *J Bone Joint Surg Br* 1996;78(6):945-950.

67. Smith JT, Novais E: Treatment of Gibbus deformity associated with myelomeningocele in the young child with use of the vertical expandable prosthetic titanium rib (VEPTR): A case report. *J Bone Joint Surg Am* 2010; 92(12):2211-2215.

    Myelokyphosis can be improved with the use of bilateral VEPTR to the pelvis. The instrumentation can be lengthened to allow growth. The scarred midline tissues can be avoided.

68. Ko AL, Song K, Ellenbogen RG, Avellino AM: Retrospective review of multilevel spinal fusion combined with spinal cord transection for treatment of kyphoscoliosis in pediatric myelomeningocele patients. *Spine (Phila Pa 1976)* 2007;32(22):2493-2501.

    Nine children with myelomeningocele underwent planned spinal cord transection along with treatment of their spine deformity. Two had late-onset hydrocephalus treated with shunt externalization. Level of evidence: IV.

69. Dunn DK: A higher powered view of the myelomeningocele defect. *Wis Med J* 1975;74(2):S17-S20.

70. Shapiro F, Specht L: The diagnosis and orthopaedic treatment of childhood spinal muscular atrophy, peripheral neuropathy, Friedreich ataxia, and arthrogryposis. *J Bone Joint Surg Am* 1993;75(11):1699-1714.

71. Phillips DP, Roye DP Jr, Farcy JP, Leet A, Shelton YA: Surgical treatment of scoliosis in a spinal muscular atrophy population. *Spine (Phila Pa 1976)* 1990;15(9):942-945.

72. Granata C, Merlini L, Magni E, Marini ML, Stagni SB: Spinal muscular atrophy: Natural history and orthopaedic treatment of scoliosis. *Spine (Phila Pa 1976)* 1989; 14(7):760-762.

73. Brown JC, Zeller JL, Swank SM, Furumasu J, Warath SL: Surgical and functional results of spine fusion in spinal muscular atrophy. *Spine (Phila Pa 1976)* 1989; 14(7):763-770.

74. King WM, Ruttencutter R, Nagaraja HN, et al: Orthopedic outcomes of long-term daily corticosteroid treatment in Duchenne muscular dystrophy. *Neurology* 2007;68(19):1607-1613.

    At a minimum 3-year follow-up, 75 of 143 boys with Duchenne muscular dystrophy had been treated with steroids for at least 1 year, and 68 had received minimal or no steroids. The prevalence of scoliosis was 31% in the treated patients and 91% in the untreated patients. The average curve size was 11° in the treated patients and 33° in the untreated patients. Level of evidence: IV.

75. Houde S, Filiatrault M, Fournier A, et al: Deflazacort use in Duchenne muscular dystrophy: An 8-year follow-up. *Pediatr Neurol* 2008;38(3):200-206.

    At 8-year follow-up of 79 boys with Duchenne muscular dystrophy, 37 had been treated with deflazacort for an average of 66 months. Their average scoliosis curve was 14°, compared with 46° in the untreated patients. Level of evidence: IV.

76. Yamashita T, Kanaya K, Kawaguchi S, Murakami T, Yokogushi K: Prediction of progression of spinal deformity in Duchenne muscular dystrophy: A preliminary report. *Spine (Phila Pa 1976)* 2001;26(11):E223-E226.

77. Yamashita T, Kanaya K, Yokogushi K, Ishikawa Y, Minami R: Correlation between progression of spinal deformity and pulmonary function in Duchenne muscular dystrophy. *J Pediatr Orthop* 2001;21(1):113-116.

78. Kurz LT, Mubarak SJ, Schultz P, Park SM, Leach J: Correlation of scoliosis and pulmonary function in Duchenne muscular dystrophy. *J Pediatr Orthop* 1983; 3(3):347-353.

79. Fox HJ, Thomas CH, Thompson AG: Spinal instrumentation for Duchenne's muscular dystrophy: Experience of hypotensive anaesthesia to minimise blood loss. *J Pediatr Orthop* 1997;17(6):750-753.

80. Alman BA, Kim HK: Pelvic obliquity after fusion of the spine in Duchenne muscular dystrophy. *J Bone Joint Surg Br* 1999;81(5):821-824.

81. Aparicio LF, Jurkovic M, DeLullo J: Decreased bone density in ambulatory patients with Duchenne muscular dystrophy. *J Pediatr Orthop* 2002;22(2):179-181.

82. Ramirez N, Richards BS, Warren PD, Williams GR: Complications after posterior spinal fusion in Duchenne's muscular dystrophy. *J Pediatr Orthop* 1997; 17(1):109-114.

83. Bentley G, Haddad F, Bull TM, Seingry D: The treatment of scoliosis in muscular dystrophy using modified Luque and Harrington-Luque instrumentation. *J Bone Joint Surg Br* 2001;83(1):22-28.

84. Bridwell KH, Baldus C, Iffrig TM, Lenke LG, Blanke K: Process measures and patient/parent evaluation of surgical management of spinal deformities in patients with progressive flaccid neuromuscular scoliosis (Duchenne's muscular dystrophy and spinal muscular atrophy). *Spine (Phila Pa 1976)* 1999;24(13):1300-1309.

5: Spine

Chapter 27

Adolescent Idiopathic Scoliosis

Burt Yaszay, MD

Introduction

All orthopaedic surgeons who take care of children encounter adolescent idiopathic scoliosis (AIS) and become involved in the diagnosis, decision making, and nonsurgical treatment, in addition to possible surgical treatment. Most patients do not require surgery to correct the deformity during adolescence or young adulthood. There have been recent advances in understanding the etiology of AIS as well as its classification and management.

Spine Alignment

The normal radiographic alignment of the spine in the coronal plane is straight, with the head, trunk, and pelvis centered on the midline. Scoliosis is defined as a coronal Cobb angle greater than 10°. The typical pattern in an AIS deformity is a right hypokyphotic thoracic curve and a left lumbar curve. In normally developing children, there is substantial variability in the sagittal plane, with thoracic kyphosis ranging from 20° to 45° and lumbar lordosis from 30° to 60°. These measurements gradually increase as the child becomes older.[1] The sagittal parameters can be increased or decreased in a child with any form of scoliosis. The typical AIS spinal curve is associated with a decrease in thoracic kyphosis, particularly within the apical zone of the curve. The apical zone can be measured by rotating a three-dimensional radiographic reconstruction of the spine until a perfect lateral view of the apical vertebrae is obtained. The measurement of the apical zone is related to a possible etiology of AIS; on this true lateral view, thoracic kyphosis within the five apical vertebrae was found to average only 1°.[2]

Dr. Yaszay or an immediate family member is a member of a speakers' bureau or has made paid presentations on behalf of DePuy, a Johnson & Johnson company; serves as a paid consultant to or is an employee of Ellipse; serves as an unpaid consultant to Orthopediatrics; has received research or institutional support from DePuy, a Johnson & Johnson company; Ellipse; and KCI; and has received nonincome support (such as equipment or services), commercially derived honoraria, or other non–research-related funding (such as paid travel) from DePuy, a Johnson & Johnson company.

The true lateral view also can be used to identify the rotational deformity characteristic of AIS in the transverse plane. This deformity appears clinically as a rib hump or lumbar prominence and can be measured with a scoliometer during the Adams forward bend test. Axial rotation is suggested by pedicle asymmetry, rib-vertebra body relationships, and rib spread, as seen on two-dimensional standing PA and lateral long cassette radiographs.[3] CT is the gold standard for assessing axial rotation, although its routine use is limited by concerns related to radiation exposure and expense. Novel radiographic and computer-based techniques are increasingly used to reconstruct two-dimensional images of the spine into three-dimensional representations.[4,5] These methods offer promise for better understanding the nature of a patient's spine deformity with limited radiation exposure.

Etiology

Before a diagnosis of AIS is made, it is critical to rule out known causes of scoliosis and associations because the treatment of AIS is significantly different from that of many neuromuscular and congenital spinal curves. The cause or associations of a spine deformity usually can be deduced from a complete medical history, a thorough physical examination, and plain radiographs. The findings may be subtle, and they are numerous. The range is from axillary freckling, which suggests neurofibromatosis; to ligamentous laxity and a history of joint injuries, which suggest Marfan syndrome; to severe back pain, which suggests an intraspinal tumor. If a neural axis condition such as syringomyelia, Chiari malformation, split cord malformation, tumor, or tethered cord is suspected, the evaluation often includes MRI. In a patient with AIS, the indications for MRI include an abnormal neurologic examination; an atypical curve pattern (a left thoracic curve and increased thoracic kyphosis); a severe deformity or rapid progression of deformity, especially in a patient with early-onset AIS (before age 10 years); or significant pain. Although controversial, presurgical MRI sometimes is used to evaluate boys (because of the relative infrequency of AIS in boys, compared with girls).

Genetic factors appear to have a complex but significant role in the development of AIS. A review of the Danish Twin Registry found that monozygotic twins had a higher concordance rate than dizygotic twins.[6] An evaluation of the family pedigrees of 131 patients with AIS found a familial scoliosis connection in 127 and suggested that one or two major genes are responsible for AIS.[7] The genes under investigation encode for extracellular matrix components and hormone receptors. A genomewide screening process is being developed for use in identifying individuals at risk for severe, progressive scoliosis. These methods have not yet been validated, but it is believed that genetic marker identification may provide clues as to the mechanism of physiologic expression.

AIS develops and worsens during the adolescent growth phase. There may be a disturbance in spine development resulting from disproportionate rates of growth in different areas of the spine.[8] The discrepancy originally was believed to occur between the right and left (concave and convex) sides of the spine. More recently, it has been suggested that the disproportionate growth occurs between the anterior and posterior vertebral column; the buckling of the spine that results from anterior overgrowth causes both the coronal curvature and the vertebral rotation that can be seen on a three-dimensional reconstruction. The thoracic hypokyphosis that frequently occurs in AIS is a factor supporting this theory.[8]

Scoliosis is associated with many neurologic and muscular diseases, and there are several theories as to its etiology. The higher incidence of scoliosis in patients with myelomeningocele, Friedreich ataxia, syringomyelia, or symptomatic tethered spinal cord suggests that subtle central nervous system abnormalities are contributing factors. Abnormalities in vestibular function, postural control, and proprioceptive function also have been found in patients with AIS. Clinically silent spinal cord tethering, as identified on MRI, was suggested as a pathogenesis of AIS.[9] Children with poor muscle control or significant muscle weakness often develop spine deformities, and subtle weakness may be a contributing factor in spinal curve development and/or progression. Electromyographic activity was found to be altered in the paraspinal muscles of children with AIS,[10] but it is not clear whether this alteration is a cause or a result of the scoliosis. An association with AIS also is being investigated for vertebral disks, ligaments, ribs, melatonin, upright posture, and osteoporosis.[8] Currently, AIS is best considered as a complex genetic disorder that is influenced by multiple extrinsic factors.

Natural History

Approximately 2% to 3% of adolescents have a spinal curve greater than 10°, with an equal division among boys and girls. The prevalence of curves greater than 40° is less than 0.1% of all adolescents, and the ratio of girls to boys is approximately 10 to 1, suggesting that female gender is a risk factor for progression. The progression of scoliosis is related to several factors in addition to gender, including skeletal maturity, curve magnitude, and curve location.[11] The amount of remaining skeletal growth is the most important factor. Progression of as much as 1° to 2° per month can occur during the adolescent growth spurt, which is identified as the curve acceleration phase. A child's clinical and radiographic skeletal maturity can be estimated by determining the Tanner stage, Risser grade, and presence of pelvic triradiate cartilage, as well as a girl's age at menarche. A skeletal maturity scoring system based on the Tanner-Whitehouse–III radius, ulna, and small bones of the hand skeletal assessment method was found to be more closely correlated than earlier indicators with the onset of peak height velocity (the rapid growth phase) and, hence, maximal curve progression of the scoliosis[12] (Figure 1). Some practice is required to use this system effectively. An AP radiograph of the hand is used to evaluate the growth plates and epiphyses of the metacarpals and phalanges, with skeletal maturity estimated on the basis of the correlation between stages of physeal capping or closure and specific growth phases. In general, the patients at the highest risk for progression are girls who are premenarchal (Risser grade 0) with open triradiate cartilage and incomplete metaphyseal capping of the phalangeal epiphyses.

Among skeletally mature patients with untreated AIS, curves smaller than 30° tend not to progress.[11] Thoracic curves greater than 50° and lumbar curves greater than 35° with substantial rotational abnormality were found to progress most rapidly, at an average 1° to 2° per year. A 50-year follow-up of patients with untreated AIS and significant curvature found that they had a greater risk of mild to moderate back pain than age-matched control subjects, and they tended to be less active because of shortness of breath.[13] Objectively, curve magnitude was found to be negatively correlated with pulmonary function; however, a pulmonary function deficit did not always lead to a functional deficit in daily activities.[14]

Classification

AIS classification systems have been developed for use in selecting the appropriate curve or levels to include in a fusion. The first such widely used system, the King-Moe classification, is based on coronal radiographs and is intended for identification of specific curve types that are amenable to selective thoracic fusion so that the lumbar spine can be spared from fusion[15] (Figure 2). The limitations of the King-Moe system are an inability to assess sagittal deformity, poor intraobserver and interobserver reliability, and inclusion of only some AIS curve patterns.[16]

The Lenke classification system is increasingly used in AIS treatment research.[17] The goals of this system are to include all curve types, have good to excellent intraobserver and interobserver reliability, include an assessment of sagittal alignment, and define and compare

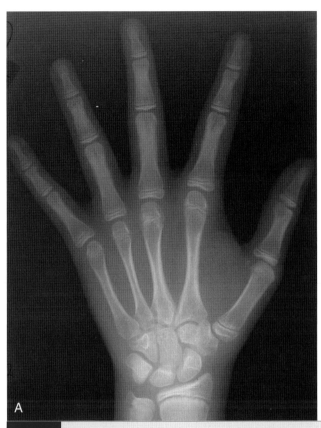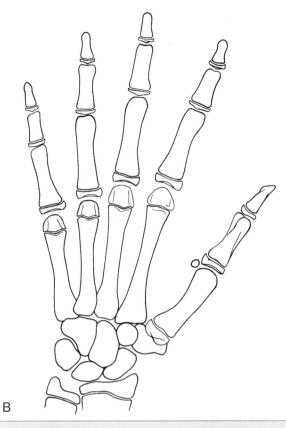

A   B

Figure 1   AP radiograph (**A**) and drawing (**B**) showing the hand of a child in stage 3 (the early adolescent rapid growth stage) on the simplified Tanner-Whitehouse–III skeletal maturity assessment. Stage 3 is correlated with peak height velocity, Risser grade 0, and open triradiate cartilage; the digital epiphyses cap the metaphyses, and the second through fifth metacarpal heads are wider than the metaphyses. (Reproduced with permission from Sanders JO, Khoury JG, Kishan S, et al: Predicting scoliosis progression from skeletal maturity: A simplified classification during adolescence. *J Bone Joint Surg Am* 2008;90[3]:544.)

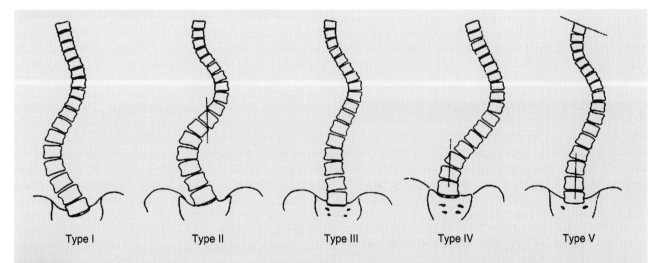

Type I   Type II   Type III   Type IV   Type V

Figure 2   The King-Moe classification of curve types. In type I, the lumbar curve is greater; in type II, the thoracic curve is greater, and the lumbar curve is flexible; in type III, the main curve is thoracic; in type IV, the thoracic curve is long; and in type V, the thoracic curve is double. (Reproduced from Grayhack J: Idiopathic scoliosis: Surgical management, in Sponseller P, ed: *Orthopaedic Knowledge Update: Pediatrics 2*. Rosemont, IL, American Academy of Orthopaedic Surgeons, 2002, p 308.)

5: Spine

Table 1

Definitions and Rules for Applying the Lenke Classification of AIS

The major curve is the curve with the largest Cobb angle.

The largest (major) curve is always structural.

A minor curve is any curve other than the major curve, with structural criteria strictly applied.

A minor curve that does not bend to less than 25° is defined as structural.

Proximal (T2-T5) and distal (T10-L2) regions of kyphosis greater than 20° are considered structural.

All structural curves and regions of the spine should be fused.

treatments. Six curve types are defined based on the structural characteristics of the major curve. The curve type is modified by the apical deviation of the lumbar curve from the central sacral vertical line and by degrees of thoracic kyphosis to yield 42 possible combinations of curve types, lumbar modifiers, and sagittal modifiers (Table 1 and Figure 3). Studies applying the Lenke classification system predicted the treatment chosen by experienced scoliosis surgeons approximately 75% to 85% of the time.[18] In clinical practice, it is difficult to determine when the classification system's surgical treatment recommendation should be ignored. If the classification system does not yield a clear recommendation, the surgeon must consider the relative sizes of the thoracic-to-lumbar and upper thoracic–to-thoracic curves, relative axial rotation, and clinical appearance. A recent three-dimensional classification system overlays a top-down representation of the major curves onto a transverse axis. This so-called da Vinci representation has yet to be validated as useful in clinical practice.[19]

Nonsurgical Treatment

Many nonsurgical treatments have been used in an attempt to prevent scoliosis progression. Exercise, electrical stimulation, and manipulation have not altered the natural history of curve progression. Bracing has long been considered the primary nonsurgical treatment for AIS, but the scientific evidence supporting its use is weak. The available studies have inconsistent indications for bracing, a lack of compliance measurement, inconsistent definitions of brace failure, and failure to account for brace design and prescriptions for wear.[20] An ongoing, multicenter randomized study of bracing is being sponsored by the National Institutes of Health in collaboration with the Canadian Institutes of Health Research.

The Scoliosis Research Society endorses bracing for patients who have significant remaining growth (Risser grade 0, 1, or 2) as well as a curve between 25° and 40° or a curve greater than 20° with documented progression of more than 5°. Bracing typically is discontinued when the patient reaches skeletal maturity or requires surgery. Many types of spine braces are available. The most commonly prescribed brace is the thoracolumbosacral orthosis, which is used for a curve with an apex no higher than T7, a thoracic curve, or a thoracolumbar curve (a double major curve). The recommended usage is 16 to 23 hours a day. For a curve with an apex above T7, a cervical extension or Milwaukee brace may be used, although evidence of brace efficacy is lacking for these curves. A cervical extension or Milwaukee brace is poorly tolerated by most patients and not routinely prescribed. A nighttime bending brace (the Charleston or Providence brace) is an option for a single curve, particularly if the curve has a thoracolumbar apex.[21] No brace has been found to permanently decrease the size of a curve in patients with AIS.

A patient who is using a brace should have an in-brace PA radiograph to determine how much the curve has been straightened by the brace. The goal for standard, full-time thoracolumbosacral orthosis use is a 50% curve correction while the patient is in the brace. The usual recommendation is for a patient with a brace to be monitored in the same manner as a patient who is not using a brace. Radiographs should be scheduled every 6 months. Follow-up radiographs should be taken with the patient out of the brace so that the deformity can be better documented. A decision to discontinue brace use or to recommend surgery is based on the curve progression as seen in out-of-brace radiographs.

Surgical Treatment

Surgery is generally considered to be indicated for a skeletally mature adolescent whose curve is greater than 50° or a skeletally immature adolescent with a curve greater than 40° to 45°. Surgery may be required for some patients with a curve below these thresholds if there is significant truncal asymmetry, especially in a thoracolumbar or lumbar curve. The goals of surgery are to prevent long-term progression into adulthood (using a solid fusion), achieve maximal deformity correction, and maintain optimal coronal and sagittal truncal balance. An anterior, posterior, or combined anterior-posterior approach is used for spinal fusion.

Anterior Fusion

An anterior approach has been recommended for a patient with a single structural thoracic curve or a thoracolumbar curve. The most important claimed advantage of anterior surgery is that fewer fusion levels may be required, in comparison with posterior surgery.[22,23] The typical anterior fusion is limited to the vertebrae that make up the measured Cobb angle. In addition, thoracic kyphosis restoration is enhanced because the anterior column is shortened by intervertebral disk

1. Criteria for Curve Classification

Classification	Structural Status		
	Proximal Thoracic	Main Thoracic	Thoracolumbar or Lumbar
1 (Main thoracic)	Nonstructural	Structural (major)	Nonstructural
2 (Double thoracic)	Structural	Structural (major)	Nonstructural
3 (Double major)	Nonstructural	Structural (major)	Structural
4 (Triple major)	Structural	Structural	Structural
5 (Thoracolumbar or lumbar)	Nonstructural	Nonstructural	Structural (major)
6 (Thoracolumbar or lumbar–main thoracic)	Nonstructural	Structural	Structural (major)

Structural Criteria for a Minor Curve

Minor Curve	Criteria
Proximal thoracic	Side-bending Cobb angle ≥ 25° T2-T5 kyphosis ≥ +20°
Main thoracic	Side-bending Cobb angle ≥ 25° T10-L2 kyphosis ≥ +20°
Thoracolumbar or lumbar	Side-bending Cobb angle ≥ 25° T10-L2 kyphosis ≥ +20°

Location of Apex*

Curve	Apex
Thoracic	T2 to T11-12 disk
Thoracolumbar	T12 to L1
Lumbar	L1-2 disk to L4

*Scoliosis Research Society definition

Modifiers

	Lumbar Spine Modifier			Thoracic Sagittal Profile (T5-T12)	
Classification	Center Sacral Vertical Line (to Lumbar Apex)	Appearance		Classification	Criterion
A	Between pedicles			− (hypo)	< 10°
B	Touching apical body/bodies			N (normal)	10° to 40°
C	Completely medial			+ (hyper)	> 40°

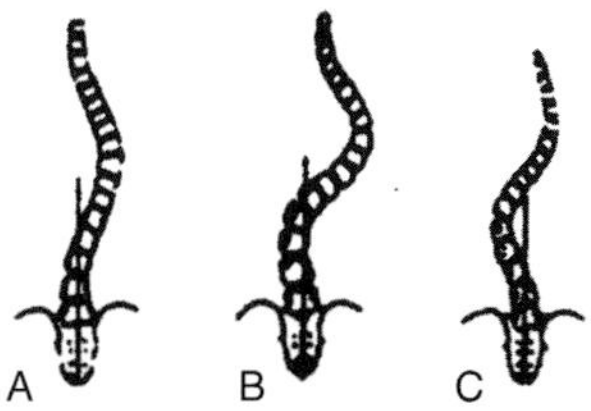

2. Classification Worksheet

Curve type (1, 2, 3, 4, 5, or 6) _____

Lumbar spine modifier (A, B, or C) _____

Thoracic sagittal modifier (−, N, or +) _____

Classification (eg, 1B+) _____

Figure 3 The Lenke classification of AIS. (Adapted with permission from Lenke LG, Betz RR, Harms J, et al: Adolescent idiopathic scoliosis: A new classification to determine extent of spinal arthrodesis. *J Bone Joint Surg Am* 2001;83[8]: 1169-1181.)

5: Spine

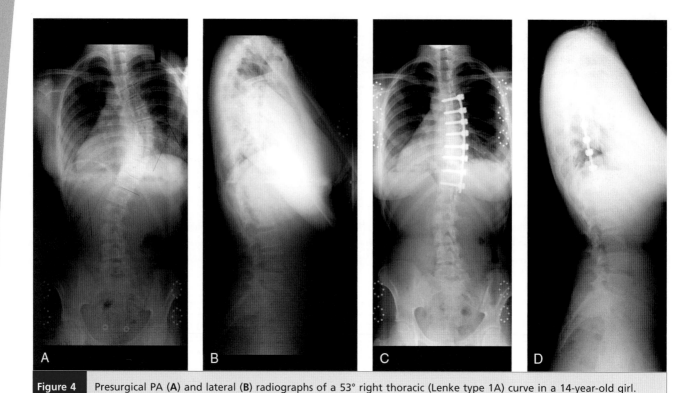

Figure 4 Presurgical PA (**A**) and lateral (**B**) radiographs of a 53° right thoracic (Lenke type 1A) curve in a 14-year-old girl. PA (**C**) and lateral (**D**) radiographs after thoracoscopic anterior spinal fusion and instrumentation. (Courtesy of Peter O. Newton, MD, San Diego, CA.)

excision, posterior paraspinal musculature injury is avoided, and the risk of crankshaft deformity is decreased in a skeletally immature patient. Anterior-only fusion is relatively contraindicated for a patient with a double or triple major curve, a large curve (greater than 70°), hyperkyphosis (T5-T12 sagittal kyphosis greater than 40°), or poor pulmonary function.

A main thoracic curve can be approached through an open thoracotomy or a thoracoscopic procedure (**Figure 4**). The open procedure has declined in popularity because of its negative effect on pulmonary function (an approximately 10% reduction, as measured by pulmonary function testing).[24] The thoracoscopic procedure has many of the advantages of the open procedure but minimizes chest wall disruption and thereby has less effect on respiratory function; baseline respiratory values are restored within 1 year after surgery.[24] The additional benefits of the minimally invasive approach include a smaller incision, decreased blood loss, and more rapid return of shoulder girdle function. The most important drawback to the thoracoscopic procedure is the learning curve required to master the technique.[25] Prominent hardware on the concave side of the deformity after thoracoscopic procedures has led to concern about aortic injury.[26] Also of concern is the possibility of rod breakage and pseudarthrosis when a single-rod construct is used in either an open or a thoracoscopic procedure.[27] Because of this risk, the use of a postoperative brace and/or autologous bone graft has been promoted.

A single thoracolumbar or lumbar curve, unlike a thoracic curve, still is frequently treated through an open anterior thoracolumbar approach. A very short fusion with overcorrection over three to four vertebral levels has been used.[28] The increased kyphosis, pseudarthrosis, and poor derotation initially associated with this technique have been remedied by using dual-rod constructs and interbody structural support. Including all vertebrae of the measured curve in the fusion results in less disk wedging below the construct. It is unclear whether the advantages of greater motion segments outweigh the increased disk angulation. Pedicle screws and posterior osteotomies recently have been used to achieve similar thoracolumbar curve correction and comparable levels of fusion, and the optimal procedure, therefore, is less clear.[29]

Posterior Fusion

Posterior spinal instrumentation and fusion is considered the standard surgical treatment for a primary thoracic curve or double or triple major curve (**Figures 5 and 6**). The options for instrumentation include sublaminar wires, hooks, pedicle screws, and hybrid constructs. The guidelines for selecting the fusion levels reflect many radiographic and clinical features and are evolving with the instrumentation. The posterior approach has significant advantages over the anterior approach: less surgical time is required, and there is a smaller risk of implant failure. Pedicle screws provide

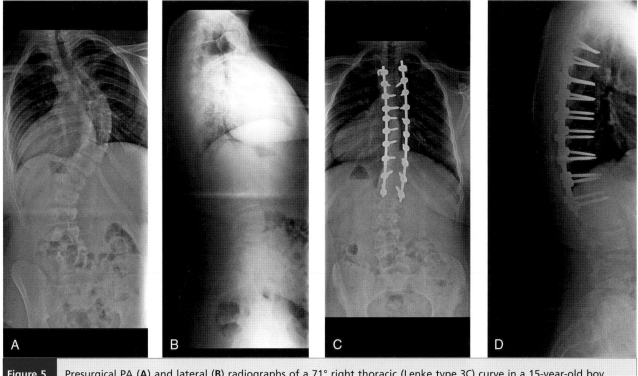

Figure 5 Presurgical PA (**A**) and lateral (**B**) radiographs of a 71° right thoracic (Lenke type 3C) curve in a 15-year-old boy. PA (**C**) and lateral (**D**) radiographs after selective thoracic fusion.

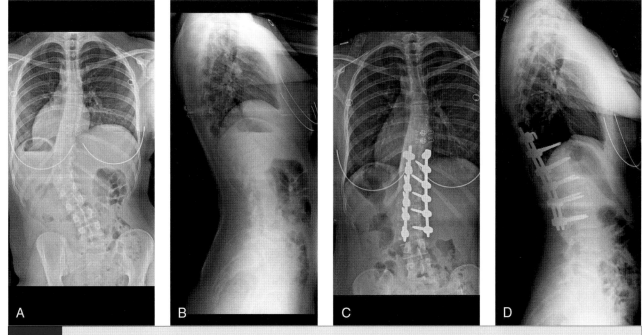

Figure 6 Presurgical PA (**A**) and lateral (**B**) radiographs of a 50° left thoracolumbar (Lenke type 5C) curve in a 14-year-old girl. PA (**C**) and lateral (**D**) radiographs after wide posterior releases and T10-L3 posterior spinal instrumentation and fusion.

greater deformity correction and minimize the number of levels fused.[30,31] Although little scientific evidence exists, it is possible that pedicle screws also minimize the risk of crankshaft deformity in skeletally immature pa-

tients by providing secure three-column fixation.

The drawbacks to a posterior procedure include a greater risk of wound complications and less ability to restore thoracic kyphosis, in comparison with anterior approaches that incorporate disk excision. The type of anchors or rods used may affect the extent of postsurgical kyphosis restoration. A loss of thoracic kyphosis may occur when segmental pedicle screws are used rather than a hybrid or hook construct.[31] This relative lordosing effect may be the result of the improved coronal and rotational correction obtained with pedicle screws, especially if direct vertebral rotation resulted in the relatively lengthened anterior column moving more completely into the sagittal plane. This hypercorrection of the coronal and axial planes unmasks the primary deformity of thoracic AIS, which is relative lordosis. The use of posterior osteotomies to lengthen the posterior column and restore thoracic kyphosis is being investigated as a means of more complete correction in all three planes of deformity. Posterior spinal fusion using an all–pedicle screw construct is popular because it leads to better curve correction, less loss of correction, and a shorter hospital stay than an anterior spinal fusion.[29]

Direct vertebral rotation and segmental pedicle screw fixation are associated with a greater reduction in rib prominence than other posterior techniques, and, therefore, the routine use of thoracoplasty has been questioned. Some of the pulmonary function morbidity associated with posterior fusion can be avoided if thoracoplasty is not done.[24] Some surgeons continue to use thoracoplasty, however, believing that it improves clinical hump correction even with pedicle screw fixation.[32]

New instrumentation and more aggressive surgical techniques have reinforced concerns about the safety of AIS treatment. The use of pedicle screws was found to be safe in the thoracic spine as long as it reflects an understanding of anatomy in the presence of deformity.[33,34] An improper medial or lateral placement can lead to a neurologic or vascular injury, respectively. Posterior osteotomy (the Ponte osteotomy, pedicle subtraction, or vertebral column resection) increasingly is used to treat large, rigid spinal curvatures, including AIS, in an attempt to limit the use of anterior release (diskectomy) procedures.[35] Posterior osteotomies vary in difficulty and risk. Intrasurgical neurologic monitoring is mandatory because of the substantial risk to the spinal cord during or after the osteotomy. Spinal cord monitoring can be done using somatosensory-evoked potentials, mixed neurogenic motor-evoked potentials, transcranial motor-evoked potentials, or H-reflexes. Changes in transcranial motor-evoked potentials were found to be more sensitive than somatosensory-evoked potentials for detecting spinal cord function deficits, especially those associated with insufficient vascular flow to the cord.[36] In addition, changes are detected more rapidly than with somatosensory-evoked potentials, thus allowing for earlier intervention. Triggered electromyographic monitoring is used to assess the placement of pedicle screws; thresholds below 6 mA have been associated with a higher incidence of medial and inferior breach of the pedicle wall, although absolute thresholds have not been established.[36,37] In general, the greater the threshold number used, the less likely they are to be in contact with neural elements. Triggered electromyographic monitoring is less useful for detecting lateral misplacement of pedicle screws.

Combined Anterior-Posterior Fusion

Combined anterior release and posterior instrumented fusion traditionally has been reserved for a large (greater than 80°) or rigid (side bending greater than 50°) curve. This procedure also has been promoted for patients younger than 10 years, who are at risk of crankshaft deformity. The anterior release procedure can be performed through an open or thoracoscopic approach. Disk excision can increase flexibility and shorten the anterior column. The use of segmental pedicle screws and more aggressive posterior surgical techniques has brought into question the need for anterior release in curves 70° to 100° or greater. These powerful correction methods may obviate the need to approach the spine anteriorly.[38] The pulmonary effects are as yet undocumented for a thoracic-level three-column osteotomy, such as a pedicle subtraction osteotomy or vertebral column resection. Further investigation is required to refine the indications for anterior release with advanced posterior methods. It may be safer and more effective to rely on the traditional indications and techniques.

The Future of AIS Treatment

Concerns about the long-term effects of spinal fusion and decreased spinal mobility have led to novel methods to manage progressive curves. There is a long-standing hope that spinal growth can be modulated and redirected from a scoliotic position to a more normal alignment with greater efficiency than external bracing allows. Internal mechanical means of achieving correction without fusion are being investigated, including vertebral body stapling and anterior spinal tethering.[39,40] The goal of these fusionless treatments is to control the patient's remaining spinal growth to achieve curve correction. The effects of the Hueter-Volkmann law are exploited by compressing and tensioning the convex growth plates to inhibit their growth, allowing the convex growth plates to continue to grow and thus straighten the spine. Although these methods are clinically in use, no controlled or large cohort studies have determined their effectiveness or longer term risk in comparison with brace treatment or no treatment. Ideally, methods that consistently attain correction without fusion will lead to a cure for scoliosis, allowing relatively normal spine mobility and function.

Summary

AIS is a three-dimensional deformity of the spine with an undetermined etiology. Most patients with a small curvature will never require active treatment. Young, skeletally immature girls are most at risk of curve progression, and they require close monitoring. The physician, patient, and family decide together whether bracing should be considered. If the curvature becomes so severe that surgery is recommended, many treatments can provide a solid fusion, achieve maximal deformity correction, and maintain optimal coronal and sagittal balance. Posterior spinal fusion is the current gold standard treatment, with increasingly greater use of pedicle screw instrumentation. In the future, treatment may allow scoliosis correction without fusion and its associated morbidity.

Annotated References

1. Cil A, Yazici M, Uzumcugil A, et al: The evolution of sagittal segmental alignment of the spine during childhood. *Spine (Phila Pa 1976)* 2005;30(1):93-100.

   An evaluation of 151 normally developing children between ages 3 and 15 years found that sagittal spinal alignment changes as a child grows.

2. Hayashi K, Upasani VV, Pawelek JB, et al: Three-dimensional analysis of thoracic apical sagittal alignment in adolescent idiopathic scoliosis. *Spine (Phila Pa 1976)* 2009;34(8):792-797.

   In this retrospective review of AIS, three-dimensional models of the spine were created from biplanar radiographic reconstructions. The reconstructions were rotated to obtain a true lateral view of the apical vertebrae. The sagittal profile was measured and compared with the standard lateral view. The standard lateral view was found to overestimate the apical kyphosis by approximately 10°.

3. Kuklo TR, Potter BK, Lenke LG: Vertebral rotation and thoracic torsion in adolescent idiopathic scoliosis: What is the best radiographic correlate? *J Spinal Disord Tech* 2005;18(2):139-147.

   The techniques for measuring vertebral rotation on preoperative and postoperative radiographs and CT were compared.

4. Kadoury S, Cheriet F, Dansereau J, Labelle H: Three-dimensional reconstruction of the scoliotic spine and pelvis from uncalibrated biplanar x-ray images. *J Spinal Disord Tech* 2007;20(2):160-167.

   A technique is described for reconstructing a three-dimensional image of a scoliotic spine from uncalibrated two-dimensional radiographs. The purpose is to retrospectively evaluate a patient's radiographs without using a calibration tool.

5. Humbert L, De Guise JA, Aubert B, Godbout B, Skalli W: 3D reconstruction of the spine from biplanar X-rays using parametric models based on transversal and longitudinal inferences. *Med Eng Phys* 2009;31(6):681-687.

   A method is described for three-dimensional reconstruction of the spine from biplanar radiographs using low-dosage radiation with the patient in a standing position.

6. Andersen MO, Thomsen K, Kyvik KO: Adolescent idiopathic scoliosis in twins: A population-based survey. *Spine (Phila Pa 1976)* 2007;32(8):927-930.

   The Danish Twin Registry was used to compare the AIS concordance rate among monozygotic and dizygotic twins. The greater concordance among monozygotic twins suggests a genetic etiology in scoliosis.

7. Ogilvie JW, Braun J, Argyle V, Nelson L, Meade M, Ward K: The search for idiopathic scoliosis genes. *Spine (Phila Pa 1976)* 2006;31(6):679-681.

   A genealogic database review of 131 patients with AIS found that 127 had a familial connection to others with scoliosis. These data may support the existence of one or two major scoliosis genes.

8. Kouwenhoven JW, Castelein RM: The pathogenesis of adolescent idiopathic scoliosis: Review of the literature. *Spine (Phila Pa 1976)* 2008;33(26):2898-2908.

   This is a review of the literature on the pathogenesis of AIS.

9. Chu WC, Man GC, Lam WW, et al: Morphological and functional electrophysiological evidence of relative spinal cord tethering in adolescent idiopathic scoliosis. *Spine (Phila Pa 1976)* 2008;33(6):673-680.

   MRI was used to evaluate the morphology and relative positioning of the spinal cord in patients with AIS. The ratio of spinal cord to vertebral length was less than that of normal control subjects, suggesting that tethering of the spinal cord is a cause of AIS.

10. Cheung J, Halbertsma JP, Veldhuizen AG, et al : A preliminary study on electromyographic analysis of the paraspinal musculature in idiopathic scoliosis. *Eur Spine J* 2005;14(2):130-137.

    Paraspinal EMG activity was examined on the convexity and concavity of patients with AIS. The significantly greater differences found in patients with curve progression suggests the usefulness of this method for predicting scoliosis progression.

11. Weinstein SL, Ponseti IV: Curve progression in idiopathic scoliosis. *J Bone Joint Surg Am* 1983;65(4): 447-455.

12. Sanders JO, Khoury JG, Kishan S, et al: Predicting scoliosis progression from skeletal maturity: A simplified classification during adolescence. *J Bone Joint Surg Am* 2008;90(3):540-553.

    A new staging system based on the Tanner-Whitehouse–III radius, ulna, and small bones of the hand score is correlated with the risk of scoliosis progression. An AP radiograph of the hand is used to evaluate the growth plates and epiphyses of the metacarpals and phalanges. Different stages of capping or closure are correlated with specific points in the growth phase.

13. Weinstein SL, Dolan LA, Spratt KF, Peterson KK, Spoonamore MJ, Ponseti IV: Health and function of patients with untreated idiopathic scoliosis: A 50-year natural history study. *JAMA* 2003;289(5):559-567.

14. Newton PO, Faro FD, Gollogly S, Betz RR, Lenke LG, Lowe TG: Results of preoperative pulmonary function testing of adolescents with idiopathic scoliosis: A study of six hundred and thirty-one patients. *J Bone Joint Surg Am* 2005;87(9):1937-1946.

    The magnitude of the thoracic curve, the number of vertebrae involved in the thoracic curve, thoracic hypokyphosis, and coronal imbalance were found to have a minimal but significant effect on the pulmonary function of 631 patients with AIS.

15. King HA, Moe JH, Bradford DS, Winter RB: The selection of fusion levels in thoracic idiopathic scoliosis. *J Bone Joint Surg Am* 1983;65(9):1302-1313.

16. Lenke LG, Betz RR, Bridwell KH, et al: Intraobserver and interobserver reliability of the classification of thoracic adolescent idiopathic scoliosis. *J Bone Joint Surg Am* 1998;80(8):1097-1106.

17. Lenke LG, Betz RR, Harms J, et al: Adolescent idiopathic scoliosis: A new classification to determine extent of spinal arthrodesis. *J Bone Joint Surg Am* 2001;83(8): 1169-1181.

18. Richards BS, Sucato DJ, Konigsberg DE, Ouellet JA: Comparison of reliability between the Lenke and King classification systems for adolescent idiopathic scoliosis using radiographs that were not premeasured. *Spine (Phila Pa 1976)* 2003;28(11):1148-1157.

19. Sangole AP, Aubin CE, Labelle H, et al : Three-dimensional classification of thoracic scoliotic curves. *Spine (Phila Pa 1976)* 2009;34(1):91-99.

    A new method, the da Vinci representation, is reported for describing the three-dimensional deformity seen in AIS. By using this method, the authors found two distinct subgroups of Lenke type 1 curves.

20. Dolan LA, Weinstein SL: Surgical rates after observation and bracing for adolescent idiopathic scoliosis: An evidence-based review. *Spine (Phila Pa 1976)* 2007; 32(19, suppl):S91-S100.

    This systematic review of the literature assesses the frequency of surgery after bracing or observation. No clear advantage was found to either approach.

21. Katz DE, Richards BS, Browne RH, Herring JA: A comparison between the Boston brace and the Charleston bending brace in adolescent idiopathic scoliosis. *Spine (Phila Pa 1976)* 1997;22(12):1302-1312.

22. Betz RR, Harms J, Clements DH III, et al: Comparison of anterior and posterior instrumentation for correction of adolescent thoracic idiopathic scoliosis. *Spine (Phila Pa 1976)* 1999;24(3):225-239.

23. Lonner BS, Kondrachov D, Siddiqi F, Hayes V, Scharf C: Thoracoscopic spinal fusion compared with posterior spinal fusion for the treatment of thoracic adolescent idiopathic scoliosis. *J Bone Joint Surg Am* 2006;88(5): 1022-1034.

    This retrospective study compared thoracoscopic fusion in 28 patients and posterior spinal fusion in 23 patients for treating a main thoracic curve. There was no difference in curve correction, sagittal contour, rates of complications, or patient outcomes. The patients with thoracoscopic fusion had less blood loss and fewer fused levels, but the surgical time was twice that of the patients with posterior fusion.

24. Newton PO, Perry A, Bastrom TP, et al: Predictors of change in postoperative pulmonary function in adolescent idiopathic scoliosis: A prospective study of 254 patients. *Spine (Phila Pa 1976)* 2007;32(17):1875-1882.

    The postoperative pulmonary function of 254 patients with AIS was evaluated at a minimum 2-year follow-up. Open anterior procedures and thoracoplasty were found to result in significantly decreased pulmonary function.

25. Lonner BS, Scharf C, Antonacci D, Goldstein Y, Panagopoulos G: The learning curve associated with thoracoscopic spinal instrumentation. *Spine (Phila Pa 1976)* 2005;30(24):2835-2840.

    A significant but acceptable learning curve is required for thoracoscopic spinal instrumentation and fusion for main thoracic curves.

26. Sucato DJ, Kassab F, Dempsey M: Analysis of screw placement relative to the aorta and spinal canal following anterior instrumentation for thoracic idiopathic scoliosis. *Spine (Phila Pa 1976)* 2004;29(5):554-559.

27. Newton PO, Upasani VV, Lhamby J, Ugrinow VL, Pawelek JB, Bastrom TP: Surgical treatment of main thoracic scoliosis with thoracoscopic anterior instrumentation: A five-year follow-up study. *J Bone Joint Surg Am* 2008;90(10):2077-2089.

    The 5-year outcomes of 41 consecutive patients treated with thoracoscopic anterior instrumentation were comparable to those of patients treated with an open anterior or posterior approach. The risks of the procedure include pseudarthrosis, hardware failure, and surgical revision. Level of evidence: IV.

28. Bernstein RM, Hall JE: Solid rod short segment anterior fusion in thoracolumbar scoliosis. *J Pediatr Orthop B* 1998;7(2):124-131.

29. Geck MJ, Rinella A, Hawthorne D, et al: Comparison of surgical treatment in Lenke 5C adolescent idiopathic scoliosis: Anterior dual rod versus posterior pedicle fixation surgery. A comparison of two practices. *Spine (Phila Pa 1976)* 2009;34(18):1942-1951.

    This retrospective review compared patients with Lenke type 5 AIS who underwent anterior or posterior spinal fusion. At 2-year follow-up, patients who underwent posterior fusion had significantly better curve correction, a shorter hospital stay, and less loss of correction over time. These patients had instrumentation of an average 5.9 levels. The patients who underwent anterior fusion had instrumentation of an average 4.3 levels.

30. Potter BK, Kuklo TR, Lenke LG: Radiographic outcomes of anterior spinal fusion versus posterior spinal fusion with thoracic pedicle screws for treatment of

Lenke Type I adolescent idiopathic scoliosis curves. *Spine (Phila Pa 1976)* 2005;30(16):1859-1866.

A retrospective study compared 40 matched patients with Lenke type 1 AIS after anterior or posterior spinal fusion with all pedicle screws. The posterior fusion was an average 1.2 levels longer than the anterior fusion. Posterior fusion led to better coronal correction, spontaneous lumbar curve correction, and better rib hump correction than anterior fusion.

31. Kim YJ, Lenke LG, Kim J, et al: Comparative analysis of pedicle screw versus hybrid instrumentation in posterior spinal fusion of adolescent idiopathic scoliosis. *Spine (Phila Pa 1976)* 2006;31(3):291-298.

A retrospective review found that pedicle screws improve curve correction better than hybrid instrumentation but cause a significantly greater loss of thoracic kyphosis.

32. Suk SI, Kim JH, Kim SS, Lee JJ, Han YT: Thoracoplasty in thoracic adolescent idiopathic scoliosis. *Spine (Phila Pa 1976)* 2008;33(10):1061-1067.

A retrospective study found improved rib hump correction in patients undergoing thoracoplasty, even with the use of an all–pedicle screw construct.

33. Kim YJ, Lenke LG, Bridwell KH, Cho YS, Riew KD: Free hand pedicle screw placement in the thoracic spine: Is it safe? *Spine (Phila Pa 1976)* 2004;29(3):333-342.

34. Suk SI, Lee CK, Kim WJ, Chung YJ, Park YB: Segmental pedicle screw fixation in the treatment of thoracic idiopathic scoliosis. *Spine (Phila Pa 1976)* 1995;20(12):1399-1405.

35. Lenke LG, O'Leary PT, Bridwell KH, Sides BA, Koester LA, Blanke KM: Posterior vertebral column resection for severe pediatric deformity: Minimum two-year follow-up of thirty-five consecutive patients. *Spine (Phila Pa 1976)* 2009;34(20):2213-2221.

The results and safety of 35 patients treated with posterior vertebral column resection are reported. The use of spinal cord monitoring is strongly recommended, especially motor-evoked potentials. Two patients had reversible intraoperative events; there were no postoperative spinal cord complications.

36. Schwartz DM, Auerbach JD, Dormans JP, et al: Neurophysiological detection of impending spinal cord injury during scoliosis surgery. *J Bone Joint Surg Am* 2007;89(11):2440-2449.

The neuromonitoring results of 1,121 consecutive surgically treated patients with AIS are reported. Motor-evoked potentials were found to be sensitive to vascular insult. The changes were detected earlier than changes to somatosensory-evoked potentials, thereby allowing for a more rapid intervention.

37. Raynor BL, Lenke LG, Kim Y, et al: Can triggered electromyograph thresholds predict safe thoracic pedicle screw placement? *Spine (Phila Pa 1976)* 2002;27(18):2030-2035.

38. Dobbs MB, Lenke LG, Kim YJ, Luhmann SJ, Bridwell KH: Anterior/posterior spinal instrumentation versus posterior instrumentation alone for the treatment of adolescent idiopathic scoliotic curves more than 90 degrees. *Spine (Phila Pa 1976)* 2006;31(20):2386-2391.

Patients with AIS curves greater than 90° had no difference in curve correction or complications after anterior or posterior instrumentation. The posterior approach may be a safe alternative, especially in patients with compromised pulmonary function.

39. Guille JT, D'Andrea LP, Betz RR: Fusionless treatment of scoliosis. *Orthop Clin North Am* 2007;38(4):541-545, vii.

The recent advances in fusionless treatment of scoliosis are reviewed.

40. Newton PO, Upasani VV, Farnsworth CL, et al: Spinal growth modulation with use of a tether in an immature porcine model. *J Bone Joint Surg Am* 2008;90(12):2695-2706.

The use of a tether in a porcine model is reviewed as a method for the fusionless treatment of AIS.

5: Spine

Chapter 28

Kyphosis

Steven Hwang, MD   Amer Samdani, MD   Suken A. Shah, MD

Normal Spine Kyphosis and Development

Children usually are born with mild spine kyphosis. As the child begins to elevate the head and ambulate, thoracic kyphosis increases and lumbar and cervical lordosis develops. The overall curvature of the spine in the sagittal plane permits the head to be centered over the pelvis. Spine curvature is inferred to be neutral when a plumb line from C7 intersects the posterior edge of the sacral end plate.[1,2] Cervical alignment, thoracic kyphosis, lumbar lordosis, pelvic tilt, and sacral slope interact to maintain postural alignment.

Thoracic kyphosis ideally should be measured from the end plate of T2 to T12. Frequently, however, radiographic obscuration from the shoulders requires that the kyphosis from T2 to T5 be inferred from the T5 to T12 measurement. Normal thoracic kyphosis generally is 20° to 40°,[3] but it can be greater because of a physiologic or pathologic process. In children, these processes are commonly related to postural, Scheuermann, iatrogenic, or congenital kyphosis.

Postural Kyphosis

Postural kyphosis, or familial round-back deformity, is a flexible kyphosis that does not have the sharp, angulated, rigid pattern of deformity characteristic of Scheuermann kyphosis.[4] Postural kyphosis should be included in the differential diagnosis for a patient with

Dr. Hwang or an immediate family member has received research or institutional support from DePuy, a Johnson & Johnson company. Dr. Samdani or an immediate family member is a member of a speakers' bureau or has made paid presentations on behalf of DePuy, a Johnson & Johnson company and Spinevision; serves as a paid consultant to or is an employee of DePuy, a Johnson & Johnson company, Spinevision, and Synthes; and has received research or institutional support from DePuy, a Johnson & Johnson company. Dr. Shah or an immediate family member has received royalties from DePuy, a Johnson & Johnson company; is a member of a speakers' bureau or has made paid presentations on behalf of DePuy, a Johnson & Johnson company; serves as a paid consultant to or is an employee of DePuy, a Johnson & Johnson company; serves as an unpaid consultant to K Spine, Inc.; has received research or institutional support from DePuy, a Johnson & Johnson company and Axial Biotech, Inc.; and owns stock or stock options in Globus Medical.

thoracic kyphosis, although this condition does not have pathologic connotations. With forward bending, the patient has a gradual, gentle kyphosis in the sagittal plane that is easily corrected by standing erect or lying prone. Radiographs do not reveal anterior vertebral wedging or end plate irregularities. Although the patient may have mild back pain, the natural history of postural kyphosis is benign. Observation is recommended for an asymptomatic child. Nonsteroidal anti-inflammatory drugs and physical therapy with postural training exercises, hamstring stretching, and back extensor strengthening form the basis of treatment for back pain accompanying postural kyphosis.

Scheuermann Kyphosis

Scheuermann kyphosis, historically called idiopathic kyphosis, is a pathologic developmental process in which vertebral wedging causes increased kyphosis.[4-6] The condition originally was described as a rigid thoracic kyphosis with wedging of vertebral bodies. The radiographic definition remains controversial; the most common definition includes at least 5° of anterior wedging at each of three consecutive vertebrae, end plate irregularity, and Schmorl nodes.[5] However, radiographic findings of irregular end plates, loss of disk height, anterior wedging of more than 10°, and overall hyperkyphosis also have been attributed to Scheuermann kyphosis.[6] The pathophysiology of Scheuermann kyphosis remains unclear. The proposed etiologies include osteonecrosis of the vertebral ring, weakening of the cartilaginous end plate, juvenile osteoporosis, abnormal cartilaginous matrix, abnormal growth hormone levels, and genetic predisposition.

Scheuermann kyphosis is the most common cause of hyperkyphosis in adolescents, in whom the reported prevalence ranges from 0.4% to 10%.[5,7] Boys age 10 to 15 years are most commonly affected, although some studies report an equal incidence among girls and boys.[8] Often the child's physical appearance is attributed to poor posture. As a result an affected child is likely to develop postural concerns, a poor self-image, or back pain. Some patients have scoliosis or contractures of the pectoralis, hip flexor, or hamstring muscles. The patient may avoid participating in athletic activities. Typically there is a well-demarcated angular thoracic or thoracolumbar kyphosis, which is accentuated

5: Spine

by forward bending, and a compensatory hyperlordosis of the lumbar spine. The apex is at T7 to T9. The compensatory hyperlordosis produces the head and neck thrust characteristic of Scheuermann kyphosis. The kyphosis is relatively rigid and cannot be corrected to the normal range with hyperextension.

The treatment is based on the severity and progression of the deformity as well as the presence of pain, cosmetic disfigurement, or, rarely, neurologic compromise. Approximately 50% of pediatric patients with Scheuermann kyphosis have concurrent thoracic back pain.[5] The prevalence decreases to 25% in skeletally mature patients,[5] although untreated Scheuermann kyphosis in adults is associated with a higher rate of disabling back pain.[9] Pain is only a relative indication for surgical intervention.

Bracing for Scheuermann kyphosis remains controversial. There is little evidence as to its effect on the natural history of kyphosis progression. Some studies have suggested that bracing leads to vertebral remodeling in immature patients.[10,11] However, all available studies of bracing for kyphosis were small, retrospective, and limited to level IV evidence.[12] The criteria for bracing are a 50° to 75° curve and passive correction of 40% or more. Patients with a curve greater than 75° may respond less favorably to bracing, and surgical intervention can be considered for these patients.[13,14] With or without a bracing program, a rigorous schedule of exercise may be helpful, emphasizing thoracic extensor strengthening and endurance as well as hamstring stretching. Initial bracing achieves an almost 50% reduction in the kyphosis in many patients, but some correction often is lost when the patient is weaned from brace wearing.[14] Bracing is routinely recommended for 16 to 23 hours per day until apical wedging is corrected or until skeletal maturity.

The current indications for surgical treatment are progressive kyphosis despite brace compliance, intractable pain, related neurologic deficit, or a persistent, significant deformity in a skeletally mature patient. The critical threshold of deformity for which surgery is recommended has not been defined. Current research recommendations on surgical indications and surgical approaches are limited to level IV evidence from retrospective cohort studies without control subjects.[12,15]

With earlier instrumentation constructs, surgical correction was followed over time by junctional kyphosis and loss of correction. These results led to interest in concomitant anterior diskectomies. However, combined anteroposterior and posterior-only constructs have had good radiographic results.[15] The anterior-posterior approach led to slightly better maintenance of kyphosis at follow-up, but the complication rate was higher than with the posterior-only approach. Proximal junctional kyphosis occurred in 32% of all patients and was related to arthrodesis below the cephalad end vertebra, a higher magnitude of residual kyphosis, and a high pelvic incidence. Distal junctional kyphosis occurred in 5% of patients and always was associated

with fusion below the sagittal stable vertebra.[15] Posterior-only instrumentation and fusion have become popular, with complete facetectomies and partial excision of the inferior lamina (a so-called Ponte osteotomy). Anterior-posterior and posterior-only procedures without extensive resection have not been compared in a research study. The selection of fusion levels is important and challenging; overcorrection should be avoided (**Figure 1**).

In the type II and lumbar subtypes, as well as pseudo-Scheuermann disease, the predominant deformity is in the thoracolumbar or lumbar spine. These conditions are most commonly seen in adolescent boys who are physically active or do heavy lifting.[16] The patient initially has localized back pain, with or without a clinical or cosmetic deformity. Radiographs reveal vertebral end plate irregularities and Schmorl nodes at and below the thoracolumbar junction, with a loss of lumbar lordosis. The etiology is unknown, although the epidemiology suggests a mechanical cause. Despite their radiographic similarity, thoracic and lumbar Scheuermann disease may be different pathophysiologic entities. Lumbar Scheuermann disease appears to be non-progressive, and its symptoms usually resolve over time with the use of nonsteroidal anti-inflammatory drugs and activity modification.[11]

Iatrogenic Kyphosis

Acquired kyphosis has been widely reported after laminectomy of the cervical or thoracic spine in children.[16,17] Most studies of pediatric iatrogenic spine deformity pertain to the cervical spine. The reported risk of cervical postlaminectomy kyphosis in the pediatric population ranges from 14% to 100%.[16-19] The risk of pediatric deformity has been linked to C2 involvement, relatively young patient age, preoperative malalignment, and irradiation. After surgery for Chiari malformation, the risk of kyphosis appears to increase when the cervical decompression extends below C2.[20]

Although most studies suggest that iatrogenic deformity is most likely in the cervical spine, one study found that the thoracic-thoracolumbar spine had a greater incidence of deformity (60% versus 25%, $P = 0.07$).[21] There was a 16.6% risk of kyphotic deformity after laminectomies at two or more levels in the thoracolumbar region. Patients younger than 18 years had a 50% incidence of deformity, but the risk was only 9% in those age 18 to 30 years.[22] The reported incidence of iatrogenic deformity in the pediatric lumbar spine varies considerably, but deformity appears to occur less frequently in the lumbar spine than in either the thoracic or cervical segments. The lordotic curvature of the lumbar spine may protect it against the development of kyphotic deformity. The current understanding of this pathology in children is limited. It is reasonable to suppose that their lower incidence of iatrogenic lumbar deformity is related to anatomic and physiologic differ-

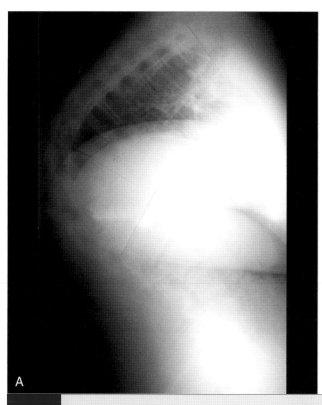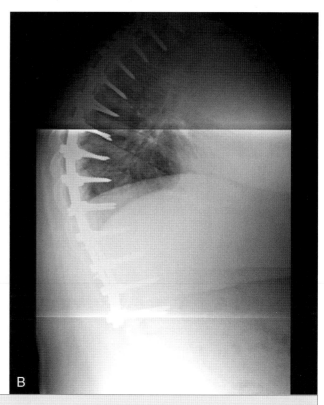

A

B

| Figure 1 | Lateral radiographs of a patient with Scheuermann kyphosis. **A**, Preoperative 90° thoracic kyphosis with prominent wedging of the apical vertebra. **B**, Correction of the kyphosis to 50° after an anterior release and posterior spine fusion. |

ences from adults (in head size, center of gravity, facet orientation, and ligamentous laxity, which predispose children to traumatic cervical spine injury), as well as the biomechanical changes in the spine after laminectomy.

Bracing appears to have a limited role in the long-term management of iatrogenic kyphosis. Although bracing has not been shown to prevent iatrogenic kyphosis after surgery, it can allow surgical intervention to be postponed until the patient reaches skeletal maturity.

During the initial surgical procedure, the surgeon should attempt to minimize the exposure and preserve as much of the facet capsule and facet joint as possible. The surgeon also should avoid involving C2, limit the exposure to as few levels as necessary, and consider performing laminoplasties.[23] The same techniques are used in the cervical and thoracic spine to limit the risk of iatrogenic kyphosis. A concurrent instrumented fusion should be considered when junctional levels are to be bridged or the patient has a preexisting deformity, significant remaining growth potential (generally in a prepubertal patient), planned adjuvant radiation therapy, or a neuromuscular compromise. A variety of osteoplastic laminoplasty techniques have been designed to preserve the dorsal structures. Little comparative research has been reported for the pediatric population, however. In a retrospective comparison of patients treated with laminectomy or laminoplasty after intramedullary tumor resection, the rate of deformity was lower after laminoplasty.[24] After tumor resection, the rate of moderate to severe deformity development was significantly lower in patients who received instrumentation than in patients with laminectomies at four or more levels (10% versus 56%).[25]

The deformity may be diagnosed immediately after the initial surgery or up to 74 months later. Early intervention and frequent follow-up may help limit the severity of deformity. Not all patients require surgical intervention. Progressive deformity, neurologic symptoms, or excessive pain warrant surgical correction, however. A ventral approach is often preferred to correct a severe iatrogenic kyphotic deformity of the cervical spine and stabilize the spine. In some patients, a combined ventral and dorsal stabilization procedure may be required. A thoracolumbar deformity can be treated using an anterior-posterior approach or a corrective technique such as a Ponte osteotomy, pedicle subtraction osteotomy, or vertebral column resection.[26,27]

Congenital Kyphosis

Congenital scoliosis is rare and of unclear etiology; it is estimated to occur in 0.1% of births and is related to

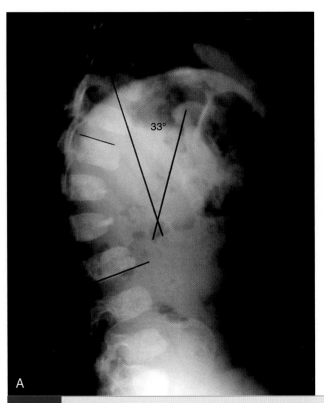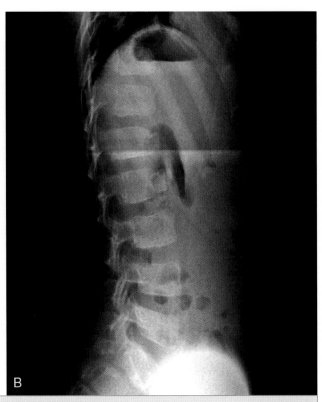

Figure 2 Lateral standing radiographs of a boy with lumbar hypoplasia. **A**, At age 2 years, the child has a 33° kyphosis. The abnormalities are limited to L1 and L2 and have a beaked appearance. **B**, At age 7 years, the child has a 10° kyphosis.

hemivertebra formation. Congenital kyphosis is even less common. Of 584 patients with a congenital spine abnormality, 112 had kyphoscoliosis and only 36 had pure kyphosis.[28] These anomalies can arise at any spine level but are most likely in the thoracolumbar junction between T10 and L1.

A type I anomaly (the most common) is caused by anterior failure of vertebral body formation. The subtypes are posterolateral quadrant vertebra, posterior hemivertebra, butterfly (sagittal cleft) vertebra, and anterior and anterolateral wedged vertebrae. A type II anomaly is derived from an anterior failure of vertebral body segmentation; its subtypes are distinguished by the presence of anterior or anterolateral unsegmented bars. A type III anomaly has characteristics of both type I and type II. A type IV anomaly is otherwise unclassifiable and typically has a larger curve than the other types. The most rapid curve progression is in type III (a mean of 5° to 8° per year, depending on patient age), and the second most rapid progression is in type I. Most neurologic deficits were found in patients with a sharp, angulated curve from a type I malformation.[28]

Congenital kyphoscoliotic deformities can progress rapidly, especially during growth spurts, and they should be monitored closely. Most of these deformities require surgical intervention; only 14 of 112 patients reached skeletal maturity without undergoing surgical intervention.[28] Surgical correction typically is recom-

mended for a significantly progressive curve or after the development of a neurologic deficit. Curve progression typically is defined as more than 10° of change, as radiographic landmarks are difficult to define in these patients. A critical threshold for surgery has not been defined. The surgical intervention typically entails short-segment instrumented fusion; a posterior asymmetric pedicle subtraction osteotomy or anteroposterior vertebral resection may be included. With a pedicle subtraction osteotomy, 10° to 24° of correction per level can be expected, depending on the level.[27]

The preoperative planning should include MRI to detect any intraspinal abnormality that would require neurosurgical intervention before the deformity correction. CT and radiographs are used to visualize the complicated osseous anatomy. The general evaluation should include an echocardiogram and a renal ultrasonogram to detect any associated congenital abnormalities.[29] Although little has been published on the surgical risks for patients with congenital kyphosis, a congenital abnormality of the cervical spine probably entails the greatest risk because of the possibility of injuring the vertebral arteries. Surgery in the thoracic spine carries a risk of neurologic compromise. The least risk is in the lumbar spine.

The available surgical techniques for treating congenital kyphosis include pedicle subtraction osteotomies, vertebrectomies, costotransversectomies, anterior approaches, and combinations.[30-33] A comparison of anteroposterior and posterolateral approaches for treating congenital scoliosis found a higher rate of minor complications in the patients treated through a posterolateral approach (40% versus 8%, P = 0.14). The sample size was relatively small, however.[32] The clinical outcomes, quality of life, and radiographic measures of patients in the two groups were otherwise comparable.[32] The surgical priorities remain restoration of sagittal and coronal balance followed by correction of the curve magnitude. Some further correction can be expected in younger patients as a result of growth and surgical fusion.

Thoracolumbar kyphosis secondary to lumbar hypoplasia is rare but should be differentiated from other etiologies. In seven normal, healthy patients, a mean kyphosis of 34.2° was normalized to −0.4° with no treatment. All patients had a wedge-shaped vertebra at L1 or L2 with an anterosuperior indentation (a beaked appearance)[34] (**Figure 2**). The diagnosis was based on radiographic appearance, lack of anomalies in the posterior elements, and improvement of the kyphosis with bipedal development. Such patients initially should be closely monitored to avoid an incorrect diagnosis, but they do not require bracing. Myelodysplasia, achondroplasia, endocrine abnormality, genetic metabolic disturbance, and other possible etiologies should be excluded from the differential diagnosis.

Summary

Postural kyphosis, Scheuermann kyphosis, iatrogenic kyphosis, and congenital kyphosis are the most common kyphotic deformities in children. However, many other pathologies can give rise to pediatric kyphoscoliosis. The possibility of a spinal cord injury, myelodysplasia, posttuberculous infection, achondroplasia, or inherited metabolic storage disease should be kept in mind during evaluation of a patient with a kyphotic deformity. The appropriate diagnosis is necessary for determining the natural history of the disease and deciding on the management options, based on the severity and progression of the deformity, its clinical presentation, the presence of a neurologic deficit, any cosmetic disfigurement, and the patient's skeletal maturity. The surgeon must carefully balance the expected course of the deformity against the risks and benefits of surgical intervention.

Annotated References

1. Jackson RP, McManus AC: Radiographic analysis of sagittal plane alignment and balance in standing volunteers and patients with low back pain matched for age, sex, and size: A prospective controlled clinical study. *Spine (Phila Pa 1976)* 1994;19(14):1611-1618.

2. Glassman SD, Bridwell K, Dimar JR, Horton W, Berven S, Schwab F: The impact of positive sagittal balance in adult spinal deformity. *Spine (Phila Pa 1976)* 2005; 30(18):2024-2029.

   Retrospective review of a multicenter database identified 352 adult patients with a positive sagittal balance. There was a strong correlation between positive sagittal balance and pain as well as decreased functional ability.

3. Bradford DS, Lonstein JE, Ogilvie JW, Winter RB: *Scoliosis and Other Spinal Deformities*, ed 2. Philadelphia, PA, WB Saunders, 1987.

4. Ascani E, La Rosa G, Ascani C: Scheuermann kyphosis, in Weinstein SL, ed: *The Pediatric Spine: Principles and Practice*, ed 2. Philadelphia, PA, Lippincott Williams & Wilkins, 2001.

5. Sorensen KH: *Scheuermann's Juvenile Kyphosis: Clinical Appearances, Radiography, Aetiology and Prognosis*. Copenhagen, Denmark, Munksgaard, 1964.

6. Bradford DS: Vertebral osteochondrosis (Scheuermann's kyphosis). *Clin Orthop Relat Res* 1981;158:83-90.

7. Bradford DS, Moe JH, Montalvo FJ, Winter RB: Scheuermann's kyphosis and roundback deformity: Results of Milwaukee brace treatment. *J Bone Joint Surg Am* 1974;56(4):740-758.

8. Winter R: The treatment of spinal kyphosis. *Int Orthop* 1991;15(3):265-271.

9. Bradford DS, Ahmed KB, Moe JH, Winter RB, Lonstein JE: The surgical management of patients with Scheuermann's disease: A review of twenty-four cases managed by combined anterior and posterior spine fusion. *J Bone Joint Surg Am* 1980;62(5):705-712.

10. Tribus CB: Scheuermann's kyphosis in adolescents and adults: Diagnosis and management. *J Am Acad Orthop Surg* 1998;6(1):36-43.

11. Wenger DR, Frick SL: Scheuermann kyphosis. *Spine (Phila Pa 1976)* 1999;24(24):2630-2639.

12. Lowe TG, Line BG: Evidence based medicine: Analysis of Scheuermann kyphosis. *Spine (Phila Pa 1976)* 2007; 32(19, suppl):S115-S119.

    A review of the literature on managing Scheuermann kyphosis found that current treatment recommendations are based on level III, IV, and V evidence.

13. Riddle EC, Bowen JR, Shah SA, Moran EF, Lawall HJ Jr: The duPont kyphosis brace for the treatment of adolescent Scheuermann kyphosis. *J South Orthop Assoc* 2003;12(3):135-140.

14. Sachs B, Bradford DS, Winter R, Lonstein J, Moe J, Willson S: Scheuermann kyphosis: Follow-up of Milwaukee-brace treatment. *J Bone Joint Surg Am* 1987;69(1):50-57.

5: Spine

15. Lonner BS, Newton P, Betz R, et al: Operative management of Scheuermann's kyphosis in 78 patients: Radiographic outcomes, complications, and technique. *Spine (Phila Pa 1976)* 2007;32(24):2644-2652.

    A retrospective, multicenter study compared anteroposterior and posterior-only fusion in patients with Scheuermann kyphosis. Level of evidence: IV.

16. de Jonge T, Slullitel H, Dubousset J, Miladi L, Wicart P, Illés T: Late-onset spinal deformities in children treated by laminectomy and radiation therapy for malignant tumours. *Eur Spine J* 2005;14(8):765-771.

    This is a study of patients who developed spine deformity after undergoing a surgical procedure or radiation treatment. Level of evidence: IV.

17. Yasuoka S, Peterson HA, Laws ER Jr, MacCarty CS: Pathogenesis and prophylaxis of postlaminectomy deformity of the spine after multiple level laminectomy: Difference between children and adults. *Neurosurgery* 1981;9(2):145-152.

18. Bell DF, Walker JL, O'Connor G, Tibshirani R: Spinal deformity after multiple-level cervical laminectomy in children. *Spine (Phila Pa 1976)* 1994;19(4):406-411.

19. Sim FH, Svien HJ, Bickel WH, Janes JM: Swan-neck deformity following extensive cervical laminectomy: A review of twenty-one cases. *J Bone Joint Surg Am* 1974; 56(3):564-580.

20. Gangemi M, Renier D, Daussange J, Hirsch JF, Rigault P: Children's cervical spine instability after posterior fossa surgery. *Acta Neurol (Napoli)* 1982;4(1):39-43.

21. Yeh JS, Sgouros S, Walsh AR, Hockley AD: Spinal sagittal malalignment following surgery for primary intramedullary tumours in children. *Pediatr Neurosurg* 2001;35(6):318-324.

22. Papagelopoulos PJ, Peterson HA, Ebersold MJ, Emmanuel PR, Choudhury SN, Quast LM: Spinal column deformity and instability after lumbar or thoracolumbar laminectomy for intraspinal tumors in children and young adults. *Spine (Phila Pa 1976)* 1997;22(4):442-451.

23. Ratliff JK, Cooper PR: Cervical laminoplasty: A critical review. *J Neurosurg* 2003;98(3, suppl):230-238.

24. McGirt MJ, Chaichana KL, Atiba A, et al: Incidence of spinal deformity after resection of intramedullary spinal cord tumors in children who underwent laminectomy compared with laminoplasty. *J Neurosurg Pediatr* 2008; 1(1):57-62.

    The incidence of spine deformity is compared in children who underwent laminectomy or laminoplasty. Level of evidence: IV.

25. Simon SL, Auerbach JD, Garg S, Sutton LN, Telfeian AE, Dormans JP: Efficacy of spinal instrumentation and fusion in the prevention of postlaminectomy spinal deformity in children with intramedullary spinal cord tumors. *J Pediatr Orthop* 2008;28(2):244-249.

    This is a retrospective comparison of the rates of spine deformity in children who underwent laminectomy or concurrent spine fusion–laminectomy. Level of evidence: IV.

26. Sciubba DM, Gallia GL, McGirt MJ, et al: Thoracic kyphotic deformity reduction with a distractible titanium cage via an entirely posterior approach. *Neurosurgery* 2007;60(4, suppl 2):223-231.

    A posterior-only approach was used for modified bilateral costotransversectomy to correct kyphotic deformity in seven patients. The mean correction of focal kyphosis was from 28.6° to 12.1°.

27. O'Shaughnessy BA, Kuklo TR, Hsieh PC, Yang BP, Koski TR, Ondra SL: Thoracic pedicle subtraction osteotomy for fixed sagittal spinal deformity. *Spine (Phila Pa 1976)* 2009;34(26):2893-2899.

    A retrospective review of 25 thoracic pedicle subtraction osteotomies found that the procedure can be safely performed in the thoracic spine. The maximal correction of sagittal deformity was obtained in the lower thoracic vertebrae.

28. McMaster MJ, Singh H: Natural history of congenital kyphosis and kyphoscoliosis: A study of one hundred and twelve patients. *J Bone Joint Surg Am* 1999;81(10): 1367-1383.

29. Chan G, Dormans JP: Update on congenital spinal deformities: Preoperative evaluation. *Spine (Phila Pa 1976)* 2009;34(17):1766-1774.

    Recommendations for the preoperative evaluation of patients with a congential spine deformity are summarized in this literature review.

30. Smith JT, Gollogly S, Dunn HK: Simultaneous anterior-posterior approach through a costotransversectomy for the treatment of congenital kyphosis and acquired kyphoscoliotic deformities. *J Bone Joint Surg Am* 2005; 87(10):2281-2289.

    Fifteen of 16 patients with congenital kyphosis or kyphoscoliosis had anteroposterior arthrodesis through a costotransversectomy. Overall results were good, with a mean correction of 31°. Four patients had complications. Level of evidence: IV.

31. Lenke LG, O'Leary PT, Bridwell KH, Sides BA, Koester LA, Blanke KM: Posterior vertebral column resection for severe pediatric deformity: Minimum two-year follow-up of thirty-five consecutive patients. *Spine (Phila Pa 1976)* 2009;34(20):2213-2221.

    Thirty-five patients were treated with vertebral column resection to correct a significant deformity. The results were good. Four patients had complications. The authors recommend a posterior-only approach for this procedure.

32. Jalanko T, Rintala R, Puisto V, Helenius I: Hemivertebra resection for congenital scoliosis in young children. *Spine (Phila Pa 1976)* 2010;36(1):41-49.

Retrospective comparison of 12 anterior-posterior and 11 posterior-only procedures for congenital scoliosis found a 40% rate of minor complications in the patients treated using a posterior-only approach and an 8% rate in those treated using an anterior-posterior approach.

33. Ruf M, Jensen R, Letko L, Harms J: Hemivertebra resection and osteotomies in congenital spine deformity. *Spine (Phila Pa 1976)* 2009;34(17):1791-1799.

A posterior-only approach was used to treat 41 patients with congenital scoliosis. The compensatory curves improved after correction. Early intervention is recommended.

34. Campos MA, Fernandes P, Dolan LA, Weinstein SL: Infantile thoracolumbar kyphosis secondary to lumbar hypoplasia. *J Bone Joint Surg Am* 2008;90(8):1726-1729.

All patients with thoracolumbar kyphosis secondary to lumbar hypoplasia had resolution without intervention. Level of evidence: IV.

5: Spine

Cervical Abnormalities, Back Pain, and the Surgical Treatment of Spondylolysis and Spondylolisthesis

Firoz Miyanji, MD, FRCSC

5: Spine

Introduction

The anatomy and biomechanics of the pediatric cervical spine are unique. Patterns of injury and nontraumatic instability as well as osseoligamentous anomalies are significantly different in the pediatric and adult populations. In children, the cervical spine frequently has an important role in the diagnosis of skeletal dysplasias and congenital syndromes. The pattern of involvement of the cervical spine in these children needs to be carefully evaluated to avoid any serious neurologic sequelae.

Back pain in children and adolescents formerly was considered rare and sinister, but more recent research suggests that back pain is relatively common in the pediatric population. Often there is no identifiable pathologic cause, but a focused assessment will help identify patients requiring further evaluation.

Spondylolysis and spondylolisthesis in children have a relatively benign course. In some patients, however, surgical intervention is warranted. Several different surgical options are available; they have the common goal of resolving symptoms and restoring the sagittal profile. No consensus exists on the surgical management of these patients, but interest is emerging in developing and applying newer classification schemes that can be useful in surgical decision making.

Cervical Abnormalities

Developmental Anatomy of the Pediatric Cervical Spine

By the fourth week of gestation, there are 42 to 44 pairs of somites (4 occipital, 8 cervical, 12 thoracic, 5 lumbar, 5 sacral, and 8 to 10 sacrococcygeal), each of which differentiates into a dermatome, myotome, and

Dr. Miyanji or an immediate family member serves as a paid consultant to or is an employee of DePuy, a Johnson & Johnson company; and has received research or institutional support from DePuy, a Johnson & Johnson company.

medial sclerotome. After the division of each sclerotome, the individual vertebral body is formed by the union of the superior half of one sclerotome to the lower half of its neighbor.

The occiput, atlas, and axis are formed by different mechanisms. The first spinal sclerotome gives rise to the atlas. The atlas is formed from three ossification centers: the anterior arch and two lateral masses. The anterior arch may not be ossified at birth, but it becomes visible as one or two ossification centers during the first year of life. The lateral masses must be present at birth, however. The lateral masses remain posteriorly separated by a remnant cartilaginous cleft, which usually ossifies by age 3 to 4 years to complete the ring. The axis is formed from three separate sclerotomes: the terminal portion of the dens is formed by the fourth occipital sclerotome (the proatlas), the dens is formed from the first spinal sclerotome, and the axis body is formed by the second spinal sclerotome. At birth, the body of the axis and the dens are separated by a vestigial disk called the neural central synchondrosis. It is important to recognize that the synchondrosis is located below the anatomic base of the dens and does not represent the anatomic base of the dens. The synchondrosis is present in most children younger than 3 to 4 years but disappears by age 8 years. The tip of the dens is not ossified at birth but is represented by a separate ossification center, which usually is apparent by age 3 years. The tip fuses to the remainder of the dens by age 12 years (**Figure 1**).

Radiographic Parameters

Several radiographic parameters are useful in interpreting pediatric cervical radiographs and avoiding the potentially devastating consequences of an undiagnosed abnormality. These parameters include measurements of the craniocervical junction, defined as the region from the basiocciput to the second cervical interspace (**Figure 2**). Atlanto-occipital instability can be assessed on plain radiographs using the Powers ratio, the basion-axial interval (BAI), the basion-dens interval (BDI), and the atlanto-occipital joint space. A Powers ratio of less than or equal to 1 is considered normal.

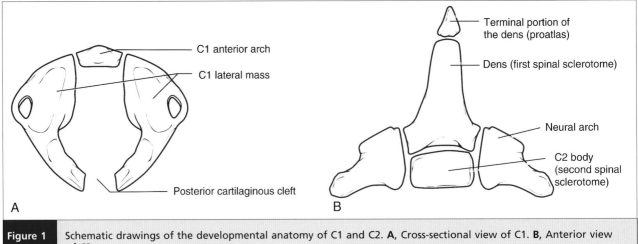

Figure 1 Schematic drawings of the developmental anatomy of C1 and C2. **A**, Cross-sectional view of C1. **B**, Anterior view of C2.

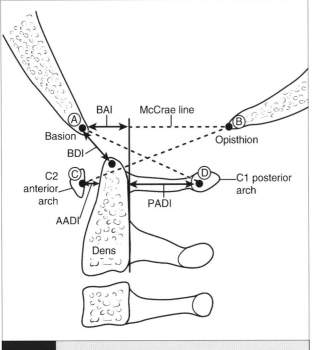

Figure 2 Schematic drawing of the upper cervical spine showing a lateral view of common radiographic parameters. The Powers ratio = AD/BC. AADI = anterior atlantodens interval, BAI = basion-axial interval, BDI = basion-dens interval, PADI = posterior atlantodens interval.

BAI and BDI values less than or equal to 12 mm are considered normal. Although one researcher specified that the atlanto-occipital joint space in children should measure less than 5 mm at any point in the joint,[1] others arbitrarily chose 2 mm as normal.[2] The reported sensitivity of the Powers ratio is 33% to 60%, and that of the BDI is 50%. The BAI is reported to be as sensitive as 100% for detecting true atlanto-occipital injury.[3] In children in particular, these radiographic parameters have been difficult to assess because of the difficulty of accurately observing the involved anatomic structures. A comparison of the interobserver and intraobserver reliability of three different techniques used to measure atlanto-occipital instability found that measurement of atlanto-occipital translation by any of the methods was not reproducible in children with Down syndrome, and the authors challenged the reliability of plain radiographs for quantifying instability at the craniocervical junction.[4] A recent study encouraged the use of CT for revealing the craniocervical junction anatomy[5] (**Figure 3**). Improved sensitivity, specificity, and positive and negative predictive values were reported with CT for the radiographic parameters commonly used in diagnosing atlanto-occipital instability. A BDI of more than 10 mm on CT was recommended as the diagnostic test of choice for confirming atlanto-occipital dissociation because of its ease of use and accuracy for this purpose.[6]

Atlantoaxial instability has commonly been assessed using the anterior atlantodens interval (AADI). In addition to its wide use as a tool for evaluating motion, the AADI is valuable as a marker for predicting cord compression at the atlantoaxial junction. The AADI was found to average 1.9 mm in very young children and to reach 2.45 mm in adolescents.[7] An AADI of less than 3 mm is considered normal between flexion and extension excursion in patients older than 8 years; in younger patients the limit is 5 mm. It is important to note that all of these values were obtained from patients with normal cervical anatomy. No current literature has determined whether AADI values beyond these are predictive of cord compression or subluxation. Some authors have suggested that minimal sagittal diameter is an important factor in developing myelopathy, but others believe that the degree of instability is more significant.[8] Although cord compression in adults has been reported when the canal diameter is 14 mm or less, no similar age-related criteria exist for children.[9]

The posterior atlantodens interval (PADI), particularly in flexion, may be more useful than the AADI for

5: Spine

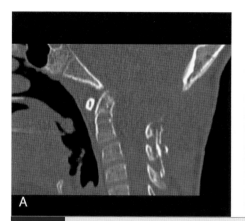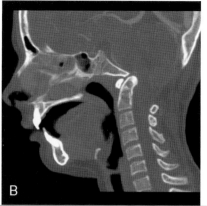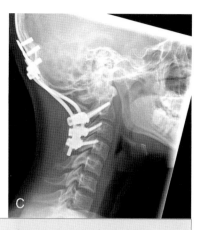

Figure 3 Progressive craniocervical instability in an 11-year-old girl. **A,** Midsagittal CT showing craniocervical instability. **B,** Midsagittal CT showing basilar invagination with increasing acuity of the clivodentate angle. **C,** Lateral cervical spine radiograph showing an occipitocervical fusion for stabilization.

identifying an increased risk of significant neurologic symptoms, particularly in patients with a chronic condition. The PADI represents the space available for the spinal cord (SAC) at the atlantoaxial junction. Absolute stenosis is defined as flexion PADI of less than 10 mm, and relative stenosis is reported to be 10 to 13 mm. In children, there is uncertainty as to the narrowing of the canal diameter beyond which cord compression occurs, but this measurement can be inferred from the age-related diameter of the cord. The AP cord diameter was reported to range from 4.5 mm in newborns to a maximum of 9 mm in older children.[10] A longitudinal prospective study found average canal diameters in the upper cervical spine of approximately 13 mm at age 6 months and 16 mm in adolescence.[7]

The use of CT or MRI is the best means of confirming basilar invagination and spinal stenosis. Spinal stenosis is represented by the direct measurement of the SAC. CT and MRI are static examinations; because patients most often have dynamic instability, an emphasis on flexion-extension views should be maintained. There is an emerging interest in using dynamic MRI for assessing cervical instability.[11]

Craniocervical Junction Abnormalities

Craniocervical junction instability of nontraumatic origin represents approximately 27% of all craniocervical instability in children. Os odontoideum, Down syndrome, Klippel-Feil syndrome, skeletal dysplasias, and mucopolysaccharidosis are commonly associated with symptomatic craniocervical instability.

Os Odontoideum

The os odontoideum probably is an independent bone lying cranial to the body of the axis; it should not be considered as an isolated dens but exists apart from a small hypoplastic dens.[12] The borders are smooth on radiographs, and a small dens is always present. The os is located near the basiocciput, where it may fuse with the clivus. The os can be orthotopic if it maintains its normal relationship with the clivus and moves in unison with the axis and atlas. A dystrophic os lies close to the base of the clivus and moves as an extension of the clivus, thus increasing the risk of neurologic injury. The cruciate ligament usually is incompetent, and atlantoaxial instability can result. In severe chronic dislocation, the os may become fixed, with resultant basilar invagination causing compression of the cervicomedullary junction.

Os odontoideum is frequently seen in patients with Down syndrome, spondyloepiphyseal dysplasia, or Morquio-Brailsford syndrome. Although both congenital and traumatic etiologies of os odontoideum have been proposed, there is growing consensus as to the traumatic etiology of os odontoideum.[13,14] The gap between the os and the remnant odontoid rarely is seen at the level of the neurocentral synchondrosis, which is often visible beneath the gap. This observation challenges the congenital theory. More often, the gap between the remnant odontoid and the os extends above the level of the superior axis facets, and this factor suggests that the abnormality is acquired. A traumatic Salter-Harris–type physeal injury is believed to explain incidences in which the gap appears at the anatomic level of the synchondrosis.[14] The instability may be fixed or reducible. The well-established potential for sudden death or significant morbidity highlights the importance of diagnosing this lesion on the initial radiographs. Surgical stabilization of atlantoaxial instability usually is recommended in the presence of os odontoideum[14] (**Figure 4**).

Down Syndrome

Approximately 14% to 20% of patients with Down syndrome have atlantoaxial instability, and approximately 1% have symptomatic C1-C2 instability requiring surgery. Long-term studies on the natural history of craniocervical instability in this patient population are lacking, however. Routine radiographic screening for

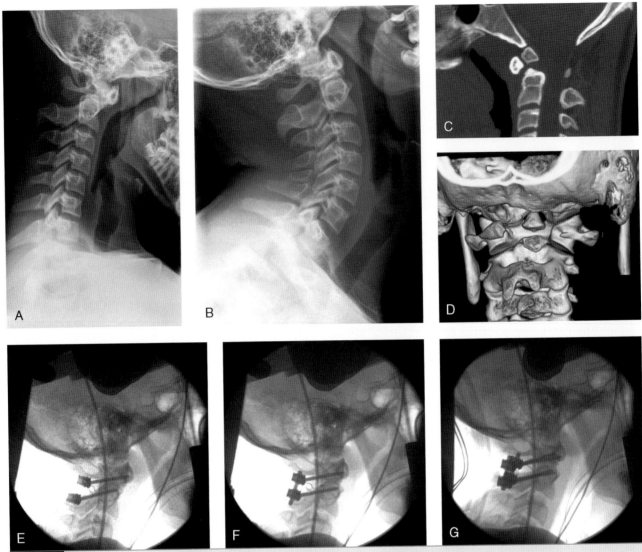

Figure 4 Atlantoaxial instability resulting from an os odontoideum in a 12-year-old boy. Lateral flexion (**A**) and extension (**B**) cervical spine radiographs showing a compromised AADI and PADI. **C**, Midsagittal CT confirming the presence of an os odontoideum. **D**, Posterior-view reformatted three-dimensional CT, revealing the absence of the posterior arch of C1. Intraoperative lateral cervical spine fluoroscopic views, showing C1 lateral mass screws and C2 pedicle screws before rod placement, with anterior subluxation of C1 on C2 (**E**); and the reduction of deformity-instability of C1-C2, with the rod in situ (**F**). **G**, Postoperative lateral cervical spine fluoroscopic view of the segmental C1 lateral mass and C2 pedicle screw fixation, which allowed preservation of occiput-C1 motion.

atlantoaxial instability remains controversial. The American Academy of Pediatrics concluded that screening radiographs for children with Down syndrome are of "potential but unproven value" in detecting individuals at risk for sports injury.[15] The American Academy of Pediatrics Committee on Genetics recommends that one set of cervical spine radiographs be taken when the child is age 3 to 5 years.[16] If the results are normal, some authors recommend repeating the radiographs every 5 years.[17,18] Radiographic studies are more important for participants in contact sports or for children who have symptoms of craniocervical or upper cervical instability.

The optimal management of patients with asymptomatic atlantoaxial subluxation remains controversial, as it is difficult to predict whether a patient with radiographic instability will develop symptoms. Patients with an ADI of at least 7 mm may be at particular risk of developing symptomatic instability.[17] If a patient has an ADI of more than 4.5 mm or a PADI of less than 14 mm, MRI should be obtained to assess for cord injury. Close observation is recommended for asymptomatic patients with abnormal radiographs, a benign clinical examination, and normal MRI findings. These patients should avoid high-risk activities such as contact sports, gymnastics, or diving. Surgery is indicated if a patient has more than 8 to 10 mm of subluxation at the occiput-C1 level, MRI findings of cord compression or myelopathy, abnormal neurology, or concomitant osseous abnormalities such as os odontoideum, odontoid hypoplasia, or abnormal ossification of the C1 arch.[18,19] Fusion rates as low as 40% have been reported in children with Down syndrome, but these findings are being challenged by the use of modern techniques.[18,20,21]

Klippel-Feil Syndrome

Congenital vertebral fusion of at least two cervical vertebrae (most commonly at C2-C3), leading to a limited neck range of motion, is one of the classic clinical symptoms of Klippel-Feil syndrome. Long-term sequelae including radiculopathy, pain, spasticity, quadriplegia, and sudden death occur in 22% to 43% of patients.[22,23] Basilar invagination and instability and hypermobility at the motion segment adjacent to the fused vertebrae may be the mechanisms of neurologic sequelae. Pathologic changes within the spinal cord itself also have been documented in the literature.[24]

Atlantoaxial hypermobility is associated with occipitalization of C1 and fusion of the C2-C3 segment. Reports of hypermobility at the atlantoaxial joint leading to neurologic symptoms were refuted by a finding that an increased AADI was not associated with developing neurology and that the greatest atlantoaxial motion occurred in the presence of occipitalization of C1 with concomitant fusion of C2-C3.[25] Other studies documented that children with Klippel-Feil syndrome have smaller cross-sectional spinal cord dimensions than age-matched control subjects[26] and that smaller vertebral body widths in the fused segments contribute to an increase in the SAC.[27]

Achondroplasia

Spine involvement in patients with achondroplasia commonly includes foramen magnum stenosis with cervicomedullary compression. In older children, multisegment spinal stenosis of the subaxial cervical spine or the lumbar spine may also be seen. Foramen magnum stenosis in these patients is a direct result of defective enchondral bone growth and premature fusion of the two posterior basal synchondroses. In addition, patients with achondroplasia often have a posteriorly and superiorly projected odontoid process, which leads to further compression at the craniocervical junction. CT was used to confirm that 96% of patients with achondroplasia had significant narrowing of the foramen magnum compared with age-matched control subjects.[28] Neurologic sequelae include myelopathy, hydrocephalus, respiratory disorders, and sudden death. In infants, cervicomedullary compression may appear with hypotonia, poor head control, feeding or sleep disturbances, and apnea. For symptomatic patients, foramen magnum decompression can be performed with a relatively low rate of morbidity.

Spinal stenosis in patients with achondroplasia results from premature fusion of the ossification centers of the vertebral bodies and posterior neural arches, causing short, thick laminae and pedicles. The vertebral bodies have a reduced height, the neural foramina are small, and the interpedicular distance is narrowed. Projection of the superior and inferior end plates into the spinal canal causes further narrowing. The manifestations of cervical stenosis include paraparesis or quadriparesis, ataxia with frequent falls, spasticity, bladder or bowel dysfunction, intermittent claudication, or temporary spinal cord deterioration after minor trauma. Posterior decompression is a good option for a symptomatic patient, but multilevel decompressive laminectomies may require fusion for stability.

Spondyloepiphyseal Dysplasia

Cervical manifestations are relatively common in spondyloepiphyseal dysplasia, often occurring as atlantoaxial instability associated with odontoid hypoplasia or ligamentous laxity. The incidence of cervical myelopathy attributable to C1-C2 subluxation is as high as 35%.[29] Myelopathy may develop gradually and appear as delayed achievement of motor milestones, progressive weakness, spasticity, or respiratory abnormality.

A study of the risk factors for myelopathy found an ADI greater than 5 mm in most patients.[30] Progression of atlantoaxial subluxation with age and increasing AADI has been reported.[29] The sagittal canal diameter usually is small in patients with spondyloepiphyseal dysplasia. Those with a C2 diameter of 10 mm or less are at increased risk for cord compression. There is a high frequency of os odontoideum, which also is associated with a narrowed sagittal canal at C1. Narrowing of the canal may persist despite reduction, requiring laminectomy decompression of the C1 arch followed by a posterior fusion. Occipitocervical fusions previously were recommended, but a recent study suggests that newer techniques may allow isolated C1-C2 fusion that preserves occipitocervical motion.[21]

Morquio-Brailsford Syndrome

The cervical spine manifestations of Morquio-Brailsford syndrome are a combination of os odontoideum, atlantoaxial instability, and cervicothoracic abnormalities. The most common and potentially serious condition is atlantoaxial subluxation with cord compression, which occurs as a result of odontoid dysplasia (hypoplasia, aplasia, or os odontoideum) and ligamentous laxity. Regardless of the presence of symptoms, surgical intervention should be considered for patients who have neurologic involvement, an AADI greater than 8 mm, or an SAC lower than 14 mm.[31] Some authors recommend considering surgery when the child is age 3 to 8 years because skeletal maldevelopment usually is complete by this age.[32]

A patient with Morquio-Brailsford syndrome may have progressive cervical stenosis caused by thickening of the extradural soft tissues and continuous deposition of glycosaminoglycans in the adjacent soft tissues, leading to severe cord compression and neurologic involvement.[32,33] Cartilage or fibrocartilage reactive hypertrophy, dural thickening caused by glycosaminoglycan accumulation, and ligamentum flavum hypertrophy contribute to severe cervical stenosis at the atlantoaxial junction and may not be associated with clear instability.[33] Occipitocervical fusion and decompression promote regression of the cartilaginous and ligamentous hypertrophy.[32]

Trauma

Although cervical spine injury is generally uncommon, approximately half of all pediatric spine injuries occur in the cervical spine. Motor vehicles crashes are the most common cause. In neonates, obstetric complications are a common cause of cervical injury. In infants and toddlers, the leading causes of cervical injury are falls, motor vehicle crashes, and nonaccidental trauma. In children older than 3 years, sporting accidents and motor vehicle crashes are the most common causes. The injury patterns are a direct result of the unique anatomy and kinetics of the pediatric cervical spine. A large head-to-body ratio and intrinsic elasticity, especially in children younger than 8 years, commonly lead to injury between the occiput and C2. In young children, the fulcrum for flexion is at approximately C2-C3. With increasing age, the head-to-body mass ratio decreases, and the fulcrum moves caudally to the C5-C6 level. The horizontal orientation and shallow nature of the facet joints in children increase translational mobility and movement during flexion-extension. Pediatric and adult cervical spine kinematics were compared using the helical axis of motion (a three-dimensional analogue defined as an axis along which an object translates and about which it rotates).[34] Cervical spine kinematics were found to vary with both age and sex; girls had a more anterior helical axis of motion in flexion-extension and axial rotation than either adult women or adult men. These differences in cervical spine kinematics may account for the greater incidence of upper cervical spine injury in children than in adults.

Atlanto-occipital dissociation and C1-C2 injuries in children are highly unstable and pose both diagnostic and management challenges (**Figure 5**). When surgical intervention is warranted, consideration must be given to the small size as well as the growth potential of the pediatric spine.

Subaxial Instability

Pseudosubluxation

Many normal variants of the pediatric cervical spine are recognized. One of the more common is nonpathologic forward slippage of C2 on C3; this condition is termed C2-C3 pseudosubluxation. Ligamentous laxity, horizontal configuration of the apophyseal joints, a relatively high fulcrum of flexion, and lack of development of the uncovertebral joints are thought to be contributing factors. C2-C3 pseudosubluxation is most common in children younger than 8 years but has been reported in older children and young adults. The spinolaminar line has been used for differentiating physiologic and pathologic displacement; if the cortex of the posterior arch of C2 lies more than 1.5 mm beyond this line, pathologic injury should be suspected.[35] This interpretation can be difficult in an infant with indistinct cortices, a patient with a hypoplastic or unfused posterior C1 arch, or a patient with other physical or radiographic signs of injury. Pseudosubluxation is uncommon in children older than 10 years but is most likely to occur at C4-C5 or C5-C6 because of the descent of the apex of flexion from C2-C3 to more distal levels.

Syndrome-Related Abnormalities and Dysplasias

Cervical kyphosis the most serious of the wide variety of spine anomalies reported in Larsen syndrome. The incidence of cervical kyphosis is approximately 12% in patients with Larsen syndrome, usually focused at the C4-C5 level. Progressive instability, myelopathy, and sudden death can occur. The natural history remains poorly defined, and long-term studies on optimal treatment are lacking. There is ongoing debate as to surveillance, bracing, timing of surgery, and surgical approach.

Baseline radiographs with serial surveillance are recommended. Plain radiographs can be supplemented with CT and MRI if warranted. Surgical intervention usually is required. Fusion is difficult in a child younger than 1 year, and bracing may be used until surgery is planned after age 18 months.[36] Some authors favor early treatment of cervical kyphosis using posterior fusion only but caution that its use should be limited to patients with flexible deformity.[37] Others recommend combined anterior and posterior approaches, with long constructs extending beyond the affected segments for optimal outcome.[38] The latter treatment is best for patients with anteroposterior dissociation and absent pedicles, resulting in complete separation of the laminae and vertebral bodies at multiple levels.[36]

Patients with diastrophic dysplasia commonly have cervical kyphosis, anterior hypoplasia (most often at C3-C5), and hyperplasia with dysmorphism of the odontoid process. The cervical kyphosis in diastrophic dysplasia usually is present at birth, improves during growth, and seldom requires treatment. Severe progression has been reported, however, with resultant quadriplegia and death. Spontaneous resolution normally begins when children can hold the head up. This movement is believed to strengthen the extensor muscles, reducing the kyphosis and therefore the pathologic load on the cartilaginous anterior vertebral bodies. The decreased mechanical stress facilitates the growth of the vertebrae into a more normal shape. Kyphosis exceeding 60° and a round or triangular posteriorly displaced apex vertebra may be related to a poor prognosis with continued progression. MRI may reveal widening of the foramen magnum and early disk degeneration with narrowing of the spinal canal.

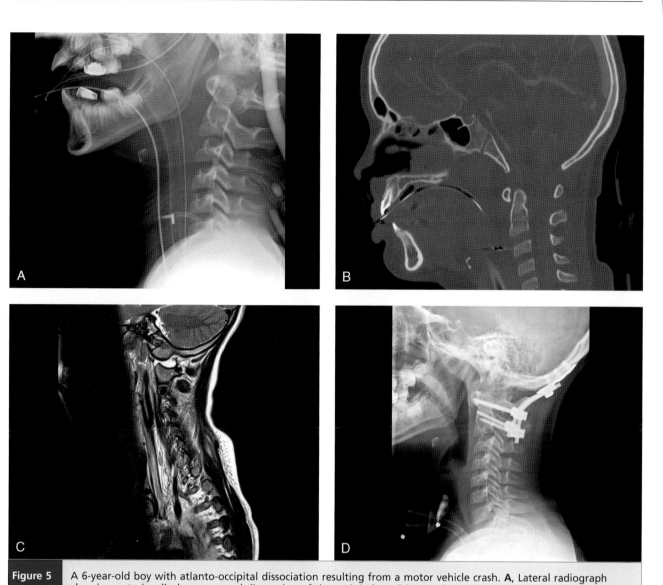

Figure 5   A 6-year-old boy with atlanto-occipital dissociation resulting from a motor vehicle crash. **A**, Lateral radiograph showing anterior displacement and distraction of the occipital condyles on the C1 lateral mass. **B**, Midsagittal CT showing a BDI of 13.3 mm. **C**, MRI of the atlanto-occiptal joint showing a distraction injury with fluid in the joint space. **D**, Lateral cervical spine radiograph showing atlanto-occipital stabilization and fusion with modern cervical instrumentation.

Trauma

The movement of the fulcrum of flexion distally from C2-C3 in infants and young children to C5-C6 in adolescents explains the distribution of traumatic subaxial spine injuries. Cervical spine injury most commonly occurs in the subaxial spine of older children because their biomechanics more closely resemble that of adults. Some authors believe that more stringent radiographic criteria than normally used should be applied for cervical instability in children.[39,40] Angulation greater than 7°, translation of more than 4.5 mm in younger children, and subluxation of more than 3.5 mm in children older than 8 years should raise suspicion of injury.

Most pediatric cervical spine injuries can be managed with external immobilization. Modern instrumentation techniques for internal fixation include the use of posterior lateral-mass screw-rod constructs. Anterior plating systems are increasingly used; they have the advantage of obviating the need for postoperative immobilization and avoiding the frequent complications of halo orthosis.

Summary

The pediatric cervical spine is commonly involved in congenital syndromes, skeletal dysplasias, and trauma. In the presence of craniocervical anomalies, atlantoaxial instability is fairly common. Spinal canal encroachment may be caused by static or dynamic factors. Plain radiographs remain a useful screening tool for assessing segmental instability, but dynamic MRI is gaining favor. The association between instability and neurologic

5: Spine

sequelae remains poorly defined. MRI is warranted in the presence of neurologic symptoms or radiographic concern about instability. Newer instrumentation techniques providing rigid fixation for stabilization and arthrodesis are increasingly popular for children because of possibly lower complication rates.

Back Pain in Children and Adolescents

Population-based studies have varied considerably in their definition of back pain in children and adolescents. Studies primarily of school-age children found a prevalence of 83% in France, 51% in Denmark, 22% in the United States, 24% in England, 17% in Iran, and 20.5% in Italy.[41-45] The incidence is reported to increase with increasing age; reports of back pain are more common in adolescents older than 15 years than in younger children.

Back pain in the pediatric population previously was considered an indicator of serious pathology; a large proportion of pediatric patients who reported back pain were found to have a diagnosable pathologic condition. However, relatively recent studies have found rates of benign unidentifiable pathology ranging from 54% to 78%.[46,47] These findings suggest that children, and especially adolescents, may not routinely require an elaborate workup but instead should receive a more limited and focused assessment.

Patient Evaluation

History

The most important elements in developing a differential diagnosis are the patient history and physical examination. The onset, duration, frequency, location, severity, and quality of pain should be recorded, as well as whether the pain is radiating. Any associated constitutional symptoms such as fever, chills, night sweats, nocturnal pain, or changes in appetite or weight should be noted. Pain exacerbated by exercise and relieved by rest is infrequently associated with pathology. Early morning stiffness can suggest an inflammatory process, and nocturnal pain is highly indicative of tumor or infection.

Alleviating or aggravating factors should be noted as well as any antecedent events such as trauma or a prodrome of flulike illness. Any infectious contacts or recent travel as well as any earlier treatments and responses should be documented. Pain related to osteoid osteoma characteristically is nocturnal and markedly improves when nonsteroidal anti-inflammatory drugs (NSAIDs) are used. Unremitting pain points to infection or malignancy. General or specific arthralgias, skin lesions, or abdominal pain can help broaden the differential diagnosis to include inflammatory arthritides. Functional impairment caused by the back pain is an important means of quantifying severity.

A general medical history, family history, and social history are important to rule out any associated conditions predisposing the child to back pain, including psychosomatic conditions. The patient's activity level and sporting endeavors may offer clues; gymnasts, football linemen, and wrestlers are at high risk for spondylolysis, commonly causing low back pain.

Physical Examination

The patient should be assessed standing, supine, and prone. The initial assessment begins with the patient's height, weight, and general health. The patient's gait and movement are evaluated; abnormalities may suggest a neuromuscular disorder. Midline skin defects or café-au-lait spots can indicate the presence of spinal dysraphism. Palpation and percussion of the spine throughout its length are useful for reproducing the pain and detecting midline or paraspinal tenderness, palpable masses, a gap or step in the posterior elements (spondylolisthesis), or paraspinal muscle spasms. Structural deformities can be ruled out by using a forward bend test to look for asymmetric rib prominence, which suggests a scoliosis, or a focal gibbus, as in Scheuermann kyphosis. The active range of motion of the lumbar spine should be documented. Pain aggravated by forward flexion or pain during extension-recovery suggests, respectively, a discogenic or posterior arch pathology (such as spondylosis). Pain with single-leg hyperextension can be specific to the side of a spondylolytic stress fracture.

A complete neurologic examination is mandatory, with assessment of motor, sensory, deep-tendon, and superficial reflexes. Nerve root tension signs can reveal the presence of radiculopathy. The provocative flexion-abduction–external rotation test is useful for sacroiliac assessment. The hips should be examined. Hamstring tightness should be examined by assessing the popliteal angle, which can be diminished in spondylolisthesis, symptomatic spondylolysis, and overuse syndromes.

The probability of a specific diagnosis was analyzed based on criteria from the history and physical examination.[48] Constant pain, night pain, radicular pain, and abnormal neurologic examination were found to have high specificity for the presence of a specific diagnosis. The probability of a specific diagnosis was 100% if the patient had three of the four predictors, 86% with two predictors, 61% with one predictor, and 19% with no predictors. The presence of these clinical markers should alert the physician to a high probability of underlying pathology warranting further investigation.

Imaging

Diagnostic imaging is warranted if the patient does not respond to nonsurgical measures, the pain or functional difficulty is escalating, or the history or physical examination includes a red-flag finding such as age younger than 10 years, night pain, fever, weight loss, malaise, limp or altered gait, abnormal neurologic examination, or pain lasting several weeks.

Plain radiographs are recommended for initial imaging of back pain.[47] Most diagnoses can be made through plain radiographs in conjunction with a thorough history and physical examination. Plain radiographs are up to 68% sensitive and specific for diagnosis.[47] The choice of an additional radiographic modality is controversial. Bone scanning alone was positive only in 22% of patients, with low sensitivity and specificity.[46] Another study also found bone scanning to have low sensitivity (37% positive in the 53% of patients with pathology) and cautioned that a negative result does not rule out serious pathology.[49] For benign tumors or metastatic disease, a bone scan may be a reasonable option, but it is less reliable for infection or malignant tumors.

CT is useful for delineating an area of pathology and assessing the osseous structures. CT can be effectively used to classify fractures, monitor healing, and confirm the diagnosis of a pars defect, and it can offer valuable information regarding any associated dysplasia. CT is useful for tailoring treatment in spondylolisthesis. MRI is gaining popularity because of its soft-tissue and bony resolution without radiation.[50] MRI is mandatory in patients who have any abnormality on neurologic examination because it allows evaluation of the spinal cord, nerve roots, and disks and can provide accurate diagnosis of diskitis, sacroiliitis, herniated disk, intraspinal pathology, and tumor. Unlike CT, MRI offers a longitudinal study of the spine. It is useful in the assessment of spondylolysis and can identify prespondylolytic lesions in the pars interarticularis.

Laboratory Investigation
Laboratory studies should be included in the workup if the patient has constitutional signs or symptoms or the history suggests infection. A complete blood count and inflammatory markers such as the erythrocyte sedimentation rate and C-reactive protein level can help in the diagnosis of infection, inflammatory conditions, and certain malignancies.

Common Causes of Back Pain
Spondylolysis
Spondylolysis is a defect in the pars interarticularis, most commonly at the L5 level. Its prevalence is 4.4% in children and 6% in adults.[51] Spondylolysis is uncommon in children younger than 5 years and is most common in patients older than 8 years. The risk factors are repetitive flexion-extension and motions that accentuate lumbar lordosis. Divers, wrestlers, weightlifters, and gymnasts are most commonly affected. In general, spondylolysis is most common among Caucasian males (6.3%).[52] It is also fairly common in adolescent Alaskan Eskimos; almost half of the adults in this population have been noted to have spondylolysis.[53]

A long-term population study identified 30 children with asymptomatic spondylolysis as first graders and reexamined them 45 years later.[54] Symptomatic slip progression had occurred in 5%. The researchers concluded that the clinical course of spondylolysis for the first 50 years of life is benign and quite similar to that of the general population. Defects proximal to L5 were associated with an increased prevalence of low back disability.

Plain radiographs have an unacceptably high rate of false-negative findings. Although bone scans can be sensitive, they are nonspecific. CT best characterizes the defect and confirms the diagnosis. The role of MRI continues to evolve and shows promise for detection of prespondylolytic stress lesions.

The use of activity modification, hamstring stretching, and analgesics can be successful. Bracing also can be effective. Surgery is reserved for patients who have persistent symptoms for longer than 6 months, despite nonsurgical measures. A direct pars repair or a posterolateral fusion can be performed.

Bertolotti Syndrome
A transitional anomaly most frequently occurs at the lumbosacral junction. The fifth lumbar vertebrae may be assimilated into the sacrum (sacralization), or the first sacral vertebra may have a lumbar configuration (lumbarization). The prevalence of these anomalies is 4% to 35%.[55,56] A systematic review found a mean prevalence of 12%, with lumbarization accounting for approximately 5% and sacralization for 7%.[57] The classification is based on the degree of articulation between the transverse process and the sacrum, in which the varying degrees of articulation culminate in complete fusion[58] (**Figure 6**).

The term Bertolotti syndrome describes low back pain secondary to the presence of lumbosacral transitional vertebrae, but this association remains controversial.[59] Of 22 observational studies, 4 studies found a positive and 5 studies a negative correlation between low back pain and lumbosacral transitional vertebrae.[57] Patients with a lumbosacral transitional anomaly are at increased risk for disk degeneration or herniation above the level of the transitional vertebrae.[60] An association with altered nerve root functioning and facet arthrosis has been reported.[61,62] Patients therefore may have discogenic back pain, radiculopathy, mechanical back pain, or facetogenic back pain. Facetogenic back pain is suspected to arise from the pseudoarticulation of the enlarged transverse process and the sacral ala or ilium and is most common in patients with unilateral transitions.

MRI is indicated in patients with radiculopathy. Single photon emission CT can be useful in identifying a painful articulation between the enlarged transverse process and the sacral ala or ilium. CT seems to be most sensitive in identifying contralateral facetogenic pain.[57] Local anesthesia and hydrocortisone infiltration can be used as diagnostic and possibly therapeutic tools.

The treatment generally is nonsurgical. Steroid injections are successful for relief of acute pain but have a high rate of symptom relapse within 3 months. Small case studies of patients undergoing either posterolateral fusion or resection of the anomalous articulation have

5: Spine

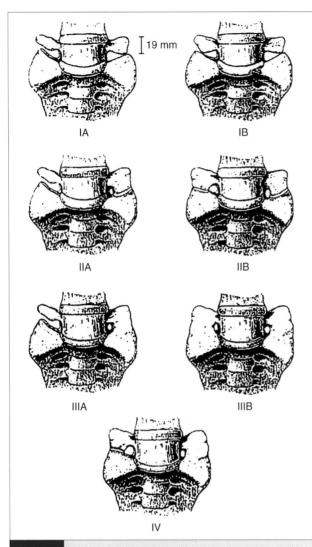

Figure 6 The Castellvi classification of lumbosacral transitional vertebrae. In type I (a dysplastic transverse process), there is a unilateral (IA) or bilateral (IB) enlarged transverse process of 19 mm or more. In type II (incomplete lumbarization or sacralization), an enlarged transverse process forms a diarthrodial joint with the sacral ala unilaterally (IIA) or bilaterally (IIB). In type III (complete lumbarization or sacralization), a bony union is formed between the transverse process and sacral ala unilaterally (IIIA) or bilaterally (IIIB). In type IV (mixed), there is a bony union on one side and an incomplete union on the other side between the enlarged transverse process and sacral ala.

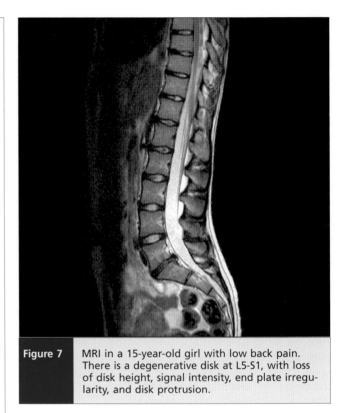

Figure 7 MRI in a 15-year-old girl with low back pain. There is a degenerative disk at L5-S1, with loss of disk height, signal intensity, end plate irregularity, and disk protrusion.

been reported. The results were similar for 16 patients with chronic back pain and radiographically diagnosed lumbosacral transitional vertebrae, regardless of whether the patient underwent a posterolateral fusion or a resection of the transitional articulation.[63]

Disk Degeneration and Intervertebral Disk Herniation

The reported prevalence of disk degeneration detected on MRI or autopsy in individuals between ages 10 and 19 years is 6% to 16%.[64,65] The association with low back pain is not fully understood, however. No significant difference was found between the incidence of degenerative disk changes in symptomatic and asymptomatic adolescents.[66] Cross-sectional and longitudinal studies found disk degeneration and herniation to be more common in young patients with low back pain than in control subjects, but the frequency of reduced disk height on MRI did not differ between the two groups. In a recent cross-sectional cohort study, MRI findings of disk protrusion, loss of disk height and irregularity of the nucleus, end plate changes, and anterolisthesis were strongly associated with low back pain in adolescents.[67]

Low back pain associated with degenerative disk disease is identified on MRI in some children (**Figure 7**). It is believed that lumbar degenerative disk disease begins before adulthood in some young patients. The incidence of recurrent low back pain associated with degenerative disk disease increases into early adulthood. Physical therapy, NSAIDs, aerobic conditioning, and attention to posture and activities usually produce a favorable response.

Disk herniations in children account for approximately 1% to 4% of all disk herniations. Disk herniation is far more common in adolescents than in younger children (**Figure 8**). The diagnosis can be delayed if the condition is not suspected or reported. Approximately two thirds of patients report localized low back pain, and one third have symptoms of radiculopathy and a positive straight-leg raise test. Usually a precipitating event such as trauma or strenuous sports

5: Spine

activity leads to the onset of symptoms. Disk herniation also occurs in patients with Scheuermann kyphosis.[68]

MRI is useful in confirming a disk herniation, defining its size and level, and determining whether it is posterolateral or far lateral. Core strengthening, a short course of NSAIDs, and activity modification usually are successful. Patients with persistent leg-dominant pain may be candidates for a diagnostic and therapeutic selective nerve root injection with a local anesthetic and steroid. Surgery is indicated for a patient whose radicular symptoms persist after nonsurgical modalities are exhausted or a patient with progressive neurology or cauda equina syndrome.

A 27-year follow-up study of children and adolescents treated with lumbar diskectomy found that 28% had one or more reoperations necessitated by recurrent low back or lower extremity pain, at an average 9.7 years after the initial procedure.[69] At final follow-up, 92% had no pain or occasional pain resulting from strenuous activities; 98% had no or mild limitation of their daily activities. The researchers concluded that although diskectomy does not always provide a permanent solution to lumbar disk disease in children, satisfactory long-term results can be expected in carefully selected patients.

Apophyseal ring injury is unique to the pediatric population. The interface of the ring apophysis and vertebral body is vulnerable to injury, and an acute flexion and axial load may result in an avulsion, usually when the posteroinferior apophysis is displaced into the spinal canal. The injury is most common in weight lifters, wrestlers, and participants in a contact sport or another sport requiring repetitive lumbar hyperflexion. The back pain is acute at onset, and radicular symptoms may be present. CT can help outline the osseus fragment, which may be excised depending on its size and the symptoms.

Diskitis and Vertebral Osteomyelitis

Childhood diskitis often is benign, self-limiting, and responsive to nonsurgical treatment. The incidence is highest in toddlers, with a second, subtler peak appearing in late childhood or early adolescence. The predisposition to diskitis in young children is thought to be related to the blood supply of the intervertebral disk and cartilaginous end plates. Pyogenic vertebral osteomyelitis and tuberculitis-related spondylitis are believed to be caused by organisms lodging in low-flow end vessels close to the end plates after hematogenous spread. In infants and young children, the numerous anastomotic blood vessels in the vertebral end plates communicate with the disk, acting as a source of nutrition but allowing hematogenous delivery of bacteria to the disk. The anastomotic channels gradually involute, leaving end arteries in the end plates by adolescence. These channels disappear by adulthood. The distinction between diskitis and vertebral osteomyelitis may be arbitrary, as the diskitis probably results from bacterial seeding within the adjacent end plates of the two vertebral bodies.

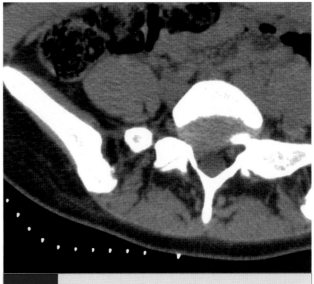

Figure 8 CT of a 16-year-old girl with back pain and right leg radiculopathy. A large posterolateral disk herniation with compression of the S1 nerve root is apparent. The patient underwent successful right-side L5-S1 microdiskectomy.

The clinical appearance often is nonspecific. In toddlers, a refusal to walk or sit is not uncommon. Limping, gait disturbances, and hip or leg pain may also be present. Back pain is typical at all ages, but adolescents are most likely to report abdominal pain and fever. The evaluation should include the complete blood count, blood cultures, erythrocyte sedimentation rate, and C-reactive protein level. Radiographic signs of diminished disk height and end plate irregularity may not appear until 3 to 8 weeks after the onset of symptoms. MRI is the imaging modality of choice. In addition to the characteristic findings of diskitis and vertebral osteomyelitis, paravertebral or epidural abscesses can be seen on MRI.

Although an infectious etiology is proposed for childhood diskitis, vertebral and disk cultures often are sterile. Some patients recover without antibiotics. Trauma and an idiopathic inflammatory process also have been implicated in the etiology. The treatment of choice remains intravenous antistaphylococcal antibiotics, with a transition to oral antibiotics after 7 to 10 days or symptom improvement. The response to treatment can be monitored with the erythrocyte sedimentation rate and C-reactive protein level, although these markers may be only mildly elevated. Rarely, surgical intervention is required to drain an abscess in the presence of instability or a progressive neurologic deficit.

If more than one disk level is affected, a diagnosis of tuberculosis or fungal spondylitis should be excluded. Tuberculosis should be suspected if the patient has an insidious onset of symptoms or is immunocompromised. Generally, diskitis in childhood has a good prognosis for recovery and no long-term complications.

5: Spine

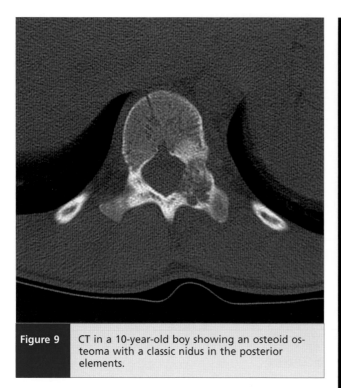

Figure 9 | CT in a 10-year-old boy showing an osteoid osteoma with a classic nidus in the posterior elements.

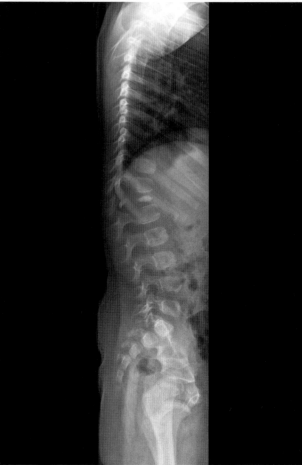

Figure 10 | Lateral radiograph showing the classic appearance of vertebra plana in an eosinophilic granuloma affecting the vertebral column.

Tumors

Spine tumors can be benign or malignant, affecting the vertebral column, spinal cord, or meninges. Malignant bone tumors of the spine are extremely rare. Nocturnal pain, progressive pain or disability, constitutional symptoms, or painful scoliosis should alert the clinician to carefully evaluate the possibility of a spine tumor. Patients often have vague symptoms that may mimic infection.

Vertebral tumors most commonly are benign. The types include osteoid osteoma, osteoblastoma, and aneurysmal bone cyst (Figure 9). Malignant lesions include Ewing sarcoma, osteosarcoma, chondrosarcoma, lymphoma, leukemia, and metastatic disease. Neuroblastoma and rhabdomyosarcoma usually occur in children younger than 7 years. In general, benign tumors are found in the posterior column, and metastatic disease and infection are found in the anterior column. Langerhans cell histiocytosis usually affects the anterior column and has a varying presentation depending on whether it is an isolated lesion or has polyostotic involvement.

Spinal cord tumors are rare in children. Astrocytoma, ependymoma, or chordoma should be considered in the differential diagnosis if weakness, a gait disturbance, a sensory abnormality, or bladder-bowel dysfunction is present, in addition to pain. Plain radiographs may detect a spine tumor, but further evaluation with CT or MRI is required. Certain tumors, such as eosinophilic granuloma, have classic vertebra plana on radiographs, and malignancies usually have lytic bone lesions (Figure 10). A bone scan has low sensitivity and specificity for detecting vertebral tumors but may be necessary for staging malignant tumors after diagnosis.

CT-guided biopsy or open biopsy may be required to confirm the diagnosis.

The treatment is dictated by the diagnosis. For a benign lesion, curettage and bone grafting or marginal excision can be considered. For a malignant primary bone tumor, surgery may be required for instability, progressive neurology, or primary treatment of disease. The surgery should involve multidisciplinary collaboration with an oncologist and a musculoskeletal tumor specialist.

Nonspecific Back Pain

The term nonspecific low back pain refers to pain in the lumbar region (with or without leg pain) that is not attributable to a recognizable, specific pathology. A recent study found than most back pain had no identifiable pathology.[47] Nonspecific low back pain may be the most common pain-related diagnosis among pediatric patients. A systematic review found strong evidence that the prevalence of low back pain increases with age and reaches a near-adult level by age 18 years.[70] Reports of low back pain were slightly more common in girls than in boys. Girls tended to report pain at an

Table 1	
The Wiltse-Neuman Classification of Spondylolisthesis	
Type	**Description**
I	Dysplastic
II	Isthmic
IIA	Pars stress fracture
IIB	Elongation of pars
IIC	Acute pars fracture
III	Degenerative
IV	Traumatic
V	Pathologic

Table 2
The Marchetti-Bartolozzi Classification of Spondylolisthesis
Developmental Type
High dysplastic
Low dysplastic
Acquired Type
Degenerative
Pathologic
Postsurgical
Stress fracture
Traumatic

earlier age, possibly corresponding to the onset of puberty.

The risk factors related to nonspecific back pain in children include poor physical conditioning, intense exercise, inadequate strength in the back-stabilizing muscles, poor abdominal muscle endurance and spine mobility, impaired flexibility in the hamstrings, a positive family history, and emotional or behavioral problems.[71] A growing body of evidence suggests that nonspecific back pain in children and adolescents is significantly associated with back pain in adult life.[70] This finding raises concern about a future adult degenerative musculoskeletal disease burden.

Postural education, spine stabilization exercise programs, and individualized physical therapy programs are the most effective modalities for treating children and adolescents with nonspecific back pain.[71-73] Treatment strategies aimed at prevention also have been successful.

Summary

Back pain in children and adolescents is more common than previously thought, and most often it has no identifiable pathologic cause. A careful history and physical examination should help identify patients requiring further evaluation. Nonspecific low back pain in the pediatric population is a significant public health issue, and it may be a risk factor for back pain in adults. Further research is needed to identify modifiable risk factors and guide interventions to prevent low back pain during childhood.

The Surgical Treatment of Spondylolysis and Spondylolisthesis

The risk of developing a progressive symptomatic spondylolisthesis in adulthood is less than 5%, although the prevalence of spondylolysis in children is 4.4%.[54] Nonsurgical management usually achieves a favorable re-sponse, but a small proportion of children remain symptomatic and require surgical treatment. Spondylolisthesis historically has been classified by the type of slippage (**Table 1**) However, there is increasing interest in the Marchetti-Bartolozzi classification, which is practical in terms of prognosis and therapy.[74] This system divides spondylolisthesis into two major groups: developmental and acquired (**Table 2**). Developmental spondylolisthesis is further divided into low-dysplastic and high-dysplastic subtypes, depending on the presence of bony dysplasia and the risk of progression. This etiology-based system emphasizes the distinction between dysplastic and spondylolytic spondylolisthesis, which have different natural histories but often are assigned an overlapping classification.

A classification system designed to guide the surgical treatment of spondylolisthesis introduced the concept of sagittal spinopelvic balance assessment, in addition to slip grade and degree of dysplasia[75] (**Figure 11**). This system emphasizes pelvic incidence, sacral slope, and pelvic tilt as measures to differentiate the types of spondylolisthesis. Surgical intervention for spondylolysis and spondylolisthesis is indicated if a pediatric patient has more than 50% of listhesis and nonsurgical treatment has been unsuccessful, the listhesis has progressed, or patient reports progressive back pain or neurologic symptoms.

Spondylolysis

Repairing the pars defect has the advantage of preserving motion. Although this procedure has a variable outcome,[76,77] spondylolytic defects treated at levels proximal to L5 appear to have a more predictably favorable response. A direct repair of the pars interarticularis defect ideally is considered for a patient with symptomatic spondylolysis with minimal slippage (grade I listhesis), a healthy intervening disk, a single-level defect, and back-dominant pain without radiculopathy. The defect should be smaller than 2 mm. Several techniques have been described, including direct fixation using a screw across the defect, wiring to bridge the defect with a compressive force, and a pedicle screw–laminar hook construct.[76] The screw-hook construct provides a larger

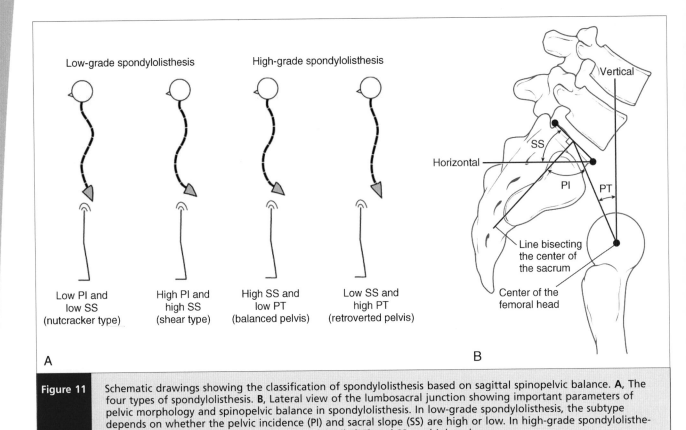

Figure 11 Schematic drawings showing the classification of spondylolisthesis based on sagittal spinopelvic balance. **A**, The four types of spondylolisthesis. **B**, Lateral view of the lumbosacral junction showing important parameters of pelvic morphology and spinopelvic balance in spondylolisthesis. In low-grade spondylolisthesis, the subtype depends on whether the pelvic incidence (PI) and sacral slope (SS) are high or low. In high-grade spondylolisthesis, the subtype depends on whether the pelvic tilt (PT) and SS are high or low.

surface area for bone healing than direct screw fixation and is more stable than a wire construct (**Figure 12**). All techniques require meticulous bone grafting of the defect for optimal healing.

Low-Grade Spondylolisthesis

The role of in situ posterolateral fusion is well established for treating spondylolysis and low-grade spondylolisthesis and, although controversial, in some centers it remains the preferred method of treating high-grade spondylolisthesis. A bilateral parasagittal approach, with iliac crest graft laid posterolaterally along the transverse processes, facet joints, and sacral alae at the L5-S1 level, can achieve fusion in more than 90% of patients and pain relief in more than 75%.[78] Postoperative immobilization in a body cast with a pantaloon extension or bracing with a leg extension is needed for 3 months.

Although instrumented in situ fusion is an option for low-grade spondylolisthesis, there appears to be no improvement in fusion rates or functional outcomes. Instrumentation may have the advantage of obviating postoperative immobilization.

High-Grade Spondylolisthesis

Although it is agreed that high-grade spondylolisthesis should be managed surgically, the type of surgical intervention is an area of ongoing debate. Solid fusion has been described after posterior in situ fusion.[79] For high-grade spondylolisthesis, this technique requires fusion to L4, with the bone graft vertically oriented to minimize tension on the fusion mass. Concerns have been raised about pseudarthrosis, progression of slip, persistent cosmetic deformity, gait disturbance, and potential neurologic injury after in situ fusion in pediatric patients with high-grade spondylolisthesis. Long-term studies of in situ fusion in children and adolescents found that degenerative changes developed earlier in life than for age-matched control subjects.[80]

Patients with severe lumbosacral kyphosis (a slip angle greater than 45°); significant dysplasia; and anatomic features that could contribute to a failed fusion, such as a trapezoidal L5 vertebral body, rounding of the sacral dome, or small transverse processes, may not be suitable for in situ fusion. Several techniques have been proposed to overcome the challenges of in situ fusion, including decompression and posterior in situ fusion, anteroposterior in situ arthrodesis, combined anteroposterior reduction and fusion, instrumented anteroposterior reduction and fusion, and instrumented posterior fusion with posterior or transforaminal interbody fusion.

In a posterior in situ interbody fusion using a transsacral approach, a wide decompression posteriorly is followed by mobilization of the thecal sac to the midline. A tunnel is then prepared through the sacrum and into the L5 vertebral body. A fibular graft is impacted

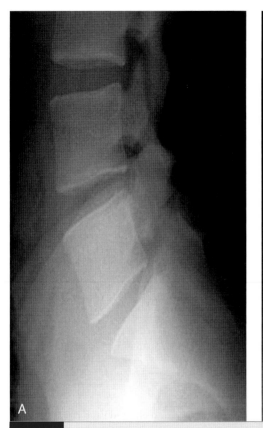
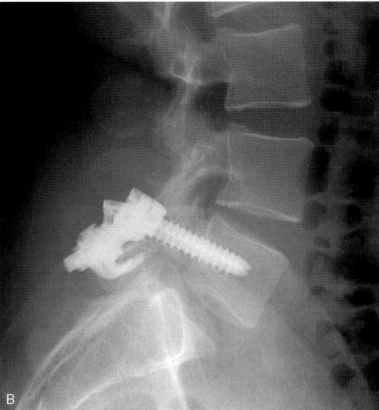

Figure 12   Lateral L5-S1 radiographs of a 16-year-old boy showing an L5 spondylolysis before (**A**) and after (**B**) direct pars repair using a screw-hook construct.

into the prepared canal.[81] Although fusion rates have been excellent, there is concern about resorption and fracture of the graft.

The use of pedicle screws has allowed surgeons to attempt to reduce the deformity and provide immediate mechanical stability, which enables faster mobilization. The risk of implant failure and pseudarthrosis may be higher in the absence of anterior column support. An anterior interbody cage resists shear forces, provides a greater surface area for fusion, restores lumbosacral lordosis, and indirectly decompresses the neural foramen. Anterior support can be achieved through an anterior or posterior approach, each of which has advantages and disadvantages. Stand-alone anterior in situ fusion carries a higher risk of pseudarthrosis compared with circumferential fusion.

The need for reduction in high-grade spondylolisthesis remains controversial. The main advantages of reduction are that it allows direct decompression of the neural elements; correction of the lumbosacral kyphosis to improve sagittal balance, cosmesis, biomechanics, and gait; and a possible decrease in the risk of acute postoperative cauda equina syndrome. Although improvement in spinopelvic sagittal balance is a goal, improvement in pelvic version after reduction for unbalanced spondylolisthesis is not correlated with the amount of translation correction or the slip angle.[82] In-

strumented posterior fusion with anterior column support is preferred by many surgeons when reduction is performed (**Figure 13**).

Reduction of high-grade spondylolisthesis has been associated with injury to the L5 nerve root in as many as 30% of patients. The injury is primarily related to translation of the L5 vertebral body. This relationship is not linear; 71% of the total strain on the nerve occurs during the second half of the reduction.[83] Partial reduction maneuvers have been considered, with emphasis on the importance of correcting the slip angle and the lumbosacral kyphosis rather than the translation. The risk of neurologic injury to the L5 nerve root also has led to consideration of a sacral dome osteotomy to further shorten the spine and prevent excess tension on the roots.[84,85] When reduction is performed, proximal fixation to L4 is preferred by most surgeons, although good results have been obtained with constructs to L5.[84]

Iliac wing screws have increased in popularity for fixation of a transitional syndrome, specifically sacral fracture, after instrumented reduction. The iliac wing fixation provides added stability of the construct, specifically in flexion-extension at the lumbosacral junction. Iliac wing screws are more biomechanically protective than interbody cages, and the addition of an interbody cage when iliac screws are used appears to

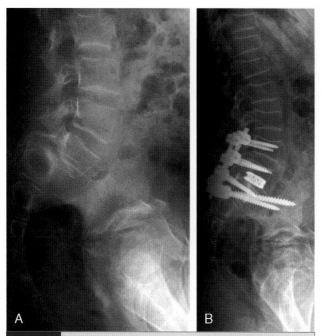

Figure 13 Lateral radiographs showing a high-grade L5-S1 dysplastic spondylolisthesis in a 9-year-old boy before (**A**) and after (**B**) instrumented reduction and circumferential fusion using an all-posterior approach.

have a small benefit. Anterior column support or fusion to L4 may not be necessary for all patients with high-grade spondylolisthesis, especially if iliac augmentation is used and the sagittal balance and biomechanics are well restored after reduction. However, the addition of anterior column support may be considered if the lumbosacral angle is less than 100° after reduction.

Spondyloptosis

The surgical options for patients with high-grade spondylolisthesis can be considered for patients with spondyloptosis. The Bohlman posterior dowel graft, gradual instrumented reduction, and posterolateral fusion have been used. An L5 vertebrectomy with reduction of L4 to the sacrum through staged anterior and posterior procedures also has been described.[86] A permanent neurologic deficit can occur in as many as one third of patients with any of these techniques.

Summary

The main goals of the surgical treatment of spondylolysis and spondylolisthesis are to resolve back pain and radicular pain, restore the sagittal profile, and achieve a solid arthrodesis while minimizing potential complications. The main controversy regarding high-grade slips is the need for reduction. Instrumented reduction should not be the routine treatment but should be reserved for patients with loss of global sagittal balance and patients requiring decompression, which may lead to further deformity. A classification system incorporat-

ing sagittal spinopelvic balance needs to be developed to guide the surgical treatment of spondylolisthesis in children and adolescents. The current treatment protocol largely depends on the degree of slip, and it overlooks the subtypes within the different grades of spondylolisthesis. This factor may explain the great variability in reported surgical outcomes and controversies regarding surgical management.

Annotated References

1. Kaufman RA, Carroll CD, Buncher CR: Atlantooccipital junction: Standards for measurement in normal children. *AJNR Am J Neuroradiol* 1987;8(6):995-999.

2. Hosalkar HS, Sankar WN, Wills BP, Goebel J, Dormans JP, Drummond DS: Congenital osseous anomalies of the upper cervical spine. *J Bone Joint Surg Am* 2008;90(2): 337-348.

    An underlying syndrome was present in 21 of 68 patients treated for upper cervical osseous anomalies. A dysmorphic C1 followed by atlantoaxial instability was most common. Thorough evaluation and advanced imaging are recommended for these children. Level of evidence: III.

3. Harris JH Jr, Carson GC, Wagner LK, Kerr N: Radiologic diagnosis of traumatic occipitovertebral dissociation: 2. Comparison of three methods of detecting occipitovertebral relationships on lateral radiographs of supine subjects. *AJR Am J Roentgenol* 1994;162(4): 887-892.

4. Karol LA, Sheffield EG, Crawford K, Moody MK, Browne RH: Reproducibility in the measurement of atlanto-occipital instability in children with Down syndrome. *Spine (Phila Pa 1976)* 1996;21:2463-2468.

5. Bertozzi JC, Rojas CA, Martinez CR: Evaluation of the pediatric craniocervical junction on MDCT. *AJR Am J Roentgenol* 2009;192(1):26-31.

    Values for the various craniocervical junction relationships were calculated using multidetector CT in 117 normal children. The values were different compared with the accepted ranges based on radiographs. The authors suggest using the values obtained on multidetector CT. Level of evidence: III.

6. Dziurzynski K, Anderson PA, Bean DB, et al: A blinded assessment of radiographic criteria for atlanto-occipital dislocation. *Spine (Phila Pa 1976)* 2005;30(12):1427-1432.

    The authors reviewed plain radiographs and CTs of the cervical spine in 104 patients. Sensitivity, specificity, and positive and negative predictive values were better when the radiographic criteria were applied to CT for most parameters used in assessing the craniocervical junction. Level of evidence: III.

7. Wang JC, Nuccion SL, Feighan JE, Cohen B, Dorey FJ, Scoles PV: Growth and development of the pediatric

cervical spine documented radiographically. *J Bone Joint Surg Am* 2001;83(8):1212-1218.

8. Watanabe M, Toyama Y, Fujimura Y: Atlantoaxial instability in os odontoideum with myelopathy. *Spine (Phila Pa 1976)* 1996;21(12):1435-1439.

9. Greenberg AD: Atlanto-axial dislocations. *Brain* 1968; 91(4):655-684.

10. Roach JW, Duncan D, Wenger DR, Maravilla A, Maravilla K: Atlanto-axial instability and spinal cord compression in children: Diagnosis by computerized tomography. *J Bone Joint Surg Am* 1984;66(5):708-714.

11. Gupta V, Khandelwal N, Mathuria SN, Singh P, Pathak A, Suri S: Dynamic magnetic resonance imaging evaluation of craniovertebral junction abnormalities. *J Comput Assist Tomogr* 2007;31(3):354-359.

    Twenty-five subjects with suspected craniovertebral junction abnormalities underwent dynamic MRI, and 20 also underwent noncontrast CT. Dynamic MRI detected atlantoaxial instability in 15 patients. Dynamic MRI was able to detect cord compression that was not seen in neutral position. Level of evidence: III.

12. Menezes AH: Craniocervical developmental anatomy and its implications. *Childs Nerv Syst* 2008;24(10): 1109-1122.

    The developmental anatomy, natural history, and treatment of a variety of craniocervical abnormalities in children are discussed. Level of evidence: I.

13. Fielding JW, Griffin PP: Os odontoideum: An acquired lesion. *J Bone Joint Surg Am* 1974;56(1):187-190.

14. Arvin B, Fournier-Gosselin MP, Fehlings MG: Os odontoideum: Etiology and surgical management. *Neurosurgery* 2010;66(3, suppl):22-31.

    In a review of the current literature on the etiology and treatment of os odontoideum, the authors conclude that there is an emerging consensus on the traumatic etiology of os odontoideum. They recommend surgical treatment in patients with an unstable or compressive os. Level of evidence: IV.

15. American Academy of Pediatrics Committee on Sports Medicine and Fitness: Atlantoaxial instability in Down syndrome: Subject review. *Pediatrics* 1995;96(1, pt 1): 151-154.

16. American Academy of Pediatrics Committee on Genetics: American Academy of Pediatrics: Health supervision for children with Down syndrome. *Pediatrics* 2001; 107(2):442-449.

17. Pueschel SM, Scola FH, Pezzullo JC: A longitudinal study of atlanto-dens relationships in asymptomatic individuals with Down syndrome. *Pediatrics* 1992;89(6, pt 2):1194-1198.

18. Brockmeyer D: Down syndrome and craniovertebral in-

stability: Topic review and treatment recommendations. *Pediatr Neurosurg* 1999;31(2):71-77.

19. Browd S, Healy LJ, Dobie G, et al: Morphometric and qualitative analysis of congenital occipitocervical instability in children: Implications for patients with Down syndrome. *J Neurosurg* 2006;105(1, suppl):50-54.

    Morphometric analysis using CT revealed an abnormal C1 superior articular surface in patients with Down syndrome and congenital occipitocervical instability, compared with 15 normal age-matched control subjects. The abnormal joint shape was thought to contribute to occipitocervical instability. Level of evidence: III.

20. Giussani C, Roux F-E, Guerra P, et al: Severely symptomatic craniovertebral junction abnormalities in children: Long-term reliability of aggressive management. *Pediatr Neurosurg* 2009;45(1):29-36.

    A retrospective review of five children with craniocervical abnormalities and spinal cord compression with severe neurologic deficits found that stable fixation and bony fusion were achieved in all patients. Each surgical technique was unique. Level of evidence: IV.

21. Miyanji F, Mulpuri K, Saravanja D, Newton PO, Reilly CW: C1 lateral mass screw fixation in children: Indications, outcomes, and technique in 11 consecutive patients. Rosemont, IL, Pediatric Orthopaedic Society of North America, 2010. http://posna.gmetonline.com/PresentationSearch.aspx?fixedkey=~im4_j.xOb9x&subscriptionpackageid=44. Accessed November 29, 2010.

    C1 lateral mass screw fixation was used to treat a variety of upper cervical pathologies in children. Radiographic and clinical union was achieved in all patients with no reported complications. The authors report significant advantages of such segmental rigid fixation over traditional techniques in children.

22. Rouvreau P, Glorion C, Langlais J, Noury H, Pouliquen JC: Assessment and neurologic involvement of patients with cervical spine congenital synostosis as in Klippel-Feil syndrome: Study of 19 cases. *J Pediatr Orthop B* 1998;7(3):179-185.

23. Theiss SM, Smith MD, Winter RB: The long-term follow-up of patients with Klippel-Feil syndrome and congenital scoliosis. *Spine (Phila Pa 1976)* 1997;22(11): 1219-1222.

24. Nagib MG, Larson DA, Maxwell RE, Chou SN: Neuroschisis of the cervical spinal cord in a patient with Klippel-Feil syndrome. *Neurosurgery* 1987;20(4):629-631.

25. Shen FH, Samartzis D, Herman J, Lubicky JP: Radiographic assessment of segmental motion at the atlantoaxial junction in the Klippel-Feil patient. *Spine (Phila Pa 1976)* 2006;31(2):171-177.

    In 33 patients with Klippel-Feil syndrome, the highest AADI values were in patients with occipitalization and a fused C2-C3 segment. The extent of AADI change was not associated with an increased risk of neurologic complications. Level of evidence: IV.

5: Spine

26. Auerbach JD, Hosalkar HS, Kusuma SK, Wills BP, Dormans JP, Drummond DS: Spinal cord dimensions in children with Klippel-Feil syndrome: A controlled, blinded radiographic analysis with implications for neurologic outcomes. *Spine (Phila Pa 1976)* 2008;33(12):1366-1371.

Plain radiographs, MRIs, and clinical records of 12 patients with Klippel-Feil syndrome were compared with those of age-matched control subjects. The Torg ratio was identical. Although the patients had a smaller spinal cord, there were no significant differences in the cerebrospinal fluid column. Level of evidence: III.

27. Samartzis D, Kalluri P, Herman J, Lubicky JP, Shen FH: 2008 Young Investigator Award: The role of congenitally fused cervical segments upon the space available for the cord and associated symptoms in Klippel-Feil patients. *Spine (Phila Pa 1976)* 2008;33(13):1442-1450.

A review of plain radiographs and the clinical records of 29 patients with Klippel-Feil syndrome revealed an increased SAC secondary to a decrease in vertebral body width caused by arrested vertebral development. This factor may delay potential neurologic and degenerative sequelae. Level of evidence: IV.

28. Wang H, Rosenbaum AE, Reid CS, Zinreich SJ, Pyeritz RE: Pediatric patients with achondroplasia: CT evaluation of the craniocervical junction. *Radiology* 1987;164(2):515-519.

29. Miyoshi K, Nakamura K, Haga N, Mikami Y: Surgical treatment for atlantoaxial subluxation with myelopathy in spondyloepiphyseal dysplasia congenita. *Spine (Phila Pa 1976)* 2004;29(21):E488-E491.

30. Nakamura K, Miyoshi K, Haga N, Kurokawa T: Risk factors of myelopathy at the atlantoaxial level in spondyloepiphyseal dysplasia congenita. *Arch Orthop Trauma Surg* 1998;117(8):468-470.

31. Ain MC, Chaichana KL, Schkrohowsky JG: Retrospective study of cervical arthrodesis in patients with various types of skeletal dysplasia. *Spine (Phila Pa 1976)* 2006;31(6):E169-E174.

Twenty-three of 25 patients with skeletal dysplasia achieved solid bony fusion after cervical arthrodesis. Five had surgery-related complications, and 14 experienced neurologic improvement. Cervical arthrodesis was found to be an effective treatment for preserving or improving neurology. Level of evidence: IV.

32. Stevens JM, Kendall BE, Crockard HA, Ransford A: The odontoid process in Morquio-Brailsford's disease: The effects of occipitocervical fusion. *J Bone Joint Surg Br* 1991;73(5):851-858.

High-definition computed cervical myelograms found extradural soft-tissue thickening. The severity of neurologic involvement was determined by the soft-tissue changes rather than by the type of odontoid hypoplasia or by subluxation. Level of evidence: III.

33. White KK, Steinman S, Mubarak SJ: Cervical stenosis and spastic quadriparesis in Morquio disease (MPS IV): A case report with twenty-six-year follow-up. *J Bone Joint Surg Am* 2009;91(2):438-442.

After 26 years, a patient surgically treated for cervical stenosis related to Morquio disease had full recovery, despite his initial neurologic condition. Level of evidence: IV.

34. Greaves LL, Van Toen C, Melnyk A, et al: Pediatric and adult three-dimensional cervical spine kinematics: Effect of age and sex through overall motion. *Spine (Phila Pa 1976)* 2009;34(16):1650-1657.

A cross-sectional study recruited 90 subjects to determine the helical axis of motion of the cervical spine. Girls had a more anterior helical axis of motion in axial rotation and flexion than adult women. The conclusion was that cervical spine kinematics vary with age and sex. Level of evidence: II.

35. Swischuk LE: Anterior displacement of C2 in children: Physiologic or pathologic. *Radiology* 1977;122(3):759-763.

36. Katz DA, Hall JE, Emans JB: Cervical kyphosis associated with anteroposterior dissociation and quadriparesis in Larsen's syndrome. *J Pediatr Orthop* 2005;25(4):429-433.

One patient with Larsen syndrome was treated nonsurgically and another was treated surgically. The authors stress the importance of searching for anteroposterior dissociation of the spine if fusion is required. Level of evidence: IV.

37. Sakaura H, Matsuoka T, Iwasaki M, Yonenobu K, Yoshikawa H: Surgical treatment of cervical kyphosis in Larsen syndrome: Report of 3 cases and review of the literature. *Spine (Phila Pa 1976)* 2007;32(1):E39-E44.

The authors review the results of surgery in three patients with Larsen syndrome and recommend that patients be screened with radiographs early. A mild kyphosis may allow a posterior fusion, whereas a rigid deformity may require an anterior decompression and circumferential fusion. Level of evidence: IV.

38. Madera M, Crawford A, Mangano FT: Management of severe cervical kyphosis in a patient with Larsen syndrome: Case report. *J Neurosurg Pediatr* 2008;1(4):320-324.

In a patient with Larson syndrome, cervical instability was treated with synchronous anterior decompression and fixation, posterior fusion and fixation, and halo placement. At 1-year follow-up, the patient had improved cervical alignment and no neurologic deficits. Level of evidence: V.

39. Pang D, Sun PP: Pediatric vertebral column and spinal cord injuries, in Winn HR, ed: *Youmans Neurological Surgery*, ed 5. Philadelphia, PA, WB Saunders, 2004, pp 3515-3557.

40. Ware ML, Gupta N, Sun PP, et al: Clinical biomechanics of the pediatric craniocervical junction and subaxial spine, in Brockmeyer DL, ed: *Advanced Pediatric Cran-*

5: Spine

iocervical Surgery. New York, NY, Thieme, 2005, pp 27-42.

41. Watson KD, Papageorgiou AC, Jones GT, et al: Low back pain in schoolchildren: Occurrence and characteristics. *Pain* 2002;97(1-2):87-92.

42. Harreby M, Nygaard B, Jessen T, et al: Risk factors for low back pain in a cohort of 1389 Danish school children: An epidemiologic study. *Eur Spine J* 1999;8(6): 444-450.

43. Olsen TL, Anderson RL, Dearwater SR, et al: The epidemiology of low back pain in an adolescent population. *Am J Public Health* 1992;82(4):606-608.

44. Mohseni-Bandpei MA, Bagheri-Nesami M, Shayesteh-Azar M: Nonspecific low back pain in 5000 Iranian school-age children. *J Pediatr Orthop* 2007;27(2):126-129.

    A cross-sectional study of 5,000 randomly recruited schoolchildren (age 11 to 14 years) used a structured questionnaire. The annual incidence of low back pain was found to be 17.4%, with no association between back pain and body mass index or sex. Level of evidence: II.

45. Masiero S, Carraro E, Celia A, Sarto D, Ermani M: Prevalence of nonspecific low back pain in schoolchildren aged between 13 and 15 years. *Acta Paediatr* 2008;97(2):212-216.

    In 7,542 school-age teenagers, nonspecific low back pain was present in 20.5%. It was more common in girls, sedentary children, and those with a positive family history. Level of evidence: II.

46. Feldman DS, Hedden DM, Wright JG: The use of bone scan to investigate back pain in children and adolescents. *J Pediatr Orthop* 2000;20(6):790-795.

47. Bhatia NN, Chow G, Timon SJ, Watts HG: Diagnostic modalities for the evaluation of pediatric back pain: A prospective study. *J Pediatr Orthop* 2008;28(2):230-233.

    Seventy-three children with back pain of at least 3 months' duration were followed prospectively. Patients were evaluated using an algorithm developed by the authors. No diagnosis was made in 78.1% of patients. No diagnosis was missed using the algorithm. Level of evidence: II.

48. Feldman DS, Straight JJ, Badra MI, Mohaideen A, Madan SS: Evaluation of an algorithmic approach to pediatric back pain. *J Pediatr Orthop* 2006;26(3):353-357.

    The authors tested an algorithm for assessment of back pain in 87 children. They found constant pain, night pain, radicular pain, and abnormal neurologic examination to have high specificity for a specific diagnosis. Level of evidence: II.

49. Sanpera I Jr, Beguiristain-Gurpide JL: Bone scan as a screening tool in children and adolescents with back pain. *J Pediatr Orthop* 2006;26(2):221-225.

    Of 142 pediatric patients who underwent bone scanning for persistent back pain, only 52 had a positive bone scan, but 75 had pathology. Bone scan was noted to have low sensitivity (0.613), high specificity (0.91), and a limited role in primary malignancies. Level of evidence: II.

50. Auerbach JD, Ahn J, Zgonis MH, Reddy SC, Ecker ML, Flynn JM: Streamlining the evaluation of low back pain in children. *Clin Orthop Relat Res* 2008;466(8):1971-1977.

    A retrospective analysis of 100 children found that a hyperextension test with radiographs had a negative predictive value of 0.81 and sensitivity of 0.90. Bone scans had perfect negative predictive value and sensitivity within 6 weeks of symptom onset. Level of evidence: II.

51. Fredrickson BE, Baker D, McHolick WJ, Yuan HA, Lubicky JP: The natural history of spondylolysis and spondylolisthesis. *J Bone Joint Surg Am* 1984;66(5):699-707.

52. Roche MB, Rowe GG: The incidence of separate neural arch and coincident bone variations: A survey of 4,200 skeletons. *Anat Rec* 1951;109(2):233-252.

53. Simper LB: Spondylolysis in Eskimo skeletons. *Acta Orthop Scand* 1986;57(1):78-80.

54. Beutler WJ, Fredrickson BE, Murtland A, Sweeney CA, Grant WD, Baker D: The natural history of spondylolysis and spondylolisthesis: 45-year follow-up evaluation. *Spine (Phila Pa 1976)* 2003;28(10):1027-1035.

55. Erken E, Ozer HT, Gulek B, Durgun B: The association between cervical rib and sacralization. *Spine (Phila Pa 1976)* 2002;27(15):1659-1664.

56. Hsieh CY, Vanderford JD, Moreau SR, Prong T: Lumbosacral transitional segments: Classification, prevalence, and effect on disk height. *J Manipulative Physiol Ther* 2000;23(7):483-489.

57. Bron JL, van Royen BJ, Wuisman PI: The clinical significance of lumbosacral transitional anomalies. *Acta Orthop Belg* 2007;73(6):687-695.

    The clinical significance of lumbosacral transitional anomalies is reviewed. There is conflicting evidence regarding an association between this condition and back pain. Some evidence of early disk degeneration was found in young patients. Level of evidence: III.

58. Castellvi AE, Goldstein LA, Chan DP: Lumbosacral transitional vertebrae and their relationship with lumbar extradural defects. *Spine (Phila Pa 1976)* 1984;9(5): 493-495.

59. Peterson CK, Bolton J, Hsu W, Wood A: A cross-sectional study comparing pain and disability levels in patients with low back pain with and without transitional lumbosacral vertebrae. *J Manipulative Physiol Ther* 2005;28(8):570-574.

    The revised Oswestry Disability Index questionnaire was administered to 353 patients with low back pain,

5: Spine

who were divided into two groups depending on the presence or absence of transitional vertebrae. No differences in pain or disability level were found. Level of evidence: III.

60. Aihara T, Takahashi K, Ogasawara A, Itadera E, Ono Y, Moriya H: Intervertebral disc degeneration associated with lumbosacral transitional vertebrae: A clinical and anatomical study. *J Bone Joint Surg Br* 2005; 87(5):687-691.

    MRI was used to study 52 patients with a transitional vertebra. Disks were significantly more degenerative immediately above the transitional vertebra than at other levels. Dissection of 70 cadavers found that a thinner and weaker iliolumbar ligament may lead to this degenerative change. Level of evidence: IV.

61. Chang HS, Nakagawa H: Altered function of lumbar nerve roots in patients with transitional lumbosacral vertebrae. *Spine (Phila Pa 1976)* 2004;29(15):1632-1635.

62. Brault JS, Smith J, Currier BL: Partial lumbosacral transitional vertebra resection for contralateral facetogenic pain. *Spine (Phila Pa 1976)* 2001;26(2):226-229.

63. Santavirta S, Tallroth K, Ylinen P, Suoranta H: Surgical treatment of Bertolotti's syndrome: Follow-up of 16 patients. *Arch Orthop Trauma Surg* 1993;112(2):82-87.

64. Powell MC, Wilson M, Szypryt P, Symonds EM, Worthington BS: Prevalence of lumbar disc degeneration observed by magnetic resonance in symptomless women. *Lancet* 1986;2(8520):1366-1367.

65. Miller JA, Schmatz C, Schultz AB: Lumbar disc degeneration: Correlation with age, sex, and spine level in 600 autopsy specimens. *Spine (Phila Pa 1976)* 1988; 13(2):173-178.

66. Tertti MO, Salminen JJ, Paajanen HE, Terho PH, Kormano MJ: Low-back pain and disk degeneration in children: A case-control MR imaging study. *Radiology* 1991;180(2):503-507.

67. Kjaer P, Leboeuf-Yde C, Sorensen JS, Bendix T: An epidemiologic study of MRI and low back pain in 13-year-old children. *Spine (Phila Pa 1976)* 2005;30(7):798-806.

    A cross-sectional cohort of 439 children underwent MRI and a structured interview. Disk degeneration was found in 33%, with changes in the upper lumbar spine corresponding to symptoms in boys and lower lumbar spine degenerative changes associated with back pain in girls. Level of evidence: IV.

68. Kapetanos GA, Hantzidis PT, Anagnostidis KS, Kirkos JM: Thoracic cord compression caused by disk herniation in Scheuermann's disease: A case report and review of the literature. *Eur Spine J* 2006;15(suppl 5):553-558.

    A patient with Scheuermann kyphosis had significant neurologic deficit caused by a thoracic disk herniation at the level of the kyphosis. He was successfully treated, with complete recovery, using a combined anterior and posterior approach. Level of evidence: V.

69. Papagelopoulos PJ, Shaughnessy WJ, Ebersold MJ, Bianco AJ Jr, Quast LM: Long-term outcome of lumbar discectomy in children and adolescents sixteen years of age or younger. *J Bone Joint Surg Am* 1998;80(5):689-698.

70. Jeffries LJ, Milanese SF, Grimmer-Somers KA: Epidemiology of adolescent spinal pain: A systematic overview of the research literature. *Spine (Phila Pa 1976)* 2007; 32(23):2630-2637.

    There is strong evidence that low back pain prevalence increases with age, reaching a near-adult level by age 18 years. Reports of low back pain are more common in girls, who have a slightly earlier onset of symptoms than boys. Level of evidence: III.

71. Ahlqwist A, Hagman M, Kjellby-Wendt G, Beckung E: Physical therapy treatment of back complaints on children and adolescents. *Spine (Phila Pa 1976)* 2008; 33(20):E721-E727.

    Forty-five patients were randomly assigned to receive individualized physical therapy, exercise, and a standardized self-training program; or the same regimen without the individualized physical therapy. Improvements were statistically significant in both groups over time. Level of evidence: I.

72. Kosseim M, Rein R, McShane C: Implementing evidence-based physiotherapy practice for treating children with low back pain: Are we there yet? *Pediatr Phys Ther* 2008;20(2):179-184.

    The authors identified best clinical practices for treating nonspecified low back pain. Fifty medical charts were critically appraised for implementation of evidence-based physical therapy practice. Strong evidence supported the effectiveness of therapeutic exercises and education. Level of evidence: II.

73. Bo Andersen L, Wedderkopp N, Leboeuf-Yde C: Association between back pain and physical fitness in adolescents. *Spine (Phila Pa 1976)* 2006;31(15):1740-1744.

    A cross-sectional study of 9,413 adolescents found that high isometric muscle endurance in the back extensors was associated with a lower risk of back pain. No associations were found with aerobic fitness, strength, flexibility, or activity level after adjusting for muscle endurance. Level of evidence: IV.

74. Marchetti PC, Bartolozzi P: Classification of spondylolisthesis as a guideline for treatment, in Bridwell KH, DeWald RL, Hammerberg KW, et al, eds: *The Textbook of Spinal Surgery*, ed 2. Philadelphia, PA, Lippincott-Raven, 1997, pp 1211-1254.

75. Mac-Thiong J-M, Labelle H: A proposal for a surgical classification of pediatric lumbosacral spondylolisthesis based on current literature. *Eur Spine J* 2006;15(10): 1425-1435.

    A classification to guide surgical treatment of L5-S1 spondylolisthesis in children and adolescents is based on

5: Spine

the degree of the slip, the degree of dysplasia, and the sagittal spinopelvic balance. Level of evidence: IV.

76. Chung C-H, Chiu H-M, Wang S-J, Hsu S-Y, Wei Y-S: Direct repair of multiple levels lumbar spondylolysis by pedicle screw laminar hook and bone grafting: Clinical, CT, and MRI-assessed study. *J Spinal Disord Tech* 2007;20(5):399-402.

Six patients with multiple-level spondylolysis were treated with segmental pedicle screw–hook fixation and autogenous bone graft. The union rate was 87% on radiographs and 75% on CT at a minimum 2-year follow-up. All patients were satisfied with the outcome. Level of evidence: IV.

77. Schlenzka D, Remes V, Helenius I, et al: Direct repair for treatment of symptomatic spondylolysis and low-grade isthmic spondylolisthesis in young patients: No benefit in comparison to segmental fusion after a mean follow-up of 14.8 years. *Eur Spine J* 2006;15(10):1437-1447.

The long-term clinical, functional, and radiographic outcomes of 25 patients with direct spondylolysis repair and 23 patients with in situ fusion were compared. The patients with direct repair had a 76% rate of very satisfactory results but a significantly lower Oswestry Disability Index score. Level of evidence: III.

78. Helenius I, Lamberg T, Osterman K, et al: Scoliosis research society outcome instrument in evaluation of long-term surgical results in spondylolysis and low-grade isthmic spondylolisthesis in young patients. *Spine (Phila Pa 1976)* 2005;30(3):336-341.

Patients treated with posterior-posterolateral fusion for low-grade isthmic spondylolisthesis were retrospectively evaluated using the Scoliosis Research Society questionnaire and Oswestry Disability Index. Long-term clinical and radiographic outcomes after posterolateral fusion of low-grade spondylolisthesis were satisfactory. Level of evidence: IV.

79. Lamberg T, Remes V, Helenius I, Schlenzka D, Seitsalo S, Poussa M: Uninstrumented in situ fusion for high-grade childhood and adolescent isthmic spondylolisthesis: Long-term outcome. *J Bone Joint Surg Am* 2007;89(3):512-518.

At a mean 17.2-year follow-up of 69 patients who underwent posterolateral, anterior, or circumferential uninstrumented fusion, circumferential fusion had better long-term results as assessed on patient-based outcomes. The differences were small when patient-based, radiographic, and functional outcomes were combined. Level of evidence: III.

80. Remes VM, Lamberg TS, Tervahartiala PO, et al: No correlation between patient outcome and abnormal lumbar MRI findings 21 years after posterior or posterolateral fusion for isthmic spondylolisthesis in children and adolescents. *Eur Spine J* 2005;14(9):833-842.

In 102 patients reviewed with clinical examination, radiographs, and MRI, in situ fusion was associated with moderate degenerative changes in the lumbar spine during the 20-year follow-up. There was no correlation between Oswestry Disability Index score and abnormal MRI findings. Level of evidence: IV.

81. Bohlman HH, Cook SS: One-stage decompression and posterolateral and interbody fusion for lumbosacral spondyloptosis through a posterior approach: Report of two cases. *J Bone Joint Surg Am* 1982;64(3):415-418.

82. Hresko MT, Hirschfeld R, Buerk AA, Zurakowski D: The effect of reduction and instrumentation of spondylolisthesis on spinopelvic sagittal alignment. *J Pediatr Orthop* 2009;29(2):157-162.

In a retrospective study of 26 adolescents with high-grade spondylolisthesis, partial surgical reduction and posterior instrumented fusion improved pelvic version. In patients with unbalanced spondylolisthesis, there was no correlation between the amount of spondylolisthesis reduction and improvement in pelvic version. Level of evidence: IV.

83. Petraco DM, Spivak JM, Cappadona JG, Kummer FJ, Neuwirth MG: An anatomic evaluation of L5 nerve stretch in spondylolisthesis reduction. *Spine (Phila Pa 1976)* 1996;21(10):1133-1139.

84. Shufflebarger HL, Geck MJ: High-grade isthmic dysplastic spondylolisthesis: Monosegmental surgical treatment. *Spine (Phila Pa 1976)* 2005;30(6, suppl):S42-S48.

In a prospective series of 18 adolescents with high-grade spondylolisthesis who were treated surgically, near-anatomic correction remained at final follow-up, with improvements in slip, slip angle, and sacral inclination. Arthrodesis was achieved in all patients without significant complications. Level of evidence: II.

85. Ruf M, Koch H, Melcher RP, Harms J: Anatomic reduction and monosegmental fusion in high-grade developmental spondylolisthesis. *Spine (Phila Pa 1976)* 2006; 31(3):269-274.

A retrospective review of 27 patients treated with temporary instrumentation of L4 and monosegmental L5-S1 fusion found that 23 patients had improved radiographic measurements and no pain at a mean 45-month follow-up. Six patients had L5 root symptoms, with two requiring reoperation. Level of evidence: IV.

86. Gaines RW: L5 vertebrectomy for the surgical treatment of spondyloptosis: Thirty cases in 25 years. *Spine (Phila Pa 1976)* 2005;30(6, suppl):S66-S70.

A retrospective review of 30 patients at an average 15-year follow-up found complications including temporary L5 root deficit in 23 patients, permanent L5 root dysfunction in 2, nonunion in 2, and retrograde ejaculation in 1. Level of evidence: IV.

5: Spine

Musculoskeletal Trauma

SECTION EDITOR:
JAMES J. McCARTHY, MD

Chapter 30

Principles of Pediatric Trauma Care

Martin J. Herman, MD

Introduction

Traumatic musculoskeletal injury is among the most common pediatric conditions requiring care from a primary care physician or emergency department. Sprains and contusions are most frequently diagnosed, but fractures account for approximately 25% of musculoskeletal injuries in children.[1] Before age 16 years, 42% of boys and 27% of girls sustain a fracture. Most fractures are isolated injuries, and the upper extremity, especially the wrist or hand, is the most common site of injury.[2] Fractures that involve the physis account for only 20% of all fractures in children.[3]

Some simple fractures can be readily managed by a primary care provider, but orthopaedic surgeons provide most fracture care. Careful evaluation and treatment following the principles of pediatric fracture care usually yield a satisfactory result. Serious complications can be prevented by early recognition and appropriate treatment of conditions such as compartment syndrome and growth disturbance.

Mechanisms of Injury

Most musculoskeletal fractures, especially those in children younger than 5 years, occur in the home. Fractures at home typically result from a low-energy mechanism such as a fall from a bed or a standing height. Relatively few pediatric fractures occur at school, and most of these are sports related.[4] A national database study found that 22,728 emergency department visits between 2002 and 2004 were necessitated by a playground equipment injury; 39% of the injuries were fractures resulting from a fall from playground equipment, and 8.5% were traumatic brain injuries.[5] Improvements in playground landing-surface materials and structural designs may reduce the incidence of such injuries.

Dr. Herman or an immediate family member serves as a board member, owner, officer, or committee member of the American Academy of Orthopaedic Surgeons and the Pediatric Orthopaedic Society of North America.

Many pediatric musculoskeletal injuries result from sports activities, particularly popular contact or collision sports such as soccer, basketball, and football.[6] Approximately one third of pediatric injuries from American football are fractures.[7] Among women's sports, gymnastics has one of the highest injury rates; sprains and fractures account for most of these injuries.[8] Cheerleading-related injuries doubled from 1990 to 2002.[9] Roller sports such as skateboarding and rollerblading cause many fractures, especially in older children and adolescents. Roller sports led to 14% of all fractures seen in one institution's fracture clinic.[10]

During the past decade, the increasing popularity of trampolines in the United States and Europe has led to a range of injuries. Fractures and head and neck injuries occur mostly in older children (average age, 8.5 years), and as many as 19% of patients require hospitalization.[11] The risk of injury is greater when more than one child jumps on a trampoline; the lightest child is most likely to be injured. The American Academy of Pediatrics advises that trampolines should be used only in a supervised training program.[12]

High-Energy Trauma

Limb- and life-threatening musculoskeletal injuries in children typically result from a high-energy mechanism. Falls from a height and motor vehicle crashes are the most common causes of death for children and adolescents in the United States. Most children involved in a motor vehicle crash are pedestrians who are struck by a vehicle; a significantly smaller number are occupants of a vehicle.[13] The increased use of child safety seats and improved compliance with the American Academy of Pediatrics' age and weight guidelines for safety seat use have contributed to the lowering of morbidity and mortality rates in children involved in a motor vehicle crash.[14]

Children and adolescents increasingly are using motorized vehicles such as all-terrain vehicles and motorcycles, with an increase in related injuries. Orthopaedic injuries are most common. Of 96 children who had injuries related to the recreational use of an all-terrain vehicle, 35% had head trauma and 20% had multisystem injuries.[15] Children older than 13 years were more

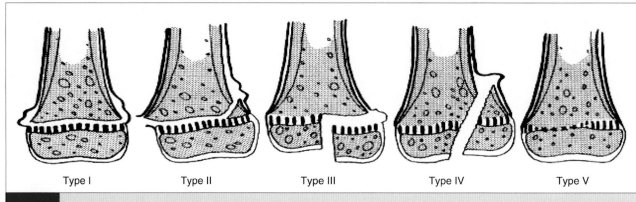

Figure 1	Schematic diagram showing the Salter-Harris classification of physeal fractures. A type I fracture traverses the physis; a type II fracture traverses the physis and the adjacent metaphysis; a type III fracture traverses the physis and the epiphysis, extending across the articular surface; and a type IV fracture extends across the metaphysis, physis, and epiphysis. A type V fracture is a crush injury to the physis; it is not radiographically apparent at the time of injury and is diagnosed retrospectively when growth disturbance appears. (Adapted with permission from Jones E: Skeletal growth and development as related to trauma, in Green NE, Swiontowski MF, eds: *Skeletal Trauma in Children.* Philadelphia, PA, WB Saunders, 2003, p 35.)

likely to sustain serious injury. There is a need for increased public awareness, improved parental supervision, and possibly legislation aimed at reducing the incidence of these injuries.

Child Abuse

The National Data Archive on Child Abuse and Neglect determined that 753,357 children were abused or neglected in the United States during 2007.[16] The death rate was 2.35 deaths per 100,000 children. Ninety percent of children who are abused have a soft-tissue injury, and fracture is the second most common injury. The fracture usually is isolated and often is of a type associated with accidental trauma. A history that is inconsistent with the injury, a lower extremity fracture in a child who is not ambulatory, a fracture of the rib or spine, or multiple fractures from a reported low-energy mechanism should lead the surgeon to suspect child abuse. Radiographic findings consistent with child abuse include multiple fractures in different stages of healing and a bucket-handle or metaphyseal corner fracture. The orthopaedic surgeon has the responsibility to report suspected abuse to the designated authorities and in some states is subject to legal action for failing to do so.

Pediatric Skeletal System and Fracture Patterns

Anatomy

Several important anatomic and physiologic features distinguish the bones of a child from those of an adult. The presence of open growth plates is the most important distinguishing feature of a child's bones. The growth plate, or physis, is composed of an expandable matrix that permits long bone growth through endochondral ossification. The metaphysis is cancellous bone adjacent to the physis; the epiphysis is a secondary ossification adjacent to the physis, at the end of the long bones, which defines the shape and size of the articular surface (**Figure 1**). In general, a child's bones are less dense and more porous than those of an adult, and they are able to absorb more energy from a traumatic mechanism before fracturing. A thick, vascular, and highly osteogenic periosteum envelops the child's bones. Largely because of this thick periosteum, a child's fracture patterns, associated soft-tissue injury, healing capacity, and ability to remodel are different from those of an adult.

Fractures

Many fracture patterns are unique to children. Compared with adults, children more commonly sustain an incomplete fracture such as a plastic deformation, torus or buckle fracture, or greenstick fracture. A complete fracture is less commonly comminuted. The thick periosteum limits fracture displacement, and its presence may be a reason that open fractures occur less frequently in children than in adults.

In a child, most joint capsules and ligaments originate and insert on the epiphysis of a long bone. These capsules and ligaments are better able to withstand traumatic forces than the adjacent physis. As a result, an injury that could cause a ligament sprain (about the knee or ankle, for example) instead is likely to cause a physeal fracture. When the physis fails, the fracture line usually traverses the hypertrophic zone, which is the weakest area of the physis. The physis is reinforced at its periphery by dense perichondrial cartilaginous tissue. The perichondrial ring diminishes in strength as the child matures and the epiphysis increases in size and density. This factor to some extent explains the increasing incidence of physeal fractures as children approach their adolescent years.

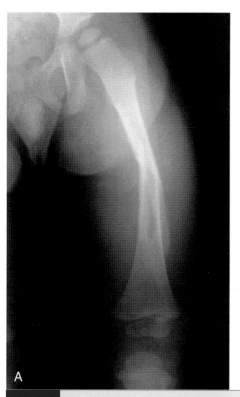 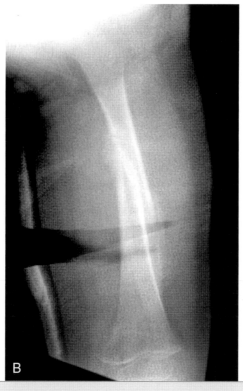 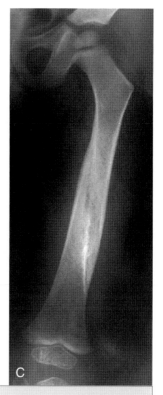

Figure 2 AP radiographs showing remodeling of a diaphyseal femur fracture in an 18-month-old child who fell from a playground slide. **A,** At the time of injury. **B,** Four weeks after spica casting; the cast wedging can be seen. **C,** Six months after cast removal. The residual angulation has been corrected and the cortical shape restored.

Classification

The Salter-Harris classification is used to describe fractures that involve the physis (**Figure 1**). In general, a Salter-Harris type I or II injury has a better prognosis than a type III or IV injury. Classifying the fracture allows the surgeon to predict the risk of growth disturbance. However, the risk of growth arrest is less reliably predicted from Salter-Harris type if the fracture is through a nonplanar physis, as in the distal femur and proximal tibia.[17,18]

Healing and Remodeling

Fractures heal more rapidly and predictably in children than in adults. Greater bone vascularity and highly osteogenic periosteum contribute to the greater capacity for healing, as does the likelihood of less soft-tissue disruption.[19] Nonunion is rare in children, occurring only in specific anatomic locations or situations, such as a displaced lateral condyle fracture or severe open tibia fracture.

Pediatric fractures have a greater capacity for remodeling than adult fractures. In children, a fracture that heals with some residual angulation is likely to become more normally aligned over time. As bone is gradually resorbed at the malunion's convexity and deposited at the concavity, the deformity is reshaped along the fractured bone's lines of stress (**Figures 2** and **3**). However, most remodeling occurs through

asymmetric longitudinal growth and physeal reorientation.[20] The factors responsible for this capacity to remodel include systemic signals for bone growth and a change in the production of growth factors at the level of the physis. The capacity to remodel is limited, however, and the surgeon must be aware of the acceptable degree of residual angulation[21] (**Table 1**).

Fracture Management

History and Examination

The emergency department assessment of a child with a possible fracture begins with a complete patient history. A thorough assessment by the trauma team is warranted if the mechanism of injury was high energy with the potential for multiple or serious injuries. However, most fractures in children are isolated and caused by a low-energy mechanism. The extremity is inspected for deformity, swelling, skin abrasions or lacerations, and exposed bone. The neurovascular examination includes motor and sensory testing, palpation of pulses, and assessment of capillary refill. The compartments are inspected for swelling and palpated for tenseness or tenderness. Despite the difficulty of examining a very young, uncooperative child who is in pain, the surgeon must obtain as complete an assessment as possible,

6: Musculoskeletal Trauma

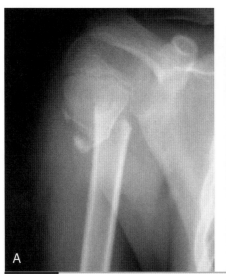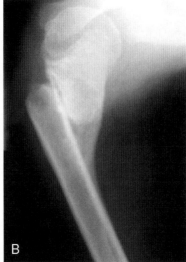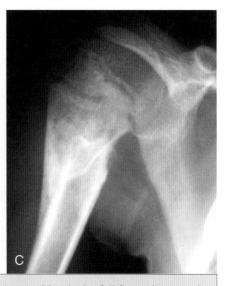

Figure 3 AP radiographs showing remodeling of a proximal humerus fracture in a 6-year-old girl who fell from playground equipment. **A**, At the time of injury. **B**, Four weeks after placement of a shoulder immobilizer. **C**, Four months after the injury, showing dramatic fracture remodeling. Remodeling was enhanced by the child's young age as well as the position of the fracture near the physis and adjacent to a joint with multiplanar mobility. (Reproduced from Khoshhal KI, Kiefer GN: Physeal bridge resection. *J Am Acad Orthop Surg* 2005;13(1):47-58.)

Table 1

Factors Affecting the Remodeling of a Malunited Fracture

General Factor	Specific Considerations
Skeletal maturity	Fracture remodeling is better if the child has at least 2 years of remaining growth. The younger the child, the more capacity there is for remodeling.
Fracture location	Fracture remodeling is better if the malunion is close to the physis. Remodeling is better for a metaphyseal malunion than a diaphyseal malunion. An interarticular deformity does not remodel.
Plane of deformity	Angulation in the plane of motion of the joint closest to the malunion remodels better than angulation in other planes. (For example, apex dorsal or volar angulation of a healed distal radius fracture is more likely to remodel than apex radial or ulnar angulation.) A rotational or multiplane deformity is relatively unlikely to remodel completely.

using age-appropriate questions, clinical observation, and patience. A grossly unstable fracture or severe deformity is best treated by gentle realignment and splinting immediately after evaluation to prevent additional vascular compromise or skin injury.

Imaging

High-quality orthogonal radiographs of the injured limb, including images of the joints above and below the site of fracture, are adequate for most fractures. Oblique radiographs of the elbow, ankle mortise radiographs, or other special views may be required. CT is not routinely used for fracture assessment but can be useful for some injuries, most commonly including pelvic and spinal injuries or intra-articular fractures of the ankle, such as the triplane fracture. CT exposes the patient to a large amount of ionizing radiation and, therefore, should be used judiciously.

Pain Control

Local and Regional Drugs

Analgesia is necessary to control pain and provide sedation during closed reduction and splinting or casting. Local anesthesia is relatively safe and easy to administer by infiltration of the fractured hematoma with a local anesthetic agent, such as lidocaine. However, local anesthesia is less frequently used for children than for adults and is best reserved for reduction of distal radius fractures in older children.[22] Intravenous regional anesthesia (the Bier block) provides satisfactory analgesia in more than 90% of patients and can be safely used in children.[23] The brachial plexus block is preferable to intravenous regional anesthesia because of its rapid onset and low complication rate. An axillary nerve block is more commonly used in the operating room but can be safely used by properly trained personnel in the emergency department.[24]

6: Musculoskeletal Trauma

Conscious Sedation and Dissociative Anesthesia

Conscious sedation, which allows the patient to protect his or her own airway, is a popular method of administering anesthesia for fracture reduction in the emergency department. Although inhalational agents such as nitrous oxide can be used to achieve conscious sedation, most emergency department personnel prefer a combination of benzodiazepines and narcotics (commonly midazolam and morphine or meperidine) to provide pain relief and a safe level of sedation.

Dissociative anesthesia, a trancelike state that combines sedation and pain relief without the risk of severe cardiovascular depression, is used in many emergency departments to facilitate fracture reduction.[25] Intravenous ketamine is frequently used to achieve dissociative anesthesia, with atropine routinely administered just before ketamine to diminish upper airway secretions. The safety of using ketamine can be further enhanced by combining it with midazolam, which reduces the risk of airway compromise as the patient emerges from anesthesia.[26] Continuous monitoring of the patient's respiratory rate, blood pressure, and pulse rate is mandatory when intravenous sedation is being used. Personnel trained in advanced cardiac life support must be present, with equipment and medication for treating airway compromise or cardiovascular complications at the bedside.

Splinting and Casting

Most fractures in children can be safely casted in the emergency department. Splinting is preferable if the injury is accompanied by severe swelling or skin lacerations or abrasions or if the child is unable to communicate or is insensate.

Casts are more reliable than splints for maintaining a fracture reduction in children, primarily because a cast is more durable and more difficult to remove. Although a cast applied by a trained person usually is safe, complications can occur. Skin irritation or breakdown and compartment syndrome from constriction are the most common cast complications.[27] Plaster is a less expensive and more easily molded material for casting than fiberglass, but it is heavier and has poor resistance to water. Plaster cures by releasing heat. To reduce the risk of thermal injury when applying a plaster cast, excessively thick wrapping and a dip water temperature exceeding 24°C should be avoided.[28] Thermal injury also can be caused by allowing the cast to cure on a pillow or overwrapping a partially dried plaster cast with fiberglass. In most institutions, fiberglass has largely replaced plaster for casting. Although fiberglass is relatively less exothermic than plaster, a fiberglass cast is stiffer and potentially more constrictive than a plaster cast. Stretching the fiberglass and allowing it to relax before rolling it around the extremity may diminish the risk that the cast will be overly tight.[29]

The use of an oscillating saw for cast removal has been associated with limb injuries. Cuts can result from excessive pressure over a bony prominence or swollen soft tissue. An excessively thick cast or the use of a dull blade for cast removal can lead to thermal injury; as the temperature of the blade increases, inadvertent contact with the skin leads to burning. The temperature of the skin increases to a greater degree during removal of a fiberglass cast, compared with a plaster cast; and during removal of a cast with two layers of padding, compared with four layers.[30] The risk of injury can be reduced by training personnel in using the cast saw, frequently changing the saw blade, cooling the blade periodically during removal of a thick cast, and applying appropriate padding during casting.

Special Situations

Polytrauma

Injury from a high-energy mechanism, such as a motor vehicle crash, is a leading cause of death in children. Fractures are common in a child with polytrauma, but 80% of the deaths associated with high-energy trauma result from traumatic brain injury. Severe thoracoabdominal and pelvic ring injuries occur less frequently in children than in adults.[31] The full recovery of a child who survives polytrauma is closely related to the effective management of fractures and other orthopaedic injuries.[32] The orthopaedic surgeon must assume that a child with polytrauma will survive and that most patients will completely recover. Aggressive, appropriate treatment of all orthopaedic injuries and careful surveillance to detect any missed injuries are necessary to ensure the best outcome.

Unlike adults, children with serious traumatic injuries rarely have a preexisting medical condition. Older children and adolescents are able to tolerate profound hypovolemia and hypoxia before cardiovascular collapse.[33] In the emergency department, outcomes can be improved for the most seriously injured children by aggressive resuscitation as well as careful, thorough examination by a pediatric trauma team or other pediatrics-trained personnel.

Emergency Orthopaedic Management

The orthopaedic surgeon who is caring for a child with polytrauma first must identify limb- or life-threatening orthopaedic injuries, such as a spinal cord injury or open fracture with a vascular injury. Spinal immobilization and application of a pediatric spine board with an occipital recess to prevent neck flexion in younger children is mandatory if the patient is unconscious or has an observable spine injury. Provisional splinting of an obvious extremity fracture increases the patient's comfort and protects the limb from further injury during resuscitation and imaging.

Damage Control

When a damage control orthopaedic treatment strategy is followed, emergency orthopaedic surgery is limited

Table 2

Principles of Pediatric Orthopaedic Polytrauma Management

1. Damage control orthopaedics is indicated if the patient has any of the following: a severe head injury, with intracranial pressure higher than 30 mm Hg or uncontrolled by medication; profound hypothermia; or persistent hypovolemia and hypotension despite resuscitation.
2. Delay of definitive management until the child is medically stable does not affect the outcome of most orthopaedic injuries.
3. Definitive treatment of all musculoskeletal injuries should allow early mobilization whenever possible.
4. It is assumed that the child will fully recover from the nonmusculoskeletal injuries. Repeated orthopaedic evaluation for occult injuries and appropriate treatment of all orthopaedic injuries improves the overall outcome.

Table 3

Sample Guidelines for Infection Prophylaxis of Open Fractures

Drug Class	Dosage	Gustilo-Anderson Fracture Types	Notes
First-generation cephalosporin	100 mg/kg/day divided into doses administered every 8 hours	All types	Consider substituting clindamycin or vancomycin if the patient has a history of methicillin-resistant *Staphylococcus aureus* infection.
Aminoglycoside	5 to 7.5 mg/kg/day divided into doses administered every 8 hours	Types II and III	Added for a severely contaminated wound.
Penicillin	150,000 units/kg/day divided into doses administered every 6 hours	All types	Added for a farm injury, other soil or fecal contamination, or risk of infection from *Clostridium* or an anaerobe.
Tetanus toxoid	0.5 mL administered intramuscularly	All types	Components are determined by the child's age. Used if immunization history is unknown or last booster was more than 5 years ago. Consider tetanus immune globulin for unknown immunization status and high-risk injury.

until the patient's condition is stable (**Table 2**). External skeletal fixation and splinting are the only procedures done until cardiovascular stabilization is achieved. The intention of the damage control strategy is to avoid the secondary physiologic stress resulting from orthopaedic surgery during the first 24 to 48 hours after injury, thereby decreasing the likelihood of acute respiratory distress syndrome and multiorgan system failure.[34] Definitive orthopaedic treatment takes place within the first week after the patient's condition significantly improves. Although damage control orthopaedic treatment has not been directly studied in children, it can be considered for a child who has a severe head injury, with intracranial pressure greater than 30 mm Hg; a child whose condition is unstable and not easily controlled medically; a child with profound hypothermia upon admission; or a child who has hypovolemia and hypotension despite ongoing resuscitation.

Limb-preserving surgery or a short surgical procedure associated with minimal blood loss, such as fasciotomy or supracondylar humerus fracture pinning, can be done on an emergency basis. Definitive surgical management typically is delayed until the entire care

team has cleared the child for surgery. This delay rarely has a detrimental effect on the long-term outcome.[35] The fracture treatment of a child with polytrauma ideally should allow early mobilization to a chair.

Open Fractures

The principles of treatment for an open fracture in children and adults do not differ significantly. Open fractures typically result from a high-energy or penetrating trauma. The Gustilo-Anderson system is used to classify pediatric open fractures, the most common of which is in the tibia. Absolute wound size is used in determining the severity of the fracture, particularly in a child's small limb. However, the extent of soft-tissue injury and periosteal stripping are more useful for determining injury severity and predicting outcome. A complete assessment often can best be done in the operating room rather than the emergency department.

Timing of Irrigation and Débridement

The emergency department treatment includes limited irrigation of grossly contaminated wounds, application of a sterile dressing, and provisional splinting. Intravenous antibiotics are administered and tetanus status is confirmed during the initial assessment, if possible (Table 3). A cephalosporin or clindamycin is administered to all children with an open fracture. An aminoglycoside is added if the wound is severely contaminated, with penicillin added if soil or fecal contamination is suspected. The decision to irrigate and débride the wound immediately or delay treatment until the next day is based on the vascular status of the limb and the severity of the bone and soft-tissue injuries. A study of more than 500 open fractures in children found that when antibiotics were administered in the emergency department upon admission, the infection rates were similar whether the wound was surgically débrided 7 to 24 hours after injury or within 7 hours of injury.[36] All open fractures should undergo irrigation and débridement within 24 hours of the injury.

Surgical Considerations

In the operating room, the bones ends are exposed, and devitalized tissue is débrided. Bone fragments stripped of periosteum and obvious debris are removed. Tissue of questionable viability is best preserved during the initial surgery and reevaluated in the operating room within 48 hours. High-pressure lavage must be used cautiously to avoid extravasation of fluid into soft-tissue compartments of the child's small limb, which can initiate compartment syndrome. The wound can be safely closed over a drain if the wound is small and has little contamination. Vacuum-assisted closure or an open dressing is useful for soft-tissue management and can diminish the risk of systemic infection associated with tight wound closure. Vacuum-assisted closure also can reduce the need for skin grafting or flap coverage of a severe injury.[37] Fracture fixation is preferable to cast immobilization alone for an unstable fracture or a fracture with a large soft-tissue injury. All children should receive intravenous antibiotic therapy for 24 to 72 hours after débridement and should be carefully assessed for signs and symptoms of a developing infection.

Outcomes

In general, children have better outcomes than adults after an open fracture, but serious complications can occur. Infection develops in approximately 3% of all pediatric open fractures, usually after a Gustilo-Anderson type III injury. Delayed union or nonunion occurs infrequently, usually after a type III open tibia fracture. Delayed healing also can occur, and its management varies with the anatomic site.

Compartment Syndrome

Compartment syndrome occurs when elevated interstitial pressure in a fixed osteofascial space leads to obstruction of venous outflow, which further increases the swelling and congestion of soft tissues. When the arteriolar pressure is exceeded, muscle ischemia develops. In children, compartment syndrome most commonly occurs in the lower extremity after a tibia fracture or in the forearm after a supracondylar fracture.[38] Compartment syndrome also can develop in the calf if traction was used while a spica cast was being applied.[39]

The classic adult compartment syndrome findings are not always readily detectable in children. A young child with a painful injury is not always able to cooperate with a detailed sensorimotor examination. Severe circumferential swelling, compartment tenseness, and pain with passive stretching of the muscles in the involved compartment are important indicators of an evolving compartment syndrome. The most reliable sign of compartment syndrome in children is escalating pain that requires an increasing amount of narcotic analgesia to control. If the diagnosis is uncertain or the child is unresponsive or uncooperative, it is useful to measure compartment pressures, using the same critical values as for adults. Measuring compartment pressures may require sedation or general anesthesia.

A compartment syndrome is treated with emergency fasciotomy using the same methods as for adults. To allow adequate decompression in the lower leg of a child, a four-compartment fasciotomy is best done through medial and lateral incisions. It is essential to adequately identify and decompress both superficial and deep flexor muscle groups. As in an adult, the deep posterior compartment often is not adequately decompressed. Volar decompression of the forearm through an extensile incision generally is adequate for release. The distal decompression always should extend to the carpal tunnel. Although obviously devitalized muscle is best débrided during the initial release, questionable muscle tissue should be preserved and reevaluated 24 to 48 hours later. After release, an open dressing or vacuum-assisted closure is used. Delayed primary closure of wounds often is possible, and skin grafting is infrequently required.

More than 90% of children who are promptly diagnosed and treated regain normal function after fasciotomies for compartment syndrome.[38] The compartments ideally should be released on an emergency basis when the diagnosis is made. However, compartment syndromes can evolve over time, and release within the first day of symptom onset usually yields a satisfactory outcome. Releasing compartments later than 48 to 72 hours after symptom onset is unlikely to improve the outcome.

Growth Disturbance

Less than 10% of physeal fractures lead to a significant disturbance of normal growth. The size and location of the physeal bar and the skeletal age of the child at the time of injury are the most important factors in determining the extent to which growth is likely to be affected. Growth arrest is most likely to occur in a young adolescent who sustains a distal femur or distal tibia fracture.[40] Complete physeal arrest may lead to limb-length inequality or a mismatch of growth between the paired bones of the forearm or lower leg. Incomplete

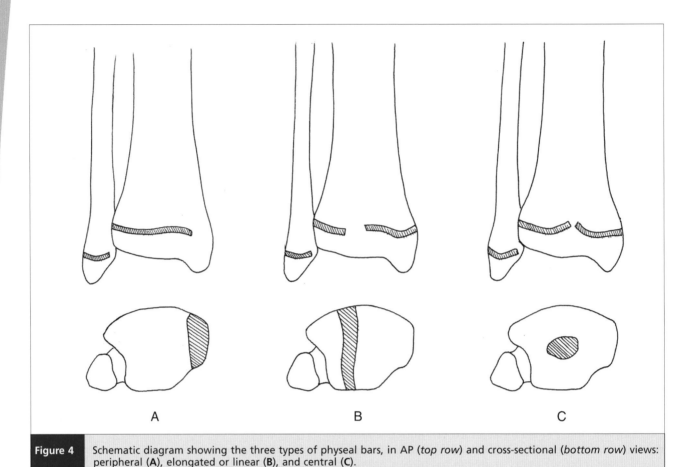

Figure 4 Schematic diagram showing the three types of physeal bars, in AP (*top row*) and cross-sectional (*bottom row*) views: peripheral (**A**), elongated or linear (**B**), and central (**C**).

physeal arrest may lead to angular limb deformities or joint surface deformation.

Etiologies of Growth Arrest

Growth arrest results from inadequate reduction of a fracture or from trauma to the physis at the time of injury. With fracture healing, an osseous bar is created that spans the physis and tethers its normal growth. Physeal arrest sometimes occurs despite anatomic reduction, however.[41] The most likely cause is damage to resting chondrocytes within the physis as a sequela of the traumatic injury. Iatrogenic injury from the surgical approach or from forceful or repeated manipulation of the physeal fracture can cause physeal arrest. Screw fixation spanning the physis also can result in growth disturbance. Vascular damage to the physis and epiphysis, such as occurs after a severe burn or infection, is an uncommon etiology.

Patterns of Bar Formation

Three patterns of bar formation have been described[42] (**Figure 4**). The most common is a peripheral bar at the physeal edge, which generally causes angular limb deformity. A central bar occurs within the physis away from the periphery and acts as a tether to growth. This type of bar may result in limb-length discrepancy but more commonly causes distortion of the articular sur-

face. The elongated or linear bar is a narrow band of physeal bridging along the healed fracture line that often causes both angular and joint surface deformities.

Treatment

Physeal growth disturbance typically is diagnosed within 6 months of injury, but bar formation or incomplete return of normal growth may not be apparent until several years after the injury. Therefore, surveillance for growth arrest is necessary after most physeal fractures for at least 2 years; ideally, a younger child with an injury having a high risk of growth disturbance, such as a distal femur fracture, should be followed until skeletal maturity. Angular growth changes and limb-length inequality may signal a growth disturbance but often are late manifestations of bar formation. Many physeal bars are evident on plain radiographs, but MRI with fat-suppressed three-dimensional spoiled gradient-recalled echo sequencing is the best modality for identifying early physeal bar formation.[43] It is useful to map the precise location and extent of the bar preoperatively using multiplanar CT and MRI.

For a child with a complete growth arrest, the surgical procedure is chosen based on the extent of the projected limb-length discrepancy. Contralateral epiphysiodesis is done if the anticipated discrepancy is less than 5 cm, and lengthening of the short limb is done for an anticipated discrepancy greater than 5 cm. If the affected bone is paired, epiphysiodesis of the unaffected bone may be necessary to prevent joint incongruity, such as ulnar impingement after a distal radial growth arrest or fibular overgrowth after a distal tibial arrest.

If partial growth arrest is diagnosed before the development of angular deformity, the best treatment is to complete the arrest by epiphysiodesis. This procedure can be done in combination with osteotomies and lengthening procedures, depending on the extent of deformity or the anticipated limb-length discrepancy. Bar resection is indicated if less than 50% of the physis is bridged, the angular deformity is less than 20°, and at least 2 years of growth remain. The best results occur after resection of a central bar; a bar bridging less than 25% of the physis; or a bar that did not result from an infection, vascular injury, or Salter-Harris type IV fracture.

Summary

Fractures and other musculoskeletal injuries are common in children, most frequently resulting from a low-energy mechanism, such as a fall from a low height or a sports activity. The anatomy and physiology of a child with open growth plates influences the types of injury the child sustains as well as the fracture management options. The surgeon should understand the child's capacity for fracture remodeling when deciding whether surgical intervention is needed. Most fractures can be adequately treated by closed manipulation and cast immobilization. Emergency departments can offer several options for safe, effective analgesia during fracture reduction. Deep sedation with ketamine and other agents is most frequently used, although many centers routinely use regional anesthesia. Careful cast application and removal reduces the likelihood of complications associated with fracture immobilization, such as pressure sores and thermal injury. A high-energy mechanism, such as a motor vehicle crash, frequently causes serious injury to the head, thorax, and abdomen as well as the musculoskeletal system. The involvement of a coordinated care team skilled in pediatric care can improve the outcome for a polytraumatized child. Infection after an open fracture, compartment syndrome, and premature physeal arrest are some important complications of children's fractures. To minimize the risk of infection, an open fracture is best treated by antibiotic administration in the emergency department, followed by irrigation and débridement within 24 hours of injury. The most reliable sign of compartment syndrome in a child is an increasing need for medication to control pain. Emergency fasciotomies yield good results if compartment syndromes are diagnosed in a timely fashion. Growth disturbance related to physeal bar formation or physeal arrest can result from a physeal fracture. Bar resection, epiphyseodeses, osteotomies, and limb lengthening or shortening procedures may be appropriate, depending on the amount of growth re-

maining, the presence of angular deformity, and the predicted limb-length discrepancy.

Annotated References

1. Landin LA: Epidemiology of children's fractures. *J Pediatr Orthop B* 1997;6(2):79-83.

2. Cheng JC, Shen WY: Limb fracture pattern in different pediatric age groups: A study of 3,350 children. *J Orthop Trauma* 1993;7(1):15-22.

3. Mann DC, Rajmaira S: Distribution of physeal and nonphyseal fractures in 2,650 long-bone fractures in children aged 0-16 years. *J Pediatr Orthop* 1990;10(6):713-716.

4. Worlock P, Stower M: Fracture patterns in Nottingham children. *J Pediatr Orthop* 1986;6(6):656-660.

5. Loder RT: The demographics of playground equipment injuries in children. *J Pediatr Surg* 2008;43(4):691-699.

   The National Electronic Injury Surveillance System (NEISS) database was used to investigate playground equipment injuries from 2002 to 2004. Most injuries occurred on swings, slides, and monkey bars. There were 22,728 emergency department visits, and 39.3% of the injuries were diagnosed as fractures.

6. Leininger RE, Knox CL, Comstock RD: Epidemiology of 1.6 million pediatric soccer-related injuries presenting to US emergency departments from 1990 to 2003. *Am J Sports Med* 2007;35(2):288-293.

   The NEISS database was used to examine pediatric soccer-related injuries seen in US emergency departments from 1990 to 2003. Most injuries involved the hand or wrist, ankle, or knee. The proportion of head and neck injuries was highest in young children.

7. Mello MJ, Myers R, Christian JB, Palmisciano L, Linakis JG: Injuries in youth football: National emergency department visits during 2001-2005 for young and adolescent players. *Acad Emerg Med* 2009;16(3):243-248.

   The NEISS database was used to analyze pediatric football injuries. Most injuries were fractures, sprains or strains, or contusions. Older players had a significantly higher risk of injury; the greatest disparity between older and younger players was in traumatic brain injury.

8. Singh S, Smith GA, Fields SK, McKenzie LB: Gymnastics-related injuries to children treated in emergency departments in the United States, 1990-2005. *Pediatrics* 2008;121(4):e954-e960.

   The NEISS database was used to analyze gymnastics injuries from 1990 to 2005. The annual injury rate was 4.8 per 1,000 participants. Most of the injuries were to an extremity. Gymnastics has one of the highest injury rates among girls' sports.

6: Musculoskeletal Trauma

9. Shields BJ, Smith GA: Cheerleading-related injuries to children 5 to 18 years of age: United States, 1990-2002. *Pediatrics* 2006;117(1):122-129.

    The NEISS database was used to analyze cheerleading injuries. The injury rate doubled over the 13-year study period. Most injuries were simple extremity fractures or dislocations. The head or neck was injured in 18.8% of patients.

10. Zalavras C, Nikolopoulou G, Essin D, Manjra N, Zionts LE: Pediatric fractures during skateboarding, roller skating, and scooter riding. *Am J Sports Med* 2005;33(4):568-573.

    A level I trauma center's fracture clinic records were used to study skateboard, roller-skating, and scooter fractures, which represented 13% of all fractures. Skateboarding accounted for 5.2% of all forearm open fractures. Level of evidence: IV.

11. Hurson C, Browne K, Callender O, et al: Pediatric trampoline injuries. *J Pediatr Orthop* 2007;27(7):729-732.

    An emergency room in Ireland evaluated 101 trampoline-related injuries during 3 summer months. Most were fractures, and 19.8% required hospital admission. The highest risk for injury was found to be for a relatively light child who was jumping with a heavier child.

12. American Academy of Pediatrics, Committee on Injury and Poison Prevention, Committee on Sports Medicine and Fitness: Trampolines at home, school, and recreational centers. *Pediatrics* 1999;103(5, pt 1):1053-1056.

13. Derlet RW, Silva J Jr, Holcroft J: Pedestrian accidents: Adult and pediatric injuries. *J Emerg Med* 1989;7(1):5-8.

14. Rice TM, Anderson CL: The effectiveness of child restraint systems for children aged 3 years or younger during motor vehicle collisions: 1996 to 2005. *Am J Public Health* 2009;99(2):252-257.

    A matched cohort study using the Fatality Reporting System determined that the use of child safety seats reduces the risk of death during a severe collision and that safety seats outperform safety belts for children younger than 3 years.

15. Kellum E, Creek A, Dawkins R, Bernard M, Sawyer JR: Age-related patterns of injury in children involved in all-terrain vehicle accidents. *J Pediatr Orthop* 2008;28(8):854-858.

    Among all-terrain vehicle–related injuries seen at a level I trauma center, orthopaedic and head injuries were most common. Twenty percent of patients had multisystem injuries, and 68% required hospital admission. Most younger children sustained a lower extremity fracture, and older children had a pelvic fracture.

16. Gaudiosi JA: Child Maltreatment 2007. http://www.acf.hhs.gov/programs/cb/stats_research/index.htm. Accessed Dec 31, 2009.

    The US Department of Health and Human Services Administration for Children and Families provides up-to-date statistics on child maltreatment, including abuse. The latest comprehensive national data are from 2007.

17. Arkader A, Warner WC Jr , Horn BD, Shaw RN, Wells L: Predicting the outcome of physeal fractures of the distal femur. *J Pediatr Orthop* 2007;27(6):703-708.

    In this study of the outcomes of displaced distal femoral physeal fractures treated at two trauma centers, most children had a Salter-Harris type II fracture. Forty percent had a complication, most commonly a growth disturbance. Displaced fractures and fixation across the physis were correlated with complications.

18. Barmada A, Gaynor T, Mubarak SJ: Premature physeal closure following distal tibia physeal fractures: A new radiographic predictor. *J Pediatr Orthop* 2003;23(6):733-739.

19. Jacobsen FS: Periosteum: Its relation to pediatric fractures. *J Pediatr Orthop B* 1997;6(2):84-90.

20. Murray DW, Wilson-MacDonald J, Morscher E, Rahn BA, Käslin M: Bone growth and remodelling after fracture. *J Bone Joint Surg Br* 1996;78(1):42-50.

21. Wilkins KE: Principles of fracture remodeling in children. *Injury* 2005;36(suppl 1):A3-A11.

    Basic principles of fracture physiology are included in this outstanding review of fracture remodeling in children. The expected remodeling capacity for common fractures can serve as a guideline for fracture management.

22. Constantine E, Steele DW, Eberson C, Boutis K, Amanullah S, Linakis JG: The use of local anesthetic techniques for closed forearm fracture reduction in children: A survey of academic pediatric emergency departments. *Pediatr Emerg Care* 2007;23(4):209-211.

    Pediatric emergency departments were surveyed to determine local anesthesia techniques (hematoma block, nerve block, intravenous) used for treating fractures. The responding departments routinely used sedation. Only 17% frequently used local anesthesia, mostly as hematoma block.

23. McCarty EC, Mencio GA, Green NE: Anesthesia and analgesia for the ambulatory management of fractures in children. *J Am Acad Orthop Surg* 1999;7(2):81-91.

24. Kriwanek KL, Wan J, Beaty JH, Pershad J: Axillary block for analgesia during manipulation of forearm fractures in the pediatric emergency department: A prospective randomized comparative trial. *J Pediatr Orthop* 2006;26(6):737-740.

    A prospective, randomized, unmasked, controlled comparison of axillary block and deep sedation for analgesia during fracture reduction found that pain scores did not statistically differ. No patient had a complication. The use of axillary block required training.

25. McCarty EC, Mencio GA, Walker LA, Green NE: Ketamine sedation for the reduction of children's fractures

in the emergency department. *J Bone Joint Surg Am* 2000;82-A(7):912-918.

26. Migita RT, Klein EJ, Garrison MM: Sedation and analgesia for pediatric fracture reduction in the emergency department: A systematic review. *Arch Pediatr Adolesc Med* 2006;160(1):46-51.

 In this meta-analysis of randomized, controlled studies of sedation and analgesia for pediatric fracture reduction, ketamine-midazolam was found to be more effective and have fewer adverse effects than fentanyl-midazolam or propofol-fentanyl. Other forms of pain control were not studied.

27. Halanski M, Noonan KJ: Cast and splint immobilization: Complications. *J Am Acad Orthop Surg* 2008; 16(1):30-40.

 Tips for avoiding complications are provided in this excellent review of the art of cast application. The highest risk of complications is in a patient who is comatose or under anesthesia or and who has an intellectual disability or neuromuscular disease.

28. Gannaway JK, Hunter JR: Thermal effects of casting materials. *Clin Orthop Relat Res* 1983;181:191-195.

29. Davids JR, Frick SL, Skewes E, Blackhurst DW: Skin surface pressure beneath an above-the-knee cast: Plaster casts compared with fiberglass casts. *J Bone Joint Surg Am* 1997;79(4):565-569.

30. Shuler FD, Grisafi FN: Cast-saw burns: Evaluation of skin, cast, and blade temperatures generated during cast removal. *J Bone Joint Surg Am* 2008;90(12):2626-2630.

 A cadaver model was used to measure skin temperatures during cast removal with an oscillating saw. The risk of thermal and other types of injuries was determined.

31. Jawadi AH, Letts M: Injuries associated with fracture of the femur secondary to motor vehicle accidents in children. *Am J Orthop (Belle Mead NJ)* 2003;32(9):459-462.

32. Sullivan T, Haider A, DiRusso SM, Nealon P, Shaukat A, Slim M: Prediction of mortality in pediatric trauma patients: New injury severity score outperforms injury severity score in the severely injured. *J Trauma* 2003; 55(6):1083-1088.

33. Armstrong PF: Initial management of the multiply injured child: The ABC's. *Instr Course Lect* 1992;41:347-350.

34. Pape HC, Tornetta P III , Tarkin I, Tzioupis C, Sabeson V, Olson SA: Timing of fracture fixation in multitrauma patients: The role of early total care and damage control surgery. *J Am Acad Orthop Surg* 2009;17(9):541-549.

 The principles of damage control orthopaedics are discussed. A patient who is hemodynamically unstable or multiply injured should be stabilized before definitive orthopaedic treatment. Pediatric care is not specifically discussed.

35. Loder RT: Pediatric polytrauma: Orthopaedic care and hospital course. *J Orthop Trauma* 1987;1(1):48-54.

36. Skaggs DL, Friend L, Alman B, et al: The effect of surgical delay on acute infection following 554 open fractures in children. *J Bone Joint Surg Am* 2005;87(1): 8-12.

 In patients who received antibiotics in the emergency department, the risk of infection was not correlated with the timing of irrigation and débridement within 6 hours or 24 hours of an open fracture.

37. Mooney JF III, Argenta LC, Marks MW, Morykwas MJ, DeFranzo AJ: Treatment of soft tissue defects in pediatric patients using the V.A.C. system. *Clin Orthop Relat Res* 2000;376:26-31.

38. Bae DS, Kadiyala RK, Waters PM: Acute compartment syndrome in children: Contemporary diagnosis, treatment, and outcome. *J Pediatr Orthop* 2001;21(5):680-688.

39. Large TM, Frick SL: Compartment syndrome of the leg after treatment of a femoral fracture with an early sitting spica cast: A report of two cases. *J Bone Joint Surg Am* 2003;85-A(11):2207-2210.

40. Khoshhal KI, Kiefer GN: Physeal bridge resection. *J Am Acad Orthop Surg* 2005;13(1):47-58.

 This outstanding review includes technical tips and up-to-date thinking on the evaluation and surgical treatment of physeal bars in children. The use of novel interposition materials, such as cultured chondrocytes, is discussed.

41. Wattenbarger JM, Gruber HE, Phieffer LS: Physeal fractures: Part I. Histologic features of bone, cartilage, and bar formation in a small animal model. *J Pediatr Orthop* 2002;22(6):703-709.

42. Peterson HA: Partial growth plate arrest and its treatment. *J Pediatr Orthop* 1984;4(2):246-258.

43. Ecklund K, Jaramillo D: Patterns of premature physeal arrest: MR imaging of 111 children. *AJR Am J Roentgenol* 2002;178(4):967-972.

6: Musculoskeletal Trauma

Chapter 31

Shoulder and Elbow Trauma

Maya E. Pring, MD   C. Douglas Wallace, MD

Introduction

Many pediatric injuries about the shoulder and elbow can be treated nonsurgically or with closed reduction and pin fixation. It is critical to understand which fractures can be treated nonsurgically and which require surgical intervention to prevent future growth disruption, deformity, arthrosis, motion limitation, refracture or dislocation, or loss of function. Many pediatric fractures have the ability to remodel, but research is needed to determine which fractures can adequately remodel and which must be anatomically realigned and fixed. The patient age at which a specific fracture should be treated as an adult fracture varies because the physes close at different times, and each physis has a different remodeling potential.

Shoulder Injuries

Clavicle Fractures

The etiology of pediatric clavicle fractures ranges from birth trauma in a newborn, to child abuse in a toddler, to a simple fall or a sports injury in an adolescent. Clavicle fracture is the most common orthopaedic injury in a newborn; the risk factors include large birth size, shoulder dystocia, mechanically assisted delivery, and prolonged gestational age. A birth fracture may be mistaken for or associated with a brachial plexus injury. The infant may have pseudoparalysis of the extremity secondary to pain or true paralysis secondary to brachial plexus palsy. One of every 11 newborns with a clavicle fracture also has a brachial plexus injury, but it is difficult to evaluate motor function in the upper extremity until the fracture pain resolves. Other signs of a clavicle fracture sustained during delivery include an absent Moro reflex on the affected side, sterno-

cleidomastoid spasm or apparent torticollis, crepitus at the fracture site, and palpable or visible bony irregularity of the clavicle. Ultrasonography is useful for diagnosis because it does not expose the infant to radiation and shows a fracture involving the physis or epiphysis, which may not be seen on radiographs. A clavicle fracture in a newborn typically heals quickly and uneventfully. Strict immobilization is not required, but pinning the sleeve to the front of the infant's clothing can remind caretakers to avoid moving the arm unnecessarily while it heals.

In rare instances, infants are born with pseudarthrosis of the clavicle. Unlike an acute fracture, a pseudarthrosis is characterized on radiographs by smooth ends. This condition typically is not tender and does not heal. Surgical intervention may be required if symptoms develop later in life. The pseudarthrosis almost always occurs in the middle portion of the right side of the clavicle. It can run in families but more commonly is sporadic.

A traumatic clavicle fracture in a child or adolescent is classified based on whether it is medial, diaphyseal, or distal. Medial fractures and sternoclavicular dislocations put the mediastinal structures at risk if the clavicle translates posteriorly. If there is any question about the medial alignment, a serendipity radiograph or, preferably, CT can reveal the position of the clavicle and the structures at risk. A posteriorly translated fracture or dislocation should be reduced and fixed if it is unstable, if the patient is having difficulty breathing or swallowing, or if neurovascular examination of the involved extremity reveals any changes. Because of the risk to the vascular and mediastinal structures, it is recommended that a vascular surgeon be available during surgical intervention for a medial clavicle fracture. Suture fixation to the sternum usually is adequate.

Historically, pediatric diaphyseal clavicle fractures have been treated nonsurgically in the absence of neurovascular compromise, open fracture, or risk to the skin. The nonsurgical treatment, which consists of using a sling or figure-of-8 brace for 4 to 6 weeks, is adequate for most diaphyseal fractures. A large callus often forms during healing. Because the clavicle is a subcutaneous structure, the callus may be visible or palpable.

For a teenager, some surgeons recommend surgical fixation of a displaced clavicle fracture. Studies of adult patients have found better functional outcomes and lower rates of malunion and nonunion in fractures

Dr. Pring or an immediate family member is a board member, owner, officer, or committee member of the American Academy for Cerebral Palsy and Developmental Medicine and the United Cerebral Palsy Association of San Diego and has received research or institutional support from DePuy, Ellipse, KCI, Axial Biotech, and Alphatec Spine. Dr. Wallace or an immediate family member has received research or institutional support from DePuy, KCI, Alphatec Spine, Ellipse, and Axial Biotech.

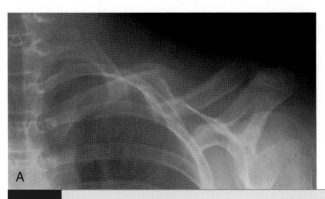
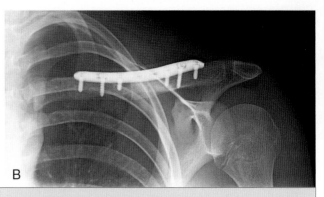

Figure 1 AP radiographs showing a clavicle shaft fracture. **A**, The fracture before fixation. **B**, Fixation of the fracture with a plate contoured to the clavicle. This type of plate is acceptable for adolescents but probably is not useful or necessary for younger children.

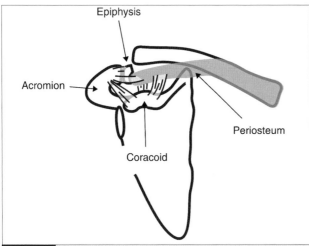

Figure 2 Schematic drawing showing an intact periosteum under a lateral physeal clavicle fracture. Because the periosteum remains intact, the remodeling potential is tremendous.

treated with plate fixation than in fractures treated nonsurgically. Surgical treatment of a completely displaced clavicle fracture has been shown to be safe in children.[1,2] A recent current-concepts review of adult clavicle fractures cautioned that, although nonsurgical treatment of displaced shaft fractures may be associated with a higher rate of nonunion and functional deficit, it remains difficult to predict which patients will have these complications; furthermore, a satisfactory functional outcome can be obtained after surgical treatment of a clavicular nonunion or malunion.[3] Thus, nonsurgical treatment remains the primary treatment for children unless the neurovascular structures are at risk, the fracture is open, or the skin is at risk.

Several types of precontoured plates can be used for surgical fixation of a diaphyseal clavicle fracture (Figure 1). A Kirschner wire can migrate[4] and, therefore, is contraindicated for clavicle fixation unless the wire is threaded to prevent migration and/or secured by an acute bend that remains outside the body. Other in-

tramedullary implants, such as a titanium elastic nail, have been successfully used in both pediatric and adult patients.[5]

The distal end of the clavicle contains the last physis to close, and many pediatric distal clavicle fractures are actually physeal injuries. At first glance, such an injury may appear to be an acromioclavicular (AC) dislocation. However, typically the AC joint is not disrupted; the epiphysis, inferior periosteum, and coracoclavicular (CC) ligaments remain intact. The fracture, therefore, heals with no instability (**Figure 2**). Surgical intervention usually is not required for a distal physeal fractures in pediatric patients.

AC Joint Injuries

The AC joint is supported medially by the CC ligaments, which attach the clavicle to the coracoid and prevent superior migration of the clavicle. The CC ligaments include the trapezoid (lateral) and the conoid (more medial). The AC ligaments attach the clavicle to the acromion and prevent anterior-posterior motion of the clavicle (**Figure 3**). An AC injury typically produces elevation of the clavicle, which may require reconstruction. If there is uncertainty as to the nature of the injury, an AP radiograph of both shoulders taken while the patient is holding a weight in each hand can accentuate the distance between the coracoid and the clavicle on the injured side. An AC separation is unusual in prepubertal or pubertal children. Most injuries of the distal clavicle in these children are physeal fractures, with a treatment and prognosis that differ from those of a true AC injury. MRI can be useful in establishing the zone of injury if it cannot be clearly seen on radiographs.

AC joint injuries are classified using the criteria listed in **Table 1**.[6] Only a high-grade AC injury (Rockwood type IV, V, or VI) is recommended for surgical fixation. As many as 18% of high-grade AC injuries are accompanied by intra-articular glenohumeral pathology such as a superior labrum anterior and posterior lesion;[7] presurgical MRI or diagnostic arthroscopy therefore should be considered. The many options for fixation of a high-grade AC injury include the use of a CC screw, a CC sling with 5-mm tape, or a hook plate; suture anchor fixation; or arthroscopic techniques. For late reconstruction, semitendinosus tendon graft was found to have better long-term results for CC ligament reconstruction than the modified Weaver-Dunn procedure.[8] A proximally based transfer of the lateral half of the conjoined tendon to the distal aspect of the clavicle, with additional CC fixation, was found to have satisfactory results for a Rockwood type III, IV, or V AC dislocation.[9]

Shoulder Dislocations

Although shoulder dislocation has been reported in children as young as 2 years,[10] the relative weakness of the physis in children makes a proximal humerus physeal fracture more likely to occur than a dislocation of the shoulder joint. Shoulder dislocations become more common as adolescents mature and the physes close, especially in athletes who are involved in a contact sport such as wrestling, football, or hockey. More than 90% of shoulder dislocations are anterior or anteroinferior, and they occur when the abducted arm is forcefully externally rotated. There is no inherent bony stability of the shoulder joint; it relies on soft-tissue stabilization. Therefore, the dislocation may be associated with significant soft-tissue disruption detectable only with MRI or magnetic resonance arthrography. Patients younger than 30 years have a high incidence of extensive labral injury (**Table 2**). Because labral injury may have a better prognosis with early intervention, early magnetic resonance arthrography sometimes is recommended after shoulder dislocation.[11]

Radiographs are recommended for evaluating a shoulder dislocation and reduction. The AP, Y lateral, and axillary lateral views are used to assess glenohumeral position, and the West Point and Stryker notch views can help in detecting a Hill-Sachs lesion or glenoid rim fracture. Adequate reduction is confirmed using radiographs. MRI or magnetic resonance arthrography is recommended for detecting injury to the labrum, capsule, glenohumeral ligaments, articular cartilage, or rotator cuff tendons.

Children and adolescents have a 66% to 94% rate of recurrence after nonsurgical treatment of an anterior shoulder dislocation.[12] The rate of recurrent dislocation was thought to be lower if the shoulder was immobilized in external rotation.[13] However, a recent prospective study found no difference in redislocation rates based on position of immobilization.[14]

Delaying glenohumeral joint reconstruction (for example, to allow the patient to complete the sports season) does not appear to be detrimental to the ultimate functional outcome of the shoulder. Because later reconstruction can be successful, the initial treatment of a first shoulder dislocation often is nonsurgical. Surgery is recommended for recurrent dislocations or if there is a large Bankart lesion or labral tear. The goal of surgery is to correct injury to the labrum, capsule, and/or

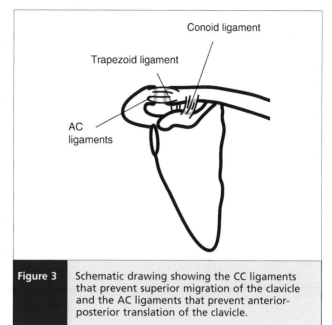

Figure 3 Schematic drawing showing the CC ligaments that prevent superior migration of the clavicle and the AC ligaments that prevent anterior-posterior translation of the clavicle.

ligaments (the static stabilizers of the shoulder). Subsequent physical therapy is directed toward improving the dynamic stabilizers of the shoulder. The results of arthroscopic and open procedures have been similar when suture anchors were used.[15] At 3-year follow-up after arthroscopic treatment, patients younger than 22 years had a 13% redislocation rate, compared with a 6% rate in older patients.[16]

Proximal Humerus Fractures

An infant sometimes sustains a proximal humerus fracture during delivery. The fracture can be diagnosed using ultrasonography or MRI. It is important to ensure that the patient's shoulder pain and decreased range of motion are caused by the fracture and not by infection, as an untreated infection can permanently damage the physis and articular cartilage. A proximal humerus fracture in a newborn heals quickly. The typical treatment is splinting for 2 to 3 weeks, which can be done by softly wrapping the broken arm and securing it to the chest or pinning the sleeve to the front of the infant's clothing.

A proximal humerus fracture in a child younger than 3 years should alert the physician to the possibility of child abuse. These fractures usually heal uneventfully because of the tremendous remodeling potential of the proximal humeral physis. Simple immobilization using a sling and swathe usually is adequate.

Proximal humerus fractures in pediatric patients are classified based on the location (physis, metaphysis, lesser tuberosity, greater tuberosity) and extent of displacement. A physeal fracture (Salter-Harris type I or II) is most common in skeletally immature patients. Because of the tremendous remodeling potential around the shoulder, anatomic reduction is not necessary if the child has more than 2 years of remaining growth. The

Table 1

The Classification of Acromioclavicular Joint Injuries

Type	Injury	Clavicle Position	Treatment
I	Stretch of AC ligaments	Normal	Nonsurgical
II	Disruption of AC ligaments Injury to CC ligaments	Slight elevation	Nonsurgical
III	Disruption of AC and CC ligaments	As much as 100% displacement above acromion	Nonsurgical or surgical (controversial)
IV	Disruption of AC and CC ligaments	Posterior displacement (buttonholed through trapezius)	Surgical fixation (usually recommended)
V	Disruption of AC and CC ligaments and muscle attachments	More than 100% superior displacement	Surgical fixation (usually recommended)
VI	Disruption of AC and CC ligaments and muscle attachments	Inferior displacement below coracoid process	Surgical fixation (usually recommended)

(Adapted with permission from Nguyen V, Williams G, Rockwood C: Radiography of acromioclavicular dislocation and associated injuries. *Crit Rev Diagn Imaging* 1991;32[3]:191-228.)

Table 2

Injuries Commonly Sustained With Anterior Shoulder Dislocation

Bankart lesion (anteroinferior labral tear)

Perthes lesion (variant of the Bankart lesion, with anterior periosteal sleeve avulsion; anterior labral tear with inferior displacement)

Anterior labral periosteal sleeve avulsion (ALPSA)

Superior labrum anterior and posterior (SLAP) lesion (tear of the superior labrum from anterior to posterior)

Glenolabral articular disruption (GLAD)

Humeral avulsion of glenohumeral ligament (HAGL)

Avulsion of inferior glenohumeral ligament (often accompanying a Bankart lesion)

Glenoid rim fracture (osteochondral injury)

Hill-Sachs lesion (depression of the posterior humeral head)

Brachial plexus injury (typically a nerve stretch injury)

use of a sling and swathe generally is adequate for treatment.

A displaced fracture in a teenager may have some ability to remodel, but the residual deformity can cause impingement during overhead sports and other activities. A varus deformity, which can be caused by malunion or premature physeal arrest, can limit abduction and flexion. This deformity and the resulting loss of motion can be corrected by a later valgus osteotomy.[17] An initial reduction and fixation often can be done percutaneously, precluding the need for later reconstructive surgery. No evidence-based criteria are available to establish a threshold for closed or open reduction of a proximal humerus fracture in a child with open growth plates. Neer classified proximal humerus

fractures by relative displacement of the humeral head and shaft (**Table 3**). If remodeling potential is inadequate (as in a Neer type III or IV fracture in a patient older than 11 years), the advantages of reduction and fixation must be considered. Percutaneous pin fixation can be used if closed reduction can be obtained, provided that the pins are bent to prevent migration. The pins can be bent and buried under the skin or left outside the skin for later removal (**Figure 4**). Pins left outside the skin must be carefully monitored for infection and removed within 3 to 4 weeks. Intramedullary rod fixation also can be used to stabilize a proximal humerus fracture that is distal to the physis.

Entrapment of soft tissue such as the biceps tendon, periosteum, or glenohumeral joint capsule sometimes prevents closed reduction and necessitates open reduction.[18] If open reduction is required, cannulated screw fixation and pin fixation both have excellent long-term results.[19]

Proximal humerus metaphyseal fractures are commonly associated with a unicameral bone cyst (UBC). A UBC tends to form in a juxtaphyseal location and migrate away from the physis as the arm grows (**Figure 5**). A large cyst or an active cyst next to the physis is at high risk of fracture.[20] Most cysts that fracture occupy 85% of the bone, as seen on two orthogonal plain radiographs.[21] The fracture risk is affected by the size of the cyst, thinning of the cortex, location of the cyst in the bone, and the patient's body mass index and activity level. The interplay of these variables needs to be better defined by research. The best treatment for a pathologic fracture through a cyst is a subject of debate. Often the fracture can be allowed to heal. The cyst is treated if radiographs or CT reveal that it is persistently large so that there is a high risk of refracture. A UBC can be treated with several methods, including aspiration and injection of steroids or a bone graft substitute (α-BSM; Etex, Cambridge, MA), open curettage and grafting with bone graft or bone graft substitute, decompression with intramedullary fixation, and cannulated screw placement. The benefit of using any one method rather than another has not been established. It is critical to confirm that the proximal humerus lesion is benign before treating it because a malignant lesion also can occur in the proximal humerus of a skeletally immature patient (**Figure 6**).

Elbow Injuries

Supracondylar Humerus Fractures

Supracondylar humerus fractures are the most common type of fracture about the pediatric elbow. The mechanism of injury typically is a fall onto an outstretched hand. More than 90% of supracondylar fractures are classified as extension type, with fewer than 10% classified as a flexion fracture (**Table 4**). Extension fractures are further classified as type I (minimally displaced), II (extended, with intact posterior periosteum), or III (completely displaced). Cast treatment can be used for a type I fracture, in which the anterior humeral line still intercepts the capitellum and no varus or valgus malalignment is present. Type II and III fractures should be aligned as anatomically as possible with either closed or open reduction and should be fixed to maintain alignment. A supracondylar fracture should not be reduced and casted without pinning because the flexion necessary to maintain a reduction risks neurovascular compromise. After the fracture is pinned, the elbow can be extended and splinted or casted in a safe

position (less than 90° of flexion) without losing the reduction.

Neurovascular injury can be sustained during the injury, the reduction, and/or the pin fixation of a displaced supracondylar fracture. The radial pulse and neurologic status of the hand must be checked before and after treatment. An extension fracture tents the brachial artery and median nerve over the metaphyseal spike of bone, and these structures may become entrapped during reduction (**Figure 7**). A compartment syndrome may be missed if the median nerve is injured; because of decreased sensation, the patient will not have the pain typically associated with a compartment syndrome. A missed compartment syndrome can have devastating long-term consequences.

A flexion injury has the potential to trap the ulnar nerve in the fracture site on the medial side of the

Table 3		
The Neer Classification of Pediatric Proximal Humerus Fractures		
Type	**Displacement**	
I	Less than 5 mm	
II	Less than one third of the shaft diameter	
III	One third to two thirds of the shaft diameter	
IV	More than two thirds of the shaft diameter	

(Adapted from Neer CS III: Displaced proximal humeral fractures: Classification and evaluation. *J Bone Joint Surg Am* 1970;52[6]:1077-1089.)

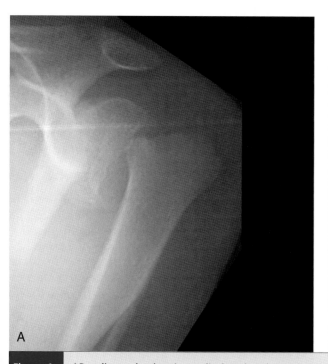

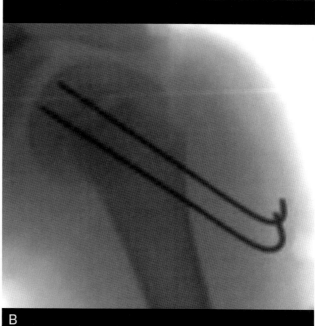

Figure 4 AP radiographs showing a displaced and angulated proximal humerus fracture in an adolescent. **A**, The fracture before fixation. **B**, Closed reduction and percutaneous pin fixation of the fracture.

6: Musculoskeletal Trauma

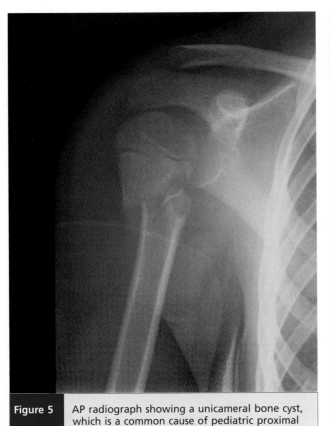

Figure 5   AP radiograph showing a unicameral bone cyst, which is a common cause of pediatric proximal humerus fracture.

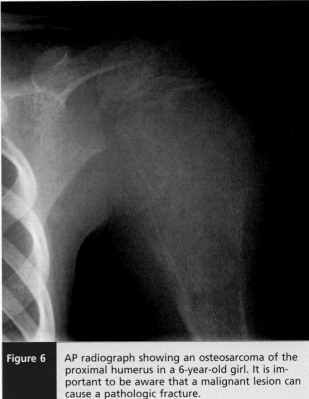

Figure 6   AP radiograph showing an osteosarcoma of the proximal humerus in a 6-year-old girl. It is important to be aware that a malignant lesion can cause a pathologic fracture.

elbow (**Figure 8**).[22] Open reduction is more commonly required for a flexion than for an extension injury, and the incidence of ulnar nerve symptoms is higher.[23] It is important to consider the possibility of ulnar nerve entrapment if the medial column is not anatomically aligned after closed reduction.

Ischemic injury from a supracondylar fracture can lead to a devastating complication such as Volkmann contracture. If the hand is poorly perfused, emergency reduction and pinning should be done to remove tension from the brachial artery. If the hand continues to be poorly perfused after reduction, the cause may be a brachial artery spasm, artery disruption, or thrombus. If the hand is pulseless and white, immediate exploration of the fracture or an arteriogram is recommended before the surgery is concluded. Subsequent required treatments include vasodilating agents if the artery is in spasm; thrombolytics if thrombus is present; or exploration (usually with a vascular surgeon) if the vessel is caught in the fracture or disrupted. If the pulse was lost during the surgery, surgical exploration usually is recommended to determine whether the artery is caught in the reduced fracture. If the pulse is not palpable but the hand is pink after reduction, it can be monitored; collateral circulation usually is adequate to maintain perfusion.[24] Although recent studies recommended aggressive vascular evaluation and possible brachial artery exploration if the pulse fails to return after reduction,

Table 4

The Classification of Supracondylar Humerus Fractures

Type	Radiographic Finding	Treatment
Extension		
I	Minimal displacement	Casting
II	Extension with intact posterior periosteum	Closed reduction and percutaneous pinning
III	Complete periosteal disruption	Closed or open reduction and pin fixation
Flexion	Flexion of distal fragment	Closed or open reduction and pin fixation

this recommendation is controversial and in need of further investigation.[25,26] A pink but pulseless hand must be monitored extremely carefully, with intervention considered if perfusion to the hand decreases.

An extension supracondylar fracture typically can be reduced with traction in extension followed by flexion and pronation. Alignment can vary with the age and gender of the child, and radiographs of the uninjured side can help determine the appropriate alignment.[27] Several studies have attempted to determine the optimal pinning configuration to obtain biomechanical stability for the reduction while minimizing the risk to the ulnar nerve.[28,29] The use of multiple lateral entry pins

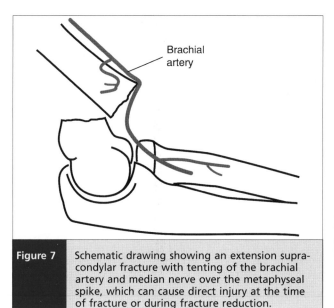

Figure 7 | Schematic drawing showing an extension supracondylar fracture with tenting of the brachial artery and median nerve over the metaphyseal spike, which can cause direct injury at the time of fracture or during fracture reduction.

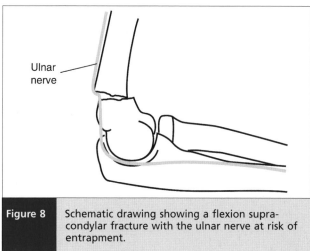

Figure 8 | Schematic drawing showing a flexion supracondylar fracture with the ulnar nerve at risk of entrapment.

and the use of medial and lateral crossed pins were found to lead to similar stability. Orthopaedic surgeons treating unstable pediatric supracondylar humerus fractures should be prepared to place either medial or lateral pins because anatomic constraints may dictate the use of one method rather than the other[30] (**Figure 9**). Ulnar nerve injury has been reported after crossed pinning; to protect the ulnar nerve during placement of the medial pin, the recommended method is to place two lateral pins and extend the elbow for placement of the medial pin, with or without a small incision.[31]If the ulnar nerve is injured, the medial pin should be removed as soon as possible, while maintaining fracture stability; if two lateral pins and a cast were used, the medial pin can be removed through a small window in the cast with only minimal risk of loss of reduction. Refixation may be necessary if only one lateral pin was used. Because nerve function often returns, some authors believe the offending pin should be left in place and the fracture allowed to heal. However, research results vary as to the rate of full recovery after iatrogenic ulnar nerve injury. Prevention of injury and prompt treatment are recommended whenever possible. Pins can be bent and cut outside the skin because they will be protected by the cast. These pins should be removed within 3 to 4 weeks after surgery; later removal is associated with a greater risk of infection. After closed reduction and percutaneous pinning of a supracondylar humerus fracture, 94% of the child's normal elbow range of motion returns within 6 months, with further improvement as late as 1 year after surgery.[32]

Cubitus varus and hyperextension are the most common deformities after inadequate reduction of a supracondylar fractures. These deformities may increase the risk of lateral condyle fracture.[33] Cubitus varus deformity from malunion of a supracondylar fracture can be treated with a simple closing wedge osteotomy. However, the standard closing wedge osteotomy leaves a

prominent lateral condyle, may cause instability, and may not correct rotational deformity. Several modified distal humerus osteotomies have been proposed to better correct distal humerus malunions, including the dome, lateral invaginating peg, reverse V, and equal limbs closing wedge osteotomies.[34-37] These four osteotomies have a better cosmetic outcome than the standard closing wedge osteotomy.

Transphyseal Fractures
A Salter-Harris type I or II fracture can extend through the unossified epiphysis of the distal humerus in a young child. Sometimes there is no ossification distal to the fracture, and as a result the fracture may be missed or confused with an elbow dislocation. In a transphyseal fracture, the distal fragment usually translates posteromedially; in an elbow dislocation, in contrast, the radius and ulna typically translate posterolaterally. It is important to remember that elbow dislocation is rare in young children, and the initial assumption should be that the injury is a fracture. Ultrasonography or arthrography can be used to confirm a transphyseal fracture. A transphyseal fracture is a classic sign of child abuse, and detecting it is therefore especially important. The fracture can be treated with closed reduction and pinning in a manner similar to a supracondylar fracture.

Lateral Condyle Fractures
A lateral condyle fracture, the second most common fracture about the elbow, often involves disruption of the articular surface. The most critical factor in treating a lateral condyle fracture is to anatomically align the joint surface and the articular cartilage. An internal oblique radiograph is the best indicator of the maximal displacement of a lateral condyle fracture.[38] A substantial part of the epiphysis is cartilage and cannot be well seen on radiographs, however. Arthrography is the gold standard for evaluating step-off or gap at the joint surface before closed treatment of a borderline lateral condyle fracture. MRI also can be used to evaluate the con-

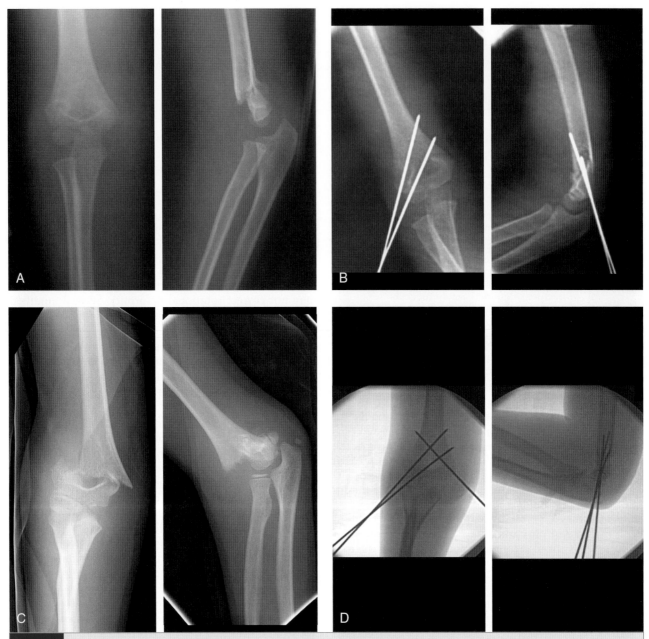

Figure 9 AP (*left*) and lateral (*right*) radiographs showing fixation of two types of supracondylar fractures. A type II fracture before (**A**) and after (**B**) fixation with closed reduction and pinning. A type III fracture before (**C**) and after (**D**) fixation using a crossed-pin technique.

gruity of the joint surface and alignment of the cartilaginous epiphysis. Weekly radiographs are important during the first 2 to 3 weeks after nonsurgical treatment of a minimally displaced lateral condyle fracture because the fracture may further displace in the cast and require surgical intervention.

The Milch classification of lateral condyle fractures formerly was used, but two other systems may be more useful for developing a treatment plan. The Jakob-Skaggs classification system is more prognostic and treatment based[39,40] (**Table 5**). The risk of complications is predicted to be three times greater after a type

III fracture than after a type II fracture. The Song classification identifies five groups of lateral condyle fractures based on degree of displacement and fracture pattern, as determined from four radiographic views. This system includes an algorithm for treating each type of fracture[41] (**Table 6**). An attempt at closed reduction and percutaneous pinning is recommended before opening the fracture; standard open reduction is recommended if the fracture gap remains greater than 2 mm.[42]

For open reduction, it is important to remember that the arterial supply to the capitellum enters posteriorly. A lateral condyle fracture should be exposed through a

6: Musculoskeletal Trauma

direct lateral approach. Dissection should remain anterior to the capitellum to avoid disrupting the blood supply to the capitellum and trochlea, exposing only the anterior joint surface. Osteonecrosis, nonunion, malunion (cubitus varus), infection, and development of a lateral prominence are potential complications after treating a pediatric lateral condyle fracture. Arthroscopic reduction and percutaneous fixation has been used as an alternative to open treatment of lateral condyle fracture; the purpose is to decrease soft-tissue stripping and the risk of malunion and osteonecrosis.[43]

Two Kirschner wires typically are used to fix a lateral condyle fracture. The first pin traverses the capitellum and exits through the anterior aspect of the medial epicondyle. The second pin is placed at an angle of approximately 45° to the first pin, exiting through the distal humeral metaphysis (Figure 10). A third divergent pin can be added if greater stability is needed. The pins are left in place for 4 weeks. As determined by radiographic healing, the elbow may need to be recast for 2 to 4 weeks after pin removal. An intra-articular lateral condyle fracture requires more time to heal than a metaphyseal fracture or a fracture that did not disrupt the joint surface.

Medial Epicondyle Fractures

Medial epicondyle fracture is the third most common type of fracture about the elbow in children and frequently is associated with elbow dislocation. The flexor-pronator mass attaches to the apophysis of the medial epicondyle just proximal to the distal humeral physis. The medial epicondyle does not ossify until a child is approximately 7 years old and therefore may not be visible on plain radiographs in a younger patient. Significant force can cause the medial epicondyle to be avulsed from the metaphysis. Medial epicondyle avulsion fractures occur in athletes, particularly in baseball pitchers, who throw with a valgus stress on the elbow combined with wrist flexion and pronation. When more forceful valgus stress is applied to the elbow (as with a fall onto an outstretched hand), the elbow may dislocate, with the medial epicondyle being pulled into the joint. It is important to ensure that the medial epicondyle is not entrapped in the joint during or after reduction of an elbow dislocation (Figure 11).

A minimally displaced fracture can be treated in a cast. There is debate as to the extent of displacement that necessitates surgical treatment. The fragment displaces distal and anterior, and the anterior displacement is difficult to accurately measure on plain radiographs. CT may provide a better indication of the displacement. Although 5 to 15 mm of displacement may be acceptable for nonsurgical treatment,[43] a recent study suggests that fractures with more than 5 mm of

---

Table 5

The Jakob-Skaggs Classification of Lateral Condyle Fractures

Type	Displacement	Treatment
I	Less than 2 mm	Casting
II	2 mm or more, with intact articular cartilage seen on arthrogram	Casting or closed reduction and percutaneous pinning
III	2 mm or more, with disruption of the articular surface	Open reduction and pinning

(Adapted with permission from Weiss JM, Graves S, Yang S, Mendelsohn E, Kay RM, Skaggs DL: A "new" classification system predictive of complications in surgically treated pediatric humeral lateral condyle fractures. *J Pediatr Orthop* 2009;29[6]:602-605.)

Table 6

The Song Classification of Lateral Condyle Fractures

Stage	Displacement	Fracture Pattern	Treatment
1	2 mm or less	Limited fracture line in metaphysis	Long arm casting
2	2 mm or less	Lateral gap	Casting or in situ fixation
3	2 mm or less	Gap as wide laterally as medially	In situ fixation or closed reduction and percutaneous pinning
4	More than 2 mm	No rotation of fragment	Closed reduction and percutaneous pinning or open reduction and internal fixation
5	More than 2 mm	Rotation of fragment	Closed reduction and percutaneous pinning or open reduction and internal fixation

(Adapted with permission from Song KS, Kang CH, Min BW, Bae KC, Cho CH, Lee JH: Closed reduction and internal fixation of displaced unstable lateral condylar fractures of the humerus in children. *J Bone Joint Surg Am* 2008;90[12]:2673-2681.)

6: Musculoskeletal Trauma

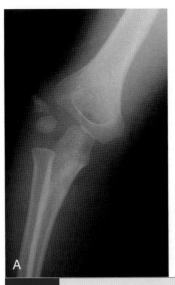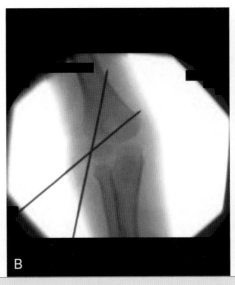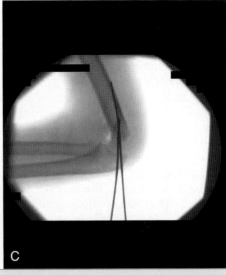

Figure 10 **A**, AP radiograph showing a displaced lateral condyle fracture. AP (**B**) and lateral (**C**) radiographs showing open reduction and internal fixation of the fracture.

displacement should be fixed.[44] A recent meta-analysis found that surgical treatment of medial epicondyle fractures results in a significantly higher union rate than nonsurgical management.[45] However, no difference in pain was found at final follow-up after surgical or nonsurgical treatments; this finding suggests that nonunion may not be predictive of pain or loss of function. Further studies are required to determine how much displacement is tolerable and for which patients surgery should be recommended. High-demand athletes may not tolerate a change in elbow biomechanics. Throwing athletes and gymnasts with open physes may have a better prognosis if the fracture is fixed, even if there is no significant displacement, because their sport activity tends to displace the medial epicondyle unless there is a solid bony union.

A medial epicondyle fracture associated with an elbow dislocation must be reduced immediately. A persistently displaced medial epicondyle or a fracture fragment caught in the joint should be treated with open reduction and internal fixation to reestablish joint congruity and stability. An external Esmarch bandage can be used in open reduction of a medial epicondyle fracture to minimize soft-tissue dissection and protect the vascularity of the fracture fragment.[46] In a child younger than 6 years, the medial epicondyle can be fixed with diverging smooth pins; in an older child, it can be fixed with a screw through the medial epicondyle and into the medial column of the distal humerus (**Figure 11**). The screw should not enter the olecranon fossa, and care needs to be taken to ensure the ulnar nerve is not in the fracture bed. Percutaneous smooth pins can be removed 4 weeks after surgery. The medial epicondyle is an apophysis, and leaving a screw in place does not affect the longitudinal growth of the humerus. However, there is very little soft-tissue coverage near the screw head, and a screw often must be removed because it has

become symptomatic. Patients with an associated elbow dislocation have a tendency to develop stiffness and may have a better result if the fragment is well fixed to allow earlier range-of-motion exercises.

Elbow Dislocations

Elbow dislocations are classified by evaluating the proximal radioulnar joint (PRUJ). Type I is a dislocation in an intact PRUJ; the most common type I dislocation is posterior, but anterior, lateral, and medial dislocation also can occur. Type II involves a disruption of the PRUJ and is relatively rare. A type II dislocation is further classified as anteroposterior PRUJ divergence, mediolateral divergence, or radioulnar translocation. It is important to evaluate neurovascular status before and after reduction because the blood vessels and nerves around the elbow can be stretched or disrupted.

Most pediatric elbow dislocations are associated with a fracture. Medial epicondyle fracture is most common with an elbow dislocation, but concomitant lateral condyle, capitellum, coronoid, olecranon, radial head and neck, osteocartilaginous, and shear fracture of the articular cartilage also can occur.[47,48] Elbow dislocations associated with a displaced fracture should generally undergo anatomic fracture fixation to stabilize the elbow and prevent long-term complications.

Closed reduction should be done as soon as possible. It is critical to ensure that the elbow is concentrically reduced and there is no crepitus during range of motion after reduction. MRI is useful for evaluating the articular cartilage. Shear injuries to the cartilage can block concentric reduction and lead to early arthrosis and limited range of motion. Nonconcentric reduction is an indication for surgical intervention.

The elbow is splinted for 2 to 3 weeks after reduction of the elbow dislocation and confirmation that

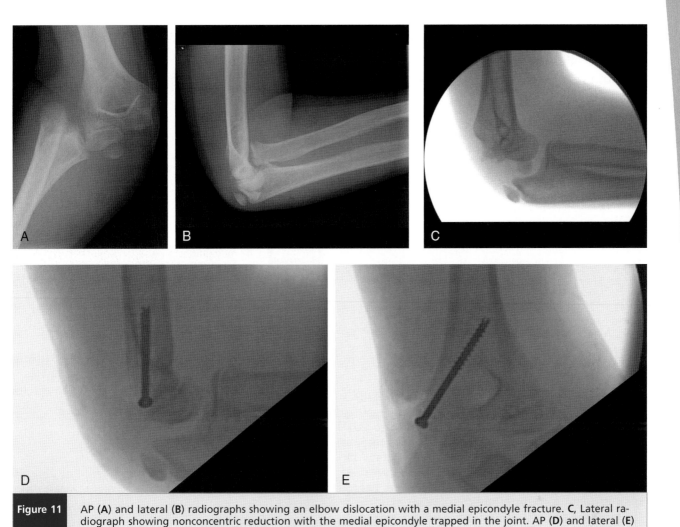

Figure 11 AP (**A**) and lateral (**B**) radiographs showing an elbow dislocation with a medial epicondyle fracture. **C**, Lateral radiograph showing nonconcentric reduction with the medial epicondyle trapped in the joint. AP (**D**) and lateral (**E**) radiographs showing open reduction and internal fixation of the fracture.

there is no fracture or cartilage injury. Early range-of-motion exercises prevent stiffness. Elbow stability should be checked after a period of rest; a hinged brace can be used to allow motion within the range of stability. If the elbow is not stable within 6 weeks, MRI should be done to evaluate soft-tissue injury. Ligamentous reconstruction is rarely necessary in pediatric patients.

Pulled Elbow (Nursemaid's Elbow)

In a child age 1 to 4 years, the annular ligament may become subluxated relative to the radial head if a traction force is applied to the extended elbow (for example, if the arm is pulled or the child hangs from a bar). The subluxation, often called pulled elbow or nursemaid's elbow, is very painful, and the child will not want to move the elbow. The elbow is usually held in slight flexion and pronation. It is important to confirm that there is no elbow fracture before attempting a reduction maneuver. If the radiographs are normal, the elbow can be flexed and supinated to reduce the subluxation; a small click is often felt during the reduction.

The elbow immediately feels better, and the child begins to use the arm if the diagnosis and treatment were correct. Parents can be taught to do this maneuver at home. It is important to teach the child and parents how to prevent the injury as well as how to reduce it.

For a recurrent pulled elbow, the arm can be casted in hyperflexion and supination for 3 weeks to decrease the risk of another recurrence. A pulled elbow rarely occurs in a child older than 5 years.

Radial Head and Neck Fractures

A radial head and neck fracture typically is caused by a valgus compression force such as a fall onto the elbow, and it can be associated with medial soft-tissue injury from the valgus force. The classification of proximal radius fractures is shown in **Table 7**. Pediatric intra-articular fractures of the radial head are rare in children, but they occasionally occur in teenagers and should be reduced anatomically to prevent arthrosis. An intra-articular step-off or gap can be fixed through a Kocher approach using a low-contour miniplate and/or headless compression screws; bioabsorbable

6: Musculoskeletal Trauma

Table 7

The Classification of Pediatric Proximal Radius Fractures

Group I. Primary displacement of the radial head

    A. Valgus fracture
1. Type A: Salter-Harris type I or II
2. Type B: Salter-Harris type IV
3. Type C: Metaphyseal

    B. Fracture associated with elbow dislocation
1. Type D: Reduction injury
2. Type E: Dislocation injury

Group II. Primary displacement of the radial neck

    A. Angular (Monteggia type III variant)

    B. Torsional injury

Group III. Stress injury

    A. Osteochondritis dissecans

    B. Physeal injury with neck angulation

(Adapted with permission from Chambers H: Fractures of the proximal radius and ulna, in Beaty JH, Kasser JR, eds: *Rockwood and Wilkins Fractures in Children*, ed 5. Philadelphia, PA, Lippincott, Williams and Wilkins, 2001, p 486.)

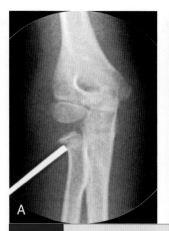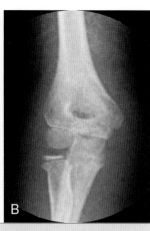

Figure 12   AP radiographs showing an angulated radial neck fracture. **A**, Percutaneous use of a Steinmann pin to correct the alignment. **B**, The fracture after reduction. Because the fracture was stable, no fixation was necessary. The fracture was placed in a cast for 4 weeks.

pins can also be used effectively.[49] A low-profile fixation technique using screws obliquely oriented from the radial head into the shaft has been developed to avoid distal dissection and keep implants away from the constrained area adjacent to the annular ligament and lateral ligamentous structures.[50] In pediatric patients, every attempt should be made to maintain the natural joint. In contrast to the treatment of adult injuries, radial head replacement or excision is almost never considered.

Radial neck fracture angulation as great as 30° is well tolerated and will remodel in a patient with open physes. These fractures can be treated with simple casting. Angulation of more than 30° should be reduced, with closed reduction attempted first. The maneuvers to reduce the displaced radial head include the Israeli, Patterson, Columbus, and Esmarch bandage techniques.[46] If closed reduction is unsuccessful, a Kirschner wire or Steinmann pin can be used percutaneously in a joystick fashion to push the radial head back onto the shaft (**Figure 12**). Translation of the radial head in relation to the shaft may create a cam effect that limits pronation and supination if the fracture is left to heal in this position. If the radial shaft is translated toward the ulna, a periosteal elevator can be inserted between the radius and the ulna from the posterior aspect so as to lever the radial shaft away from the ulna and thereby move the shaft into line with and under the radial head. Reduction of the displaced radial head and fixation with an intramedullary nail also has been shown to be an effective technique.[51]

The PRUJ is stabilized by the annular ligament. The annular ligament can become trapped in a displaced radial head and neck fracture, thus preventing reduction. Open reduction with annular ligament reconstruction becomes necessary to regain elbow stability and obtain adequate reduction. If the reduction is unstable, a smooth Kirschner wire can be used to temporarily fix the fracture (**Figure 13**), with care to avoid injuring the posterior interosseous nerve. The pins should be removed after 3 weeks because they are intra-articular and can lead to infection if not removed. The Kirschner wire should engage the radial head and shaft but not the capitellum. The complications of open treatment of radial head and neck fractures include stiffness, osteonecrosis, infection, premature physeal arrest, nerve injury, and nonunion.

Radial Head Dislocations

Radial head dislocation is discussed in Chapter 32 as a Monteggia fracture or variant.

Olecranon Fractures

Apophysitis or complete avulsion of the olecranon apophysis often occurs in throwing athletes secondary to overpulling of the triceps. With complete fracture, contraction of the triceps tends to pull the fracture fragment proximally. The alignment therefore may worsen in a cast or splint. If nonsurgical management is attempted, weekly radiographs are necessary for 2 to 3 weeks to ensure the fracture does not pull apart. Casting in relative extension (20° to 30° of flexion) decreases the tendency toward loss of alignment. Olecranon fractures are intra-articular, and anatomic joint reduction is important to maintain concentric joint motion and prevent arthrosis. CT or MRI can be used to confirm articular alignment and ensure there are no chondral injuries requiring attention. Unfixed osteochondral or pure cartilage injuries will impair long-term joint function.

The olecranon can be fixed with a tension band construct (**Figure 14**). In a child younger than 6 years, a su-

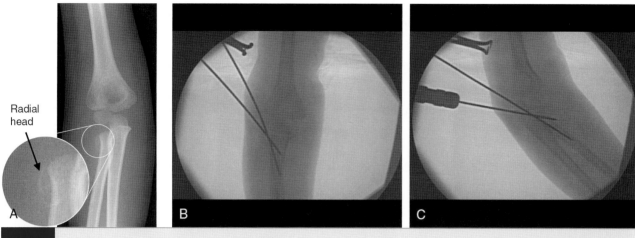

Figure 13 **A,** AP radiograph showing a radial neck fracture with complete displacement of the epiphysis, which can be difficult to detect if the epiphysis is not ossified. AP (**B**) and lateral (**C**) radiographs showing open reduction and pin fixation of the fracture.

ture tension band can be used with Kirschner wires buried under the skin or bent outside the skin to facilitate later removal.[52] However, sutures have a lower ultimate load to failure and offer less compression at the fracture site than conventional pin-and-wire techniques.[53] A suture tension band is unlikely to be adequate for an adolescent. In a skeletally immature child, it is important to remove the hardware after fracture healing to allow continued apophyseal growth.

Summary

Injuries to the shoulder and elbow are very common in pediatric patients, and many can be treated nonsurgically. It is important to identify a fracture that will not remodel adequately and a joint injury that can lead to long-term complications if not realigned appropriately. The goals of treating shoulder and elbow trauma in a pediatric patient are to obtain alignment and joint congruity while preventing neurovascular complications, stiffness, growth disruption, and loss of function. The shoulder is a more forgiving joint than the elbow and has tremendous remodeling potential, but the closer the child is to skeletal maturity, the more attention must be paid to appropriate alignment to prevent impingement and loss of motion.

Joint surfaces must be realigned and allowed to heal in anatomic alignment to prevent arthrosis. Lateral condyle, olecranon, and radial head fractures are the most common intra-articular fractures of the elbow that require surgical intervention. Supracondylar fractures are the most common fracture around the elbow; although extra-articular, they must be near-anatomically aligned with prevention of neurovascular compromise. An arthrogram or MRI should be considered if there is any concern about joint alignment and cartilage congruity. A displaced osteochondral fracture should be treated with open reduction and fixation. Ev-

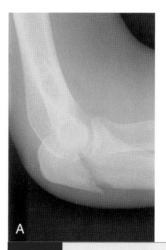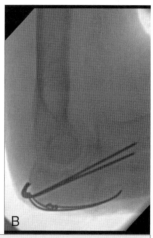

Figure 14 Lateral radiographs showing an intra-articular olecranon fracture. **A,** The fracture before fixation. **B,** Open reduction and internal fixation of the fracture with a tension band construct.

ery pediatric orthopaedic surgeon must be able to reconstruct the articular surfaces of the elbow to ensure the joint is protected over the long term.

Annotated References

1. Mehlman CT, Yihua G, Bochang C, Zhigang W: Operative treatment of completely displaced clavicle shaft fractures in children. *J Pediatr Orthop* 2009;29(8):851-855.

   Of 24 patients age 7 to 16 years treated with open reduction and internal fixation for a displaced clavicle fracture, 2 had scar sensitivity. No other complications were reported, and all fractures healed. Level of evidence: IV.

2. Kubiak R, Slongo T: Operative treatment of clavicle fractures in children: A review of 21 years. *J Pediatr Orthop* 2002;22(6):736-739.

3. Khan LA, Bradnock TJ, Scott C, Robinson CM: Fractures of the clavicle. *J Bone Joint Surg Am* 2009;91(2): 447-460.

   This is a current concepts review of adult clavicle fractures.

4. Nakayama M, Gika M, Fukuda H, et al: Migration of a Kirschner wire from the clavicle into the intrathoracic trachea. *Ann Thorac Surg* 2009;88(2):653-654.

   A 70-year-old man had a rare complication related to the insertion of Kirschner wires for fixation of a clavicle fracture. The wire migrated into the trachea.

5. Mueller M, Rangger C, Striepens N, Burger C: Minimally invasive intramedullary nailing of midshaft clavicular fractures using titanium elastic nails. *J Trauma* 2008;64(6):1528-1534.

   Thirty-one midshaft clavicular fractures were treated using an intramedullary titanium elastic nail. There were no nonunions or refractures. The complications included medial migration, perforation of the lateral cortex, secondary shortening, and a broken nail.

6. Nguyen V, Williams G, Rockwood C: Radiography of acromioclavicular dislocation and associated injuries. *Crit Rev Diagn Imaging* 1991;32(3):191-228.

7. Tischer T, Salzmann GM, El-Azab H, Vogt S, Imhoff AB: Incidence of associated injuries with acute acromioclavicular joint dislocations types III through V. *Am J Sports Med* 2009;37(1):136-139.

   All 77 patients surgically treated for acute AC joint dislocation underwent diagnostic glenohumeral joint arthroscopy. Intra-articular injury was found in 14 patients (18%), and a superior labrum anterior and posterior lesion was found in 11 (14%).

8. Tauber M, Gordon K, Koller H, Fox M, Resch H: Semitendinosus tendon graft versus a modified Weaver-Dunn procedure for acromioclavicular joint reconstruction in chronic cases: A prospective comparative study. *Am J Sports Med* 2009;37(1):181-190.

   Twenty-four patients with painful, chronic AC joint dislocation had surgical reconstruction. Autogenous semitendinosus tendon graft led to significantly better clinical and radiologic outcomes than a modified Weaver-Dunn procedure. Level of evidence: II.

9. Jiang C, Wang M, Rong G: Proximally based conjoined tendon transfer for coracoclavicular reconstruction in the treatment of acromioclavicular dislocation: Surgical technique. *J Bone Joint Surg Am* 2008;90(suppl 2, pt 2): 299-308.

   A retrospective review found acceptable short-term outcomes after 38 AC dislocations were treated with transfer of the lateral half of the conjoined tendon to the distal aspect of the clavicle in a proximally based fashion, with additional CC fixation.

10. Seybold D, Schildhauer TA, Muhr G: Rare anterior shoulder dislocation in a toddler. *Arch Orthop Trauma Surg* 2009;129(3):295-298.

    The treatment of a 2-year-old child with traumatic shoulder dislocation caused by a pull on an abducted arm included gentle closed reduction with the Milch maneuver and short sling immobilization. At 2.5-year follow-up, the shoulder was stable, with free range of motion. A Hill-Sachs lesion was still present.

11. Antonio GE, Griffith JF, Yu AB, Yung PS, Chan KM, Ahuja AT: First-time shoulder dislocation: High prevalence of labral injury and age-related differences revealed by MR arthrography. *J Magn Reson Imaging* 2007;26(4):983-991.

    After a first shoulder dislocation, magnetic resonance arthrography of 66 patients revealed that those younger than 30 years (34 patients) were more likely to have extensive labral injury.

12. Robinson CM, Howes J, Murdoch H, Will E, Graham C: Functional outcome and risk of recurrent instability after primary traumatic anterior shoulder dislocation in young patients. *J Bone Joint Surg Am* 2006;88(11): 2326-2336.

    In a prospective study, 252 anterior glenohumeral dislocations in patients age 15 to 35 years were treated with sling immobilization followed by physical therapy. Instability developed in 67% by the fifth year after the dislocation; younger, male patients were most at risk of instability.

13. Itoi E, Hatakeyama Y, Sato T, et al: Immobilization in external rotation after shoulder dislocation reduces the risk of recurrence: A randomized controlled trial. *J Bone Joint Surg Am* 2007;89(10):2124-2131.

    In 198 patients with anterior shoulder dislocation who were randomly assigned to immobilization in internal or external rotation, recurrence occurred significantly less often in those assigned to external rotation. In patients 30 years or younger, the relative risk reduction was 46.1%.

14. Finestone A, Milgrom C, Radeva-Petrova DR, et al: Bracing in external rotation for traumatic anterior dislocation of the shoulder. *J Bone Joint Surg Br* 2009;91(7): 918-921.

    In a prospective study, 51 men age 17 to 27 years with anterior shoulder dislocation were randomly assigned to immobilization in internal or external rotation. The rates of redislocation were not statistically different.

15. Brophy RH, Marx RG: The treatment of traumatic anterior instability of the shoulder: Nonoperative and surgical treatment. *Arthroscopy* 2009;25(3):298-304.

    This literature review compares surgical and nonsurgical treatments of traumatic anterior shoulder instability in patients younger than 24 years, most of whom were in their teens or early 20s. The rate of recurrent instability was significantly lower after surgical treatment; the rate was similar after arthroscopic or open stabilization with anchors.

16. Porcellini GC, Campi F, Pegreffi F, Castagna A, Paladini P: Predisposing factors for recurrent shoulder dislocation after arthroscopic treatment. *J Bone Joint Surg Am* 2009;91(11):2537-2542.

When 385 patients with anterior unidirectional instability were evaluated 36 months after arthroscopic Bankart surgery, 31 (8.1%) had had redislocation. The rate was 13.3% among patients age 22 years or younger and 6.3% among older patients. Age at the time of the first dislocation, male sex, and time from first dislocation to surgery were significant risk factors for recurrence.

17. Ugwonali OF, Bae DS, Waters PM: Corrective osteotomy for humerus varus. *J Pediatr Orthop* 2007;27(5):529-532.

Six patients with humerus varus were treated with a proximal humerus valgus osteotomy. Mean forward flexion and abduction improved significantly.

18. Bahrs C, Zipplies S, Ochs BG, et al: Proximal humeral fractures in children and adolescents. *J Pediatr Orthop* 2009;29(3):238-242.

In this evaluation of 43 proximal humerus fractures, closed reduction was impossible in 9 because of entrapment of the periosteum or biceps tendon. Level of evidence: IV.

19. Dobbs MB, Luhmann SL, Gordon JE, Strecker WB, Schoenecker PL: Severely displaced proximal humeral epiphyseal fractures. *J Pediatr Orthop* 2003;23(2):208-215.

20. Tey IK, Mahadev A, Lim KB, Lee EH, Nathan SS: Active unicameral bone cysts in the upper limb are at greater risk of fracture. *J Orthop Surg (Hong Kong)* 2009;17(2):157-160.

In a retrospective review of 22 patients with UBC, fractured cysts were found to be larger than unfractured cysts (cyst index, 4.5 and 2.2, respectively). Active cysts in the upper extremity were most likely to fracture.

21. Ahn JI, Park JS: Pathological fractures secondary to unicameral bone cysts. *Int Orthop* 1994;18(1):20-22.

22. Steinman S, Bastrom TP, Newton PO, Mubarak SJ: Beware of ulnar nerve entrapment in flexion-type supracondylar humerus fractures. *J Child Orthop* 2007;1(3):177-180.

Of 1,650 supracondylar fractures, 30 required open reduction and internal fixation. All 30 had muscle or periosteum entrapped in the medial fracture gap, 6 were flexion fractures, and 3 also had an entrapped ulnar nerve.

23. Mahan ST, May CD, Kocher MS: Operative management of displaced flexion supracondylar humerus fractures in children. *J Pediatr Orthop* 2007;27(5):551-556.

In this retrospective review, flexion supracondylar fractures were more likely to require open reduction (31%) than extension fractures (10%). The flexion fractures had a significantly greater incidence of ulnar nerve symptoms with a need for ulnar nerve decompression.

24. Sabharwal S, Tredwell SJ, Beauchamp RD, et al: Management of pulseless pink hand in pediatric supracondylar fractures of humerus. *J Pediatr Orthop* 1997;17(3):303-310.

25. Luria S, Sucar A, Eylon S, et al: Vascular complications of supracondylar humeral fractures in children. *J Pediatr Orthop B* 2007;16(2):133-143.

A retrospective review found that exploration and repair of the brachial artery were undertaken in 11 of 24 children with supracondylar humeral fracture and vascular compromise because the pulse did not resume after fracture reduction.

26. Schoenecker PL, Delgado E, Rotman M, Sicard GA, Capelli AM: Pulseless arm in association with totally displaced supracondylar fracture. *J Orthop Trauma* 1996;10(6):410-415.

27. Herman MJ, Boardman MJ, Hoover JR, Chafetz RS: Relationship of the anterior humeral line to the capitellar ossific nucleus: Variability with age. *J Bone Joint Surg Am* 2009;91(9):2188-2193.

The position of the anterior humeral line was radiographically defined in normal skeletally immature elbows, and the intrarater and interrater reliability of this parameter was determined.

28. Kocher MS, Kasser JR, Waters PM, et al: Lateral entry compared with medial and lateral entry pin fixation for completely displaced supracondylar humeral fractures in children: A randomized clinical trial. *J Bone Joint Surg Am* 2007;89(4):706-712.

A prospective, randomized clinical study found that pin fixation with either lateral or mediolateral entry is effective for treating completely displaced (type III) extension supracondylar fractures of the humerus in children. Level of evidence: I.

29. Brauer CA, Lee BM, Bae DS, Waters PM, Kocher MS: A systematic review of medial and lateral entry pinning versus lateral entry pinning for supracondylar fractures of the humerus. *J Pediatr Orthop* 2007;27(2):181-186.

A meta-analysis of mediolateral pin and lateral pin fixation of pediatric supracondylar humerus fractures found that mediolateral entry pinning is the most stable configuration.

30. Tripuraneni KR, Bosch PP, Schwend RM, Yaste JJ: Prospective, surgeon-randomized evaluation of crossed pins versus lateral pins for unstable supracondylar humerus fractures in children. *J Pediatr Orthop B* 2009;18(2):93-98.

A surgeon-randomized study compared crossed-pin and lateral-only pin fixation for displaced supracondylar fractures. Some of the fractures were not amenable to the randomly assigned treatment. Surgeons should be able to use both techniques as needed.

31. Eidelman M, Hos N, Katzman A, Bialik V: Prevention of ulnar nerve injury during fixation of supracondylar fractures in children by 'flexion-extension cross-pinning' technique. *J Pediatr Orthop B* 2007;16(3):221-224.

6: Musculoskeletal Trauma

A retrospective comparison of 67 displaced supracondylar fractures treated with two lateral pins placed with the elbow in flexion and one medial pin placed with the elbow in extension found no complications related to the ulnar nerve. The technique is described.

32. Zionts LE, Woodson CJ, Manjra N, Zalavras C: Time of return of elbow motion after percutaneous pinning of pediatric supracondylar humerus fractures. *Clin Orthop Relat Res* 2009;467(8):2007-2010.

   In a retrospective review of 63 supracondylar fractures treated with two or three lateral entry pins, elbow range of motion was found to return to 72% of contralateral elbow motion within 6 weeks after pinning, with a progressive increase to 98% within 52 weeks

33. Davids JR, Maguire MF, Mubarak SJ, Wenger DR: Lateral condylar fracture of the humerus following posttraumatic cubitus varus. *J Pediatr Orthop* 1994;14(4): 466-470.

34. Pankaj A, Dua A, Malhotra R, Bhan S: Dome osteotomy for posttraumatic cubitus varus: A surgical technique to avoid lateral condylar prominence. *J Pediatr Orthop* 2006;26(1):61-66.

   A retrospective review of 12 patients treated with dome osteotomy to correct posttraumatic cubitus found it to be a simple, safe, and technically sound procedure that prevents lateral condyle prominence and yields an excellent cosmetic outcome

35. Butt MF, Dhar SA, Farooq M, Kawoosa AA, Mir MR: Lateral invaginating peg (LIP) osteotomy for the correction of post-traumatic cubitus varus deformity. *J Pediatr Orthop B* 2009;18(5):265-270.

   Four patients treated with the authors' technique had good results, with correction of cubitus varus and internal rotation deformities.

36. Yun YH, Shin SJ, Moon JG: Reverse V osteotomy of the distal humerus for the correction of cubitus varus. *J Bone Joint Surg Br* 2007;89(4):527-531.

   A retrospective review of 22 children with cubitus varus treated with a reverse V osteotomy and fixation by cross pinning and wiring found absence of a prominent lateral condyle after correction and firm fixation allowing early movement. The technique is described.

37. El-Adl W: The equal limbs lateral closing wedge osteotomy for correction of cubitus varus in children. *Acta Orthop Belg* 2007;73(5):580-587.

   This is a review and technique description of malunion of the distal humerus treated with an equal limbs lateral closing wedge osteotomy of the distal humerus in 12 patients. The cosmetic outcome was excellent, with a low complication rate.

38. Song KS, Kang CH, Min BW, Bae KC, Cho CH: Internal oblique radiographs for diagnosis of nondisplaced or minimally displaced lateral condylar fractures of the humerus in children. *J Bone Joint Surg Am* 2007;89(1): 58-63.

   In a prospective study, 54 lateral condyle fractures were evaluated using AP, lateral, and internal and external oblique radiographs; 7 fractures also received three-dimensional CT. The internal oblique radiograph was most accurate for revealing the fracture gap and fracture pattern.

39. Jakob R, Fowles JV, Rang M, Kassab MT: Observations concerning fractures of the lateral humeral condyle in children. *J Bone Joint Surg Br* 1975;57(4):430-436.

40. Weiss JM, Graves S, Yang S, Mendelsohn E, Kay RM, Skaggs DL: A new classification system predictive of complications in surgically treated pediatric humeral lateral condyle fractures. *J Pediatr Orthop* 2009;29(6): 602-605.

   A retrospective review of 316 patients with lateral condyle fracture was used to develop a treatment-based classification system predictive of complication risk.

41. Song KS, Kang CH, Min BW, Bae KC, Cho CH, Lee JH: Closed reduction and internal fixation of displaced unstable lateral condylar fractures of the humerus in children. *J Bone Joint Surg Am* 2008;90(12):2673-2681.

   In a prospective treatment study, closed reduction was attempted in 63 unstable lateral condyle fractures; 46 fractures were reduced in a closed fashion to a gap of less than 2 mm, then pinned percutaneously. If the gap remained greater than 2 mm, the fracture underwent open reduction and internal fixation. The classification system is presented.

42. Hausman MR, Qureshi S, Goldstein R, et al: Arthroscopically-assisted treatment of pediatric lateral humeral condyle fractures. *J Pediatr Orthop* 2007; 27(7):739-742.

   Of six patients treated with arthroscopic reduction and percutaneous fixation of lateral condyle fractures, one developed radiolucency of the capitellum. There were no other complications. Level of evidence: IV.

43. Farsetti P, Potenza V, Caterini R, Ippolito E: Long-term results of treatment of fractures of the medial humeral epicondyle in children. *J Bone Joint Surg Am* 2001; 83(9):1299-1305.

44. Lee HH, Shen HC, Chang JH, Lee CH, Wu SS: Operative treatment of displaced medial epicondyle fractures in children and adolescents. *J Shoulder Elbow Surg* 2005;14(2):178-185.

   A retrospective review of 25 patients with medial epicondylar fractures (displacement greater than 5 mm) found good to excellent results with a variety of surgical treatments.

45. Kamath AF, Baldwin K, Horneff J, Hosalkar HS: Operative versus non-operative management of pediatric medial epicondyle fractures: A systematic review. *J Child Orthop* 2009;3(5):345-357.

   In this literature review, surgical treatment was found to offer a significantly higher union rate than nonsurgical management of medial epicondyle fractures. There was no difference in pain at final follow-up.

46. Kamath AF, Cody SR, Hosalkar HS: Open reduction of medial epicondyle fractures: Operative tips for technical ease. *J Child Orthop* 2009;3(4):331-336.

An Esmarch bandage was used to reduce medial epicondyle fractures, with provisional needle fixation to decrease the need for soft-tissue release and, theoretically, to maintain the soft-tissue vascularity of fracture fragments. The technique is described.

47. Eksioglu F, Uslu MM, Gudemez E, Cetik O: Medial elbow dislocation associated with a fracture of the lateral humeral condyle in a child. *Orthopedics* 2008;31(1):93.

Open reduction and internal fixation led to a good result in a 5-year-old boy with a medial elbow dislocation associated with a Milch type II lateral condyle fracture.

48. Sharma H, Sibinski M, Sherlock DA: Outcome of lateral humeral condylar mass fractures in children associated with elbow dislocation or olecranon fracture. *Int Orthop* 2009;33(2):509-514.

In a retrospective review of 20 lateral condylar mass fractures of the humerus associated with elbow dislocation or olecranon fracture, the result was poor in 3 (25%) of the 12 surgically treated patients because of a terminal 20° to 30° loss of extension.

49. Givissis PK, Symeonidis PD, Ditsios KT, Dionellis PS, Christodoulou AG: Late results of absorbable pin fixation in the treatment of radial head fractures. *Clin Orthop Relat Res* 2008;466(5):1217-1224.

In a retrospective review of 21 patients with an intra-articular radial head fracture fixed with absorbable pins, outcomes were comparable to those in earlier studies of radial head arthroplasty. There were no adverse reactions to the implant.

50. Smith AM, Morrey BF, Steinmann SP: Low profile fixation of radial head and neck fractures: Surgical technique and clinical experience. *J Orthop Trauma* 2007;21(10):718-724.

The technique is described for low-profile fixation using obliquely oriented screws from the radial head into the shaft to avoid distal dissection of the soft tissues and placement of hardware into an already-constrained area adjacent to the annular ligament and lateral ligamentous structures.

51. Metaizeau JP, Lascombes P, Lemelle JL, Finlayson D, Prevot J: Reduction and fixation of displaced radial neck fractures by closed intramedullary pinning. *J Pediatr Orthop* 1993;13(3):355-360.

52. Gortzak Y, Mercado E, Atar D, Weisel Y: Pediatric olecranon fractures: Open reduction and internal fixation with removable Kirschner wires and absorbable sutures. *J Pediatr Orthop* 2006;26(1):39-42.

Six patients were treated with a fixation technique for pediatric olecranon fractures using percutaneous Kirschner wires and absorbable suture. Subsequent surgery to remove hardware was avoided.

53. Parent S, Wedemeyer M, Mahar AT, et al: Displaced olecranon fractures in children: A biomechanical analysis of fixation methods. *J Pediatr Orthop* 2008;28(2):147-151.

Synthetic ulnae were randomly assigned to suture or wire tension band fixation. Compression was measured after fixation and during cyclic loading with a load cell at the articular surface. Suture tension bands had lower ultimate failure loads and less compression at the fracture.

6: Musculoskeletal Trauma

Chapter 32

Fractures of the Forearm, Wrist, and Hand

Dan A. Zlotolow, MD   Scott H. Kozin, MD

Introduction

Fractures of the upper extremity are extremely common in children. Children incur physeal injuries, unicortical (greenstick or buckle) fractures, and plastic deformation, in addition to the types of injuries that also occur in adults. Avulsion fractures are common because children's ligaments and tendons tend to be more robust than their bone. The growing limb is capable of remodeling most fractures, but the remodeling potential depends on the amount of remaining growth at the nearest physis, the proximity of the injury to the physis, and the plane of motion of the nearest joint. For example, a fracture at the distal radial metaphysis with substantial volar-dorsal angulation in a 2-year-old child has a much greater likelihood of fully remodeling than an apex ulnar proximal radial diaphyseal fracture in a 15-year-old child. The factors to be considered before treating an individual fracture include remodeling potential; a comparison of the risks of closed, percutaneous, and open management; and the likelihood that long-term disability will result from a nonanatomic reduction. Although guidelines are available for the treatment of younger children (as old as 8 years) and older children, the treatment decision should be based on the individual circumstances of the patient.

Monteggia Fracture-Dislocations

Assessment

An isolated ulnar shaft fracture results in dislocation of the radiocapitellar joint if there is sufficient angulation and/or shortening at the ulna. The mechanism varies but is suggested by the fracture type. The Bado classification is based on the direction of displacement and the status of the radius[1] (Table 1). Although anterior dislocation is most common, lateral dislocation may be more common in children than in adults and is difficult to see on lateral radiographs alone. The pediatric variants of the adult Monteggia fracture include greenstick fracture and plastic deformation (Figure 1). All fractures of the ulna should be evaluated for radial head subluxation-dislocation, no matter how minimally displaced they appear to be on initial radiographs. The radial shaft should point to the center of the capitellum in all radiographic views. Scrutiny should be given to the shape of the radial head; a convex radial head suggests congenital or long-standing radiocapitellar dislocation. The physical examination should include a neurovascular and compartment assessment. Transient ulnar nerve and posterior interosseous nerve dysfunction can occur but rarely lead to long-term nerve palsy.[2,3]

Treatment

Closed reduction and casting has been recommended for an incomplete fracture or plastic deformation; intramedullary fixation for a transverse or short oblique fracture; and plate-and-screw fixation for a comminuted or long oblique fracture[4] (Figure 2). The reduction can be difficult, and it should not be attempted in an office setting. The use of general anesthesia or conscious sedation is recommended. Caution is required with circumferential casting, particularly for a higher energy fracture, because the cumulative edema and soft-tissue injury from the mechanism of injury and the reduction can lead to a compartment syndrome. Splitting the cast and maintaining elbow flexion at less than 90° can reduce the risk, but close monitoring during the first 1 to 2 days is nonetheless necessary. Serial radiographs are necessary at the end of the first and sec-

Table 1		
The Bado Classification of Monteggia Fractures		
Type	**Radiographic Description**	
I	Anterior radial dislocation	
II	Posterior radial dislocation	
III	Lateral radial dislocation	
IV	Radius fracture and dislocation	

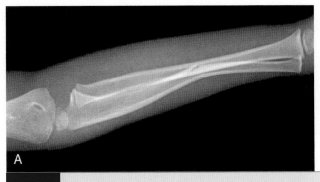

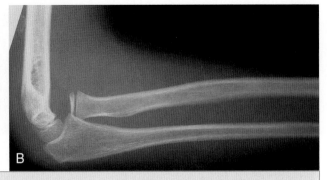

Figure 1 The pediatric variants of Monteggia fracture-dislocation. **A,** Oblique radiograph showing a greenstick fracture. **B,** Lateral radiograph showing a plastic deformation. The severity of the injury often is underestimated, and radial head dislocation can be missed.(Reproduced with permission from Shriners Hospital for Children, Philadelphia, PA.)

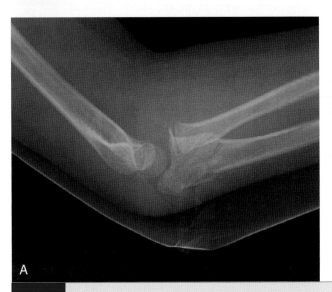

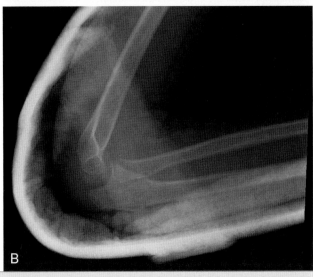

Figure 2 Lateral radiographs showing a proximal ulna fracture with radial head dislocation (a Monteggia fracture variant) before treatment **(A)** and after **(B)** closed reduction of the ulna leading to spontaneous reduction of the radiocapitellar joint. (Reproduced with permission from Shriners Hospital for Children, Philadelphia, PA.)

ond weeks to ensure that reduction is maintained as the edema subsides. The indications for surgery include loss of reduction, irreducibility of the fracture-dislocation, and questionable patient or family compliance. In both open and closed treatment, reduction of the ulna usually causes reduction of the radiocapitellar dislocation. In older children with minimal remodeling potential, plate-and-screw fixation is preferred.

Complications

Monteggia fractures are commonly missed, especially if there is plastic deformation of the ulna. Persistent radial head dislocation can lead to elbow instability with loss of motion, pain, and tardy ulnar nerve palsies. Early intervention is recommended if there is an impending or recent malunion of the ulna.[5] An anatomic reduction of the ulna is critical, followed by closed or open reduction of the radial head. A corrective osteotomy is needed after the ulnar malunion has become established. Some authors recommend overcorrection of

the ulnar malunion with a posterior bending-elongation ulnar osteotomy to assist the radiocapitellar alignment.[6] If the radial head is stable after reduction, ligament reconstruction may not be necessary. An annular ligament reconstruction should be added if there is any suggestion of instability[7] (**Figure 3**).

A radial head that has been dislocated for a long time may become deformed, precluding a reduction.[8] The ulna fracture may have remodeled, and it may be difficult to identify the malunion site. Nonsurgical treatment may be the best option if the child is minimally symptomatic (**Figure 4**).

Diaphyseal Forearm Fractures

Assessment

Diaphyseal forearm fractures are common in children of all ages. The fracture can involve one or both bones.

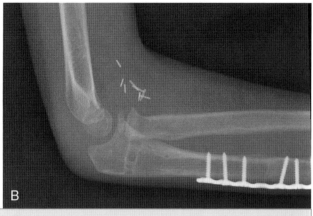
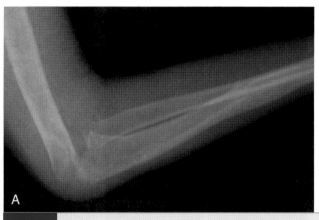

Figure 3 Lateral radiographs showing ulnar shaft malunion and radial head dislocation in a missed Monteggia fracture before treatment (**A**) and after an osteotomy of the ulna and annular ligament reconstruction (**B**). (Reproduced with permission from Shriners Hospital for Children, Philadelphia, PA.)

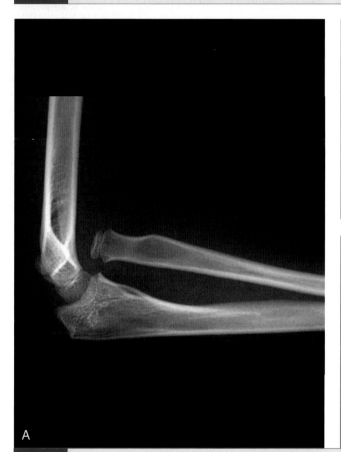
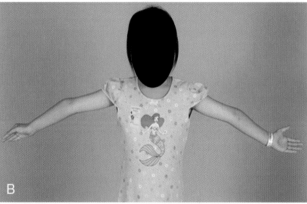
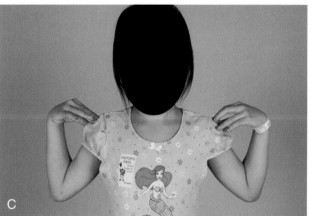

Figure 4 **A**, Lateral radiograph showing a late-presenting Monteggia fracture. **B** and **C**, Photographs showing excellent range of motion in a child who was asymptomatic and best treated with interval observation. (Reproduced with permission from Shriners Hospital for Children, Philadelphia, PA.)

If a single bone is fractured, a concomitant joint injury at the elbow (the Monteggia fracture) or the wrist (the Galeazzi fracture) must be ruled out by examining the areas above and below the joint. The mechanisms of injury are as varied as the types of fractures, with rotational injuries being most common. The inherent rotational motion of the radius means that the rotational component of the fracture typically is in the radius; the predominant direction of force is in the ulna fracture. The symptoms range from mild pain and loss of forearm rotation with plastic deformation to severe pain and deformity with a complete fracture. Neurovascular injuries and open fractures are rare.

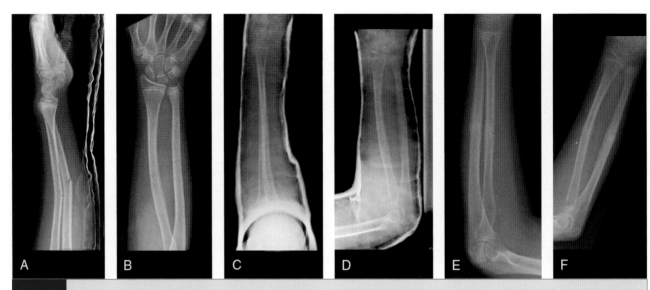

Figure 5 Lateral and PA radiographs showing a greenstick fracture of the forearm. **A** and **B**, The fracture before treatment. **C** and **D**, The fracture responded well to closed reduction and casting in a well-molded plaster cast. **E** and **F**, Regular follow-up ensured that the fracture remained reduced until union was achieved. (Reproduced with permission from Shriners Hospital for Children, Philadelphia, PA.)

Treatment

An anatomic reduction generally is preferred, regardless of the patient's age. However, the risks of achieving an anatomic reduction, such as those associated with anesthesia and compartment syndrome, must be weighed against the risks of a malunited fracture. The younger the child, the greater the deformity that can be accepted. The characteristics of the fracture should be considered: type of fracture (plastic deformation, greenstick, complete, or comminuted), level (proximal, middle, distal third, or mixed), position (displaced, angulated, shortened, or rotated), and personality (stable, reducible-stable, reducible-unstable, or irreducible). The algorithm also should be influenced by social aspects including the child's compliance, activity level, and caretaker support. A long arm cast with a good interosseous mold always is used, unless the condition of the soft tissue precludes circumferential casting or rigid skeletal stabilization negates the need for cast immobilization.

In children younger than 8 years, most fractures can be treated with closed reduction and casting. Plastic deformation of more than 20° is likely to limit forearm rotation and typically requires closed reduction under conscious sedation or general anesthesia. However, any fracture that limits functional forearm rotation should be reduced regardless of its strict angular measurement. The reduction is achieved with a three-point bend, and it may require a strong, steady force (as much as 30 kg) sustained over several minutes.[9] Sometimes the deformation is so severe that a greenstick or complete fracture of the diaphysis unavoidably occurs during the reduction. Because the periosteum remains intact, fracture displacement and rotation are minimal. A greenstick fracture is amenable to closed reduction and casting (**Figure 5**). The reduction maneuver should follow the rotation of the fracture, following the principle of bringing the distal fragment to the proximal fragment. Fracture completion during the reduction can be destabilizing if the periosteum is disrupted. Bayonet apposition and 20° of angulation are acceptable in younger children.[10] Rotational deformities of as much as 30° are well tolerated because of compensatory rotation at the wrist, but they do not remodel over time.[11]

The indications for intramedullary or rigid fixation in a young child include the presence of an open, irreducible, or segmental fracture; a floating elbow injury; loss of reduction; and an evolving neurovascular injury. Intramedullary fixation has several advantages. It is a relatively percutaneous technique requiring no soft-tissue stripping at the fracture site, it can be performed relatively quickly, and no permanent hardware is left in place.[12] The risk of a compartment syndrome is increased by multiple passes of the nail and extended tourniquet time.[13] The disadvantages of intramedullary fixation include the need for postoperative casting, the inability to control rotation in a transverse fracture or to control length in a comminuted or segmental fracture, and the difficulty of re-creating an anatomic bow at the radius. Plate-and-screw fixation is rigid, obviates the need for casting in some patients, allows for control of both length and rotation, and can be achieved in a late-presenting nascent malunion. However, it is necessary to expose the fracture site, and a secondary procedure may be required to remove the plate. The current trend is in favor of intramedullary fixation unless the fracture is open, segmental, or comminuted; there is neurovascular injury requiring exploration and repair; or the child is within 1 year of skeletal maturity.[14]

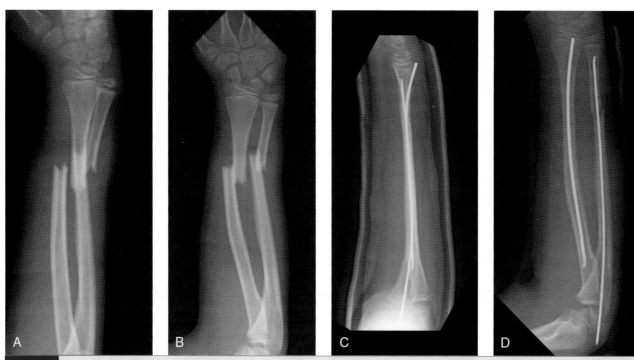

Figure 6 Oblique radiographs showing a displaced complete fracture of a both-bone forearm fracture in a skeletally immature child before treatment (**A** and **B**) and after intramedullary fixation (**C** and **D**), which can be done if a closed reduction is inadequate. Care must be taken to restore the radial bow and to minimize the number of passes with the intramedullary device. (Reproduced with permission from Shriners Hospital for Children, Philadelphia, PA.)

The choice of intramedullary implant depends on the size of the canal at the isthmus. A larger implant is preferred for enhancing construct rigidity, but it can be difficult to pass such an implant or to re-create the radial bow. Generally, the ulna is treated first in an antegrade fashion. A retrograde pin or rod is then inserted into the radius just proximal to the distal radial physis (**Figure 6**). In plate-and-screw fixation, a common mistake is to attempt to minimize the surgical exposure and the need for later plate removal by using a plate that is too short or insufficiently rigid. If casting is planned for a highly compliant young child with a low activity level, four cortices on either side of the fracture with a properly sized one-third tubular plate may be sufficient. For other patients, a rigid compression or reconstruction plate with at least six holes is recommended. The closer the child is to skeletal maturity, the greater the need for an anatomic reduction with rigid fixation. In older children, fixation is recommended for any fracture that limits functional forearm rotation or has more than 10° of angulation (**Figure 7**).

Complications

Nonunions are rare, but malunions with persistent loss of forearm motion are more common.[15] Overgrowth also can contribute to deformity. Corrective osteotomy of one or both forearm fractures within 1 year of the original fracture can improve forearm rotation dramatically, as long as length and an anatomic bow are restored to the radius and length and angulation are corrected at the ulna. After the first year, recovery of forearm rotation is less predictable because of secondary soft-tissue contractures.[16] Synostosis of the radius and ulna is a more rare and difficult complication than nonunion or malunion. The risk of synostosis is increased if both bones fractured at the same level, the fracture resulted from a high-energy injury, or a single incision was used to treat both fractures.[17,18] Once radioulnar synostosis occurs, it is difficult to treat. Resection of the heterotopic bone and soft-tissue interposition has had inconsistent results. Single-dose radiation therapy is not recommended in children with open physes.[19,20] If an attempt to take down the synostosis fails, a rotational osteotomy can be considered.

Refracturing can occur at any time but is most likely soon after removal of the cast or hardware. The incidence may be as high as 5%, and it is inversely proportional to the length of time the cast was used.[21] Activity modification and splinting for as long as 2 months after union may limit the risk, but no firm guidelines exist.

Compartment syndrome is the most worrisome complication of forearm fracture. The common signs of pain, paresthesias, pulselessness, and pallor typically are not encountered until irreversible injury has occurred. In children, increased analgesia, agitation, and anxiety are the indications of a compartment syndrome. A child often is irritable and disoriented after a procedure under general anesthesia and may be less articulate than an adult. It is difficult to differentiate between an unhappy child with a cast and an unhappy

6: Musculoskeletal Trauma

child with a cast and an impending compartment syndrome, particularly in the absence of information about the child's personality. A low threshold for treatment is critical to avert disaster. Increasing analgesic needs after cast placement, pain with motion or unwillingness to actively move the digits, and worsening digital edema should prompt bivalving and removal of the anterior shell of the cast to examine the compartments. The value of measuring compartment pressures is controversial, and the decision to perform a fasciotomy is largely made on clinical grounds. If a compartment syndrome is suspected, emergency fasciotomy is required. The typical claw of a Volkman ischemic contracture is seen in a late-presenting compartment syndrome; release of the entire flexor compartment can restore some muscle function if viable muscle persists, and a neurolysis may allow for some nerve recovery (Figure 8). Tendon transfers may be required to augment hand function.

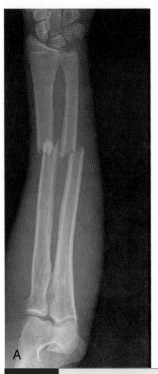
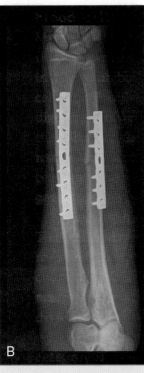

Figure 7 AP radiographs showing a both-bone forearm fracture before treatment (**A**) and after open reduction and internal fixation (**B**). Open reduction and internal fixation should be considered if the child is nearing skeletal maturity or fracture stability cannot be achieved using intramedullary rods alone. (Reproduced with permission from Shriners Hospital for Children, Philadelphia, PA.)

Distal Radius and Ulna Fractures

Assessment

Fractures of the distal end of the radius, with or without a distal ulna fracture, are among the most common pediatric injuries. The typical mechanism is a fall onto an outstretched hand, usually from a bicycle, bunk bed, or scooter. Children tend to tolerate these injuries, especially if the fracture is minimally displaced or incomplete; therefore, delays in seeking treatment are common. The diagnosis is simple if gross displacement with deformity is present, but it is more subtle for a buckle (torus) fracture, plastic deformation, or physeal injury. Point tenderness over the bone is presumed a fracture until proved otherwise. Radiographs should be obtained out of plaster whenever feasible. If the patient already has a splint or cast in place, an attempt should be made to acquire the original radiographs and office notes. The splint or cast should not be removed if there

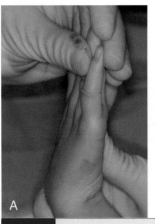
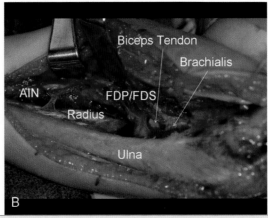
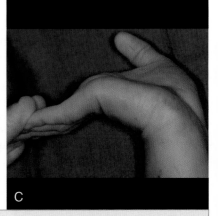

Figure 8 Photographs showing compartment syndrome, which is the most devastating complication of forearm fractures. **A**, A child's hand with a tight flexor compartment and limited wrist extension (an Eaton angle of 45°). **B**, An ulnar-side release of the entire forearm flexor compartment. AIN = anterior interosseous nerve, FDP/FDS = flexor digitorum profundus/flexor digitorum superficialis. **C**, Full passive motion was restored, with almost-full restoration of active motion. (Reproduced with permission from Shriners Hospital for Children, Philadelphia, PA.)

is any uncertainty about the type of injury. After radiographs are obtained, the limb is more extensively examined. A concomitant distal radioulnar joint (DRUJ) disruption should be suspected, particularly with a fracture of the radius at the distal diaphysis or metadiaphysis. A true lateral radiograph with the pisiform overlapping the distal pole of the scaphoid may reveal the dislocation (Figure 9).

Treatment

In young children, all but the most severely displaced and angulated fractures can remodel because of the proximity of the fracture to the distal ulnar and radial physes. The remodeling potential is highest along the plane of motion of the joint. As much as 20° to 25° of sagittal plane angulation is acceptable in children younger than 12 years, and 10° to 15° is permissible in older children. Little remodeling can be expected in the coronal plane, and more than 10° of angulation should be corrected. Rotational deformities will not remodel and should be accepted with caution. Buckle fractures and plastic deformation are inherently stable, and they respond well to 3 weeks in a removable splint. Most bicortical or greenstick fractures can be reduced and casted. Recent studies indicate that a well-molded short arm cast is just as effective as a long arm cast.[22,23] After a reduction maneuver, weekly radiographs should be obtained during the first 3 weeks to monitor for redisplacement. Completely displaced fractures and fractures with high obliquity are more likely to become redisplaced, but the risk of redisplacement can be decreased by minimizing the cast padding around the fracture site.[24] If redisplacement occurs, repeat reduction of the fracture with percutaneous pin fixation is recommended.

Although percutaneous pin fixation minimizes the risk of redisplacement, approximately one third of 34 patients had pin-related complications in a 2005 study.[25] Open reduction and internal fixation is effective and allows earlier motion, but a larger surgical approach and soft-tissue stripping are required. Percutaneous fixation is preferred for an unstable fracture unless the child is nearing or has achieved skeletal maturity. No consensus exists as to the optimal fixation method in young adults.

A suspected Galeazzi fracture requires an anatomic reduction, sometimes with plate fixation; one study found good to excellent outcomes.[26] The DRUJ spontaneously reduces when the radius is anatomically reduced, unless the injury is nonacute or there is soft-tissue interposition. Postoperative DRUJ immobilization remains controversial. A removable, forearm-based splint may be sufficient for a cooperative child if stable fixation was achieved at the radius and the DRUJ was stable under examination in the operating room. If only relative stability was achieved at the radius fracture and the DRUJ is unstable, it is preferable to use a long arm cast with the forearm held in the position of DRUJ reduction closest to neutral.

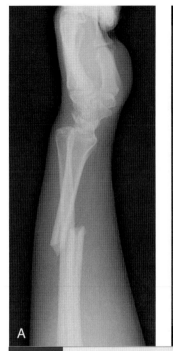
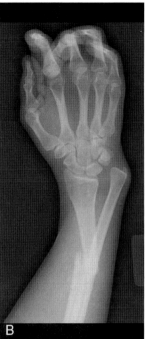

Figure 9 Radiographs showing a distal radial diaphyseal fracture, which can result in a dislocation of the DRUJ (a Galeazzi fracture). **A,** A true lateral radiograph of the wrist showing the dislocation, with overlay of the pisiform and distal pole of the scaphoid. **B,** In some fractures, the dislocation can be seen on a PA radiograph. (Reproduced with permission from Shriners Hospital for Children, Philadelphia, PA.)

Unlike distal radial physeal fractures, distal ulnar physeal fractures carry a high risk of growth disturbance.[27] An early anatomic reduction should be attempted by closed, percutaneous, or open means, although the quality of the reduction has not been correlated with the risk of growth arrest. Distal radial injuries are both more common and more forgiving. A gentle closed reduction can be attempted within 7 to 10 days of the injury. After that time, the risks to the physis from the reduction itself outweigh the benefits; it is better to accept the deformity and perform a late extraphyseal osteotomy if remodeling is incomplete. If fixation is needed, every attempt should be made to avoid crossing the physis. An unstable Salter-Harris type I fracture or a fracture with a small Thurston-Holland fragment requires transphyseal fixation; the risk of bar formation can be decreased by placing smooth pins with a minimal number of passes.

Complications

Physeal arrest occurs after almost 5% of distal radial physeal injuries and in 50% of distal ulnar physeal injuries.[28] If a growth disturbance is present, serial radiographs reveal a change in ulnar variance, worsening angular deformities, and a loss of clear space at the physis. MRI is optimal for mapping the topography of

6: Musculoskeletal Trauma

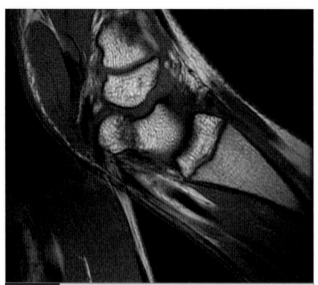

Figure 10 Sagittal MRI showing a nondisplaced fracture of the scaphoid waist that was not visible on radiographs taken 2 weeks after the injury. (Reproduced with permission from Shriners Hospital for Children, Philadelphia, PA.)

the physis and quantifying the extent of physeal bar formation. A child who is near skeletal maturity and has minimal deformity should undergo radial and ulnar epiphysiodesis. A bar excision should be attempted if substantial growth remains and more than half of the physis is viable. Other treatment options include corrective osteotomies, selective epiphysiodesis, and lengthening or shortening procedures.[29]

A late-presenting or missed Galeazzi fracture can be treated in a manner analogous to a missed Monteggia fracture. The earlier the dislocation is treated, the better the outcome is likely to be. Any relevant deformity of the radius should be corrected with an osteotomy. If the DRUJ remains irreducible or unstable, open reduction and repair or reconstruction of the volar and dorsal radioulnar ligaments becomes necessary. The presence of open physes precludes using the ligament reconstruction favored for adults.[30] If the dislocation is long-standing and the patient is only minimally symptomatic, observation may be the best course.

Scaphoid Fractures

Assessment

Most scaphoid fractures in children occur at the waist or distal pole. Because the scaphoid does not begin to ossify until age 5 years, a fracture that occurs in a child younger than 7 years is difficult to diagnose; fortunately, these fractures are rare. The progression of ossification with vascularization in a distal-to-proximal direction initially decreases the likelihood of proximal fractures. The overall incidence of scaphoid fractures is correlated with

the rate of ossification and is at its peak at age 15 years.[31] The mechanism of injury for scaphoid waist fractures is axial load and hyperextension at the wrist. The classic signs of snuff box tenderness and dorsoradial wrist edema should raise suspicion that the patient has a scaphoid fracture. Radiographs should include pronated oblique and PA ulnar deviation views, but these may not reveal a nondisplaced fracture.

Treatment

A suspected fracture should be immobilized in a forearm-based thumb spica splint or cast. New radiographs should be taken if snuff box tenderness persists after 2 weeks. If these radiographs are inconclusive, the immobilization can be continued until pain is resolved or the fracture can be seen on radiographs. A short arm–thumb spica cast is used when the definitive diagnosis is made. MRI may show an occult fracture, and it can be used to obtain an earlier diagnosis (**Figure 10**). A distal pole fracture readily unites and is treated with a cast. Two treatment options are available for a nondisplaced fracture: a long arm–thumb spica cast for the first 6 weeks, followed by a short arm–thumb spica cast until fracture healing; or percutaneous compression screw fixation and a removable splint (**Figure 11**). The two modalities are similar in efficacy and risk, and the choice can be left to the patient and family.

A displaced acute scaphoid waist fracture should be reduced and stabilized. The current trend is to attempt a closed reduction whenever possible, followed by percutaneous fixation with smooth pins or a compression screw. If closed reduction is not possible, an open reduction with pin or screw fixation is necessary.

Complications

Nonunion of an appropriately treated fracture is rare in children. Most nonunions are the result of a delay in diagnosis or a late presentation. Some evidence suggests that early nonunions without displacement are amenable to percutaneous fixation without bone grafting.[32,33] Displaced or avascular nonunions are best managed with bone grafting, with or without vascular transfer. Sources of additional vascular supply include the Zaidenberg graft,[34] the superficial volar branch of the radial artery, and the medial femoral condyle.[35]

Hand Fractures

Assessment

Most hand fractures in children occur as a result of crush injury or torsional and axial load. A child's tendency to ignore a common injury such as a jammed finger can lead to a delay in fracture diagnosis. Fractures of the phalanges are common, with the small finger ray most at risk.[36] Children have ligament avulsion fractures, transphyseal injuries, plastic deformation, buckle fractures, and greenstick fractures, in addition to the types of fractures seen in adults. It is important to obtain radio-

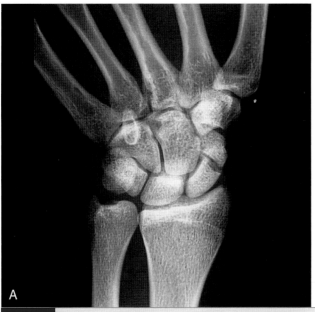
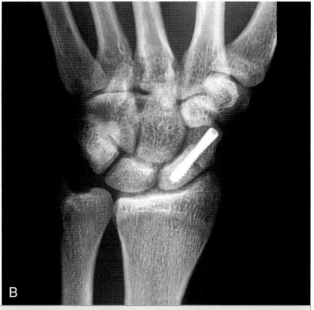

Figure 11 PA radiographs of the wrist of a 15-year-old boy. **A**, A 4-week-old nondisplaced fracture of the scaphoid; cavitary changes can be seen at the fracture site, with bony resorption and an incipient nonunion–fibrous union. **B**, Within 6 weeks of percutaneous screw fixation, the defect is filling with bone. (Reproduced with permission from Shriners Hospital for Children, Philadelphia, PA.)

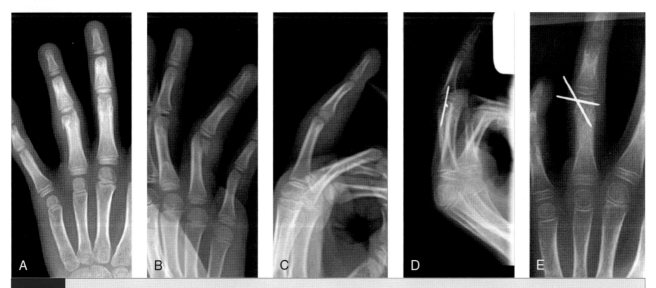

Figure 12 Radiographs showing a condylar shear fracture of the ring finger phalanx, as seen in the AP (**A**), oblique (**B**), and lateral (**C**) views. This type of fracture is inherently unstable and requires percutaneous fixation (**D** and **E**) or open fixation with at least two pins or screws. (Reproduced with permission from Shriners Hospital for Children, Philadelphia, PA.)

graphs centered over the area of interest. A phalangeal condyle fracture, for example, may be missed on standard radiographs of the hand (**Figure 12**).

Treatment

Most hand fractures can be managed with immobilization until union. Casting, splinting, or buddy strapping can be used. Metacarpal fractures and proximal and distal phalangeal fractures generally heal within 3 to 4 weeks, although the middle phalanx may require 4 to 5 weeks. For unacceptable displacement, rotation, or angulation, a closed reduction can be attempted while using a wrist or digital block, Bier block, sedation, or general anesthesia. If the reduction cannot be maintained or a risk of redisplacement can be foreseen, percutaneous pinning is recommended. There is a high risk of malunion if a displaced, angulated, or rotated fracture is located at the base of the thumb metacarpal; the

6: Musculoskeletal Trauma

base of the proximal phalanx of the thumb, with ligament avulsion; the base of the proximal phalanx of a finger; a phalangeal condyle; or the base of a distal phalanx, with nail plate avulsion proximally (the Seymour fracture) (**Table 2**).

In the Seymour fracture, eponychial fold interposition between the germinal matrix and the nail plate prevents reduction of the fracture, exposes the fracture to infection, and can lead to persistent nail deformity and chronic osteomyelitis if not appropriately treated (**Figure 13**). Treatment of this open fracture requires nail plate removal, irrigation and débridement, fracture reduction, nail bed repair, and replacement of the nail plate beneath the eponychial fold to augment fixation. If necessary, a single pin may be placed across the fracture and the distal interphalangeal joint.

A ligament-equivalent injury such as a beak ligament avulsion (the Bennett fracture) or thumb collateral ligament avulsion should be reduced and stabilized with percutaneous or internal fixation if it is displaced, particularly if the fragment is large and malrotated[37] (**Figure 14**). Malunion or nonunion of the avulsion can lead to chronic instability, deformity, and late degener-

ative changes (**Figure 15**). An epibasilar fracture or Salter-Harris type I or II fracture of the thumb metacarpal is more stable and is easier to reduce and hold in a cast, with high remodeling potential. However, close follow-up is necessary after an acceptable closed reduction and casting.[38] Surgery is indicated for an open fracture or an unstable fracture that cannot be reduced or held within an acceptable angulation of less than 30° by closed means (**Figure 16**). In children who are near skeletal maturity, an apex dorsal deformity of the metacarpal should not be accepted because it can predispose the child to basal joint arthritis later in life.

A tendinous avulsion injury can lead to long-term deformity unless it is treated acutely. Extensor mechanism avulsions such as central slip insertion and mallet fracture rarely retract, and most can be treated acutely with extension splinting at the proximal and distal interphalangeal joints, respectively. A mallet fracture often is a Salter-Harris type III fracture; it can be successfully managed with closed reduction and continuous splinting for at least 6 weeks (**Figure 17**). Surgery is not indicated even if distal interphalangeal joint subluxation is present. Jersey finger (an avulsion injury of the flexor digitorum profundus muscle, which is on the volar side of the distal phalangeal base) requires surgical repair to restore active flexion at the distal interphalangeal joint. A large bony fragment may become entrapped at the annular pulleys, maintaining some length and allowing a subacute repair. Small avulsion fragments can retract with the flexor digitorum profundus into the palm, and urgent repair is required within 10 days of the injury.[39]

A phalangeal neck or condylar fracture is prone to rotation, extension, and further displacement. Most such fractures should be treated with closed reduction and percutaneous pinning. The use of a single pin is never sufficient. Open reduction occasionally is necessary for accurately observing and reducing the fracture. However, the blood supply to the fragment must be preserved to prevent osteonecrosis. Subacute injuries may be amenable to percutaneous osteoclasis and

Table 2

High-Risk Hand Fractures

Location	Additional Feature
Base of the thumb metacarpal	Displacement, angulation, or rotation
Base of the proximal phalanx of the thumb	Ligament avulsion equivalent
Base of the proximal phalanx of a finger	
A phalangeal condyle	
Base of a distal phalanx	Proximal nail plate avulsion (Seymour fracture)

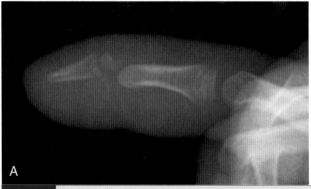
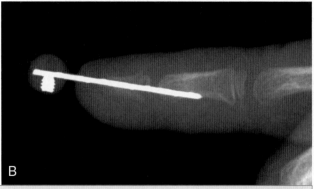

Figure 13   A variant of a Seymour fracture with retraction and dislocation of the proximal fragment in a 4-year-old girl. The fracture was missed immediately after the injury. **A**, Lateral radiograph showing the fracture 2 weeks after the injury. **B**, An open reduction and nail bed repair was stabilized with suture fixation and cross pinning. (Reproduced with permission from Shriners Hospital for Children, Philadelphia, PA.)

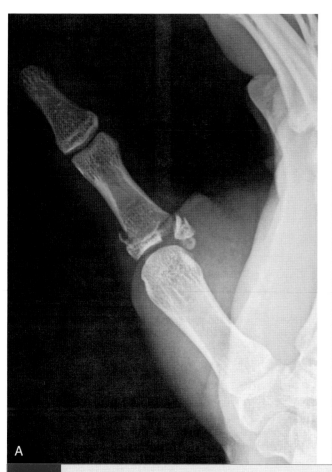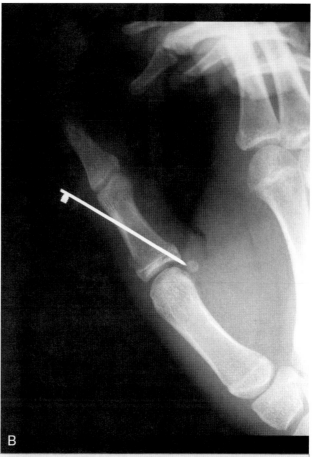

Figure 14 **A**, AP radiograph showing an avulsion fracture of the base of the proximal thumb phalanx (the pediatric equivalent of a gamekeeper or skier thumb). **B**, AP radiograph showing a closed reduction and pinning of the fracture; either this treatment or open reduction and internal fixation is recommended to restore collateral ligament function if the fracture is displaced or leads to collateral ligament instability. (Reproduced with permission from Shriners Hospital for Children, Philadelphia, PA.)

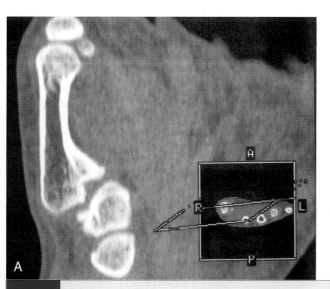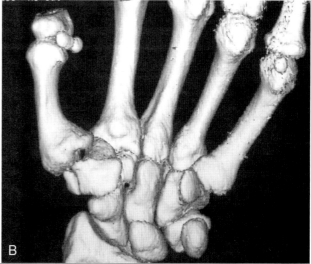

Figure 15 An untreated Bennett fracture in a 21-year-old man. CT (**A**) and three-dimensional CT reconstruction (**B**) reveal fracture malunion, articular incongruity, and joint subluxation. (Reproduced with permission from Shriners Hospital for Children, Philadelphia, PA.)

6: Musculoskeletal Trauma

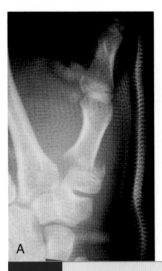
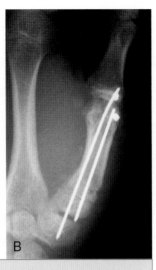

Figure 16 **A**, Oblique radiograph showing an epibasilar fracture after unsuccessful treatment with closed reduction and casting. **B**, Oblique radiograph showing subsequent closed reduction and pinning of the fracture. Many epibasilar fractures can be treated with closed reduction and casting, but if an adequate closed reduction cannot be achieved or maintained, closed reduction and pinning or open reduction and internal fixation is recommended. (Reproduced with permission from Shriners Hospital for Children, Philadelphia, PA.)

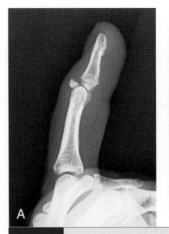
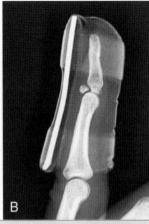

Figure 17 Lateral radiographs showing a mallet fracture before treatment (**A**) and after closed reduction and extension splinting (**B**). Closed treatment may be successful as late as 1 year after the injury, but it requires a minimum of 6 weeks' continuous immobilization. (Reproduced with permission from Shriners Hospital for Children, Philadelphia, PA.)

pinning, but a formal osteotomy at the fracture site is discouraged because of the risk of osteonecrosis of the condyles. A late-presenting injury is best treated by subcondylar fossa reconstruction.

Fractures at the base of the proximal phalanges of the fingers are difficult to see on radiographs, and the amount of angulation and rotation easily can be underestimated. Closed treatment can be accomplished by fully flexing the metacarpophalangeal joint to correct the angulation and by flexing the interphalangeal joints far enough to evaluate and correct the rotation. In a cooperative child or adolescent, a hand-based cast in the position of reduction is sufficient, but a forearm-based cast is necessary for most children. Evaluation of fracture redisplacement is almost impossible while the cast is in place. In an older child with severe angulation, a single pin through the metacarpophalangeal joint or crossed pins outside the joint may be indicated.

Carpometacarpal fracture-dislocations also are difficult to see on radiographs. A lateral radiograph with overlap of the distal pole of the scaphoid and the pisiform shows the often-subtle dorsal displacement of the base of the metacarpal, with or without a portion of the adjacent carpal bone. If a fracture is suspected, CT is recommended to confirm the diagnosis and guide the choice of treatment. Closed reduction and pinning often can be achieved acutely, but an open reduction usually is necessary 2 weeks after injury. An older fracture with joint destruction and pain is best treated with fusion.

Complications

Most fractures in the hand can be managed by immobilization alone. Serious complications usually are the result of undertreatment of the previously identified troublesome fractures. An untreated Seymour fracture can lead to chronic osteomyelitis, permanent nail deformity, and gross fingertip angulation. Phalangeal neck fracture malunion leads to loss of proximal or distal interphalangeal joint motion. Ligament avulsion injury can lead to chronic instability requiring ligament repair or reconstruction or joint fusion. Unrecognized extensor mechanism tendinous avulsion injury can lead to a swan or boutonnière deformity requiring surgical reconstruction. Malrotation in the phalanges and metacarpals does not remodel and requires osteotomy for correction.

The complications of surgical management include pin site infection, neurovascular injury, and loss of reduction that creates the need for further surgery. For each fracture, the risks of surgery should be weighed against the risks of malunion and nonunion.

Summary

The ability of severely angulated and displaced fractures to remodel in young children should not lead the treating physician to believe that all fractures in children can be managed without surgery. Although this generalization holds true for most pediatric fractures, the location and type of fracture as well as the proximity of the child to skeletal maturity must be considered in determining the best treatment. Some fractures require surgical fixation if there is any displacement, and others rarely require surgery. Any practitioner treating

6: Musculoskeletal Trauma

pediatric fractures of the forearm, wrist, and hand should be able to distinguish the high-risk fractures from more common pediatric fractures.

Annotated References

1. Bado JL: The Monteggia lesion. *Clin Orthop Relat Res* 1967;50:71-86.

2. Spinner M, Freundlich BD, Teicher J: Posterior interosseous nerve palsy as a complication of Monteggia fractures in children. *Clin Orthop Relat Res* 1968;58:141-145.

3. Stein F, Grabias SL, Deffer PA: Nerve injuries complicating Monteggia lesions. *J Bone Joint Surg Am* 1971;53(7):1432-1436.

4. Ring D, Jupiter JB, Waters PM: Monteggia fractures in children and adults. *J Am Acad Orthop Surg* 1998;6(4):215-224.

5. Fowles JV, Sliman N, Kassab MT: The Monteggia lesion in children: Fracture of the ulna and dislocation of the radial head. *J Bone Joint Surg Am* 1983;65(9):1276-1282.

6. Nakamura K, Hirachi K, Uchiyama S, et al: Long-term clinical and radiographic outcomes after open reduction for missed Monteggia fracture-dislocations in children. *J Bone Joint Surg Am* 2009;91(6):1394-1404.

   Twenty-two consecutive patients were treated with a posterior bending-elongation ulnar osteotomy and anular ligament reconstruction. The radiographic results were significantly better after surgery within 3 years of injury or in children younger than 12 years.

7. Bell Tawse AJ: The treatment of malunited anterior Monteggia fractures in children. *J Bone Joint Surg Br* 1965;47(4):718-723.

8. Seel MJ, Peterson HA: Management of chronic post-traumatic radial head dislocation in children. *J Pediatr Orthop* 1999;19(3):306-312.

9. Sanders WE, Heckman JD: Traumatic plastic deformation of the radius and ulna: A closed method of correction of deformity. *Clin Orthop Relat Res* 1984;188:58-67.

10. Ploegmakers JJ, Verheyen CC: Acceptance of angulation in the non-operative treatment of paediatric forearm fractures. *J Pediatr Orthop B* 2006;15(6):428-432.

    Expert opinion and a meta-analysis of the literature were used in determining acceptable levels of angulation for eight types of pediatric forearm fractures.

11. Price CT, Scott DS, Kurzner ME, Flynn JC: Malunited forearm fractures in children. *J Pediatr Orthop* 1990;10(6):705-712.

12. Garg NK, Ballal MS, Malek IA, Webster RA, Bruce CE: Use of elastic stable intramedullary nailing for treating unstable forearm fractures in children. *J Trauma* 2008;65(1):109-115.

    Twenty-one patients were treated with intramedullary nailing and long arm casting for unstable forearm fractures. The results were good, with only one delayed union and one nonunion.

13. Yuan PS, Pring ME, Gaynor TP, Mubarak SJ, Newton PO: Compartment syndrome following intramedullary fixation of pediatric forearm fractures. *J Pediatr Orthop* 2004;24(4):370-375.

14. Reinhardt KR, Feldman DS, Green DW, Sala DA, Widmann RF, Scher DM: Comparison of intramedullary nailing to plating for both-bone forearm fractures in older children. *J Pediatr Orthop* 2008;28(4):403-409.

    This retrospective study compared the results of intramedullary fixation in 19 patients and plating in 12 patients. No significant between-group differences were found except for surgical time.

15. Schmittenbecher PP, Fitze G, Gödeke J, Kraus R, Schneidmüller D: Delayed healing of forearm shaft fractures in children after intramedullary nailing. *J Pediatr Orthop* 2008;28(3):303-306.

    A retrospective study of 10 patients found that open fracture, open reduction, and ulna fracture were more common in patients who had nonunion or delayed union than in patients with union. Union occurred as late as 13 months after surgery.

16. Trousdale RT, Linscheid RL: Operative treatment of malunited fractures of the forearm. *J Bone Joint Surg Am* 1995;77(6):894-902.

17. Vince KG, Miller JE: Cross-union complicating fracture of the forearm: Part II. Children. *J Bone Joint Surg Am* 1987;69(5):654-661.

18. Bauer G, Arand M, Mutschler W: Post-traumatic radio-ulnar synostosis after forearm fracture osteosynthesis. *Arch Orthop Trauma Surg* 1991;110(3):142-145.

19. Cullen JP, Pellegrini VD Jr, Miller RJ, Jones JA: Treatment of traumatic radioulnar synostosis by excision and postoperative low-dose irradiation. *J Hand Surg Am* 1994;19(3):394-401.

20. Abrams RA, Simmons BP, Brown RA, Botte MJ: Treatment of posttraumatic radioulnar synostosis with excision and low-dose radiation. *J Hand Surg Am* 1993;18(4):703-707.

21. Schwarz N, Pienaar S, Schwarz AF, Jelen M, Styhler W, Mayr J: Refracture of the forearm in children. *J Bone Joint Surg Br* 1996;78(5):740-744.

22. Bohm ER, Bubbar V, Yong Hing K, Dzus A: Above and below-the-elbow plaster casts for distal forearm fractures in children: A randomized controlled trial. *J Bone Joint Surg Am* 2006;88(1):1-8.

A well-executed randomized controlled study found that short and long arm casts were equally efficacious for treating distal forearm fractures. The factors associated with loss of reduction included persistent angulation after reduction and combined radius and ulna fracture.

23. Webb GR, Galpin RD, Armstrong DG: Comparison of short and long arm plaster casts for displaced fractures in the distal third of the forearm in children. *J Bone Joint Surg Am* 2006;88(1):9-17.

   A well-executed randomized, controlled study found that short and long arm casts were equally efficacious for treating displaced distal forearm fractures. The quality of the mold was found to be critical in maintaining the reduction.

24. Alemdaroğlu KB, Iltar S, Cimen O, Uysal M, Alagöz E, Atlihan D: Risk factors in redisplacement of distal radial fractures in children. *J Bone Joint Surg Am* 2008; 90(6):1224-1230.

   In a prospective study of 75 fractures of the distal radius after a closed reduction and casting, complete displacement and degree of angulation were found to be most closely correlated with redisplacement.

25. Miller BS, Taylor B, Widmann RF, Bae DS, Snyder BD, Waters PM: Cast immobilization versus percutaneous pin fixation of displaced distal radius fractures in children: A prospective, randomized study. *J Pediatr Orthop* 2005;25(4):490-494.

   This prospective randomized study followed 34 patients with a distal radius fracture who underwent closed reduction and casting or closed reduction and pinning. In both groups, complications occurred in approximately one third of the patients (those with a cast, redisplacement requiring remanipulation, or a pin).

26. Eberl R, Singer G, Schalamon J, Petnehazy T, Hoellwarth ME: Galeazzi lesions in children and adolescents: Treatment and outcome. *Clin Orthop Relat Res* 2008; 466(7):1705-1709.

   In a retrospective study of 26 patients with Galeazzi fracture who were treated with modalities including short and long arm casting and surgery, most patients were found to have a good or excellent outcome.

27. Golz RJ, Grogan DP, Greene TL, Belsole RJ, Ogden JA: Distal ulnar physeal injury. *J Pediatr Orthop* 1991; 11(3):318-326.

28. Cannata G, De Maio F, Mancini F, Ippolito E: Physeal fractures of the distal radius and ulna: Long-term prognosis. *J Orthop Trauma* 2003;17(3):172-180.

29. Waters PM, Bae DS, Montgomery KD: Surgical management of posttraumatic distal radial growth arrest in adolescents. *J Pediatr Orthop* 2002;22(6):717-724.

30. Adams BD, Berger RA: An anatomic reconstruction of the distal radioulnar ligaments for posttraumatic distal radioulnar joint instability. *J Hand Surg Am* 2002; 27(2):243-251.

31. Simmons BP, Lovallo JL: Hand and wrist injuries in children. *Clin Sports Med* 1988;7(3):495-512.

32. Jeon IH, Kochhar H, Micic ID, Oh SH, Kim SY, Kim PT: Clinical result of operative treatment for scaphoid non-union in the skeletally immature: Percutaneous versus open procedure. *Hand Surg* 2008;13(1):11-16.

   This retrospective study of 13 patients included 3 who had a fibrous union with no displacement or angulation after treatment with percutaneous screw fixation alone. The average time to union in these 3 patients was 9 weeks.

33. Jeon IH, Kochhar H, Lee BW, Kim SY, Kim PT: Percutaneous screw fixation for scaphoid nonunion in skeletally immature patients: A report of two cases. *J Hand Surg Am* 2008;33(5):656-659.

   Two patients with an early nondisplaced nonunion of the scaphoid were successfully treated with percutaneous screw fixation alone.

34. Larson AN, Bishop AT, Shin AY: Dorsal distal radius vascularized pedicled bone grafts for scaphoid nonunions. *Tech Hand Up Extrem Surg* 2006;10(4):212-223.

   The technique for vascularized bone grafting of the scaphoid using the 1,2 intercompartmental supraretinacular artery is described.

35. Jones DB Jr, Bürger H, Bishop AT, Shin AY: Treatment of scaphoid waist nonunions with an avascular proximal pole and carpal collapse: A comparison of two vascularized bone grafts. *J Bone Joint Surg Am* 2008; 90(12):2616-2625.

   This retrospective study found that scaphoid avascular nonunions had a higher union rate when a medial femoral condylar vascularzed bone graft was used rather than a distal radial pedicle graft.

36. Vadivelu R, Dias JJ, Burke FD, Stanton J: Hand injuries in children: A prospective study. *J Pediatr Orthop* 2006; 26(1):29-35.

   A prospective evaluation of 360 children with a hand injury in one emergency department determined that the small finger was most commonly injured, followed by the thumb.

37. Griffiths JC: Bennett's fracture in childhood. *Br J Clin Pract* 1966;20(11):582-583.

38. Kozin SH: Fractures and dislocations along the pediatric thumb ray. *Hand Clin* 2006;22(1):19-29.

   This review article describes the common fractures and dislocations of the thumb.

39. Leddy JP, Packer JW: Avulsion of the profundus tendon insertion in athletes. *J Hand Surg Am* 1977;2(1):66-69.

6: Musculoskeletal Trauma

Chapter 33

Fractures of the Femur, Hip, and Pelvis

William L. Hennrikus, MD

Introduction

Pediatric fractures of the femur, hip, and pelvis can be treated using a variety of available and acceptable methods. The treatment decision should be based on the evidence-based literature, individual patient needs, available resources, and the experience of the orthopaedic surgeon.

Femur Fractures

Subtrochanteric Fractures

Subtrochanteric fractures of the femur are uncommon in children.[1] These fractures most often result from high-energy trauma, are more common in boys than in girls, and tend to occur in children younger than 10 years.[2] The subtrochanteric area of the femur is commonly defined either as the area extending 3 cm below the lesser trochanter or as the proximal 10% of total femur length below the lesser trochanter.[2,3]

An accurate closed reduction of a subtrochanteric fracture can be difficult. The proximal fragment displaces into flexion, abduction, and external rotation because of the unopposed forces of the adductors and gluteus maximus.[1,2] Advocates of nonsurgical treatment suggest that traction and casting are acceptable for children younger than 10 years who have less than 2 cm of shortening and less than 30° of angulation.[2,4] In these children, remodeling and overgrowth usually lead to a satisfactory long-term outcome, despite an imperfect reduction. Early spica casting for subtrochanteric femur fractures has been used in children younger than 10 years. The reduction is lost in approximately 25% of patients, however, and remanipulation or a different treatment is required.[4]

Surgical treatment is recommended for a subtrochanteric fracture if the patient is age 10 years or older

or has multiple injuries, an open fracture, or a closed head injury. Surgery also is needed if a satisfactory reduction cannot be achieved with traction, regardless of the child's age.[1,4] Rates of leg-length inequality and varus angulation are unacceptably high after nonsurgical treatment in children age 10 years or older.[1] The surgical treatment options include flexible nailing, with or without a one-leg spica cast;[1,3] open reduction and internal fixation with submuscular plating; dynamic screw and side plate or locked plating (Figure 1); and rigid intramedullary nailing.[1,3] The reported complications of surgery include heterotopic ossification, delayed union, transient peroneal nerve palsy, persistent incisional pain, and osteonecrosis of the femoral head.[1,4] Because of the risk of osteonecrosis, a rigid intramedullary nail is used only in skeletally mature adolescents.[1]

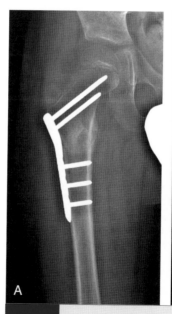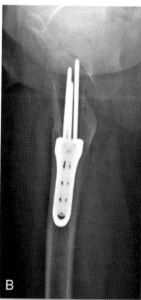

| Figure 1 | AP (A) and lateral (B) radiographs showing a healing subtrochanteric femur fracture in an 11-year-old boy after stabilization with a locking plate. The locking plate acts as a fixed-angle device. |

Dr. Hennrikus or an immediate family member serves as a board member, owner, officer, or committee member of the Society of Military Orthopaedic Surgeons, the Pediatric Orthopaedic Society of North America, and the American Academy of Pediatrics.

6: Musculoskeletal Trauma

Table 1

Age-Based Treatment of a Pediatric Femoral Shaft Fracture

Patient Age	Treatment Options
Younger than 1 year	Pavlik harness use Early spica casting
1 to 5 years	Early spica casting Traction followed by spica casting
6 to 10 years	Flexible nailing External fixation Submuscular plating Traction and casting
11 years to age of skeletal maturity	Greater trochanter entry nailing Submuscular plating Flexible nailing
Skeletal maturity	Reamed antegrade nailing through the piriformis fossa

Femoral Shaft Fractures

The incidence of femoral shaft fractures is approximately 19 per 100,000 children, and they account for approximately 1.4% of all pediatric fractures.[5] The distribution pattern is bimodal, with peaks at ages 2 and 17 years. Boys sustain this injury more commonly than girls.[6] An isolated femoral shaft fracture is the most common pediatric orthopaedic cause of extended hospitalization.[7]

Multiple treatment methods are available for pediatric femur fractures, including the use of a Pavlik harness, early spica casting, traction followed by spica casting, external fixation, flexible intramedullary nailing, submuscular plate fixation, and lateral-entry rigid intramedullary nailing. Each of these methods has a role in pediatric fracture treatment. The treatment decision is based on the individual needs of the patient and is influenced by the age of the patient, mechanism of injury, fracture location and pattern, and whether the fracture is open or closed. Other important factors include the presence of a concomitant ipsilateral tibial fracture, head injury, multitrauma, or pathologic fracture; the home environment; parental preference; and the experience of the surgeon.[8] The general age-based guidelines for treating an isolated closed femoral shaft fracture are outlined in **Table 1**. The patient's care and treatment always should be based on the clinician's independent medical judgment concerning the clinical circumstances.[8]

Pavlik Harness

A femur fracture in an infant heals rapidly and remodels completely. The possibility of nonaccidental trauma should be considered in an infant younger than 1 year with a femur fracture. A femur fracture in these infants can be treated using a spica cast or a Pavlik harness.[9] The advantages of the Pavlik harness over the spica cast in this age group include fewer skin complications,

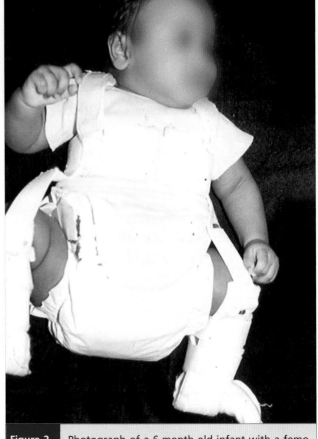

Figure 2   Photograph of a 6-month-old infant with a femoral shaft fracture treated with a Pavlik harness.

simplicity of application, ease of diaper changing, minimal cost, and better infant-to-mother bonding[9,10] (**Figure 2**).

Early Spica Casting

Spica casting on the day of injury or within the first few days is indicated for an otherwise healthy child as old as 6 years who has an isolated femoral shaft fracture stemming from a low-energy injury, with intact soft tissue, no evidence of a compartment syndrome, and a suitable home environment. Early spica casting is not recommended if the child is obese, the fracture is the result of a high-energy trauma, or the child has multitraumatic injuries or a floating knee injury. This method can be successful for a thin child as old as approximately 10 years. Early spica cast treatment minimizes the length of the hospital stay, allowing the child to return home in 1 to 2 days.

Early spica casting is an undervalued but demanding technique that can be used in the emergency department, the clinic, or the ward with the patient under sedation; or in the operating room under general anesthesia.[11,12] Follow-up radiographs should be obtained approximately 10 days after cast application to assess the angulation and shortening. Angulation of 20° in the

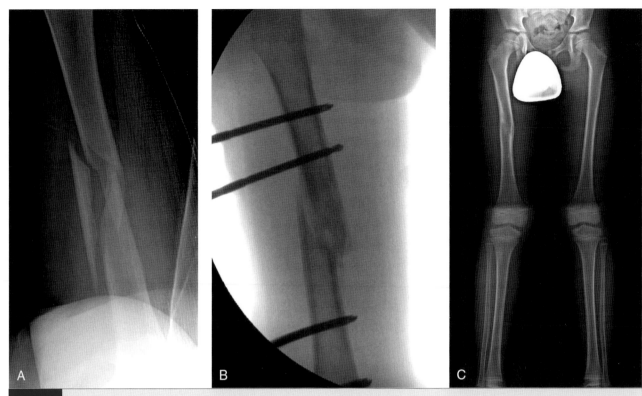

Figure 3 AP radiographs showing a comminuted femur fracture with a butterfly piece in an 8-year-old boy at the time of injury (**A**), during treatment with an external fixator (**B**), and at 9-month follow-up (**C**).

frontal and sagittal planes is considered reasonable, although the limit of acceptable angulation is a controversial topic. Greater angulation can be treated in the clinic by using a cast wedge approximately 10 days after cast application.[13] As much as 25° of malrotation is acceptable.[14] The limit of acceptable shortening in the cast is controversial, but shortening of 2 to 2.5 cm usually is acceptable in a child younger than 10 years. In these children, overgrowth of the femur averages 10 mm, and overgrowth of the uninjured tibia is as much as 0.5 cm. Shortening of as much as 1 cm is usually well tolerated at maturity.

Compartment syndrome and soft-tissue pressure injuries at the anterior ankle and posterior calf can occur with an early spica cast applied in the sitting position with the hip and knee flexed to 90°. The injury most commonly occurs when traction is applied to a short or long leg cast, and the cast is then incorporated into a spica cast with 90° hip and knee flexion.[15] Cast application with the leg in a more extended position and the foot left out of the cast can minimize these risks.

For a child younger than 6 years, the number of weeks the cast is required is estimated by adding 3 to the age of the child in years. Thus, a 5-year-old would be in the cast for approximately 8 weeks. For an older child, length of time in the cast is determined by the clinical and radiographic course; no evidence-based guidelines exist. No current studies are available to determine the efficacy of physical therapy for children with a femur fracture.

Traction Followed by Casting

Treating pediatric femur fractures with traction followed by casting has lost popularity for socioeconomic reasons.[16-18] This method remains an option for children as old as approximately 10 years who have a high-energy or comminuted fracture and for whom early spica casting or surgical treatment is deemed less appropriate. Skeletal traction is most commonly used, although skin traction can be used for a younger child.[19,20] The traction pin is best placed in the distal femoral metaphysis parallel to and about 2 cm above the physis. The use of home traction, as recently reported, has the advantage of reducing the length and expense of hospital stay.[21,22]

External Fixation

The risk of delayed union, refracture after device removal, or pin infection has diminished the former enthusiasm for routinely using external fixation to treat femur fractures in children.[23] External fixation is most likely to lead to complications when used for a diaphyseal transverse or short oblique facture. However, external fixation remains an option for children as old as approximately 10 years whose fracture is comminuted or accompanied by severe shortening, severe soft-tissue injury, head trauma, vascular injury, or life-threatening injuries[24] (**Figure 3**). Approximately 1 to 1.5 cm of shortening is acceptable, with 10° of angulation in any plane.[25] External fixation can be considered a form of portable traction that allows the child to ambulate,

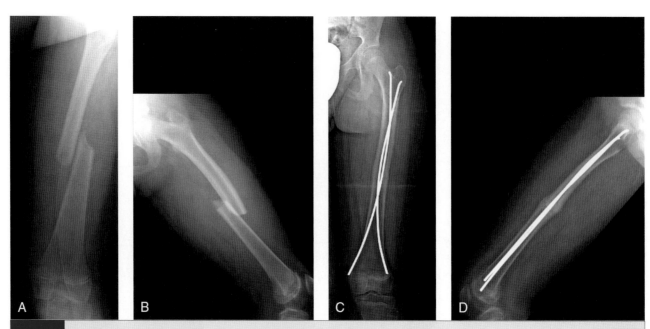

Figure 4   AP (**A**) and lateral (**B**) radiographs showing a length-stable transverse femoral shaft fracture in a 9-year-old girl. AP (**C**) and lateral (**D**) radiographs showing the fracture after treatment with flexible titanium nails.

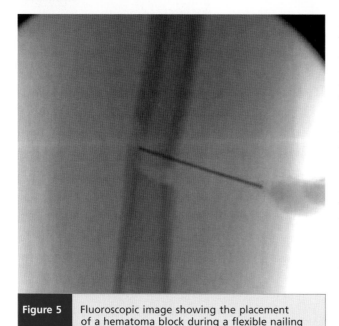

Figure 5   Fluoroscopic image showing the placement of a hematoma block during a flexible nailing procedure.

attend school, and bathe. A randomized, prospective study found that external fixation was better than spica casting for preventing malunion.[26]

Flexible Intramedullary Nailing
Flexible nailing has become the method of choice for the fixation of a transverse or short oblique femoral shaft fracture in the middle 60% of the femoral diaphysis. This technique is generally most appropriate for stable fractures (**Figure 4**). Spiral and comminuted fractures can shorten with flexible nail treatment.[27] Leg-

length inequality, excessive angulation, or malunion was found to be more likely when flexible titanium nailing was used in children who weighed more than 110 lb or were age 12 years or older.[28] Other methods of femur stabilization may be more appropriate for these children. For appropriately selected patients, flexible nailing allows a short hospitalization, early mobilization, more rapid return to function, and minimal morbidity.

The most common complication of flexible nail fixation is irritation and nail tip prominence, followed by development of a painful bursa at the insertion site at the tip of a nail.[29] The tip of the nail should be left flush with the cortex, with approximately 2 cm left outside the bone to minimize tip irritation. When the nail reaches its final position, it is backed out about 2 cm, cut at the skin level, and tapped back under the soft tissues so that only approximately 2 cm of nail extends from the bone. The use of a bupivacaine hematoma block into the fracture site can reduce the patient's need for narcotic analgesia during the first postoperative day[30] (**Figure 5**).

Because of the elastic nature of the implants, some motion occurs at the fracture site. As many as 60% of patients therefore are treated with a knee immobilizer or cast to minimize discomfort for the first 2 to 3 weeks.[31] Full weight bearing usually is delayed for approximately 4 weeks, until callus can be seen on radiographs. Nail removal is not mandatory, and it should be delayed until complete healing is seen on radiographs, typically after at least 6 months. Nail removal can be more difficult than nail insertion; it is facilitated by using specialized vise grips available from a flexible nail system manufacturer.

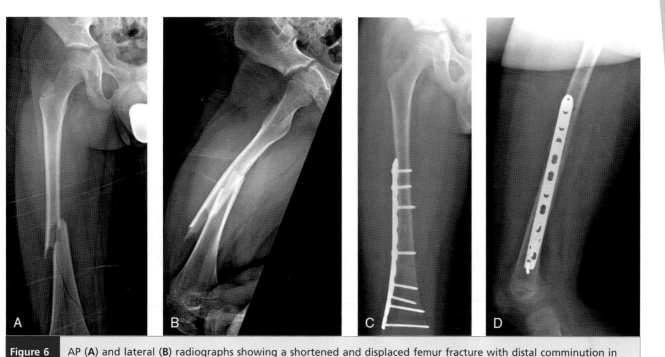

Figure 6 AP (**A**) and lateral (**B**) radiographs showing a shortened and displaced femur fracture with distal comminution in an 11-year-old boy. AP (**C**) and lateral (**D**) radiographs showing fracture stabilization with a submuscular plate.

Submuscular Plating

Submuscular bridge plating, a new technique for stabilizing femoral shaft fractures in children, can be used for a length-unstable, long spiral, comminuted, very proximal, or distal third fracture.[32,33] The technique is similar to placement of an external fixator under the skin and against the bone. A fracture table and C-arm are essential. A small incision is made to slide a 4.5-mm plate along the lateral femoral shaft. The plate is pre-contoured to fit to the lateral femur. Three screws are placed percutaneously above and below the fracture site, which is not opened. A screw is placed close to the proximal and distal ends of the fracture; these two screws reduce the femur to the plate, thus bridging the fracture. No lag screws are placed. To maximize stability, the remaining screws are placed as far apart as possible (**Figure 6**). Protected weight bearing is recommended for 6 to 12 weeks after surgery. A cast is not used.[34]

Plate removal is recommended approximately 6 to 9 months after the surgery. If follow-up radiographs show bone overgrowth at the leading edge of the plate, more extensive surgical exposure may be required to remove the hardware.[35] Sports participation is prohibited for approximately 6 weeks after plate removal. Open plate fixation remains an option, especially for a patient with a head injury or multiple injuries.[36]

Greater Trochanter Entry Intramedullary Nailing

Locked intramedullary nailing from a greater trochanter starting point is indicated for a middle third femoral shaft fracture in a child with open physes who weighs more than 110 lb or is age 11 years or older

(**Figure 7**). Insertion of a rigid intramedullary nail through the piriformis fossa risks injury to the lateral ascending branches of the medial circumflex artery, which supply blood to the femoral head.[37] New intramedullary nails designed for pediatric and adolescent patients are now available.[38,39] The insertion point of the nail is just lateral to the tip of the greater trochanter, instead of the piriformis fossa, to minimize the risk of osteonecrosis of the femoral head.[40] The femoral canal must be at least 9 mm wide to accept the nail. Greater trochanter entry intramedullary nailing has been successful in patients as young as 8 years who have a comminuted or segmental fracture at risk of shortening.[41]

The complications of greater trochanter entry intramedullary nailing include valgus overgrowth because of trochanteric arrest in children younger than 9 years, an intraoperative trochanteric fracture, and varus deformity at the fracture site. The greater trochanter entry site is not collinear with the axis of the intramedullary canal. Therefore, the proximal femur should be overreamed to prevent comminution or fracture of the proximal femur. A nail at least 1 mm smaller in diameter than the last reamer should be inserted, with a bend placed in the nail as recommended by the manufacturer.[42] Closed femoral nailing through the piriformis fossa can be used in a skeletally mature adolescent with closed physes, as in an adult.

Supracondylar Femur Fractures

Supracondylar fractures of the femur are uncommon in children.[43,44] These nonphyseal fractures occur just above the insertion of the gastrocnemius muscle on the

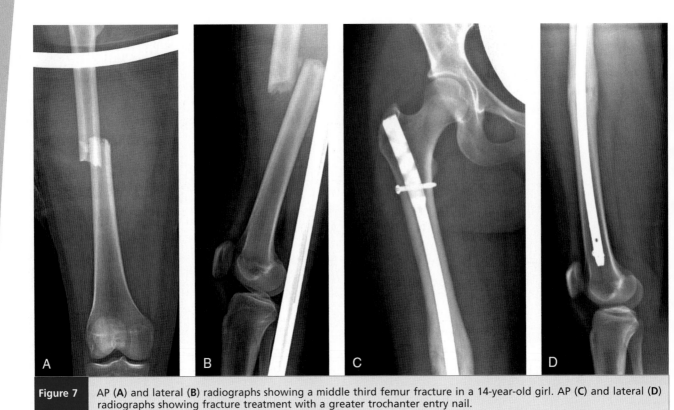

Figure 7   AP (**A**) and lateral (**B**) radiographs showing a middle third femur fracture in a 14-year-old girl. AP (**C**) and lateral (**D**) radiographs showing fracture treatment with a greater trochanter entry nail.

distal femur.[44] The gastrocnemius and adductor muscles produce apex posterior and medial angulation. In some fractures, the proximal fragment can be buttonholed through the quadriceps mechanism. Reduction can be challenging; knee flexion may help to reduce the pull of the gastrocnemius. Because of the difficulty of obtaining and maintaining a reduction, the acceptable treatment options include closed or open reduction, crossed smooth-pin fixation with a cast,[43] open reduction and internal fixation with a plate,[44] and external fixation.[45] Traction and casting are acceptable for treating children younger than 10 years. Two-pin epiphyseal-metaphyseal traction has been suggested for controlling sagittal rotation.[45] The acceptable angulation in a cast is less than 10° of varus or valgus, less than 10° of posterior bowing, and less than 20° of anterior bowing. The use of plating and external fixation is limited by the size of the metaphyseal fragment.[43] The distal femoral physis should be avoided during plate fixation (**Figure 8**); a T-plate can be helpful.[44] External fixation of a supracondylar femur fracture can lead to knee joint sepsis (caused by penetration of the knee joint capsule by the pins) or stiffness (caused by adhesions in the distal iliotibial band). Percutaneously placed pins can be buried under the skin to avoid knee joint sepsis.

Distal Femoral Physeal Fractures

Distal femoral physeal fractures are uncommon and most often result from a motor vehicle crash or football accident.[46,47] Most distal femoral physeal fractures are classified as Salter-Harris type II.[47] Growth disturbance

occurs after approximately 50% of these fractures and can lead to angulation and shortening; half of such fractures require later surgical intervention.[48] Growth arrest is believed to result from bone bridge formation after direct physeal trauma or nonanatomic reduction. Displacement of more than 2 mm and Salter-Harris types II, III, and IV are correlated with the incidence of growth arrest.

A patient with a displaced Salter-Harris type II distal femoral fracture should undergo a gentle closed or open anatomic reduction while under general anesthesia, and fixation with smooth wires or screws should be done to minimize further damage to the physis (**Figure 9**). Threaded pins or screws should not be placed across the physis, to avoid additional physeal injury. Pins used around the knee can be buried under the skin to avoid an intra-articular pin infection that can lead to septic arthritis. Fixation is recommended to prevent redisplacement, and usually it is supplemented with a cast or brace.[47,48] The postoperative use of a long leg cast or a one-leg spica cast is recommended. Pins can be removed and knee motion allowed approximately 6 weeks after the injury.[48]

A nondisplaced distal femoral Salter-Harris type II fracture can initially be treated with a cast. Radiographic follow-up is recommended after 1 week; reduction and pinning can be done if displacement is detected.[47] A displaced Salter-Harris type III or IV fracture is more likely to require open reduction. Compression screws can be placed between the two epiphyseal fragments or between the metaphyseal spike and the

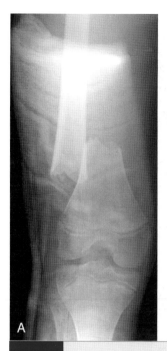
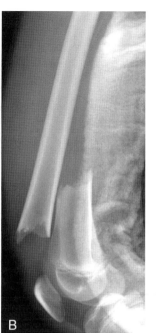
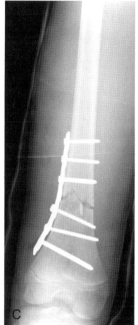
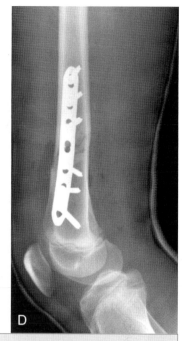

Figure 8 AP (**A**) and lateral (**B**) radiographs showing a displaced and shortened supracondylar femur fracture in an 11-year-old boy. AP (**C**) and lateral (**D**) radiographs showing fracture treatment with open reduction and plating.

femoral metaphysis. Casting for an additional 6 weeks is recommended for additional stability.

Despite appropriate treatment, partial or complete growth arrest often leads to complications including leg-length inequality and angulation.[47] Growth arrest is more common in a displaced fracture,[47,49] a Salter-Harris type III or IV fracture, or a fracture for which hardware was placed across the physis. The patient should be followed for 2 years because of the risk of a physeal bar and growth disturbance. A later bar resection, lateral hemiepiphyseodesis, contralateral epiphysiodesis, osteotomy, or lengthening procedure sometimes is needed.

Hip Fractures

Pediatric hip fractures are uncommon, accounting for fewer than 1% of all pediatric fractures.[50,51] With the exception of pathologic hip fractures (such as those associated with a unicameral bone cyst), hip fractures in children are associated with high-energy trauma.[50,52] Often there are concomitant musculoskeletal and visceral injuries. Hip fractures in children are classified using the Delbet system, which is based on the location of the fracture within the femoral neck[53] (**Table 2**). The Delbet system may have prognostic value for osteonecrosis.[50,52,54,55]

A displaced Delbet type I, II, or III fracture is considered an orthopaedic emergency because immediate treatment has the potential to reverse the injury to the blood supply of the femoral head.[56] Intracapsular hematoma also can contribute to ischemia of the femoral

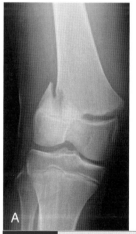
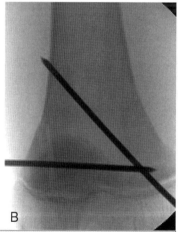

Figure 9 **A**, AP radiograph showing a displaced distal femoral fracture (Salter-Harris type II) in a 13-year-old boy. **B**, AP radiograph showing fracture treatment with gentle reduction and percutaneous pin fixation, done with the patient under general anesthesia.

head by increasing intracapsular pressure and inhibiting venous drainage.[52] Therefore, urgent reduction and decompression of the hematoma may be prudent.[56]

Transepiphyseal Fractures

A Delbet type I transepiphyseal fracture is least common, accounting for 10% of pediatric hip fractures, and it tends to occur in children younger than 2 years. A type I fracture in a child younger than 2 years may be the result of child abuse.[56] Half of type I injuries are

Table 2	
The Delbet Classification of Pediatric Hip Fractures	
Type	**Description**
I	Transepiphyseal fracture, with or without dislocation of the femoral head from the acetabulum
II	Transcervical fracture
III	Cervicotrochanteric fracture
IV	Intertrochanteric fracture

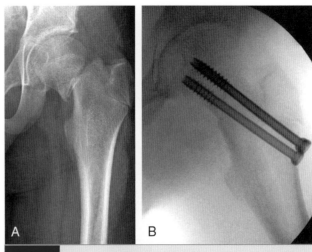

Figure 10   **A**, AP radiograph showing a Delbet type II hip fracture in a 13-year-old boy. **B**, AP radiograph showing fracture treatment with open reduction, capsulotomy, and internal fixation using cannulated screws. Screw fixation crosses the epiphysis for additional stability.

accompanied by a dislocation of the capital femoral epiphysis, and the rate of osteonecrosis approaches 100% in these rare injuries.[51] Some authors reported that spontaneous remodeling occurs in children younger than 2 years if a type I injury is treated using a spica cast without a reduction.[57] In most children, however, treatment of a type I fracture starts with an attempt at closed reduction using traction, abduction, and internal rotation followed by pin fixation and spica casting. If closed reduction is unsuccessful, open reduction is indicated. The anterolateral or anterior approach to the hip is used, although a posterior approach is used for the rarely encountered type I hip fracture associated with a posterior dislocation. By necessity, fixation of a type I fracture involves crossing the physis. Fixation can be done with smooth pins in a child younger than 4 years or screws in a child older than 4 years. The use of a spica cast is recommended for additional stability.

Epiphyseal separation caused by birth trauma stemming from a breech delivery is an even rarer Delbet type I fracture. The newborn infant usually has pseudoparalysis of the leg. Ultrasonography can help differentiate fracture from infection. Fortunately, epiphyseal separation in the newborn tends to remodel completely if the physis does not prematurely close. The recommended treatment is simple skin traction followed by casting and careful follow-up.

Transcervical and Cervicotrochanteric Fractures

Approximately 45% of pediatric hip fractures are Delbet type II transcervical hip fractures. Most of these fractures are displaced, and their rate of capital epiphyseal osteonecrosis is as high as 60%.[52] A type III cervicotrochanteric fracture is the second most common hip fracture, accounting for 30% of fractures. Osteonecrosis occurs in approximately 30% of type III fractures.[58] A nondisplaced type II or III fracture in a child younger than 6 years can be treated with spica casting and careful follow-up.[56] Percutaneous fixation and a spica cast are recommended for most children with this injury, however, to minimize the risk of secondary displacement and varus angulation.[59] A dis-

placed type II or III fracture is treated with anatomic reduction and internal fixation (**Figure 10**). Either a closed or open reduction can be done.[56,60,61] Some authors recommend an anterior capsulotomy to decompress the hip capsule and reduce the risk of osteonecrosis.[52] Other authors recommend a simple aspiration of the hip capsule, with early closed reduction and internal fixation.[56] Still other authors believe that the risk of osteonecrosis is influenced by the quality and timing of the reduction rather than by the use of capsular aspiration or decompression.[55]

In an adolescent, a type II or III injury often requires fixation across the proximal femoral physis to maximize stability. For these patients, achieving fracture stability is more important than preserving the proximal femoral physis. The resulting leg-length discrepancy usually is small (2 to 3 mm per year of remaining growth). A contralateral distal femoral epiphysiodesis can be done if the discrepancy is predicted to exceed 2 cm.

After fracture fixation, a one-leg spica cast is used in children younger than 10 years to maximize fracture stability.[56,61] Adolescents can use crutches and partial weight bearing on the injured leg; a hip-to-knee orthosis can add stability if needed.

Intertrochanteric Fractures

Delbet type IV intertrochanteric fractures account for 15% of hip fractures. This type of fracture has the lowest incidence of osteonecrosis (approximately 10%).[50,54] A type IV fracture in a child younger than 8 years can be treated using closed reduction or traction, followed by spica casting. Closed reduction that achieves angulation of less than 10° of varus is considered acceptable because of remodeling.[56] Open reduction and internal fixation with a pediatric hip screw and side plate or a pediatric blade plate is recommended for an irreducible fracture in a child of any age, a fracture in a child with multiple trauma, or a fracture in a child older than 10 years. The screw fixation can stop short of the physis in most type IV fractures.

Hip Fracture Complications

Osteonecrosis of the femoral head is the most common complication resulting from a pediatric hip fracture.[50,52,54,56] The patient's age, the fracture location, and the initial fracture displacement affect the risk of osteonecrosis.[54] Osteonecrosis can develop as late as 2 years after the injury.[56] Although some authors believe that the damage to the vascular supply of the hip occurs at the time of injury,[50,58] others believe that a delay in reduction of more than 12 hours is an important risk factor.[54] Decompression of the hip capsule at the time of fixation may lessen the risk of osteonecrosis.[52] The complications of a pediatric femoral neck fracture include varus angulation (25% of fractures),[58] nonunion (5%),[50,58] and leg-length discrepancy caused by premature physeal closure (2%). Valgus osteotomy and compression fixation are recommended for a nonunion or a union with varus angulation of more than 120° that does not correct with growth.[62] The leg-length discrepancy usually is less than 2 cm, and it can be observed. If the discrepancy is more than 2 cm, a well-timed contralateral distal femoral epiphysiodesis can be performed.

Traumatic Hip Dislocation

Traumatic hip dislocation is an uncommon injury in children.[63-66] The ligamentous laxity and resulting flexibility of the periacetabular structures in children younger than 10 years means that minor trauma, such as a fall caused by tripping while playing, can cause a hip dislocation.[63,65] In rare instances, the hip reduces spontaneously, with capsular interposition and joint incongruity.[67] In children older than 10 years, a hip dislocation usually results from high-energy trauma, such as a motor vehicle crash.[65]

Approximately 90% of pediatric hip dislocations are posterior.[63,65,68] The patient's leg is flexed, adducted, and internally rotated. A neurovascular examination should be performed, and radiographs should be obtained before reduction.[63] Closed reduction under conscious sedation or general anesthesia usually is successful.[63,65] In adolescents, epiphysiolysis of the femoral head can occur with a traumatic hip dislocation.[69] If there is any suspicion of associated physeal injury on plain radiographs, or if physeal instability is observed under fluoroscopy, open reduction and internal fixation of the epiphysis is recommended to prevent inadvertent displacement of the epiphysis during closed reduction.[51,69] During fixation, the posterolateral epiphyseal vessels and the periosteum attached to the femoral head should be protected to minimize the risk of osteonecrosis.[70] Hip stability after reduction should be determined by examination while the patient is sedated.

Reduction usually is easily achieved, although labral, capsular, or osteochondral fragment interposition may prevent reduction. Surgery is required to achieve anatomic reduction in as many as 15% of patients.[65] The postreduction radiographs should be examined carefully to confirm a concentric reduction with no evidence of intra-articular fragments. As much as 3 mm of hip joint asymmetry may be caused by hematoma or joint laxity.[65,67,68] Any suspicious area on radiographs should be studied further using CT or MRI; CT is preferable for detecting osteochondral lesions, and MRI is best for soft-tissue interposition. Open reduction is indicated for a patient with an intra-articular fragment, a nonconcentric reduction, or an unstable acetabular rim fracture.[63]

The surgical approach to the hip should be from the direction of the dislocation (posterior for a posterior dislocation, and anterior for the less common anterior dislocation). Arthroscopic treatment of an interposed fragment has been reported.[71] To prevent redislocation in a child younger than 10 years, some authors recommend postreduction spica casting for 4 to 6 weeks.[63,72] An older child or adolescent may benefit from a brace and protected ambulation with crutches for 6 weeks.[63]

Osteonecrosis has been reported in 3% to 15% of patients after a traumatic hip dislocation.[68] Reduction of the hip within 6 hours of injury may reduce the risk of osteonecrosis.[63,68] However, osteonecrosis sometimes develops after a child's dislocation was reduced within 6 hours of injury. Deficiency in the growing child's arterial blood supply to the epiphysis may explain the occurrence of osteonecrosis despite the urgent reduction.[65] In an older child, high-energy injury may be a risk factor for osteonecrosis.[66]

Postreduction bone scanning or MRI does not appear to reliably predict the later development of osteonecrosis.[65,68] Asymptomatic coxa magna develops over time in approximately 20% of patients.[65] Rarely, a sciatic or superior gluteal nerve palsy may stem from a pediatric hip dislocation. Prompt reduction of the hip dislocation and observation of the nerve for spontaneous recovery are recommended.[63]

In rare instances, a hip dislocation may be unrecognized for days or weeks in a pediatric patient with multiple trauma.[63] The rate of osteonecrosis in such patients approaches 100%.[73] Skeletal traction usually does not reduce a neglected dislocation.[64,73] Instead, open reduction is recommended for positioning the femoral head into the acetabulum, stimulating the growth of the femur and pelvis, and minimizing the deformity and leg-length inequality.[64]

Pelvic Fractures

Pelvic fracture is uncommon in skeletally immature patients, accounting for approximately 1% of all pediatric fractures.[74,75] The two general categories of pediatric pelvic fractures are those resulting from low-energy and

Table 3

The Torode and Zieg Classification of Pelvic Fractures

Type	Description
I	Avulsion fracture
II	Iliac wing fracture
IIA	Separation of the iliac apophysis
IIB	Fracture of the bony iliac wing
III	Simple ring fracture (stable pelvic ring)
IIIA	Fracture of the pubis and separation of the pubic symphysis, with intact posterior structures
IIIB	Fracture involving the acetabulum, with no pelvic ring fracture
IV	Fracture producing an unstable segment
IVA	Straddle fracture (bilateral inferosuperior pubic rami fracture)
IVB	Fracture involving the anterior pubic rami or pubic symphysis and posterior structures
IVC	Fracture resulting in an unstable segment between the anterior ring of the pelvis and acetabulum

high-energy trauma. A low-energy, sports-related avulsion fracture commonly occurs in the anterosuperior iliac spine because of a sartorius avulsion, in the anteroinferior iliac spine because of a rectus avulsion, in the ischium because of a hamstring avulsion, or in the lesser trochanter because of an iliopsoas avulsion. These injuries are not life threatening and usually can be treated nonsurgically with crutches, ice, and pain medication over a brief period of time.[74,76,77] Athletes with a pelvic avulsion fracture can be expected to return to sports in 6 to 8 weeks. Pediatric pelvic fracture resulting from a high-energy trauma, such as a motor vehicle crash, a motor vehicle–pedestrian collision, or a fall from a height, can be life threatening.[75,76] Emergency stabilization and surgery may be needed.

Pelvic fractures in children differ from those in adults. The triradiate cartilage closes at approximately 14 years in boys and 12 years in girls.[76] Closure of the triradiate cartilage as seen on a pelvic radiograph has been suggested as a means of distinguishing a pediatric pelvic fracture (often treated without surgery) from an adult fracture (often treated with open reduction and internal fixation).[78] Treatment of an unstable pelvic fracture in a skeletally mature adolescent should follow the principles used for an adult fracture; the indications for surgery in a skeletally immature patient are less clear.[74,79]

There are multiple classification systems for pelvic fractures. The Torode and Zieg classification often is used for patients with open triradiate cartilage[80] (Table 3). Children with open triradiate cartilage can sustain a single break to the pelvic ring because of the elasticity

of pediatric bones and the laxity of the sacroiliac and symphysis joints of the pediatric pelvis.[76,78]

The radiographic evaluation of the injured pelvis should include the AP view, supplemented by inlet and outlet views to better define the position and extent of pelvic instability. The inlet view, obtained with the x-ray beam directed from the head of the patient to the midpelvis at a 60° angle, reveals injuries to the sacral ala and pubic ramus as well as anterior-posterior pelvic displacement. The outlet view, obtained with the beam directed from the foot of the patient to the symphysis pubis at a 45° angle, reveals injuries to the sacrum, sacral foramina, and symphysis, as well as superior displacement of the injured pelvis. CT with 3-mm cuts is routinely used for displaced pelvic fractures and is extremely valuable in defining posterior ring instability, detecting visceral injuries, and planning surgery.[76,80] However, one study found that pelvic fracture classification and management in children can be reliably determined using plain radiographs alone.[78]

A pediatric pelvic fracture requires systematic, multidisciplinary initial management by a pediatric or trauma surgeon, an orthopaedic surgeon, a urologist, and an interventional radiologist.[79,81] The trauma team usually performs the initial survey and directs the patient's resuscitation and overall care. Any child with a significant pelvic fracture should have a rectal, neurologic, and genitourinary examination. Although an open pelvic fracture is rare in children,[74] laceration of the perineum, rectum, or skin may indicate an open fracture; the wounds should be explored and managed aggressively to prevent contamination of the fracture. The general surgeon decides on such issues as the need for a diverting colostomy.

The elasticity of a child's immature bones, the ability of a child's elastic arteries to undergo vasoconstriction, and the thick periosteum lead to a lower overall mortality rate after pediatric pelvic fracture than after adult fracture.[74-76] In general, orthopaedic-related bleeding from a pelvic fracture is less likely to cause hemodynamic instability in a child than in an adult. Therefore, additional sources of bleeding should be sought in a child's abdominal and head injuries.[82] Mortality after a pediatric pelvic fracture often stems from the associated injuries rather than from the fracture.[74,75,78]

Nonsurgical treatment is the mainstay for a nondisplaced or minimally displaced pelvic fracture in a child. In a child with open triradiate cartilage, definitive treatment with a spica cast is the acceptable traditional treatment.[75,76] Pediatric pelvic fractures heal rapidly, pseudarthrosis is rare, the child's thick periosteum enhances fracture stability, and remodeling corrects pelvic asymmetry with growth.[80]

The treatment of a displaced pediatric pelvic fracture in a child with closed triradiate cartilage is evolving to favor surgery to restore the pelvic anatomy and symmetry and thus limit morbidity.[75,79] A recent report suggested that the quality of the reduction may be correlated with the outcome, especially if the posterior

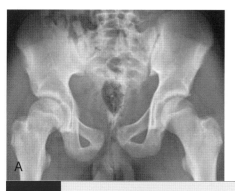
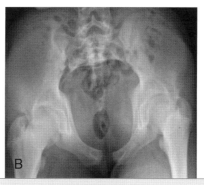
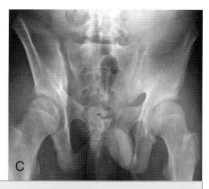

Figure 11 AP (**A**), outlet (**B**), and inlet (**C**) radiographs showing a Torode and Zieg type IV pelvic fracture at the time of injury in a 14-year-old boy. Pubic diastasis and a right sacroiliac joint disruption can be seen. (Courtesy of David Goodspeed, MD, Madison, WI.)

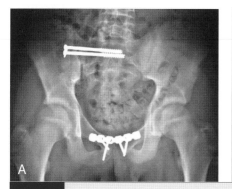
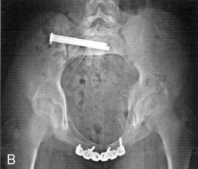
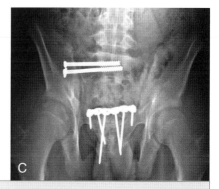

Figure 12 AP (**A**), outlet (**B**), and inlet (**C**) radiographs of the fracture shown in Figure 11 after treatment with a symphysis plate and percutaneous sacroiliac screws. (Courtesy of David Goodspeed, MD, Madison, WI.)

elements are disrupted.[81] Surgery is indicated to facilitate wound care in an open fracture and to control hemorrhage during resuscitation. The potential complications of nonsurgical treatment of a pediatric pelvic fracture include malunion, low back pain, leg-length inequality, and scoliosis.[80]

The use of a pelvic binder, pelvic traction, and/or an external fixator may be indicated for an acute, hemodynamically unstable pelvic fracture. These techniques can be used to control the pelvic fracture temporarily while the patient is stabilized, pending definitive treatment. Traction also can be used to control a vertically unstable fracture. Definitive pelvic surgery usually is deferred for several days until pelvic hemostasis is obtained.[81] A Torode and Zieg type IV unstable pelvic fracture with posterior and anterior injury is uncommon in children; when present, it may benefit from posterior percutaneous sacroiliac screw placement under C-arm guidance and anterior open reduction and fixation with a symphysis plate[81] (**Figures 11** and **12**).

The posterior pelvic ligaments in children are stronger than the adjacent bone. Fracture usually occurs in the posterior bone and is accompanied by injury to the anterior sacroiliac ligaments. Posterior injury can be treated by fixation with a small plate or lag screws. A disrupted sacroiliac joint also can be fixed with a two-

hole plate placed through an anterior retroperitoneal approach, with care to avoid injuring the L5 nerve root.[81] External fixation is considered if the symphysis is disrupted, the fracture is open, or the patient has multiple trauma. External fixation typically is not used in a patient with an unstable iliac wing fracture or a posterior injury or a patient who may require a laparotomy for abdominal injuries.[76] Children have a greater rehabilitation capacity after pelvic fracture than adults; their average functional outcomes are almost normal 6 months after the injury.[83]

Summary

The management of femur, hip, and pelvis fractures in children is evolving. Although most pediatric fractures heal without long-term sequelae, fractures of the femur, hip, and pelvis often are complex and can lead to complications. When making treatment decisions, the surgeon should consider the risks and benefits of the acceptable, age-appropriate methods and should be aware of the unique anatomic and physiologic variables related to children. Despite prompt and appropriate treatment, complications such as leg-length inequality, malunion, and osteonecrosis sometimes occur.

Annotated References

1. Jarvis J, Davidson D, Letts M: Management of subtrochanteric fractures in skeletally immature adolescents. *J Trauma* 2006;60(3):613-619.

   In a retrospective review, 10 of 13 subtrochanteric fractures were treated with multiple surgical methods. The complications included osteonecrosis (1 fracture), leg-length inequality (2), heterotopic ossification (1), and transient peroneal nerve palsy (1). Surgical care was recommended. Level of evidence: IV.

2. Jeng C, Sponseller PD, Yates A, Paletta G: Subtrochanteric femoral fractures in children: Alignment after 90 degrees-90 degrees traction and cast application. *Clin Orthop Relat Res* 1997;341:170-174.

3. Pombo MW, Shilt JS: The definition and treatment of pediatric subtrochanteric femur fractures with titanium elastic nails. *J Pediatr Orthop* 2006;26(3):364-370.

   A subtrochanteric fracture was defined as occurring within 10% of the total length of the femur below the lesser trochanter. Elastic nailing was found to be a safe and effective treatment in 13 patients. Level of evidence: IV.

4. Theologis TN, Cole WG: Management of subtrochanteric fractures of the femur in children. *J Pediatr Orthop* 1998;18(1):22-25.

5. Sahlin Y: Occurrence of fractures in a defined population: A 1-year study. *Injury* 1990;21(3):158-160.

6. Hinton RY, Lincoln A, Crockett MM, Sponseller P, Smith G: Fractures of the femoral shaft in children: Incidence, mechanisms, and sociodemographic risk factors. *J Bone Joint Surg Am* 1999;81(4):500-509.

7. Schwend RM, Werth C, Johnston A: Femur shaft fractures in toddlers and young children: Rarely from child abuse. *J Pediatr Orthop* 2000;20(4):475-481.

8. Kocher MS, Sink EL, Blasier RD, et al: Treatment of pediatric diaphyseal femur fractures. *J Am Acad Orthop Surg* 2009;17(11):718-725.

   In the American Academy of Orthopaedic Surgeons clinical practice guideline for femur fracture management, the authors conclude that there is controversy and a lack of conclusive evidence regarding the different treatment methods. Level of evidence: V.

9. Podeszwa DA, Mooney JF III, Cramer KE, Mendelow MJ: Comparison of Pavlik harness application and immediate spica casting for femur fractures in infants. *J Pediatr Orthop* 2004;24(5):460-462.

10. Stannard JP, Christensen KP, Wilkins KE: Femur fractures in infants: A new therapeutic approach. *J Pediatr Orthop* 1995;15(4):461-466.

11. Cassinelli EH, Young B, Vogt M, Pierce MC, Deeney VF: Spica cast application in the emergency room for select pediatric femur fractures. *J Orthop Trauma* 2005;19(10):709-716.

    Of 145 children younger than 7 years who had an isolated femur fracture treated with immediate spica casting without general anesthesia, one third were discharged to home from the emergency department. A later spica cast change was required in 8%. Level of evidence: IV.

12. Illgen R II, Rodgers WB, Hresko MT, Waters PM, Zurakowski D, Kasser JR: Femur fractures in children: Treatment with early sitting spica casting. *J Pediatr Orthop* 1998;18(4):481-487.

13. Martinez AG, Carroll NC, Sarwark JF, Dias LS, Kelikian AS, Sisson GA Jr: Femoral shaft fractures in children treated with early spica cast. *J Pediatr Orthop* 1991;11(6):712-716.

14. Davids JR: Rotational deformity and remodeling after fracture of the femur in children. *Clin Orthop Relat Res* 1994;302:27-35.

15. Mubarak SJ, Frick S, Sink E, Rathjen K, Noonan KJ: Volkmann contracture and compartment syndromes after femur fractures in children treated with 90/90 spica casts. *J Pediatr Orthop* 2006;26(5):567-572.

    Nine patients with an isolated femur fracture treated with a sitting spica cast developed skin loss and/or compartment syndrome. The authors believe that leg immobilization in the 90°-90° position is dangerous and suggest placing the leg in greater extension, with the foot left out of the cast to minimize complications. Level of evidence: IV.

16. Buechsenschuetz KE, Mehlman CT, Shaw KJ, Crawford AH, Immerman EB: Femoral shaft fractures in children: Traction and casting versus elastic stable intramedullary nailing. *J Trauma* 2002;53(5):914-921.

17. Sturdee SW, Templeton PA, Dahabreh Z, Cullen E, Giannoudis PV: Femoral fractures in children: Is early interventional treatment beneficial? *Injury* 2007;38(8):937-944.

    Compared with historical control subjects, 25 children treated with an early intervention (spica casting, flexible nailing, or external fixation) had a shorter hospital stay but a slightly higher malunion rate. Most of the malunions remodeled over a 2-year follow-up period. Level of evidence: III.

18. Wright JG: The treatment of femoral shaft fractures in children: A systematic overview and critical appraisal of the literature. *Can J Surg* 2000;43(3):180-189.

19. Lee YH, Lim KB, Gao GX, et al: Traction and spica casting for closed femoral shaft fractures in children. *J Orthop Surg (Hong Kong)* 2007;15(1):37-40.

    Sixty-three children (average age, 5 years) were treated with skin traction followed by spica casting. There were no malunions, nonunions, or rotational deformities; 22% had a leg-length inequality of less than 1.5 cm. This technique is simple, safe, and effective. Level of evidence: IV.

20. Flynn JM, Luedtke LM, Ganley TJ, et al: Comparison of titanium elastic nails with traction and a spica cast to treat femoral fractures in children. *J Bone Joint Surg Am* 2004;86(4):770-777.

21. Boman A, Gardell C, Janarv PM: Home traction of femoral shaft fractures in younger children. *J Pediatr Orthop* 1998;18(4):478-480.

22. Scheerder FJ, Schnater JM, Sleeboom C, Aronson DC: Bryant traction in paediatric femoral shaft fractures: Home traction versus hospitalisation. *Injury* 2008; 39(4):456-462.

    Treatment with home traction in 38 patients was compared with hospital traction in 16 patients. Home traction was simple and effective; it reduced hospital stay by more than 2 weeks and substantially reduced costs. Level of evidence: II.

23. Probe R, Lindsey RW, Hadley NA, Barnes DA: Refracture of adolescent femoral shaft fractures: A complication of external fixation. A report of two cases. *J Pediatr Orthop* 1993;13(1):102-105.

24. Barlas K, Beg H: Flexible intramedullary nailing versus external fixation of paediatric femoral fractures. *Acta Orthop Belg* 2006;72(2):159-163.

    A comparison of 40 children with a femur fracture treated using an external fixator or flexible nailing found that flexible nailing resulted in earlier weight bearing, improved range of motion, earlier return to school, and fewer complications. The authors reserve external fixation for open or comminuted fractures. Level of evidence: III.

25. Blasier RD, Aronson J, Tursky EA: External fixation of pediatric femur fractures. *J Pediatr Orthop* 1997;17(3): 342-346.

26. Wright JG, Wang EE, Owen JL, et al: Treatments for paediatric femoral fractures: A randomised trial. *Lancet* 2005;365(9465):1153-1158.

    Children age 4 to 10 years were treated with spica casting or external fixation. The rate of malunion was higher in the children treated with spica casting. The two groups had similar Rand Physical Function Questionnaire, posthospitalization questionnaire, parent satisfaction, and children's happiness scores. Level of evidence: I.

27. Sink EL, Gralla J, Repine M: Complications of pediatric femur fractures treated with titanium elastic nails: A comparison of fracture types. *J Pediatr Orthop* 2005; 25(5):577-580.

    A 60% complication rate was reported when flexible nails were used in length-unstable fractures. The use of flexible nails should be limited to short transverse fracture patterns. Level of evidence: IV.

28. Moroz LA, Launay F, Kocher MS, et al: Titanium elastic nailing of fractures of the femur in children: Predictors of complications and poor outcome. *J Bone Joint Surg Br* 2006;88(10):1361-1366.

    A multicenter study from six US and French hospitals reported that poor outcomes including leg-length inequality, unacceptable angulation, and fixation failure were related to patient age older than 11 years and weight greater than 49 kg. Level of evidence: IV.

29. Flynn JM, Hresko T, Reynolds RA, Blasier RD, Davidson R, Kasser J: Titanium elastic nails for pediatric femur fractures: A multicenter study of early results with analysis of complications. *J Pediatr Orthop* 2001;21(1): 4-8.

30. Herrera JA, Wall EJ, Foad SL: Hematoma block reduces narcotic pain medication after femoral elastic nailing in children. *J Pediatr Orthop* 2004;24(3):254-256.

31. Ho CA, Skaggs DL, Tang CW, Kay RM: Use of flexible intramedullary nails in pediatric femur fractures. *J Pediatr Orthop* 2006;26(4):497-504.

    Ninety-four fractures were treated with flexible nailing between 1998 and 2003, and 60% of patients used a postoperative cast or brace. The average time to full weight bearing was 11 weeks, and the average time to return to normal activities was 5 months. Level of evidence: IV.

32. Ağuş H, Kalenderer O, Eryanilmaz G, Omeroğlu H: Biological internal fixation of comminuted femur shaft fractures by bridge plating in children. *J Pediatr Orthop* 2003;23(2):184-189.

33. Sink EL, Hedequist D, Morgan SJ, Hresko T: Results and technique of unstable pediatric femoral fractures treated with submuscular bridge plating. *J Pediatr Orthop* 2006;26(2):177-181.

    After 27 patients from two centers were treated with submuscular plating for comminuted, unstable femur fracture, early callus formed by 8 weeks, and stable union formed by 12 weeks. No complications were reported. Level of evidence: IV.

34. Kanlic EM, Anglen JO, Smith DG, Morgan SJ, Pesántez RF: Advantages of submuscular bridge plating for complex pediatric femur fractures. *Clin Orthop Relat Res* 2004;426(426):244-251.

35. Pate O, Hedequist D, Leong N, Hresko T: Implant removal after submuscular plating for pediatric femur fractures. *J Pediatr Orthop* 2009;29(7):709-712.

    The records and radiographs of 22 patients undergoing submuscular plate removal were reviewed. Seven patients required a more extensive procedure to remove the plate than was needed for plate insertion. The presence of bone overgrowth at the leading edge of the plate required patient counseling as to the need for a more extensive exposure during implant removal. Level of evidence: IV.

36. Kregor PJ, Song KM, Routt ML Jr, Sangeorzan BJ, Liddell RM, Hansen ST Jr: Plate fixation of femoral shaft fractures in multiply injured children. *J Bone Joint Surg Am* 1993;75(12):1774-1780.

6: Musculoskeletal Trauma

37. Beaty JH, Austin SM, Warner WC, Canale ST, Nichols L: Interlocking intramedullary nailing of femoral-shaft fractures in adolescents: Preliminary results and complications. *J Pediatr Orthop* 1994;14(2):178-183.

38. Jencikova-Celerin L, Phillips JH, Werk LN, Wiltrout SA, Nathanson I: Flexible interlocked nailing of pediatric femoral fractures: Experience with a new flexible interlocking intramedullary nail compared with other fixation procedures. *J Pediatr Orthop* 2008;28(8):864-873.

    In 137 patients with open growth plates (age 7 to 18 years), flexible interlocked intramedullary nailing led to less blood loss, shorter time to weight bearing, and fewer complications than in patients treated with other fixation devices. Level of evidence: III.

39. Keeler KA, Dart B, Luhmann SJ, et al: Antegrade intramedullary nailing of pediatric femoral fractures using an interlocking pediatric femoral nail and a lateral trochanteric entry point. *J Pediatr Orthop* 2009;29(4):345-351.

    Seventy-eight older children and adolescents were successfully treated with a greater trochanter entry rigid nail. No osteonecrosis or femoral neck valgus or narrowing occurred. Level of evidence: IV.

40. Kanellopoulos AD, Yiannakopoulos CK, Soucacos PN: Closed, locked intramedullary nailing of pediatric femoral shaft fractures through the tip of the greater trochanter. *J Trauma* 2006;60(1):217-222, discussion 222-223.

    Twenty adolescents age 11 to 16 years were treated with a reamed lateral trochanteric nail. No complications were reported, and no osteonecrosis or leg-length inequality occurred. Fourteen nails were removed 10 to 18 months after the injury, without complication. Level of evidence: IV.

41. Gordon JE, Khanna N, Luhmann SJ, Dobbs MB, Ortman MR, Schoenecker PL: Intramedullary nailing of femoral fractures in children through the lateral aspect of the greater trochanter using a modified rigid humeral intramedullary nail: Preliminary results of a new technique in 15 children. *J Orthop Trauma* 2004;18(7):416-422, discussion 423-424.

42. Gordon JE, Swenning TA, Burd TA, Szymanski DA, Schoenecker PL: Proximal femoral radiographic changes after lateral transtrochanteric intramedullary nail placement in children. *J Bone Joint Surg Am* 2003;85(7):1295-1301.

43. Butcher CC, Hoffman EB: Supracondylar fractures of the femur in children: Closed reduction and percutaneous pinning of displaced fractures. *J Pediatr Orthop* 2005;25(2):145-148.

    Nine patients age 5 to 13 years were treated with closed reduction, percutaneous pinning, and casting. One patient had a resulting valgus deformity of 6°, and another developed a peroneal nerve palsy. No leg-length inequality or knee stiffness occurred. Level of evidence: IV.

44. Smith NC, Parker D, McNicol D: Supracondylar fractures of the femur in children. *J Pediatr Orthop* 2001; 21(5):600-603.

45. Canale ST, Tolo VT: Fractures of the femur in children. *Instr Course Lect* 1995;44:255-273.

46. Peterson HA, Madhok R, Benson JT, Ilstrup DM, Melton LJ III: Physeal fractures: Part 1. Epidemiology in Olmsted County, Minnesota, 1979-1988. *J Pediatr Orthop* 1994;14(4):423-430.

47. Arkader A, Warner WC Jr, Horn BD, Shaw RN, Wells L: Predicting the outcome of physeal fractures of the distal femur. *J Pediatr Orthop* 2007;27(6):703-708.

    In 73 patients from two medical centers who had a distal femoral physeal fracture, poor outcomes were related to a higher Salter-Harris classification, a displaced fracture, and the need for surgical treatment. Level of evidence: III.

48. Thomson JD, Stricker SJ, Williams MM: Fractures of the distal femoral epiphyseal plate. *J Pediatr Orthop* 1995;15(4):474-478.

49. Ilharreborde B, Raquillet C, Morel E, et al: Long-term prognosis of Salter-Harris type 2 injuries of the distal femoral physis. *J Pediatr Orthop B* 2006;15(6):433-438.

    A retrospective study of 20 patients found that 14 (70%) developed complications including growth arrest (12), overlengthening (1), and/or knee stiffness (5). Level of evidence: IV.

50. Togrul E, Bayram H, Gulsen M, Kalaci A, Ozbarlas S: Fractures of the femoral neck in children: Long-term follow-up in 62 hip fractures. *Injury* 2005;36(1):123-130.

    An 8-year follow-up of 62 patients with hip fracture found coxa vara in 8%, osteonecrosis in 14%, premature epiphyseal fusion in 8%, coxa valga in 3%, nonunion in 2%, limb shortening in 11%, and arthritis in 3%. Level of evidence: IV.

51. Canale ST: Traumatic dislocations and fracture-dislocations of the hip in children. *Hip* 1981;219-245.

52. Swiontkowski MF, Winquist RA: Displaced hip fractures in children and adolescents. *J Trauma* 1986;26(4):384-388.

53. Colonna PC: Fracture of the neck of the femur in children. *Am J Surg* 1929;6:793-797.

54. Moon ES, Mehlman CT: Risk factors for avascular necrosis after femoral neck fractures in children: 25 Cincinnati cases and meta-analysis of 360 cases. *J Orthop Trauma* 2006;20(5):323-329.

    A meta-analysis revealed that fracture type and older age were the most significant predictors of osteonecrosis after pediatric femoral neck fracture. Level of evidence: III.

55. Shrader MW, Jacofsky DJ, Stans AA, Shaughnessy WJ, Haidukewych GJ: Femoral neck fractures in pediatric patients: 30 years experience at a level 1 trauma center. *Clin Orthop Relat Res* 2007;454:169-173.

    The quality and timing of reduction, but not capsular decompression, influenced the risk of osteonecrosis in 20 patients with a pediatric femoral neck fracture. Level of evidence: IV.

56. Boardman MJ, Herman MJ, Buck B, Pizzutillo PD: Hip fractures in children. *J Am Acad Orthop Surg* 2009; 17(3):162-173.

    This detailed review discusses the treatment and complications of hip fractures in children. Level of evidence: V.

57. Forlin E, Guille JT, Kumar SJ, Rhee KJ: Transepiphyseal fractures of the neck of the femur in very young children. *J Pediatr Orthop* 1992;12(2):164-168.

58. Davison BL, Weinstein SL: Hip fractures in children: A long-term follow-up study. *J Pediatr Orthop* 1992; 12(3):355-358.

59. Forster NA, Ramseier LE, Exner GU: Undisplaced femoral neck fractures in children have a high risk of secondary displacement. *J Pediatr Orthop B* 2006;15(2): 131-133.

    Three patients age 11 to 16 years with a nondisplaced femoral neck fracture were treated nonsurgically. All three fractures were displaced and needed internal fixation. The authors recommend primary internal fixation for nondisplaced femoral neck fractures in children. Level of evidence: IV.

60. Dhammi IK, Singh S, Jain AK: Displaced femoral neck fracture in children and adolescents: Closed versus open reduction: A preliminary study. *J Orthop Sci* 2005; 10(2):173-179.

    Seventeen hip fractures treated with closed reduction and internal fixation were compared with nine fractures treated with open reduction and internal fixation. No differences in outcomes were noted. Level of evidence: III.

61. Flynn JM, Wong KL, Yeh GL, Meyer JS, Davidson RS: Displaced fractures of the hip in children: Management by early operation and immobilisation in a hip spica cast. *J Bone Joint Surg Br* 2002;84(1):108-112.

62. Min BW, Bae KC, Kang CH, Song KS, Kim SY, Won YY: Valgus intertrochanteric osteotomy for non-union of femoral neck fracture. *Injury* 2006;37(8):786-790.

    Valgus intertrochanteric osteotomy was an effective treatment of femoral neck nonunion in 11 patients. Level of evidence: IV.

63. Herrera-Soto JA, Price CT: Traumatic hip dislocations in children and adolescents: pitfalls and complications. *J Am Acad Orthop Surg* 2009;17(1):15-21.

    A detailed review discusses the management and complications of traumatic hip dislocations in children. Level of evidence: V.

64. Kumar S, Jain AK: Neglected traumatic hip dislocation in children. *Clin Orthop Relat Res* 2005;431:9-13.

    The outcomes of open reduction in 18 patients with neglected traumatic hip dislocation are reported. Traction failed to reduce the hip in all patients. The authors recommend open reduction rather than observation because an anatomically placed femoral head helps maintain the stimulus for growth of the femur and pelvis, minimizes deformity, and maintains limb length. Level of evidence: IV.

65. Vialle R, Odent T, Pannier S, Pauthier F, Laumonier F, Glorion C: Traumatic hip dislocation in childhood. *J Pediatr Orthop* 2005;25(2):138-144.

    Nine of 35 children with a traumatic hip dislocation after minor trauma required surgery to remove interposed joint capsule and/or osteochondral fragments and achieve anatomic reduction.

66. Zrig M, Mnif H, Koubaa M, Abid A: Traumatic hip dislocation in children. *Acta Orthop Belg* 2009;75(3):328-333.

    The factors predisposing patients to osteonecrosis were delayed reduction and severity of the trauma. Level of evidence: IV.

67. Price CT, Pyevich MT, Knapp DR, Phillips JH, Hawker JJ: Traumatic hip dislocation with spontaneous incomplete reduction: A diagnostic trap. *J Orthop Trauma* 2002;16(10):730-735.

68. Mehlman CT, Hubbard GW, Crawford AH, Roy DR, Wall EJ: Traumatic hip dislocation in children: Long-term followup of 42 patients. *Clin Orthop Relat Res* 2000;376:68-79.

69. Herrera-Soto JA, Price CT, Reuss BL, Riley P, Kasser JR, Beaty JH: Proximal femoral epiphysiolysis during reduction of hip dislocation in adolescents. *J Pediatr Orthop* 2006;26(3):371-374.

    Five patients with displacement of the femoral epiphysis at the time of reduction all developed osteonecrosis. The authors recommend careful examination of the hip under fluoroscopy before an attempt at closed reduction. If physeal instability is noted, an open reduction is recommended. Level of evidence: IV.

70. Mass DP, Spiegel PG, Laros GS: Dislocation of the hip with traumatic separation of the capital femoral epiphysis: Report of a case with successful outcome. *Clin Orthop Relat Res* 1980;146:184-187.

71. Kashiwagi N, Suzuki S, Seto Y: Arthroscopic treatment for traumatic hip dislocation with avulsion fracture of the ligamentum teres. *Arthroscopy* 2001;17(1):67-69.

72. Nirmal Kumar J, Hazra S, Yun HH: Redislocation after treatment of traumatic dislocation of hip in children: A report of two cases and literature review. *Arch Orthop Trauma Surg* 2009;129(6):823-826.

    Two of five children age 2 to 9 years sustained a redislocation after closed reduction. The authors recommend spica casting and protected weight bearing after a closed

6: Musculoskeletal Trauma

reduction in children younger than 10 years to prevent redislocation. Level of evidence: IV.

73. Banskota AK, Spiegel DA, Shrestha S, Shrestha OP, Rajbhandary T: Open reduction for neglected traumatic hip dislocation in children and adolescents. *J Pediatr Orthop* 2007;27(2):187-191.

    Eight children with a neglected traumatic dislocation were treated with open reduction after unsuccessful traction. The results were good in three patients, fair in three, and poor in two. All developed osteonecrosis, and the prognosis was guarded. The authors nonetheless recommend open reduction for this rare injury. Level of evidence: IV.

74. Rieger H, Brug E: Fractures of the pelvis in children. *Clin Orthop Relat Res* 1997;336:226-239.

75. Spiguel L, Glynn L, Liu D, Statter M: Pediatric pelvic fractures: A marker for injury severity. *Am Surg* 2006; 72(6):481-484.

    A retrospective review of pelvic fractures at a level I pediatric trauma center found that most were treated nonsurgically. However, more than half of the patients had concomitant injuries requiring surgery. Level of evidence: IV.

76. Holden CP, Holman J, Herman MJ: Pediatric pelvic fractures. *J Am Acad Orthop Surg* 2007;15(3):172-177.

    A detailed review discusses pediatric pelvic fracture treatment, which is individualized based on patient age, fracture classification, stability, concomitant injuries, and hemodynamic stability. Level of evidence: V.

77. McKinney BI, Nelson C, Carrion W: Apophyseal avulsion fractures of the hip and pelvis. *Orthopedics* 2009; 32(1):42.

A review article discusses the diagnosis and management of apophyseal avulsion fractures. Increased athletic participation by adolescents and improved imaging techniques have led to an increased awareness of these injuries. Level of evidence: V.

78. Silber JS, Flynn JM: Changing patterns of pediatric pelvic fractures with skeletal maturation: Implications for classification and management. *J Pediatr Orthop* 2002; 22(1):22-26.

79. Karunakar MA, Goulet JA, Mueller KL, Bedi A, Le TT: Operative treatment of unstable pediatric pelvis and acetabular fractures. *J Pediatr Orthop* 2005;25(1):34-38.

    Eighteen patients younger than 16 years were treated with surgical fixation of an unstable pelvic fracture. All fractures healed by 10 weeks. No wound complications, infections, or growth arrests occurred. Level of evidence: IV.

80. Torode I, Zieg D: Pelvic fractures in children. *J Pediatr Orthop* 1985;5(1):76-84.

81. Smith WR, Oakley M, Morgan SJ: Pediatric pelvic fractures. *J Pediatr Orthop* 2004;24(1):130-135.

82. Ismail N, Bellemare JF, Mollitt DL, DiScala C, Koeppel B, Tepas JJ III: Death from pelvic fracture: Children are different. *J Pediatr Surg* 1996;31(1):82-85.

83. Signorino PR, Densmore J, Werner M, et al: Pediatric pelvic injury: Functional outcome at 6-month follow-up. *J Pediatr Surg* 2005;40(1):107-112, discussion 112-113.

    Children have an improved functional status (self-care, mobility, and cognition) 6 months after a pelvic fracture and return to near-normal status. Level of evidence: IV.

Chapter 34

Fractures of the Tibia, Ankle, and Foot

Susan A. Scherl, MD

Introduction

Fractures of the lower leg are common in children. There are many different mechanisms of fracture. The fracture patterns vary depending on the child's age and stage of growth as well as the location of the fracture. A displaced or intra-articular fracture in the lower leg has a prognosis and treatment algorithm different from those of a less complex fracture. Surgical indications and other treatment options must be specifically considered for a fracture of the proximal, midshaft, or distal tibia or fibula; a physeal or intra-articular fracture; a fracture of the foot; or a lawn mower injury to the lower extremity.

Proximal Tibia Fractures

Intercondylar Eminence Fractures

Tibial intercondylar eminence fractures are uncommon injuries that typically occur in children age 8 to 14 years. The mechanism of injury is forced hyperextension of the knee or a direct blow to the distal femur with the knee flexed, often as a result of a fall from a bicycle. This injury creates excessive tension on the anterior cruciate ligament, leading to avulsion of the anterior tibial spine. Thus, the injury is both an intra-articular fracture and a childhood analog of anterior cruciate ligament rupture. Tibial intercondylar eminence fractures were classified as type I, a nondisplaced fracture; type II, an anterior displacement with an intact posterior hinge; or type III, a completely dis-

placed fracture.[1] Type IV, a fracture with displacement and comminution, subsequently was added[2] (Figure 1).

The treatment of a type I or II fracture usually is nonsurgical. Placement of a long leg cast with the knee in 10° to 20° of flexion generally is sufficient for a type I fracture. A type II fracture typically requires reduction by full extension of the knee, followed by placement of a long leg cast with the knee in 10° to 20° of flexion. Aspiration may aid in the reduction and decrease discomfort if a large knee hemarthrosis is present. Most authors agree that a type III fracture requires surgical reduction and fixation.[3] Open arthrotomy traditionally is used, but arthroscopic techniques were found to lead to good results.[4-7] Sutures or hardware can be used for fixation. The optimal internal fixation has not yet been defined. The options range from cannulated screws to minifragmentation plates (Figure 2). It is generally recommended that the internal fixation not cross the physis. A recent in vitro animal model biomechanical study found no significant difference in fixation with suture, metal hardware, or bioabsorbable hardware.[8] Although soft-tissue interposition at the fracture site has been cited as causing fracture irreducibility, one arthroscopic study found no soft-tissue interposition in

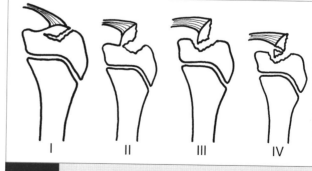

| Figure 1 | Schematic drawings showing the modified Meyers and McKeever classification of tibial intercondylar eminence fractures. (Adapted from Herman MJ, Cho RH: Fractures about the knee, in Scherl S, ed: *Surgical Management of Pediatric Long-Bone Fractures*. Rosemont, IL, American Academy of Orthopaedic Surgeons, 2009, p 117.) |

Dr. Scherl or an immediate family member serves as a board member, owner, officer, or committee member of the Orthopaedic Trauma Association and the Pediatric Orthopaedic Society of North America; has received research or institutional support from Arthrex, the National Institutes of Health (National Institute of Arthritis and Musculoskeletal and Skin Diseases, National Institute of Child Health and Human Development), Tornier, and ESKA; and has received nonincome support (such as equipment or services), commercially derived honoraria, or other non–research-related funding (such as paid travel) from Wolters Kluwer Health–Lippincott Williams & Wilkins.

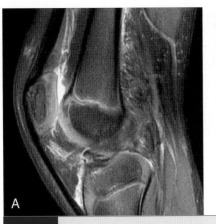
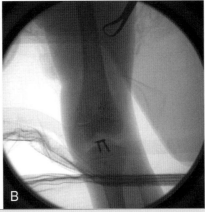
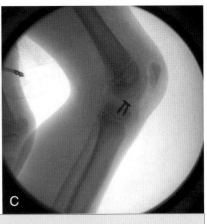

Figure 2 A, Sagittal MRI of a Meyers and McKeever type III tibial intercondylar eminence fracture. AP (**B**) and lateral (**C**) radiographs of the fracture after screw fixation.

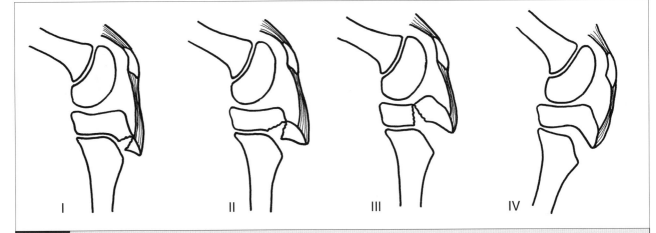

Figure 3 Schematic drawings showing the Ogden modification of the Watson-Jones classification of tibial tubercle fractures. (Adapted from Herman MJ, Cho RH: Fractures of the tibial shaft, in Scherl S, ed: *Surgical Management of Pediatric Long-Bone Fractures*. Rosemont, IL, American Academy of Orthopaedic Surgeons, 2009, p 112.)

12 irreducible type III fractures.[9] The fracture fragment instead was attached to the anterior horn of the lateral meniscus, and traction on the meniscus aided reduction. After surgery, a long leg cast in slight flexion is used for 4 weeks, followed by physical therapy to strengthen the quadriceps. Asymptomatic anterior knee laxity is a common late complication, regardless of the treatment method or quality.[10,11]

Tibial Physeal Fractures

The Salter-Harris classification is used for proximal tibial physeal fractures. A type I or II fracture often can be treated nonsurgically, as can a type I or II Salter-Harris fracture elsewhere in the skeleton. A type III or IV fracture is intra-articular and therefore usually requires open reduction and fixation. MRI may be useful in diagnosing, evaluating, and planning surgery for such a fracture.[12] Coronal split fractures of the proximal tibial epiphysis are rare;[13] the prognosis is good, although growth arrest has been reported.[14,15]

A displaced proximal tibial physeal fracture is a childhood analog of knee dislocation. A careful neurovascular examination is mandatory, and an arteriogram should be obtained if vascular injury is suspected. A high index of suspicion should be maintained for compartment syndrome, and fasciotomies should be done as needed. Proximal tibial physeal fracture occasionally is accompanied by collateral ligament tearing and meniscal injury, which can lead to clinical instability and may require surgical treatment.[16]

Tubercle Avulsion Fractures

Tibial tubercle avulsion fractures occur in adolescents who are nearing the end of skeletal growth. The mechanism of injury is passive flexion of the knee during active quadriceps contraction, and the fracture is associated with jumping sports. Tibial tubercle avulsion fractures were classified by Watson-Jones, and the classification was modified by Ogden[17] (**Figure 3**). A type I fracture occurs across the secondary ossification center

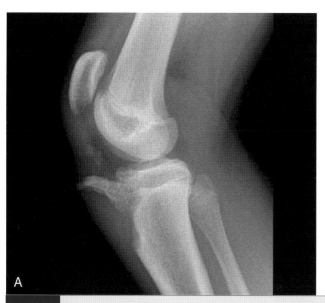
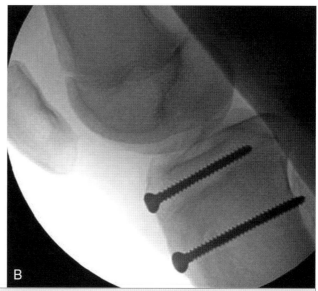

Figure 4 Lateral radiographs of a modified Watson-Jones type III tibial tubercle fracture (**A**) and the fracture after screw fixation (**B**).

in the region of the patellar tendon insertion, and a type II fracture occurs across the secondary ossification center at the level of the epiphysis. A type III fracture extends proximally and posteriorly to cross the primary ossification center; essentially, it is a Salter-Harris type III fracture of the epiphysis. A type IV fracture extends transversely and posteriorly through the proximal tibial physis toward the posterior tibial cortex. The associated injuries include quadriceps and patellar tendon avulsions, cruciate and collateral ligament tears, and meniscal tears. Tibial tubercle avulsion associated with a lateral plateau rim fracture has been reported.[18]

A type I tibial tubercle fracture with little or no displacement can be treated nonsurgically with a long leg cast in extension. Most type II, III, or IV fractures require open reduction and internal fixation (**Figure 4**). Because a type III fracture is intra-articular, it is imperative that an arthrotomy be done to observe the joint surface and menisci. Rare instances of anterior compartment syndrome have been reported secondary to bleeding from the recurrent anterior tibial arteries.[19]

Metaphyseal Fractures

A proximal tibial metaphyseal fracture, even if it is nondisplaced, has a tendency to grow into valgus. This deformity has been reported in children as old as 10 years, but it is most common in children age 3 to 6 years.[20] The deformity progresses for about 20 months after the initial fracture. The mechanism is unknown, and parents should be warned of this possibility at the time of injury. The data on spontaneous remodeling and resolution are contradictory; two studies reported that significant improvement in alignment usually occurs with growth, but a third study reported resolution only in two of seven children, both of whom were younger than 2 years.[20-22]

Tibial Shaft Fractures

Tibial shaft fractures account for approximately 15% of long bone fractures in children and adolescents;[23] they are the third most common type of pediatric long bone fracture, after forearm and femur fractures. Approximately half of tibial diaphyseal fractures occur in the distal third, 40% in the midshaft, and the remainder in the proximal third. Concomitant fibular fracturing occurs with 30% to 73% of these fractures.[23,24] Another associated musculoskeletal injury, such as floating knee, occurs with approximately 6%.[25,26]

Most pediatric tibial shaft fractures are amenable to nonsurgical treatment. A long leg cast is used with the knee in approximately 45° of flexion. No evidence-based guidelines exist for the extent of angulation or shortening correlated with an unacceptable clinical outcome. A recent report suggests that for children younger than 8 years, as much as 100% displacement, 10° of angulation, and 1 cm of shortening allow a satisfactory outcome; for children older than 8 years, as much as 50% displacement, 5° of angulation, and 5 mm of shortening had a satisfactory outcome.[27]

Several surgical interventions can be considered if an acceptable reduction cannot be achieved or maintained or if the fracture is open and accompanied by extensive soft-tissue injury, a compartment syndrome, or multiple trauma. External fixation with a straight or circular frame has been the most frequently used surgical modality. Although the results are good, complications including pin tract infection, refracture, malunion, and nonunion occasionally occur.[28-31] External fixation nonetheless is useful for an open fracture with extensive soft-tissue injury, a highly comminuted and

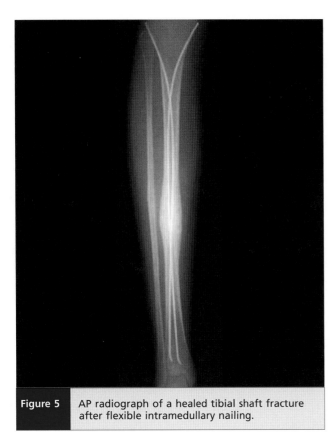

Figure 5 AP radiograph of a healed tibial shaft fracture after flexible intramedullary nailing.

unstable fracture, or a very distal or proximal shaft fracture.[31-33]

In recent years, intramedullary nailing, particularly with a flexible titanium nail, has become popular, and several studies have reported good results.[34-37] A retrospective study found that children treated with flexible nailing for a tibia fracture had a better outcome related to global function, pain, happiness, and sports than children treated with external fixation.[38] A rigid locked nail suitable for adults should be used only for adolescents whose physes have closed.

Flexible intramedullary nails are inserted anterograde through incisions made anteromedially and anterolaterally about 1.5 cm distal to the proximal tibial physis. It is recommended that the nails be of the same diameter and fill 40% of the canal at its narrowest point; the tip should have a bend and the rod should have a gentle curvature to facilitate passage (**Figure 5**). The reported complications of flexible intramedullary nailing include delayed union, nonunion, malunion, infection, refracture, and pain at the nail insertion sites.[39,40] Open reduction and fixation with a plate-and-screw construct is rarely used in children.

Ankle Fractures

Distal Tibial and Fibular Epiphyseal Fractures
Most ankle fractures in children are physeal and therefore can be classified using the Salter-Harris system. Be-

cause the physes are the weakest link in the bone and soft-tissue construct of the ankle, a growing child is more likely to sustain a physeal fracture than a sprain. The mechanism of most pediatric ankle fractures is indirect, and classification schemes for adult ankle fracture, including the Weber and Lauge-Hansen systems, have limited usefulness for children. The Dias-Tachdjian classification is a synthesis of the Salter-Harris and Lauge-Hansen schemes that is specifically designed for children; the descriptor indicates the position of the foot at the time of injury and the direction of the sustained force[41] (**Figure 6**). Many practitioners find the Dias-Tachdjian classification too complicated and difficult. The simpler Vahvanen-Aalto system, also designed to describe pediatric ankle fractures, classifies a low-risk epiphyseal separation as a group I fracture (corresponding to a Salter-Harris type I or II fracture) and a high-risk fracture through the epiphyseal plate as a group II fracture (corresponding to a Salter-Harris type III or IV fracture).[42]

A Salter-Harris type I or II fracture generally is managed with closed reduction and casting. A Salter-Harris type III or IV fracture with more than 2 mm of displacement requires surgical reduction and fixation to restore the physis and joint surface.[43-45] The exception is a distal tibial Salter-Harris type I or II fracture with a 3-mm physeal gap of more than 3 mm after an attempted closed reduction. This gap is associated with periosteal interposition. Without reduction, premature physeal closure was found to occur in 60% of such fractures; in comparison, the overall incidence of physeal closure was 12% in all distal tibial fractures and 25% in Salter-Harris type II fractures.[46,47] There was a statistically significant association among physeal closure, high-energy mechanisms of injury, and initial fracture displacement.

CT or MRI can be useful in assessing the reduction and planning any surgery. Screws or Kirschner wires can be used for surgical fixation. For a Salter-Harris type II fracture with a sufficiently large Thurston-Holland fragment, the wire or screw can be passed through the fragment parallel to the physis. Smooth pins should be used if it is necessary to cross the physis. For a Salter-Harris type III or IV fracture, it is often possible to pass the wire or screw through the epiphysis distal and parallel to the physis.[43]

Tillaux Fractures
A fracture that occurs in early adolescence when the distal tibial physis is closing, such as the Tillaux or triplane fracture, sometimes is called a transitional fracture. A Tillaux fracture is a Salter-Harris type III fracture of the distal tibial physis that occurs just before closure of the physis, when only the anterolateral portion remains open. The anterolateral fragment is avulsed secondary to the pull of the anteroinferior tibiotalar ligament. Because a Tillaux fracture occurs toward the end of growth, there is no risk of premature physeal closure. The goal of treatment is to restore the

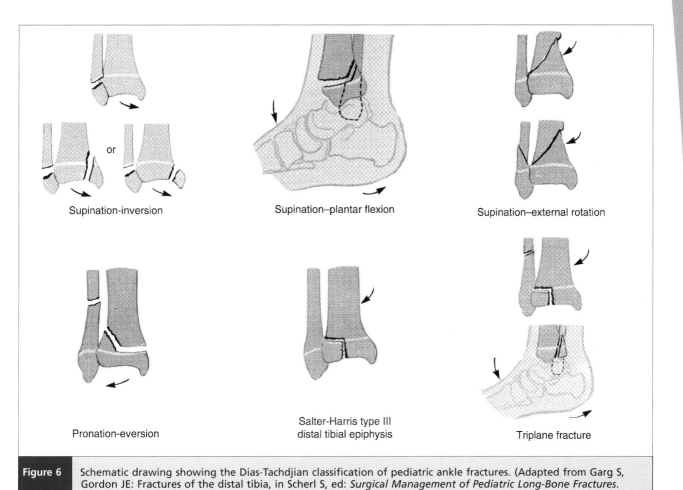

Supination-inversion

Supination–plantar flexion

Supination–external rotation

Pronation-eversion

Salter-Harris type III
distal tibial epiphysis

Triplane fracture

Figure 6 Schematic drawing showing the Dias-Tachdjian classification of pediatric ankle fractures. (Adapted from Garg S, Gordon JE: Fractures of the distal tibia, in Scherl S, ed: *Surgical Management of Pediatric Long-Bone Fractures.* Rosemont, IL, American Academy of Orthopaedic Surgeons, 2009, p 134.)

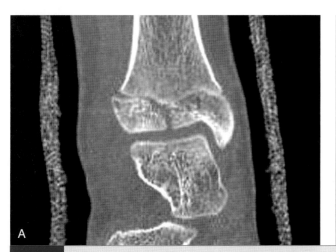
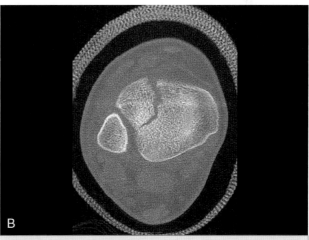

Figure 7 Coronal (**A**) and axial (**B**) CT images of a Tillaux fracture.

joint surface. CT is accurate and sensitive for revealing displacement and can be helpful in surgical planning.[48] The recommended treatment for a Tillaux fracture with more than 2 mm of displacement or step-off is open or closed reduction and internal fixation (**Figure 7**). One or two wires or screws typically are inserted tran-

sepiphyseally from medial to lateral. Other strategies, such as lateral-to-medial hardware insertion or trans-physeal fragment fixation, also are acceptable (**Figure 8**). Arthroscopically assisted reduction and fixation of a Tillaux fracture has been reported.[49]

6: Musculoskeletal Trauma

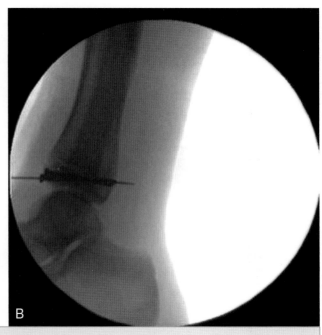
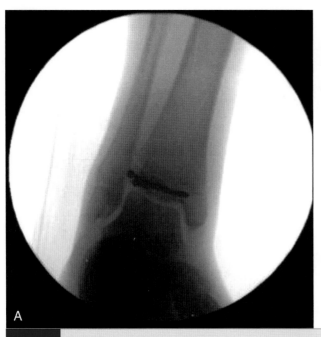

Figure 8   AP (**A**) and lateral (**B**) radiographs of transepiphyseal screw fixation of a Tillaux fracture.

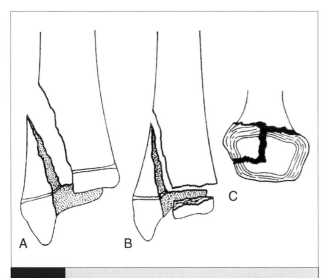

Figure 9   Schematic drawing showing triplane fractures. **A**, Two-part (Salter-Harris type IV) fracture. **B** and **C**, Three-part (Salter-Harris types II and III) fracture. (Reproduced with permission from Rockwood CA Jr, Wilkins KE, King RE, eds: *Fractures in Children*. Philadelphia, PA, JB Lippincott, 1984, pp 1021-1027.)

Triplane Fractures

Triplane fractures also are transitional, although they occur earlier in adolescence than Tillaux fractures. As with a Tillaux fracture, the primary goal of treatment is to reduce the joint surface. Growth disturbance is uncommon. A triplane fracture occurs in a complicated three-dimensional pattern of two, three, or (less commonly) four parts. A two-part triplane fracture is a Salter-Harris type IV fracture. A three-part triplane

fracture is a combined Salter-Harris type II and III fracture in which the type III component is a Tillaux fragment[50] (**Figure 9**). CT is useful in detecting a triplane fracture and planning for surgery[43,51,52] (**Figure 10**). An articular step-off or a gap of more than 2 mm is an indication for surgery, as it is in a Tillaux fracture.

An adequate closed reduction of a displaced triplane fracture sometimes can be done by internally rotating the foot under sedation or general anesthesia. A long leg cast is applied, and the reduction is confirmed by CT. Sometimes an anterolateral incision is sufficient if open reduction is necessary, but a posteromedial incision also may be required. One or two transepiphyseal screws or wires typically are used to fix the intra-articular fracture component, and one or two screws or wires are placed from anterior to posterior to fix the Thurston-Holland fragment of the metaphyseal fracture component (**Figure 11**). A prospective study found that 95% of patients were satisfied after treatment of a triplane fracture, and 67% had an objectively measured excellent outcome; 67% of the fractures had been treated nonsurgically.[51]

Foot Fractures

Pediatric foot fractures are relatively uncommon and generally have a good prognosis. Most can be successfully treated without surgery. Displaced foot fractures requiring surgical treatment typically occur in older children or adolescents; they usually are treated using the techniques and principles of adult surgery. The architecture of a growing child's foot is largely cartilaginous, and, diagnosis and identification of a fracture can

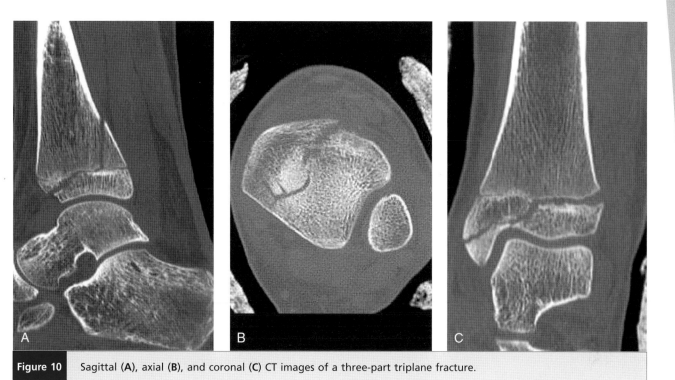

Figure 10　Sagittal (**A**), axial (**B**), and coronal (**C**) CT images of a three-part triplane fracture.

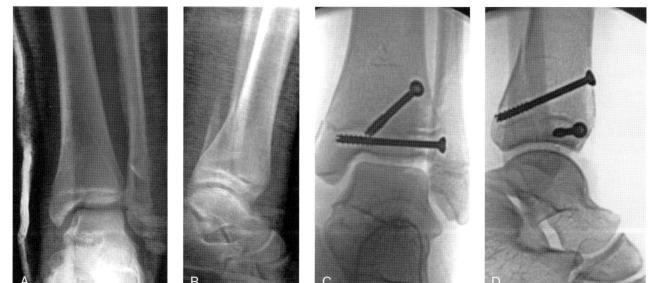

Figure 11　AP (**A**) and lateral (**B**) radiographs of a three-part triplane fracture. AP (**C**) and lateral (**D**) radiographs of the fracture after open reduction and internal fixation.

be challenging. The diagnosis usually can be made after a careful history and physical examination. Familiarity with the radiographic appearance of a child's foot at different stages of development is required, with judicious use of comparison radiographs and advanced imaging modalities.

Talar Neck Fractures

Talar neck fractures are as rare in children as they are in adults. In both children and adults, such a fracture,

particularly a displaced fracture, carries a relatively high risk of osteonecrosis of the talar body secondary to the retrograde flow of the blood supply to the talus. In a growing child, the high percentage of cartilage in the talus means that the bone is better able to absorb bending forces.[53] The talus has remodeling potential in children but not in adults.[54]

The Hawkins classification of talar neck fractures, as modified by Canale and Kelly, is used for both children and adults.[54,55] A type I fracture is nondisplaced; a type

II fracture is displaced with subluxation or dislocation of the subtalar joint; a type III fracture is displaced with subluxation or dislocation of both the subtalar and ankle joints; and a type IV fracture includes subluxation or dislocation of the talonavicular joint. The risk of osteonecrosis is minimal in a type I fracture, 41% in a type II fracture, and 90% in a type III or IV fracture.

A nondisplaced talar neck fracture can be treated using a non–weight-bearing cast for 6 to 8 weeks. A displaced fracture requires closed or open reduction. If the fracture is unstable, internal fixation typically is done with cannulated screws inserted from posterior to anterior.[56] A healing fracture should be monitored for the Hawkins sign, which is a subchondral lucency in the talar dome that indicates viability of the talar body. Usually the Hawkins sign is visible 6 to 8 weeks after the injury. An absent Hawkins sign may not be significant in a child; however, MRI can be useful if talar body viability is in question. Osteonecrosis in children typically appears within 6 months of the injury. The treatment of established osteonecrosis must be individualized because the clinical symptoms may not be correlated with the radiographic findings.[56]

Talar Osteochondritis Dissecans

Osteochondral lesions of the talus in children typically occur on the anterolateral or posteromedial aspect of the dome. Patients have pain and swelling of the ankle. The diagnosis often can be made using plain radiographs. If the lesion is confined to the subchondral bone, immobilization in a non–weight-bearing cast for 6 to 8 weeks usually is sufficient for healing. If the fracture has broached the articular cartilage and detached the lesion, open or arthroscopic débridement usually is required.[56]

The etiology of talar osteochondritis is believed to involve ischemia or, more commonly, trauma. Lateral lesions are caused by an inversion force to a dorsiflexed foot, and medial lesions are caused by an inversion force to a plantarflexed foot, with internal rotation of the tibia. A lateral lesion is more likely than a medial lesion to be preceded by trauma, and a lateral lesion is more likely to lead to persistent symptoms and degenerative changes in the joint.[57,58]

Calcaneus Fractures

Fractures of the calcaneus are less common and less severe in children than in adults. The prognosis is good, and surgical treatment rarely is required, even if the fracture is displaced.[59,60] Although calcaneus fractures often occur as a result of a fall from a height, they are not frequently associated with a vertebral fracture, as they are among adults. However, associated soft-tissue injury and fracturing of other extremities are common.[61] Stress fractures of the calcaneus have been reported in children with a neuromuscular disorder, as have occult toddler fractures of the calcaneus.[62]

Midfoot Fractures and Dislocations

Midfoot fractures are rare in children. They can be caused by direct force from a falling object or indirect force from a fall onto a plantar-flexed foot. The fracture generally is treated nonsurgically. Stress fracturing of the navicular and the cuboid has been reported.[63,64] A cuboid fracture may be associated with the Lisfranc tarsometatarsal injury. Although Lisfranc injuries are rare in children, the presence of a cuboid fracture, especially in combination with a fracture of the base of the second metatarsal, should raise the index of suspicion.[56] These injuries disrupt the articulations of the medial three metatarsals with the three cuneiforms and of the lateral two metatarsals with the cuboid. They are classified based on the direction of displacement of the metatarsals. Spontaneous reduction can occur, and therefore the initial radiographs may appear negative. Often there is considerable soft-tissue swelling and ecchymosis, and these injuries must be monitored for compartment syndrome.[56,65]

A nondisplaced Lisfranc injury can be treated with casting for approximately 4 weeks. A displaced injury requires closed or open reduction with stabilization using Kirschner wires or screws. The relationship between the second metatarsal and middle cuneiform is the keystone of the reduction; in addition, the second, first, and fifth tarsometatarsal joints should be stabilized as needed.[56] In a study of 18 pediatric Lisfranc injuries, 14 were asymptomatic at short-term follow-up.[66] Atypical pediatric Lisfranc injury has been associated with a fall from a miniscooter.[67]

Metatarsal Fractures

Metatarsal fractures are the most common type of pediatric foot fractures. The first metatarsal is most commonly injured in children younger than 5 years, and the base of the fifth metatarsal is the most common site of injury in children older than 10 years.[68] Direct trauma from a falling object typically results in a midshaft fracture; indirect torsional forces result in a neck fracture. A nondisplaced or minimally displaced metatarsal fracture can be treated symptomatically, with immobilization as needed for pain relief. A fracture at the base of the second through fifth metatarsal should be evaluated carefully for evidence of a Lisfranc injury. A fracture of the base of the first metatarsal in rare instances causes damage to the physis, with shortening of the first ray and the longitudinal arch of the foot.[56]

Avulsion fractures of the base of the fifth metatarsal result from the pull of the peroneus brevis during forceful inversion or adduction. The fracture line is perpendicular to the shaft of the bone. The secondary apophysis of the fifth metatarsal, which appears at approximately age 8 years and fuses at age 12 years in girls or age 15 years in boys, is sometimes mistaken for an avulsion fracture. However, the apophysis is oriented parallel to the fifth metatarsal shaft.

An avulsion fracture sometimes is mistaken for a Jones fracture. A Jones fracture is more distal, occur-

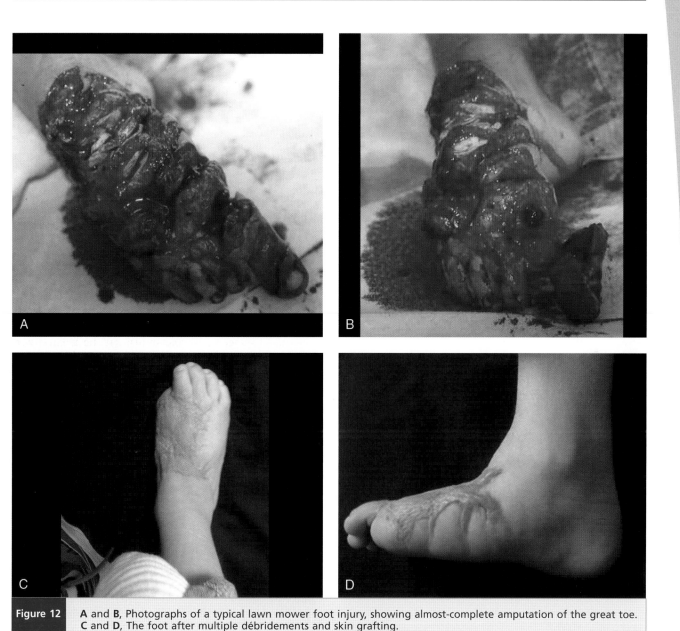

Figure 12   A and B, Photographs of a typical lawn mower foot injury, showing almost-complete amputation of the great toe. C and D, The foot after multiple débridements and skin grafting.

ring at the fifth metatarsal metaphyseal-diaphyseal junction, and it has a considerably different treatment and prognosis. A Jones fracture carries a risk of delayed union or nonunion, even in a child. The treatment is with a non–weight-bearing short leg cast for 6 weeks. An early return to weight bearing and sports activity sometimes leads to failure of nonsurgical treatment. Delayed union and nonunion are treated with internal fixation, with or without bone grafting.[69,70]

There should be a high index of suspicion for compartment syndrome of the foot, particularly in a child with a crush injury. Although a compartment syndrome of the foot often is associated with fracture or dislocation, it can occur in the absence of osseous injury. Swelling and pain with passive motion are common, but neurologic symptoms may be absent. Compartment pressure measurements can aid in the diagnosis. The treatment is

fasciotomy through two dorsal incisions, one medial incision, or a combination of the two approaches.[65,71]

Phalanx Fractures

Most pediatric phalangeal fractures can be treated with buddy taping as necessary for symptomatic relief. However, a Salter-Harris type III fracture of the proximal phalanx of the great toe that involves more than one third of the joint surface or is displaced more than 2 mm requires closed or open reduction and possibly fixation with a Kirschner wire or small screw.

A phalangeal fracture should be carefully examined for rotational deformity, which will not remodel successfully. A crush injury of the distal phalanx should be treated as an open fracture. Irrigation, débridement, and antibiotics should be used. If possible, the toenail should be preserved for use as a biologic dressing.[56,70]

6: Musculoskeletal Trauma

Lawn Mower Injuries

A 26-inch rotary lawn mower blade can produce a force equivalent to that of a 211-lb weight dropped 100 feet, and it is capable of causing significant high-energy trauma. Approximately half of all lawn mower injuries involve the lower extremity.[72] Although lawn mower injuries are largely preventable, 16,200 children sustained such injuries in the United States during 2007.[73] The incidence of traumatic amputation is 20% to 50%.[74-76] Traumatic amputation most often is at the level of the toes or midfoot, but higher level or bilateral amputation sometimes is required (**Figure 12**).

The treatment of a lawn mower injury begins with immediate administration of tetanus prophylaxis and antibiotics. Irrigation and débridement often must be repeated multiple times. Revision or completion of amputation often is necessary, as are fracture stabilization, skin grafts, and muscle flaps. It may be beneficial to use vacuum-assisted closure for such high-energy pediatric soft-tissue wounds.[77,78]

Wound infection or osteomyelitis occurs in 5% to 60% of children with a lawn mower injury.[72] A variety of organisms have been recovered, including anaerobes.[72,79,80] The initial empiric antibiotic prophylaxis should cover a broad spectrum including anaerobes, methicillin-resistant *Staphylococcus aureus*, and gram-negative organisms, and it should be administered for 5 to 10 days.[72,79]

The American Academy of Orthopaedic Surgeons and other organizations recommend that a manual lawn mower should be operated only by a person older than 12 years and that a riding mower should be operated only by a person older than 16 years. A child should never be a passenger on a riding mower and should not be allowed to play in the vicinity of any operating lawn mower.[73]

Summary

Lower leg and foot injuries are common in children. Although most of the fractures can be treated nonsurgically, the indications and options for surgical treatment are increasing. Intra-articular and physeal injuries should receive particular attention. After most types of fracture, thoughtful decision making and attention to detail usually lead to a good outcome.

Annotated References

1. Meyers MH, McKeever FM: Fracture of the intercondylar eminence of the tibia. *J Bone Joint Surg Am* 1959; 41-A(2):209-222.

2. Meyers MH, McKeever FM: Fracture of the intercondylar eminence of the tibia. *J Bone Joint Surg Am* 1970; 52(8):1677-1684.

3. Fehnel DJ, Johnson R: Anterior cruciate injuries in the skeletally immature athlete: A review of treatment outcomes. *Sports Med* 2000;29(1):51-63.

4. Jung YB, Yum JK, Koo BH: A new method for arthroscopic treatment of tibial eminence fractures with eyed Steinmann pins. *Arthroscopy* 1999;15(6):672-675.

5. Osti L, Merlo F, Liu SH, Bocchi L: A simple modified arthroscopic procedure for fixation of displaced tibial eminence fractures. *Arthroscopy* 2000;16(4):379-382.

6. Reynders P, Reynders K, Broos P: Pediatric and adolescent tibial eminence fractures: Arthroscopic cannulated screw fixation. *J Trauma* 2002;53(1):49-54.

7. Yip DK, Wong JW, Chien EP, Chan CF: Modified arthroscopic suture fixation of displaced tibial eminence fractures using a suture loop transporter. *Arthroscopy* 2001;17(1):101-106.

8. Mahar AT, Duncan D, Oka R, Lowry A, Gillingham B, Chambers H: Biomechanical comparison of four different fixation techniques for pediatric tibial eminence avulsion fractures. *J Pediatr Orthop* 2008;28(2):159-162.

   A bovine-model biomechanical comparison study of the stability of tibial eminence avulsion fractures after suture, resorbable screw, resorbable nail, or metal screw fixation found no clear biomechanical advantage to any particular technique.

9. Lowe J, Chaimsky G, Freedman A, Zion I, Howard C: The anatomy of tibial eminence fractures: Arthroscopic observations following failed closed reduction. *J Bone Joint Surg Am* 2002;84-A(11):1933-1938.

10. Wiley JJ, Baxter MP: Tibial spine fractures in children. *Clin Orthop Relat Res* 1990;255:54-60.

11. Willis RB, Blokker C, Stoll TM, Paterson DC, Galpin RD: Long-term follow-up of anterior tibial eminence fractures. *J Pediatr Orthop* 1993;13(3):361-364.

12. Close BJ, Strouse PJ: MR of physeal fractures of the adolescent knee. *Pediatr Radiol* 2000;30(11):756-762.

13. Patari SK, Lee FY, Behrens FF: Coronal split fracture of the proximal tibia epiphysis through a partially closed physis: A new fracture pattern. *J Pediatr Orthop* 2001; 21(4):451-455.

14. Gautier E, Ziran BH, Egger B, Slongo T, Jakob RP: Growth disturbances after injuries of the proximal tibial epiphysis. *Arch Orthop Trauma Surg* 1998;118(1-2): 37-41.

15. Rhemrev SJ, Sleeboom C, Ekkelkamp S: Epiphyseal fractures of the proximal tibia. *Injury* 2000;31(3):131-134.

16. Bertin KC, Goble EM: Ligament injuries associated with physeal fractures about the knee. *Clin Orthop Relat Res* 1983;177:188-195.

6: Musculoskeletal Trauma

17. Ogden JA, Tross RB, Murphy MJ: Fractures of the tibial tuberosity in adolescents. *J Bone Joint Surg Am* 1980; 62(2):205-215.

18. Ozer H, Turanli S, Baltaci G, Tekdemir I: Avulsion of the tibial tuberosity with a lateral plateau rim fracture: Case report. *Knee Surg Sports Traumatol Arthrosc* 2002;10(5):310-312.

19. Pape JM, Goulet JA, Hensinger RN: Compartment syndrome complicating tibial tubercle avulsion. *Clin Orthop Relat Res* 1993;295:201-204.

20. Müller I, Muschol M, Mann M, Hassenpflug J: Results of proximal metaphyseal fractures in children. *Arch Orthop Trauma Surg* 2002;122(6):331-333.

21. McCarthy JJ, Kim DH, Eilert RE: Posttraumatic genu valgum: Operative versus nonoperative treatment. *J Pediatr Orthop* 1998;18(4):518-521.

22. Tuten HR, Keeler KA, Gabos PG, Zionts LE, MacKenzie WG: Posttraumatic tibia valga in children: A long-term follow-up note. *J Bone Joint Surg Am* 1999;81(6): 799-810.

23. Shannak AO: Tibial fractures in children: Follow-up study. *J Pediatr Orthop* 1988;8(3):306-310.

24. Yang JP, Letts RM: Isolated fractures of the tibia with intact fibula in children: A review of 95 patients. *J Pediatr Orthop* 1997;17(3):347-351.

25. Vitale M: Fractures of the tibial shaft, in Scherl S, ed: *Surgical Management of Pediatric Long-Bone Fractures.* Rosemont, IL, American Academy of Orthopaedic Surgeons, 2009, pp 121-131.

    Indications and techniques for the surgical treatment of pediatric tibia fractures are described.

26. Setter KJ, Palomino KE: Pediatric tibia fractures: Current concepts. *Curr Opin Pediatr* 2006;18(1):30-35.

    This review article describes and compares surgical options for the treatment of pediatric tibia fractures.

27. Dwyer AJ, John B, Krishen M, Hora R: Remodeling of tibial fractures in children younger than 12 years. *Orthopedics* 2007;30(5):393-396.

    Forty-eight children (average age, 7.2 years) were examined clinically and radiographically to analyze the correction of deformity after a tibial shaft fracture. At an average 4-year follow-up, the best correction was for anterior angular deformity (53%), followed by varus (41%), valgus (24%), and posterior angular (18.5%) deformities. Acceptable angular deformity was 12° for anterior, 10° for varus, 8° for valgus, and 6° for posterior deformity. Level of evidence: IV.

28. Al-Sayyad MJ: Taylor Spatial Frame in the treatment of pediatric and adolescent tibial shaft fractures. *J Pediatr Orthop* 2006;26(2):164-170.

    Ten tibia fractures, including five open fractures, were retrospectively reviewed after treatment with a Taylor Spatial Frame. All patients were boys age 8 to 15 years (mean, 12 years). The mean healing time was 18 weeks. Five patients developed a pin tract infection. All patients were involved in sports at a mean 3.1-year follow-up. Level of evidence: IV.

29. Gregory RJ, Cubison TC, Pinder IM, Smith SR: External fixation of lower limb fractures in children. *J Trauma* 1992;33(5):691-693.

30. Myers SH, Spiegel D, Flynn JM: External fixation of high-energy tibia fractures. *J Pediatr Orthop* 2007; 27(5):537-539.

    Thirty-one consecutive high-energy tibia fractures (including 19 open fractures) were retrospectively reviewed in 22 boys and 9 girls age 4 to 17 years (mean, 11.9 years) after external fixation (mean duration, 3.2 months; time to union, 4.8 months). Skin graft was required for 3 and fasciotomy for 7 of 30 fractures. Complications included delayed union, nonunion, malunion, limb-length discrepancy, pin tract infection, wound infection, and osteomyelitis. Level of evidence: IV.

31. Schmittenbecher P: Treatment options for fractures of the tibial shaft and ankle in children. *Tech Orthop* 2000;15(1):38-53.

32. Bartlett CS III, Weiner LS, Yang EC: Treatment of type II and type III open tibia fractures in children. *J Orthop Trauma* 1997;11(5):357-362.

33. Song KM, Sangeorzan B, Benirschke S, Browne R: Open fractures of the tibia in children. *J Pediatr Orthop* 1996; 16(5):635-639.

34. Goodwin RC, Gaynor T, Mahar A, Oka R, Lalonde FD: Intramedullary flexible nail fixation of unstable pediatric tibial diaphyseal fractures. *J Pediatr Orthop* 2005;25(5):570-576.

    In a retrospective review of 19 patients and a biomechanical analysis of two implant configurations, all patients had union; 5 (26%) had complications not requiring surgery. Two patients (11%) had angular deformity (at least 10°) with a medial C-and-S construct. There was no deformity with the double C construct. Mechanical testing with axial and torsional loading found that the C-and-S construct was more stable. Level of evidence: IV.

35. O'Brien T, Weisman DS, Ronchetti P, Piller CP, Maloney M: Flexible titanium nailing for the treatment of the unstable pediatric tibial fracture. *J Pediatr Orthop* 2004;24(6):601-609.

36. Salem KH, Lindemann I, Keppler P: Flexible intramedullary nailing in pediatric lower limb fractures. *J Pediatr Orthop* 2006;26(4):505-509.

    A retrospective review studied 73 unilateral femoral or tibial shaft fractures (70 closed fractures) treated using elastic intramedullary nails in 48 boys and 25 girls (mean age, 5.7 years). All fractures were reduced by closed manipulation, and union was achieved without additional intervention. Several technical problems oc-

6: Musculoskeletal Trauma

curred. One third of the patients had an associated injury. Level of evidence: IV.

37. Srivastava AK, Mehlman CT, Wall EJ, Do TT: Elastic stable intramedullary nailing of tibial shaft fractures in children. *J Pediatr Orthop* 2008;28(2):152-158.

    A retrospective review studied 24 tibial shaft fractures (including 16 open fractures) treated over 8 years using elastic stable intramedullary nails. The average time to union was 20.4 weeks (closed, 21.5 weeks; open, 20.2 weeks). Neurovascular complication, infection, or malunion each occurred in two patients (8%), and one patient (4%) had a limb-length discrepancy. Level of evidence: IV.

38. Kubiak EN, Egol KA, Scher D, Wasserman B, Feldman D, Koval KJ: Operative treatment of tibial fractures in children: Are elastic stable intramedullary nails an improvement over external fixation? *J Bone Joint Surg Am* 2005;87(8):1761-1768.

    Clinical, radiographic, and functional outcomes were compared in a retrospective review of 31 consecutive patients with open physes who underwent surgical treatment of a tibia fracture (16 with elastic stable intramedullary nails, 15 with unilateral external fixation). Malunion, delayed union, nonunion, infection, and the need for subsequent surgical treatment occurred. Functional outcomes (pain, happiness, sports, and global function) were significantly better for patients who received intramedullary nailing. Level of evidence: III.

39. Lascombes P, Haumont T, Journeau P: Use and abuse of flexible intramedullary nailing in children and adolescents. *J Pediatr Orthop* 2006;26(6):827-834.

    The indications and techniques for flexible intramedullary nailing of pediatric long bones are described.

40. Gordon JE, Gregush RV, Schoenecker PL, Dobbs MB, Luhmann SJ: Complications after titanium elastic nailing of pediatric tibial fractures. *J Pediatr Orthop* 2007;27(4):442-446.

    Sixty diaphyseal tibia fractures were retrospectively reviewed after flexible intramedullary fixation, with 51 fractures (50 patients; mean age, 11.7 years) followed until union; 45 fractures had bony union within 18 weeks (mean, 8 weeks). The 5 patients (11%) with delayed healing had a mean age of 14.1 years. Fixation of pediatric diaphyseal tibia fractures with titanium elastic nails is effective but has a substantial rate of delayed healing, particularly in older patients. Level of evidence: IV.

41. Dias LS, Tachdjian MO: Physeal injuries of the ankle in children: Classification. *Clin Orthop Relat Res* 1978; 136:230-233.

42. Vahvanen V, Aalto K: Classification of ankle fractures in children. *Arch Orthop Trauma Surg* 1980;97(1):1-5.

43. Kay RM, Matthys GA: Pediatric ankle fractures: Evaluation and treatment. *J Am Acad Orthop Surg* 2001; 9(4):268-278.

44. Kling TF Jr, Bright RW, Hensinger RN: Distal tibial

45. Berson L, Davidson RS, Dormans JP, Drummond DS, Gregg JR: Growth disturbances after distal tibial physeal fractures. *Foot Ankle Int* 2000;21(1):54-58.

46. Barmada A, Gaynor T, Mubarak SJ: Premature physeal closure following distal tibia physeal fractures: A new radiographic predictor. *J Pediatr Orthop* 2003;23(6): 733-739.

47. Leary JT, Handling M, Talerico M, Yong L, Bowe JA: Physeal fractures of the distal tibia: Predictive factors of premature physeal closure and growth arrest. *J Pediatr Orthop* 2009;29(4):356-361.

    A retrospective review of 124 pediatric patients with a physeal fracture of the distal end of the tibia found that 15 fractures (12%) were complicated by premature physeal closure, 10 of which (67%) occurred in a Salter-Harris II fracture. Level of evidence: IV.

48. Horn BD, Crisci K, Krug M, Pizzutillo PD, MacEwen GD: Radiologic evaluation of juvenile Tillaux fractures of the distal tibia. *J Pediatr Orthop* 2001;21(2):162-164.

49. Leetun DT, Ireland ML: Arthroscopically assisted reduction and fixation of a juvenile Tillaux fracture. *Arthroscopy* 2002;18(4):427-429.

50. Cooperman DR, Spiegel PG, Laros GS: Tibial fractures involving the ankle in children: The so-called triplane epiphyseal fracture. *J Bone Joint Surg Am* 1978;60(8): 1040-1046.

51. El-Karef E, Sadek HI, Nairn DS, Aldam CH, Allen PW: Triplane fracture of the distal tibia. *Injury* 2000;31(9): 729-736.

52. Jones S, Phillips N, Ali F, Fernandes JA, Flowers MJ, Smith TW: Triplane fractures of the distal tibia requiring open reduction and internal fixation: Pre-operative planning using computed tomography. *Injury* 2003; 34(4):293-298.

53. Letts RM, Gibeault D: Fractures of the neck of the talus in children. *Foot Ankle* 1980;1(2):74-77.

54. Hawkins LG: Fractures of the neck of the talus. *J Bone Joint Surg Am* 1970;52(5):991-1002.

55. Canale ST, Kelly FB Jr: Fractures of the neck of the talus: Long-term evaluation of seventy-one cases. *J Bone Joint Surg Am* 1978;60(2):143-156.

56. Ribbans WJ, Natarajan R, Alavala S: Pediatric foot fractures. *Clin Orthop Relat Res* 2005;432:107-115.

    This review of common injuries to a child's foot includes differential diagnosis and treatment.

physeal fractures in children that may require open reduction. *J Bone Joint Surg Am* 1984;66(5):647-657.

57. Canale ST, Belding RH: Osteochondral lesions of the talus. *J Bone Joint Surg Am* 1980;62(1):97-102.

58. Wester JU, Jensen IE, Rasmussen F, Lindequist S, Schantz K: Osteochondral lesions of the talar dome in children: A 24 (7-36) year follow-up of 13 cases. *Acta Orthop Scand* 1994;65(1):110-112.

59. Brunet JA: Calcaneal fractures in children: Long-term results of treatment. *J Bone Joint Surg Br* 2000;82(2): 211-216.

60. Inokuchi S, Usami N, Hiraishi E, Hashimoto T: Calcaneal fractures in children. *J Pediatr Orthop* 1998;18(4): 469-474.

61. Schmidt TL, Weiner DS: Calcaneal fractures in children: An evaluation of the nature of the injury in 56 children. *Clin Orthop Relat Res* 1982;171:150-155.

62. Schindler A, Mason DE, Allington NJ: Occult fracture of the calcaneus in toddlers. *J Pediatr Orthop* 1996; 16(2):201-205.

63. Nicastro JF, Haupt HA: Probable stress fracture of the cuboid in an infant: A case report. *J Bone Joint Surg Am* 1984;66(7):1106-1108.

64. Spitz DJ, Newberg AH: Imaging of stress fractures in the athlete. *Radiol Clin North Am* 2002;40(2):313-331.

65. Bibbo C, Lin SS, Cunningham FJ: Acute traumatic compartment syndrome of the foot in children. *Pediatr Emerg Care* 2000;16(4):244-248.

66. Wiley JJ: Tarso-metatarsal joint injuries in children. *J Pediatr Orthop* 1981;1(3):255-260.

67. Bibbo C, Davis WH, Anderson RB: Midfoot injury in children related to mini scooters. *Pediatr Emerg Care* 2003;19(1):6-9.

68. Owen RJ, Hickey FG, Finlay DB: A study of metatarsal fractures in children. *Injury* 1995;26(8):537-538.

69. Kavanaugh JH, Brower TD, Mann RV: The Jones fracture revisited. *J Bone Joint Surg Am* 1978;60(6):776-782.

70. Realyvasquez J: Fractures and dislocations: Foot, in Cramer K, Scherl SA, eds: *Orthopaedic Surgery Essentials: Pediatrics*. Philadelphia, PA, Lippincott Williams & Wilkins, 2004, pp 165-170.

71. Silas SI, Herzenberg JE, Myerson MS, Sponseller PD: Compartment syndrome of the foot in children. *J Bone Joint Surg Am* 1995;77(3):356-361.

72. Campbell JR: Infectious complications of lawn mower injuries. *Pediatr Infect Dis J* 2001;20(1):60-62.

73. Lawn mowing injuries common in children and teens. *Science Daily*. June 8, 2008. http://www.sciencedaily.com/releases/2008/06/080603091342.htm. Accessed November 5, 2009.

Lawn mower safety guidelines from the American Academy of Orthopaedic Surgeons and other organizations are outlined.

74. Vollman D, Smith GA: Epidemiology of lawn-mower-related injuries to children in the United States, 1990-2004. *Pediatrics* 2006;118(2):e273-e278.

A retrospective analysis of patients younger than age 21 years in the National Electronic Injury Surveillance System of the US Consumer Products Safety Commission found that 140,700 lawn mower–related injuries were treated in emergency departments from 1990 to 2004 (9,400 injuries per year, 11 injuries per 10,0000 children per year). Level of evidence: IV.

75. Loder RT, Brown KL, Zaleske DJ, Jones ET: Extremity lawn-mower injuries in children: Report by the Research Committee of the Pediatric Orthopaedic Society of North America. *J Pediatr Orthop* 1997;17(3):360-369.

76. Vollman D, Khosla K, Shields BJ, Beeghly BC, Bonsu B, Smith GA: Lawn mower-related injuries to children. *J Trauma* 2005;59(3):724-728.

Eighty-five children (65% boys; mean age, 7.6 years) were treated for a lawn mower–related injury in one emergency department over 53 months. Thirty-four (40%) were admitted to the hospital, and 30 (35%) required surgical intervention. Level of evidence: IV.

77. Mooney JF III, Argenta LC, Marks MW, Morykwas MJ, DeFranzo AJ: Treatment of soft tissue defects in pediatric patients using the V.A.C. system. *Clin Orthop Relat Res* 2000;376:26-31.

78. Shilt JS, Yoder JS, Manuck TA, Jacks L, Rushing J, Smith BP: Role of vacuum-assisted closure in the treatment of pediatric lawnmower injuries. *J Pediatr Orthop* 2004;24(5):482-487.

79. Brook I: Recovery of anaerobic bacteria from wounds after lawn-mower injuries. *Pediatr Emerg Care* 2005; 21(2):109-110.

Two children with a lawn mower foot injury developed severe wound infection. Culturing revealed heavy growth of *Clostridium bifermentans* and *Peptostreptococcus magnus* in one patient and *Clostridium perfringens* in the other child. Antimicrobial therapy directed at the pathogens and vigorous surgical irrigation and débridement led to complete recovery.

80. Gaglani MJ, Friedman J, Hawkins EP, Campbell JR: Infections complicating lawn mower injuries in children. *Pediatr Infect Dis J* 1996;15(5):452-455.

6. Musculoskeletal Trauma

Chapter 35

Spine Trauma

Suken A. Shah, MD   Jon Oda, MD

Introduction

Pediatric spine trauma accounts for only 1% to 10% of all spine trauma and approximately 5% of pediatric trauma. Although uncommon, pediatric spine trauma has significant implications; one institution reported an overall rate of neurologic injury of 66% and a mortality rate of 27%.[1] Children sustain more severe injuries than adults and are more likely to have an injury to the cervical spine (60% to 80% of young children have a cervical spine injury with spine trauma,[2,3] compared with 21% of adults[4]). Motor vehicle crashes are the most common cause of injury, followed by falls in younger children and sports accidents in older children. Spinal cord injury occurs in approximately 2 per 100,000 children and is twice as frequent in boys as in girls.[5] Older children and adolescents have a higher incidence of subaxial cervical or thoracolumbar spine injuries,[6-8] and younger children have a higher incidence of upper cervical spine injuries.[1]

Pediatric and Adult Spine Trauma

Compared with adults, children have a larger head-to-body ratio, greater ligamentous laxity, underdeveloped paraspinal musculature, and anteriorly wedged vertebrae. In the cervical region, children have horizontally oriented facet joints, and before age 10 years they lack uncinate processes. Cartilaginous vertebral apophyses and synchondroses are weaker than mature bone and ligaments, and they are more prone to injury. All of these factors contribute to an increased risk of serious spine injury with trauma in children.

The surgeon must consider the child's smaller anatomy as well as the future growth and development of

the immature spine. Children appear to have higher rates of neurologic recovery than adults. In one study, 14 of 22 patients (64%) younger than 18 years who had a spinal cord injury with neurologic deficit experienced neurologic improvement.[9] Five patients who initially had a complete spinal cord injury (American Spinal Injury Association grade A) eventually regained ambulatory status.

Evaluation and Management

Evaluation

The evaluation of pediatric spine trauma can be difficult. The physical examination of a young child may be unreliable because of the child's limited ability to cooperate.[8,10] The physician must suspect a spine injury with every pediatric trauma, and cervical spine injury should be suspected in every patient who sustains severe head trauma. To prevent excessive cervical flexion during transport, a child's large head-to-body ratio dictates the use of a special backboard with an occipital cutout or pads placed underneath the shoulders and trunk. Sandbags should be placed around the head, with an appropriate-size pediatric cervical orthosis for further stabilization. A comprehensive evaluation is necessary in the emergency department because pediatric spine trauma often is associated with trauma to other organ systems. Clinical decision-making rules for the radiographic evaluation of adult cervical spine trauma were found to have inadequate sensitivity for use in children, especially those younger than 10 years.[11] If spinal column trauma is detected, the entire spine from occiput to sacrum must be investigated because of the possibility of vertebral fractures at noncontiguous levels.[12]

The radiographic evaluation of pediatric spine trauma is complicated by multiple factors. In neonates, the spine is largely cartilaginous and ligamentous, with minimal ossification. Synchondroses can be misinterpreted as fractures. Children and adolescents may have localized kyphosis in the midcervical spine (an abnormal finding in adults).[13] A child's normal ligamentous laxity can mimic soft-tissue injury, as with pseudosubluxation or a greater-than-expected atlantodens interval; 20% of children age 1 to 7 years were found to have an atlantodens interval greater than 3 mm.[14] Crying increases swelling in the soft tissues anterior to the

Dr. Shah or an immediate family member has received royalties from DePuy Spine, Inc., a Johnson & Johnson company; is a member of a speakers' bureau or has made paid presentations on behalf of DePuy Spine; serves as a paid consultant to or is an employee of DePuy Spine; serves as an unpaid consultant to K Spine, Inc.; has received research or institutional support from DePuy Spine and Axial Biotech, Inc.; and owns stock or stock options in Globus Medical. Dr. Oda or an immediate family member serves as a board member, owner, officer, or committee member of Kuakini Hospital in Honolulu, HI; and owns stock or stock options in Smith & Nephew.

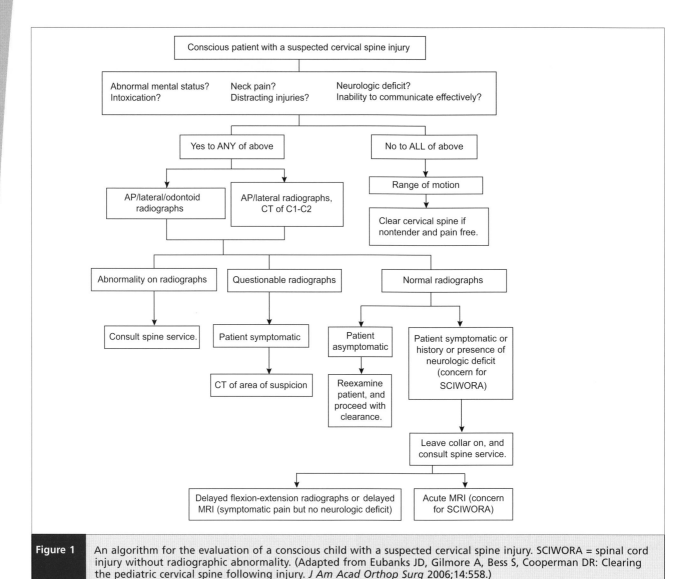

Figure 1 An algorithm for the evaluation of a conscious child with a suspected cervical spine injury. SCIWORA = spinal cord injury without radiographic abnormality. (Adapted from Eubanks JD, Gilmore A, Bess S, Cooperman DR: Clearing the pediatric cervical spine following injury. *J Am Acad Orthop Surg* 2006;14:558.)

vertebral column, making the interpretation of soft-tissue anatomy less reliable.[15] A child often does not report neck tenderness, especially in the setting of multiple injuries.

Plain radiographs should be the initial step in evaluating pediatric spine trauma. CT is more accurate than plain radiographs,[16] and it should be used if plain radiographs are inadequate. However, even the combination of plain radiographs and CT can be difficult to interpret, especially in a child with trauma.[17] Therefore, MRI is the imaging modality of choice in evaluating a child for spine trauma. The ability to assess soft tissues on MRI means that the spinal cord can be evaluated, and ligamentous injuries, disk herniations, apophyseal avulsions, and physeal fractures can be detected. Although no national consensus protocols are available to guide physicians on pediatric cervical spine clearance or imaging indications, general guidelines are provided in **Figures 1** and **2.**

Nonsurgical and Surgical Treatment

Most pediatric spine trauma injuries can be adequately treated with nonsurgical methods such as the use of an orthosis, halo vest, or Minerva cast. A noninvasive pinless halo vest was recently developed to avoid the complications associated with halo pins.[18] The use of methylprednisolone in pediatric acute spinal cord injury is controversial and based on anecdotal evidence only. Approximately one third of children with spine trauma require surgical stabilization.[3]

Recent developments in spine instrumentation have led to more widespread use of hardware in treating pediatric spine trauma. Pedicle screws have been used off-label in the thoracolumbar spine of children as young as 8 months.[19] There has been concern about the potential of precipitating spinal stenosis by using pedicle screws in young children. However, a study of 91 pedicle screws placed in children age 1 to 2 years found no evidence of growth retardation or spinal stenosis at intermediate-term follow-up.[20] A study of modern cer-

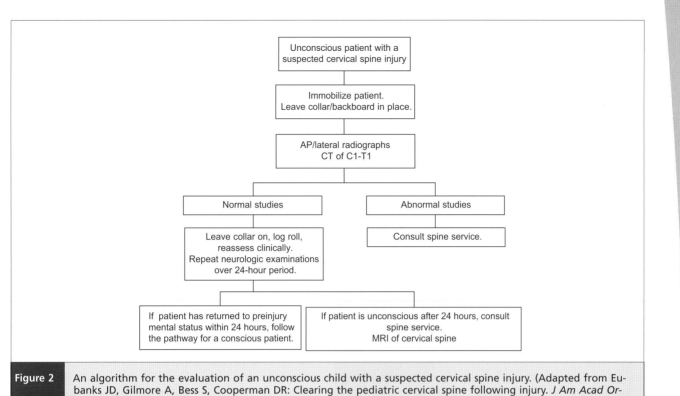

Figure 2 An algorithm for the evaluation of an unconscious child with a suspected cervical spine injury. (Adapted from Eubanks JD, Gilmore A, Bess S, Cooperman DR: Clearing the pediatric cervical spine following injury. *J Am Acad Orthop Surg* 2006;14:563.)

vical instrumentation used in pediatric patients found no implant-related complications and a 100% union rate.[21] Although bone morphogenetic protein (BMP) has been used to enhance spinal fusion in young children, the exact indications and complications have yet to be defined.[22] A recent study of the use of recombinant human BMP-2 in 81 pediatric patients (mean age, 11.3 years) found a possible association with dural fibrosis.[23] BMP and anti-BMP antibodies have been found to cross the placenta in animal models;[24] the use of BMP is therefore contraindicated for pregnant women and not recommended by the manufacturer for female patients of childbearing age. Other fusion techniques that may be helpful in very young children include spinous process and sublaminar fixation with wires or polyester fiber tape (**Figure 3**) and supplementation of fixation with an external orthosis or body cast.

Types of Pediatric Spine Trauma

Spinal Cord Injury Without Radiographic Abnormality

Spinal cord injury without radiographic abnormality (SCIWORA) primarily occurs in children and usually is in the cervical spine. The cause is believed to be the greater ligamentous laxity in children, which allows the spinal column to stretch beyond the tolerance of the spinal cord. SCIWORA represents between 5% and 67% of all pediatric spinal cord injuries.[25] The wide range probably is the result of differing definitions of SCIWORA. The original description of SCIWORA was based on plain radiography, CT, and myelography.[26] MRI subsequently allowed physicians to identify spinal cord pathologies such as epidural hematoma, hematomyelia, disk herniation, spinal cord contusion, and spinal cord transection. These conditions are now recognized as distinct entities with separate treatments and prognoses, but earlier they were inconsistently labeled as SCIWORA. Some authors have suggested the use of the term "spinal cord injury without neuroimaging abnormality" to distinguish SCIWORA from spinal cord injuries with MRI-identified pathology. Spinal cord injury without neuroimaging abnormality has a much better prognosis than is suggested by the older literature on SCIWORA; as many as 80% of patients have a good clinical outcome.[27] The treatment of spinal cord injury without neuroimaging abnormality is conservative, consisting of immobilization for 3 months with close follow-up for detection of residual instability.[25]

Birth Spine Trauma

Spine injuries resulting from birth trauma are rare and are believed to be the result of excessive traction applied during a difficult delivery with fetal head entrapment. Injury can occur in both the cervical and thoracic spine. Birth spine trauma should be suspected in a neonate with hypotonia or flaccid paralysis. Evaluation is with plain radiographs and MRI. The long-term prognosis is poor, with neurologic recovery being the exception rather than the rule.[28]

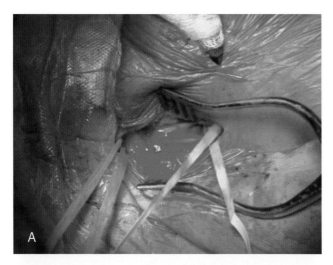

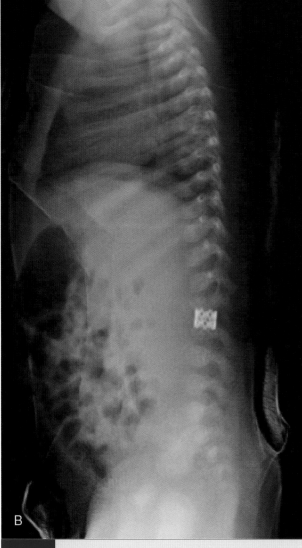

Figure 3 Photograph (**A**) and lateral spine radiograph (**B**) showing the use of polyester fiber tape to stabilize the posterior elements in a 14-day-old infant with congenital dislocation of the spine. An external body cast was used postoperatively.

Spine Trauma From Child Abuse

Spine injury can result from severe shaking, and it should be a part of the differential diagnosis for an infant or toddler with sudden flaccid paralysis. Other indicators of child abuse, such as retinal or cerebral hemorrhage, may or may not be present. The spine injuries associated with child abuse include hangman's fracture, cervical fracture-dislocation, thoracolumbar fracture-dislocation, fracture through the neurocentral junction, and meningeal hemorrhage.

Airbag and Seatbelt Injuries

The use of airbags and seatbelts in motor vehicles has dramatically decreased the mortality rate from crashes. However, improper use of these devices poses specific risks to the pediatric spine. Seatbelts have been identified as a risk factor in severe and fatal pediatric spine injuries in motor vehicle crashes.[29,30] Airbags deploy at the level of a young child's head and neck, and this combination can be lethal.[31] In older children and adolescents, seatbelts have been linked to lumbar Chance fractures and other intra-abdominal injuries. These injuries probably occur because of a child's large head-to-body ratio and small iliac crest, which allows the lap belt to ride up into the abdominal area. Misuse of a vehicle's three-point restraint system also can be a factor.

Sports-Related Injuries

Spine trauma related to a sport or another recreational activity is a common mechanism of injury in children older than 10 years. Children and adolescents participating in a high-risk sport or other recreational activity always should wear protective gear and should be taught appropriate techniques for injury prevention, such as training for strength and flexibility or avoidance of spear tackling or hockey checks from behind.

Occipitocervical Junction Injuries

Atlanto-occipital injury is associated with a high-energy mechanism of injury and frequently is fatal. However, recent advances in trauma management are increasing the survival rate. Children are twice as likely as adults to sustain this injury. Detection can be difficult; often there is spontaneous reduction, and the patient usually is noncommunicative because of the severity of the trauma. The diagnosis should be suspected in patients with agonal respirations, an irregular heart rate, lower cranial nerve deficits, asymmetric motor deficits, or the moaning sign.[32] Various radiographic measurements have been used in defining the injury (**Figure 4**). Adequate radiographs can be difficult to obtain in children, especially if the patient has multiple traumatic injuries, and an MRI should be obtained if an atlanto-occipital injury is suspected. Retroclival hematomas and tectorial membrane injuries may indicate occipitocervical trauma.[34,35] These injuries are highly unstable, and immobilization with halo-thoracic traction should be instituted expeditiously, with surgical stabilization performed as soon as the patient is clinically stable.

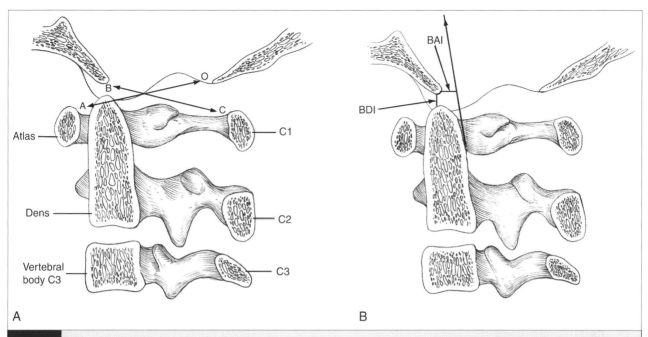

Figure 4 The radiographic analysis of the pediatric upper cervical spine. **A**, The Powers ratio is used to detect anterior atlanto-occipital instability. A = anterior arch of the atlas, B = basion, C = posterior arch of the atlas, O = opisthion. Anterior instability is suspected if BC/AO is greater than 1.0. The Powers ratio does not detect posterior instability. **B**, The basion-dental interval (BDI) and the basion-axial interval (BAI) each should measure less than 12 mm. Values greater than 12 mm imply occipitocervical instability. In a child younger than 13 years, the BDI may be an unreliable measurement because of variable ossification of the dens; however, the BDI should be less than 12 mm in all children. (Adapted from Eubanks JD, Gilmore A, Bess S, Cooperman DR: Clearing the pediatric cervical spine following injury. *J Am Acad Orthop Surg* 2006;14:561.)

Occiput-C2 fusion with structural autologous bone grafting usually is recommended. C1 lateral mass screws, C2 pars screws, C2 pedicle screws, and C2 laminar screws all have been used with success in pediatric patients.[36-38] Occipitocervical and atlantoaxial fusions were found to alter the normal lordosis of the cervical spine in children,[39,40] and their long-term consequences are unknown.

Atlantal and Atlantoaxial Injuries

Atlantoaxial instability can be assessed radiographically using the atlantodens interval (**Figure 5**). Younger children may have an atlantodens interval as great as 5 mm without injury[41]; in older children and adults, an interval greater than 3 mm indicates injury. A fracture of the ring of C1 (a Jefferson fracture) can be confused with a normal synchondrosis, and a fracture can occur through a synchondrosis. Most fractures of the ring of C1 are minimally displaced and not associated with neurologic compromise; they can be treated with immobilization in a soft collar or a halo vest.[42] If the anterior arch is significantly displaced, transoral reduction can be attempted.[43] Transarticular screws provide rigid fixation of C1 on C2 and are useful in managing atlantoaxial instability resulting from a hypoplastic posterior arch, trauma, os odontoideum, or pathologic ligamentous laxity (as in Down syndrome).[44,45] Atlantoaxial rotary subluxation can occur as a result of infection or trauma. The treatment is soft-collar immobiliza-

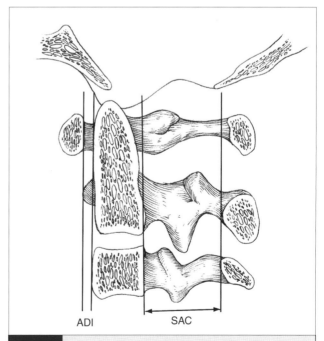

Figure 5 The atlantodens interval (ADI) and space available for the cord (SAC) in the upper cervical spine. An ADI of more than 10 mm may result in spinal cord compression. (Reproduced from Eubanks JD, Gilmore A, Bess S, Cooperman DR: Clearing the pediatric cervical spine following injury. *J Am Acad Orthop Surg* 2006;14:561.)

6: Musculoskeletal Trauma

tion or head-halter traction, with anti-inflammatory drugs. Surgery is reserved for a chronic or recurrent condition.

C2 Fractures (Odontoid and Hangman's Fractures)

Hangman's fracture is rare in children and can be associated with child abuse. This fracture generally is not associated with neurologic compromise and can be treated with halo immobilization or Minerva casting. Fracture through the odontoid synchondrosis typically is treated with cast immobilization or a halo vest. The presence of an os odontoideum in adults may be the result of an odontoid fracture above the synchondrosis that evolved into a chronic nonunion, and the long-term instability may increase the risk of late neurologic degeneration.[46]

Injuries to the Subaxial Cervical Spine

The spectrum of injury to the subaxial spine includes vertebral and facet fracture-dislocation, burst fracture, compression fracture, ligamentous injury, physeal fracture, and avulsion fracture. In older children, injury to the subaxial spine usually involves high-energy trauma; the most commonly involved levels are C5-C7.[6] A subaxial cervical spine injury is less likely to be associated with head trauma than an upper cervical injury and therefore has a more favorable prognosis. Anterior instrumentation and fusion generally are not used in children younger than 8 years to avoid interfering with growth; however, case reports of successful anterior cervical fusion in young children have been published.[47,48] Laminar screws have been gaining in popularity as a method of instrumentation for the posterior elements of the cervical spine.[49] Laminar thickness in the subaxial cervical spine of pediatric patients is in the range of 2 to 3 mm;[50] it should be determined with preoperative CT before this technique is used.

Thoracic and Lumbar Spine Injuries

Thoracic and lumbar injuries are most common among adolescent boys. Typically the trauma is from a motor vehicle crash, a recreational activity accident, or a fall from a height. The evaluation and treatment are similar to those for an injury in an adult. A fracture involving two or three columns should be treated with stabilization.[51] A one-column injury (a compression fracture) generally can be treated nonsurgically. Complete restoration of vertebral height and sagittal alignment can be expected in a patient younger than 12 years who has a compression fracture with a compression deformity of less than 20° to 30°.[52] Stable compression fractures without neurologic injury have a benign long-term outcome, with no increased incidence of disk degeneration at adjacent levels, even in the absence of significant remodeling.[53] Stable burst fractures can be successfully treated nonsurgically but must be monitored for progressive kyphosis. In general, thoracic and lumbar vertebral fractures without neurologic compromise have a favorable long-term prognosis.[53]

Chance Fractures

A Chance flexion-distraction fracture usually is the result of a seatbelt injury sustained in a motor vehicle crash. A high index of suspicion should be maintained for other intra-abdominal injuries. Small bowel or colon perforation or transection, diaphragmatic rupture, ureteral transection, abdominal aortic injury, or pancreatic injury occurs with approximately 40% of Chance fractures.[54] The Chance fracture involves the physis in one third of skeletally immature patients.[55] MRI is useful in defining the pattern of injury. A Chance fracture in a skeletally immature patient has a less favorable long-term outlook than a compression fracture; a significant number of patients reported pain and disability at intermediate-term follow-up.[56]

Disk Herniation and Ring Apophyseal Fractures

Ossification of the vertebral ring apophysis begins at approximately 6 years, and fusion with the vertebral body at approximately 17 years. Until fusion, the junction of the apophysis and the vertebral body is a relatively weak point (**Figure 6**). Ring apophyseal fractures were found to be associated with 28% of adolescent disk herniations and were correlated with more severe symptoms and a greater risk of chronic back pain.[57] True disk herniations are rare in children. The outcomes of surgical disk excision are similar to those of adults.

Spondylolysis

True traumatic spondylolysis is uncommon in children. This high-energy injury usually responds well to nonsurgical treatment. The use of bracing is controversial, and its clinical outcomes are not correlated with fracture healing.[58] Unilateral spondylolysis that is detectable using single photon emission computed tomography, but not plain radiography, responds well to conservative therapy. A patient with spina bifida occulta, however, may be at increased risk of incomplete resolution of symptoms.[59] If nonsurgical measures fail, most authors recommend an attempt at pars repair in adolescents and young adults instead of an L5-S1 fusion.[60] The surgical methods include in situ bone grafting, pedicle screw and hook instrumentation, Scott wiring, and pars intra-articularis screw fixation.

Summary

Pediatric spine trauma is rare but can have catastrophic results. Children with spine trauma, especially those younger than 10 years, require evaluation and management that differs from the evaluation and management of adult patients. Most pediatric spine injuries are amenable to nonsurgical treatment. Recent advances in understanding pathoanatomy, imaging, surgical techniques, and instrumentation should lead to improved outcomes after these injuries.

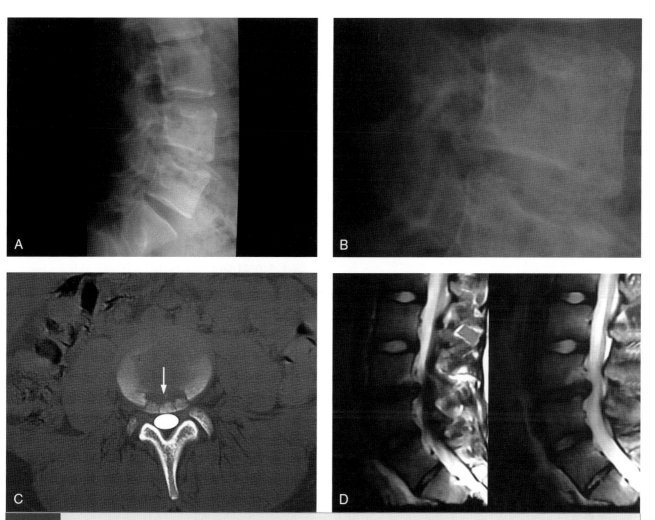

Figure 6 A ring apophyseal fracture in a 16-year-old boy. **A** and **B**, Lateral spine radiographs showing a subtle fracture of the posteroinferior corner of the vertebral body. **C**, Axial CT showing a fracture of the posterior aspect of the vertebral body *(arrow)*. **D**, T2-weighted sagittal MRI studies showing disk herniation *(left)* and posteroinferior vertebral body fracture *(right)*.

Annotated References

1. Platzer P, Jaindl M, Thalhammer G, et al: Cervical spine injuries in pediatric patients. *J Trauma* 2007;62(2):389-396.

   A retrospective analysis of all 56 pediatric cervical spine injuries at one institution between 1980 and 2004 found that 37 patients (66%) had neurologic deficits, and 15 (27%) died.

2. Bilston LE, Brown J: Pediatric spinal injury type and severity are age and mechanism dependent. *Spine (Phila Pa 1976)* 2007;32(21):2339-2347.

   A retrospective review of all 340 spine injuries at two major pediatric trauma centers over a 5-year period examined the relationships among patient age, injury mechanism, spine level, and injury severity.

3. Puisto V, Kääriäinen S, Impinen A, et al: Incidence of spinal and spinal cord injuries and their surgical treatment in children and adolescents: A population-based study. *Spine (Phila Pa 1976)* 2010;35(1):104-107.

   Data were examined for all pediatric spinal and spinal cord injuries treated in one Finnish hospital between 1997 and 2006.

4. Leucht P, Fischer K, Muhr G, Mueller EJ: Epidemiology of traumatic spine fractures. *Injury* 2009;40(2):166-172.

   This is a retrospective analysis of 562 patients with a traumatic fracture of the spine who were treated in one level I trauma center between 1996 and 2000.

5. Vitale MG, Goss JM, Matsumoto H, Roye DP Jr: Epidemiology of pediatric spinal cord injury in the United States: Years 1997 and 2000. *J Pediatr Orthop* 2006;26(6):745-749.

   All pediatric spinal cord injuries identified from two national pediatric databases during 1997 and 2000 were examined to identify their incidence and mechanisms.

6: Musculoskeletal Trauma

6. Dogan S, Safavi-Abbasi S, Theodore N, Horn E, Rekate HL, Sonntag VK: Pediatric subaxial cervical spine injuries: Origins, management, and outcome in 51 patients. *Neurosurg Focus* 2006;20(2):E1.

    A retrospective review of all 51 pediatric subaxial cervical spine injuries at one institution between 1999 and 2005 found that the injuries were more common among older children; 51% were successfully treated using nonsurgical measures.

7. Dogan S, Safavi-Abbasi S, Theodore N, et al: Thoracolumbar and sacral spinal injuries in children and adolescents: A review of 89 cases. *J Neurosurg* 2007;106(6, suppl):426-433.

    A retrospective review of all 89 pediatric admissions for thoracic, lumbar, or sacral spine trauma between 1997 and 2005 found that these injuries were more common in older children and that multilevel injuries were common.

8. Santiago R, Guenther E, Carroll K, Junkins EP Jr: The clinical presentation of pediatric thoracolumbar fractures. *J Trauma* 2006;60(1):187-192.

    A retrospective case-controlled study of all 96 thoracolumbar fractures at a pediatric level I trauma center between 1997 and 2001 found that the injuries occurred in adolescents. The physical examination sensitivity for thoracolumbar spine fractures was 87%.

9. Wang MY, Hoh DJ, Leary SP, Griffith P, McComb JG: High rates of neurological improvement following severe traumatic pediatric spinal cord injury. *Spine (Phila Pa 1976)* 2004;29(13):1493-1497.

10. Junkins EP Jr, Stotts A, Santiago R, Guenther E: The clinical presentation of pediatric thoracolumbar fractures: A prospective study. *J Trauma* 2008;65(5):1066-1071.

    A prospective case-controlled study examined the sensitivity and specificity of clinical examination in detecting pediatric thoracolumbar spine fractures. A sensitivity of 81% and a specificity of 68% were found.

11. Ehrlich PF, Wee C, Drongowski R, Rana AR: Canadian C-spine rule and the national emergency X-radiography utilization low-risk criteria for C-spine radiography in young trauma patients. *J Pediatr Surg* 2009;44(5):987-991.

    A 2-year retrospective case-matched study of 1,307 trauma patients younger than 10 years found that the sensitivity and specificity of two separate adult clinical decision-making protocols were inadequate for evaluating young children.

12. Mahan ST, Mooney DP, Karlin LI, Hresko MT: Multiple level injuries in pediatric spinal trauma. *J Trauma* 2009;67(3):537-542.

    A retrospective analysis identified 195 patients with spine injuries from a level I pediatric trauma center between 1994 and 2004. One third of the patients sustained multiple spine injuries at contiguous levels, and 6% sustained an injury to a noncontiguous level.

13. Loder RT: The cervical spine, in Morrissy RT, Weinstein SL, eds: *Lovell and Winter's Pediatric Orthopaedics*, ed 4. Philadelphia, PA, Lippincott-Raven, 1996, pp 739-779.

14. Cattell HS, Filtzer DL: Pseudosubluxation and other normal variations in the cervical spine in children: A study of one hundred and sixty children. *J Bone Joint Surg Am* 1965;47(7):1295-1309.

15. Hedequist D: Pediatric spine trauma, in Abel MF, ed: *Orthopaedic Knowledge Update: Pediatrics 3*. Rosemont, IL, American Academy of Orthopaedic Surgeons, 2006, pp 323-331.

16. Rana AR, Drongowski R, Breckner G, Ehrlich PF: Traumatic cervical spine injuries: Characteristics of missed injuries. *J Pediatr Surg* 2009;44(1):151-155.

    A retrospective review of all pediatric trauma patients with cervical spine imaging between 2004 and 2006 found that CT was more sensitive than plain radiography.

17. Avellino AM, Mann FA, Grady MS, et al: The misdiagnosis of acute cervical spine injuries and fractures in infants and children: The 12-year experience of a level I pediatric and adult trauma center. *Childs Nerv Syst* 2005;21(2):122-127.

    This is a retrospective review of all pediatric cervical spine injuries misdiagnosed between 1985 and 1997 during initial emergency department imaging evaluation.

18. Skaggs DL, Lerman LD, Albrektson J, Lerman M, Stewart DG, Tolo VT: Use of a noninvasive halo in children. *Spine (Phila Pa 1976)* 2008;33(15):1650-1654.

    The use of a noninvasive pinless halo vest orthosis is described in 30 children.

19. Bode KS, Newton PO: Pediatric nonaccidental trauma thoracolumbar fracture-dislocation: Posterior spinal fusion with pedicle screw fixation in an 8-month-old boy. *Spine (Phila Pa 1976)* 2007;32(14):E388-E393.

    This is a case report of the successful use of pedicle screws in an infant.

20. Ruf M, Harms J: Pedicle screws in 1- and 2-year-old children: Technique, complications, and effect on further growth. *Spine (Phila Pa 1976)* 2002;27(21):E460-E466.

21. Hedequist D, Hresko T, Proctor M: Modern cervical spine instrumentation in children. *Spine (Phila Pa 1976)* 2008;33(4):379-383.

    Modern segmental cervical spine instrumentation was successfully used in 25 children and young adolescents.

22. Oluigbo CO, Solanki GA: Use of recombinant human bone morphogenetic protein-2 to enhance posterior cervical spine fusion at 2 years of age: Technical note. *Pediatr Neurosurg* 2008;44(5):393-396.

    This is a case report of the use of recombinant human BMP-2 (rhBMP-2) in a 2-year-old child.

23. Oetgen ME, Richards BS: Complications associated with the use of bone morphogenetic protein in pediatric patients. *J Pediatr Orthop* 2010;30(2):192-198.

   In a retrospective review of 81 patients younger than 18 years, 16 complications were identified after rhBMP-2 was used. Only one complication was believed to be directly attributable to the use of rhBMP-2.

24. Harwood PJ, Giannoudis PV: Application of bone morphogenetic proteins in orthopaedic practice: Their efficacy and side effects. 2005;4:75-89.

   This is a review of the use of BMP in orthopaedic surgery.

25. Pang D: Spinal cord injury without radiographic abnormality in children, 2 decades later. *Neurosurgery* 2004;55(6):1325-1343.

26. Pang D, Wilberger JE Jr: Spinal cord injury without radiographic abnormalities in children. *J Neurosurg* 1982;57(1):114-129.

27. Yucesoy K, Yuksel KZ: SCIWORA in MRI era. *Clin Neurol Neurosurg* 2008;110(5):429-433.

   A review of the English-language research literature on SCIWORA and MRI revealed that MRI-negative SCIWORA has a better prognosis than SCIWORA with an MRI-defined abnormality such as hematomyelia, disk herniation, or epidural hematoma.

28. Vialle R, Piétin-Vialle C, Ilharreborde B, Dauger S, Vinchon M, Glorion C: Spinal cord injuries at birth: A multicenter review of nine cases. *J Matern Fetal Neonatal Med* 2007;20(6):435-440.

   This is a retrospective review of nine spinal cord birth injuries.

29. Stawicki SP, Holmes JH, Kallan MJ, Nance ML: Fatal child cervical spine injuries in motor vehicle collisions: Analysis using unique linked national datasets. *Injury* 2009;40(8):864-867.

   Two large national mortality datasets were used to identify 176 fatal cervical spine injuries in children between 1999 and 2002. The identified risk factors included female sex, use of passenger restraints, and traumatic brain injury.

30. Brown J, Bilston LE: Spinal injury in motor vehicle crashes: Elevated risk persists up to 12 years of age. *Arch Dis Child* 2009;94(7):546-548.

   Seventy-two children with spine trauma from a motor vehicle crash were identified at two major children's hospitals between 1999 and 2004. The risk of serious spinal injury was greater in children younger than 12 years. The authors postulate that adequacy of seatbelt fit may have a role.

31. Quiñones-Hinojosa A, Jun P, Manley GT, Knudson MM, Gupta N: Airbag deployment and improperly restrained children: A lethal combination. *J Trauma* 2005;59(3):729-733.

   This is a retrospective analysis of 263 injuries associated with airbag deployment between 1993 and 2002 in patients younger than 19 years.

32. Hosalkar HS, Cain EL, Horn D, Chin KR, Dormans JP, Drummond DS: Traumatic atlanto-occipital dislocation in children. *J Bone Joint Surg Am* 2005;87(11):2480-2488.

   This is a retrospective case study of 16 patients with atlanto-occipital dislocation who were treated at a major children's hospital between 1986 and 2003.

33. Harris JH Jr, Carson GC, Wagner LK: Radiologic diagnosis of traumatic occipitovertebral dissociation: 1. Normal occipitovertebral relationships on lateral radiographs of supine subjects. *AJR Am J Roentgenol* 1994;162(4):881-886.

34. Farley FA, Gebarski SS, Garton HL: Tectorial membrane injuries in children. *J Spinal Disord Tech* 2005;18(2):136-138.

   Of three children with tectorial membrane injury diagnosed by MRI, two were treated with halo immobilization and one underwent occiput-C2 fusion.

35. Guillaume D, Menezes AH: Retroclival hematoma in the pediatric population: Report of two cases and review of the literature. *J Neurosurg* 2006;105(4, suppl):321-325.

   Two patients were diagnosed with posttraumatic retroclival hematoma on MRI. Both were treated nonsurgically, with resolution of the hematoma.

36. Haque A, Price AV, Sklar FH, Swift DM, Weprin BE, Sacco DJ: Screw fixation of the upper cervical spine in the pediatric population: Clinical article. *J Neurosurg Pediatr* 2009;3(6):529-533.

   A retrospective analysis of 17 pediatric patients who underwent screw fixation involving the atlas or axis between 2003 and 2008 found no nonunions, neurovascular injury, or hardware revisions. The authors assert that this technique is viable in children.

37. Heuer GG, Hardesty DA, Bhowmick DA, Bailey R, Magge SN, Storm PB: Treatment of pediatric atlantoaxial instability with traditional and modified Goel-Harms fusion constructs. *Eur Spine J* 2009;18(6):884-892.

   This is a retrospective case review of five pediatric patients who underwent a Goel-Harms fusion (with C1 lateral mass screws and C2 pedicle screws) performed by one surgeon.

38. Hedequist D, Proctor M: Screw fixation to C2 in children: A case series and technical report. *J Pediatr Orthop* 2009;29(1):21-25.

   All 17 patients who underwent surgical fixation to C2 had preoperative CT, and 16 had postoperative CT. The authors believe that screw fixation can be accomplished safely, even in young children.

39. Moorthy RK, Rajshekhar V: Changes in cervical spine curvature in pediatric patients following occipitocervical fusion. *Childs Nerv Syst* 2009;25(8):961-967.

6: Musculoskeletal Trauma

In 14 patients who underwent occipitocervical fusion between 1995 and 2006, follow-up at a mean 16 months revealed an increase in the lordotic curvature of the spine caused by the crankshaft phenomenon.

40. Ishikawa M, Matsumoto M, Chiba K, Toyama Y, Kobayashi K: Long-term impact of atlantoaxial arthrodesis on the pediatric cervical spine. *J Orthop Sci* 2009;14(3): 274-278.

   In eight children who underwent atlantoaxial arthrodesis, follow-up at a mean 11.9 years revealed that the development of postoperative malalignment was common, although most children had spontaneous realignment with growth.

41. Pennecot GF, Gouraud D, Hardy JR, Pouliquen JC: Roentgenographical study of the stability of the cervical spine in children. *J Pediatr Orthop* 1984;4(3):346-352.

42. AuYong N, Piatt J Jr: Jefferson fractures of the immature spine: Report of 3 cases. *J Neurosurg Pediatr* 2009; 3(1):15-19.

   This is a case report of three young children with a Jefferson fracture through the anterior synchondrosis.

43. Reilly CW, Leung F: Synchondrosis fracture in a pediatric patient. *Can J Surg* 2005;48(2):158-159.

   A displaced anterior synchondrosis fracture of C1 was treated with transoral reduction and immobilization in a halo vest.

44. Reilly CW, Choit RL: Transarticular screws in the management of C1-C2 instability in children. *J Pediatr Orthop* 2006;26(5):582-588.

   This is a retrospective review of 12 patients with C1-C2 instability treated with transarticular screw fixation.

45. Gluf WM, Brockmeyer DL: Atlantoaxial transarticular screw fixation: A review of surgical indications, fusion rate, complications, and lessons learned in 67 pediatric patients. *J Neurosurg Spine* 2005;2(2):164-169.

   A retrospective review of 67 pediatric patients who underwent C1-C2 transarticular screw fixation (using 127 screws) found that all patients had successful fusion. There were two vertebral artery injuries.

46. Klimo P Jr, Kan P, Rao G, Apfelbaum R, Brockmeyer D: Os odontoideum: Presentation, diagnosis, and treatment in a series of 78 patients. *J Neurosurg Spine* 2008; 9(4):332-342.

   In a retrospective review, 3 of 78 pediatric and adult patients were found to have neurologic injury after attempted conservative management of known os odontoideum. The authors recommend an aggressive surgical approach to os odontoideum, even in asymptomatic patients.

47. Dickerman RD, Morgan JT, Mittler M: Circumferential cervical spine surgery in an 18-month-old female with traumatic disruption of the odontoid and C3 vertebrae: Case report and review of techniques. *Pediatr Neurosurg* 2005;41(2):88-92.

An 18-month-old girl with traumatic C2-C3 disruption with neurologic compromise was treated with C2-C4 anterior cervical corpectomy and plating and occiput-C3 posterior spinal fusion.

48. Ozer E, Yucesoy K, Kalemci O: Temporary anterior cervical plating in a child with traumatic cervical ligamentous instability. *Pediatr Neurosurg* 2005;41(5):269-271.

   A 7-year-old child with C2-C3 and C3-C4 traumatic instability was treated with anterior cervical fusion and plating. The plate was removed 1 year after surgery.

49. Chamoun RB, Relyea KM, Johnson KK, et al: Use of axial and subaxial translaminar screw fixation in the management of upper cervical spinal instability in a series of 7 children. *Neurosurgery* 2009;64(4):734-739.

   This is a retrospective review of seven pediatric patients who underwent upper cervical translaminar screw fixation for instability.

50. Chern JJ, Chamoun RB, Whitehead WE, Curry DJ, Luerssen TG, Jea A: Computed tomography morphometric analysis for axial and subaxial translaminar screw placement in the pediatric cervical spine. *J Neurosurg Pediatr* 2009;3(2):121-128.

   Cervical spine CT in 69 pediatric patients was used to determine the feasibility of translaminar screw fixation. Although C2 translaminar fixation was deemed anatomically appropriate in 50%, only rarely could the subaxial spine accept translaminar screws.

51. Denis F: The three column spine and its significance in the classification of acute thoracolumbar spinal injuries. *Spine (Phila Pa 1976)* 1983;8(8):817-831.

52. Clark P, Letts M: Trauma to the thoracic and lumbar spine in the adolescent. *Can J Surg* 2001;44(5):337-345.

53. Möller A, Maly P, Besjakov J, Hasserius R, Ohlin A, Karlsson MK: A vertebral fracture in childhood is not a risk factor for disc degeneration but for Schmorl's nodes: A mean 40-year observational study. *Spine (Phila Pa 1976)* 2007;32(22):2487-2492.

   In a retrospective analysis of 20 children who sustained a lumbar or thoracic vertebral fracture without neurologic deficit, the mean follow-up was 40 years. Stable vertebral fractures in childhood did not increase the incidence of disk degeneration, although the incidence of Schmorl nodes was increased.

54. Choit RL, Tredwell SJ, Leblanc JG, Reilly CW, Mulpuri K: Abdominal aortic injuries associated with Chance fractures in pediatric patients. *J Pediatr Surg* 2006;41(6):1184-1190.

   This is a case report of three patients with a Chance fracture associated with abdominal aortic injury, with a review of the literature.

55. de Gauzy JS, Jouve JL, Violas P, et al: Classification of Chance fracture in children using magnetic resonance imaging. *Spine (Phila Pa 1976)* 2007;32(2):E89-E92.

   In a retrospective analysis of 18 flexion-distraction fractures evaluated by MRI in children between 1995 and 2005, the intervertebral disk was intact in all 18. The fracture propagated through the vertebral body in 6 patients, the superior end plate in 8, and the inferior end plate in 4.

56. Mulpuri K, Jawadi A, Perdios A, Choit RL, Tredwell SJ, Reilly CW: Outcome analysis of Chance fractures of the skeletally immature spine. *Spine (Phila Pa 1976)* 2007; 32(24):E702-E707.

A retrospective outcome analysis of 25 skeletally immature patients with a Chance fracture found that patients had low scores on a pain and disability scale at a mean 6.4-year follow-up.

57. Chang CH, Lee ZL, Chen WJ, Tan CF, Chen LH: Clinical significance of ring apophysis fracture in adolescent lumbar disc herniation. *Spine (Phila Pa 1976)* 2008; 33(16):1750-1754.

A retrospective review of 96 adolescents with disk bulging or displacement diagnosed by CT found that 28% had a ring apophyseal fracture, which was hypothesized to be associated with more severe symptoms.

58. Klein G, Mehlman CT, McCarty M: Nonoperative treatment of spondylolysis and grade I spondylolisthesis in children and young adults: A meta-analysis of observational studies. *J Pediatr Orthop* 2009;29(2):146-156.

Symptoms resolved after 1 year in 84% of pediatric patients with spondylolysis and grade I spondylolisthesis, although most did not have radiographic healing. The use of a brace did not affect the outcome.

59. Takemitsu M, El Rassi G, Woratanarat P, Shah SA: Low back pain in pediatric athletes with unilateral tracer uptake at the pars interarticularis on single photon emission computed tomography. *Spine (Phila Pa 1976)* 2006;31(8):909-914.

In a retrospective analysis of 22 patients with spondylolysis that was radiographically negative but positive on single photon emission computed tomography, 82% of patients had an excellent outcome after activity modification and use of a lumbosacral orthosis.

60. Hu SS, Tribus CB, Diab M, Ghanayem AJ: Spondylolisthesis and spondylolysis. *J Bone Joint Surg Am* 2008; 90(3):656-671.

The pathogenesis and treatment options for spondylolisthesis and spondylolysis are reviewed.

Section 7

Sports-Related Topics

SECTION EDITOR:
MININDER S. KOCHER, MD, MPH

Chapter 36

Anterior Cruciate Ligament Injuries

Allen F. Anderson, MD

Introduction

Tears to the anterior cruciate ligament (ACL) are relatively uncommon in pediatric patients. Anatomic factors predispose a skeletally immature patient to an avulsion injury rather than a ligament tear. However, a growing body of evidence indicates that the incidence of ACL tears in children and adolescents is increasing, primarily because of increased sports participation.[1-13] The management of these injuries is both challenging and controversial.

The published evidence indicates that nonsurgical treatment of pediatric ACL tears has a poor outcome[3,14-19] but that reconstruction can cause iatrogenic physeal injury.[8-12] Management decisions are complicated by a deficiency in basic science studies on physeal injury and by the methodologic limitations of clinical studies documenting the results of surgical treatment.

Biomechanics

The ACL is the central part of a unique viscoelastic chain that can fail at different sites, depending on the magnitude and rate of load application as well as the patient's level of skeletal maturity. An ACL tear is more common at a lower load application rate, and an ACL avulsion fracture is more likely at a higher load application rate. The physes are relatively viscoelastic in younger children. As the physes become stiffer with maturity, the incidence of ACL tears increases and that of physeal injury decreases. The transition from predominantly ACL avulsion fractures to predominantly ACL intrasubstance tears occurs before complete physeal closure. One study found that ACL avulsion fracture occurs three times as often in children age 12 years or younger than in older children and adolescents.[4] Another study found that 80% of ACL avulsion fractures occur in children younger than 12 years, and 90% of intrasubstance

tears occur in older children and adolescents.[20] Whether an ACL tear in a child or adolescent is partial or complete depends on a myriad of factors. Partial tears are more common in skeletally immature children than in adults.

Epidemiology and Natural History

The prevalence of ACL tears in children and adolescents is unknown. ACL tears were found in 10% to 65% of skeletally immature patients with acute hemarthrosis of the knee.[1,18] The natural history of pediatric ACL tears has not been clearly documented. A growing body of evidence shows that partial ACL tears without an associated pivot shift have a generally favorable natural history in both skeletally immature and adult patients.[14] In contrast, studies found that the natural history of complete ACL tears is unfavorable in skeletally immature patients, for behavioral and other reasons.[3,14-19] Children and adolescents with an ACL deficiency tend to be noncompliant with activity restrictions, rehabilitation, and bracing. Consequently, recurrent instability, meniscal injury, and articular cartilage damage frequently occur.

Surgical reconstruction of an ACL tear in a skeletally immature patient ideally should be postponed until skeletal maturity. The only published evidence on nonsurgical treatment is from small case studies that included patients of different ages and lacked control subjects. These studies suggest that the risk of nonsurgical treatment of the knee may exceed that of surgical reconstruction.[14-19]

Maturity Assessment

The most important concern in the surgical treatment of an ACL tear in a child or adolescent is the patient's stage of skeletal maturity, which determines the severity of consequences of any iatrogenic injury. The effect of a physeal injury may be severe in a child who has a great deal of growth remaining, but it may be inconsequential in a teenager with minimal growth remaining in the distal femoral and proximal tibial physes.

Dr. Anderson or an immediate family member serves as a board member, owner, officer, or committee member of the American Orthopaedic Society for Sports Medicine; and serves as a paid consultant to or is an employee of Genzyme.

Table 1

The Tanner Staging of Secondary Sexual Characteristics, With Peak Height Velocity and Menarche

	Characteristics	
Stage or Event	Male	Female
Tanner I (prepubescent)	No pubic hair	No breast development No pubic hair
Tanner II (prepubescent)	Minimal pubic hair	Breast buds Minimal pubic hair
Tanner III (pubescent)	Pubic hair over penis Voice change Muscle mass increase	Enlargement of breasts and areola Pubic hair on mons Axillary hair
Tanner IV	Adult pubic hair Axillary hair	Areola enlargement Adult pubic hair
Tanner V (postpubescent)	Adult maturation	Adult maturation
Peak height velocity	Average age, 13.5 years	Average age, 11.5 years
Menarche		Average age, 12.7 years

The concept of skeletal maturity represents a wide spectrum. Chronologic age is an excellent predictor of skeletal maturity in large populations, but individual patients may significantly vary from the average. Therefore, chronologic age alone is not sufficient for determining the potential consequences of physeal injury. Instead, it is necessary to estimate the patient's skeletal and physiologic age. The most common method of estimating skeletal age is to compare an AP radiograph of the patient's left hand and wrist to an age-specific radiograph in the Greulich and Pyle atlas of normal standards.[21] Physiologic age can be classified using the Tanner staging of sexual maturation[22] (Table 1). Preliminary staging of physiologic age is done before surgery by questioning the patient about the date of menarche or the growth of axillary and pubic hair. The Tanner staging can be confirmed after induction of anesthesia in the operating room. A prepubescent patient is categorized into Tanner stage I or II (Figure 1), a pubescent patient into Tanner stage III or IV (Figures 2 and 3), and a postpubescent patient into Tanner stage V (Figure 4).

Normal Growth

The most rapidly growing physis is in the distal femur, and the second most rapidly growing physis is in the proximal tibia. The growth of the distal femur is 1.3 cm per year until the last 2 years before skeletal maturity, when the growth rate decreases to 0.65 cm per year. The distal femoral physis contributes 40% of the lower extremity length. The proximal tibial physis contributes 0.9 cm of growth per year until the last 2 years before skeletal maturity, when the rate decreases to 0.5 cm per year.[23] The proximal tibial physis contributes 27% of the overall lower extremity length.[24]

Peak height velocity in boys on average occurs at age 13.5 years, usually at Tanner stage IV. However, 20% of boys do not reach peak height velocity until Tanner stage V. Peak height velocity occurs approximately 2 years earlier in girls, at age 11.5 years and in Tanner stage III. Peak height velocity in girls precedes menarche by approximately 1 year.

The severity of an iatrogenic growth disturbance can be predicted by the patient's skeletal maturity when the injury occurred. A 3-cm limb-length discrepancy (almost three times the normal limb-length variance) can occur if complete closure of the proximal tibial physis occurs in a 12-year-old boy with average development, if complete closure of the distal femoral physis occurs in an average 13-year-old boy, or if complete closure of both physes occurs in an average 14-year-old boy.

Angular deformity is an even greater concern than limb-length discrepancy. A valgus flexion deformity can be caused by an over-the-top femoral groove if the perichondral ring of LaCroix is damaged. Recurvatum can occur if the anterior tibial physis is injured. In the worst-case scenario, an average 14-year-old boy with 2 cm of growth remaining could develop a 14° valgus deformity or an 11° recurvatum.[25] Prepubescent patients (Tanner stage I or II) are at greatest risk, followed by early pubescent patients (Tanner stage III). Patients at the lowest risk are nearing skeletal maturity (Tanner stage IV or V).

Risk Factors for Growth Disturbance

Evidence from basic science research on physeal injuries, although incomplete and not entirely generalizable to humans, is useful in assessing the risk factors for growth disturbance. The risk generally is associated

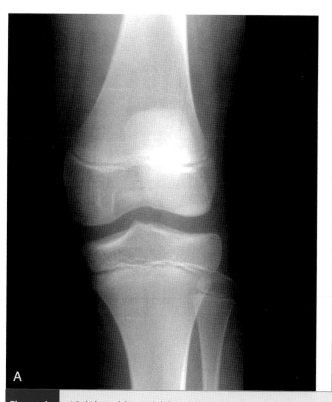
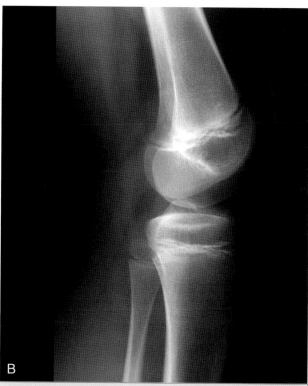

Figure 1 AP (**A**) and lateral (**B**) radiographs showing the left knee of a prepubescent boy (Tanner stage I) with a chronologic age and a bone age of 10 years 6 months. He is at high risk for growth disturbance and should be treated with a transepiphysis-sparing procedure or a modified physis-sparing procedure.

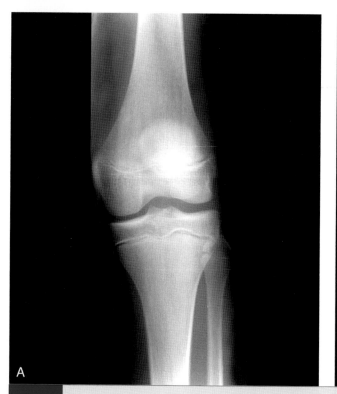
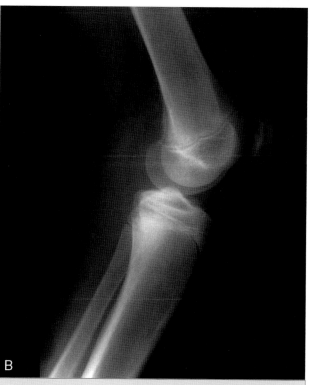

Figure 2 AP (**A**) and lateral (**B**) radiographs showing the left knee of a pubescent boy (Tanner stage III) with a chronologic age and a bone age of 13 years 7 months. He is at intermediate risk of growth disturbance. The treatment of such a patient is controversial. Pending the availability of high-level evidence, the safest treatment may be a transepiphyseal or modified physis-sparing procedure.

7: Sports-Related Topics

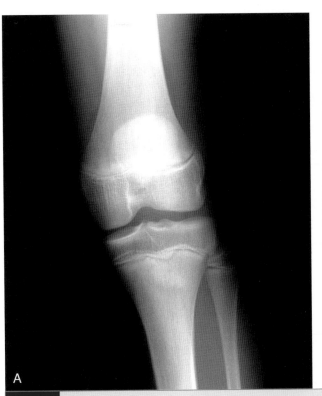
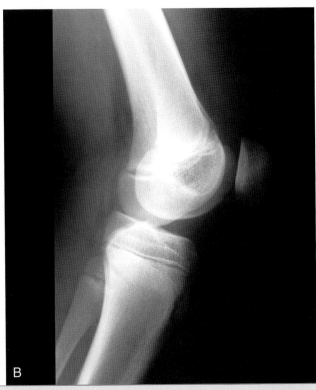

Figure 3 AP (**A**) and lateral (**B**) radiographs showing the left knee of a pubescent boy (Tanner stage III) with a chronologic age of 13 years 3 months and a bone age of 14 years 6 months. Because of his higher bone age, this patient is at lower risk for growth disturbance than the patient shown in Figure 2. He was treated with a transphyseal reconstruction using quadruple hamstring tendon grafts.

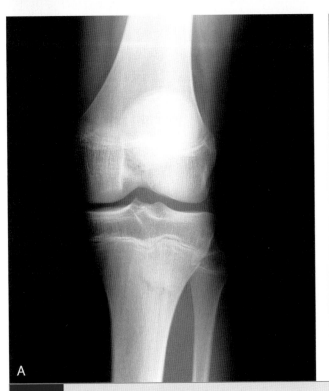
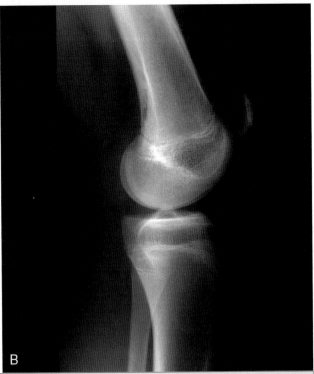

Figure 4 AP (**A**) and lateral (**B**) radiographs showing the left knee of a postpubescent boy nearing skeletal maturity, with a chronologic age of 14 years 3 months and a bone age of 16 years. He was treated with a standard adult ACL reconstruction.

with the extent of damage to the cross-sectional area of the physis. In animal models, the threshold for growth disturbance appears to be 3% to 4% of the cross-sectional area.[26-28] However, neither animal studies nor clinical studies of children have determined the drill hole size or orientation that can be used without risking growth disturbance.

Studies designed to evaluate the safety of placing a soft-tissue graft through a transphyseal hole have not had uniform results. Three animal model studies found that the soft tissue provided no protection,[27-29] but two other studies found that a soft-tissue graft across the physis prevented growth disturbance.[30,31] Despite these mixed animal study results, it is quite likely that soft-tissue grafts placed across the physis are protective against bone bridging and growth arrest in adolescents.

Researchers have determined that graft tensioning across an open physis can cause valgus femoral and varus tibial deformities.[32,33] These results indicate that the physis responds to the Hueter-Volkmann principle, which states that compressive forces applied perpendicular to the physis can inhibit longitudinal growth. The implication is that even physis-sparing procedures can pose a risk in pediatric patients.

Treatment

There is no consensus on the best method of treating complete ACL tears in children and adolescents. The lack of consensus primarily relates to the paucity of basic science research on physeal response to injury and the poor methodology and data quality of the clinical studies. However, the current pediatric literature can be used to develop a reasonable treatment plan based on the consequences of iatrogenic growth disturbance.

Nonsurgical Management

Nonsurgical management is especially appealing for the treatment of ACL tears in children and adolescents. The advantages of treating patients with bracing, rehabilitation, and activity modification include psychological maturation of the patient, which improves compliance with postoperative rehabilitation; and greater skeletal maturity, which permits less risky and more traditional ACL reconstructions. For these reasons, some surgeons still recommend a nonsurgical approach. Noncompliance with nonsurgical treatment is an important concern, however. Prohibiting sports participation, sometimes for years, is onerous for children. In addition, a child may be injured during free play.

A large body of evidence in the literature provides compelling evidence that nonsurgical treatment of an ACL tear in children carries a high probability of long-term knee impairment.[3,14-19]

Surgical Procedures

Some surgical procedures, such as primary repair and extra-articular replacement, have led to poor outcomes in pediatric patients.[5,16,17] It is possible to minimize the risk of physeal injury, improve stability, and thus avoid long-term knee impairment by performing a modified physis-sparing interarticular replacement.[1,7,13] Placing the iliotibial band or hamstring tendons over the top of the lateral femoral condyle and through a groove in the tibia has been done in a modified ACL replacement. Although the over-the-top position has not caused growth disturbance, the graft is not isometric. The over-the-top femoral position results in 10 mm of graft elongation with knee extension.[34] Transepiphyseal reconstruction of the ACL using quadruple hamstring tendons has been recommended as a more anatomic intra-articular ACL replacement in children and adolescents. This procedure adheres to the well-accepted principles of ACL replacement in adults, and theoretically it minimizes the risk of physeal injury without transgressing on the tibial or femoral physis.[13]

Intra-articular transphyseal replacement with quadruple hamstring grafts also has been used to reconstruct the ACL.[2] This procedure remains controversial because of the deficiencies in the basic science and clinical studies. Basic science studies have not determined the protective effects of using soft-tissue graft, the safe drill hole size, or the safe graft tension. The clinical studies showing the safety of transphyseal replacements primarily included postmenarchal girls and postpubescent boys nearing skeletal maturity, who have a relatively low risk of angular deformity or limb-length discrepancy.[10-13,33]

Current Recommendation

The scientific rigor that can be provided by multicenter research is necessary to clarify the contradictions in the literature and help determine the best method of surgically treating pediatric patients with a torn ACL. Until high-level evidence is available, most surgeons modify the procedure to suit the patient's physiologic and skeletal age, which determines the severity of any growth disturbance. The patients at highest risk are in Tanner stage I or II, which represent prepubescent boys younger than 12 years and girls younger than 11 years. These patients can be treated effectively and with relative safety using a transepiphyseal procedure with quadruple hamstring tendon grafts (**Figure 5**) or a modified physis-sparing technique with iliotibial band grafts (**Figure 6**). The treatment of intermediate-risk patients in early Tanner stage III is more controversial. Until high-level evidence is available to clarify the optimal procedure, a physis-sparing procedure may be safest for these patients. Later pubescent patients at Tanner stage III or IV (13 to 16 years in boys and 12 to 14 years in girls) are nearing skeletal maturity and, therefore, are

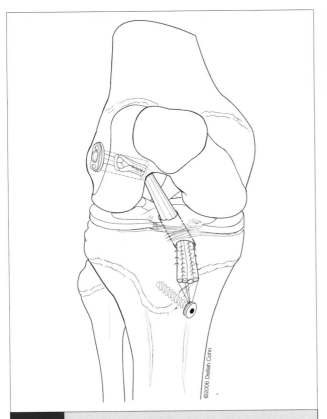

Figure 5 Schematic drawing showing a transepiphyseal physis-sparing ACL reconstruction with a quadruple hamstring tendon graft secured proximally with an Endobutton (Smith & Nephew, Memphis, TN) and distally with a screw and post. (©2006 Delilah Cohn, Nashville, TN.)

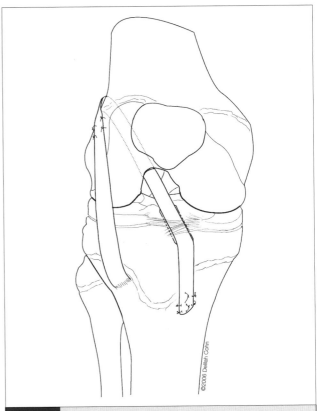

Figure 6 Schematic drawing showing a modified physis-sparing procedure in which a strip of iliotibial band graft is passed over the lateral femoral condyle and through a groove in the tibia, then sutured to the tibial periosteum. (©2006 Delilah Cohn, Nashville, TN.)

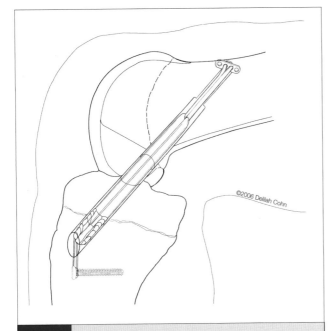

Figure 7 Schematic drawing showing a transphyseal reconstruction with a quadruple hamstring tendon graft secured proximally with an Endobutton and distally with a screw and post. (©2006 Delilah Cohn, Nashville, TN.)

at lower risk for growth disturbance. These patients can be safely treated using a transphyseal reconstruction with small, centrally placed perpendicular drill holes and quadruple hamstring grafts (**Figure 7**). Patients at Tanner stage V (boys older than 16 years and girls older than 14 years) can be treated with a standard adult ACL reconstruction.

Summary

The incidence of ACL injuries in children and adolescents is increasing, primarily because of increased sports participation. For behavioral or other reasons, nonsurgical treatment often leads to instability, meniscal tears, and cumulative degenerative changes. Current research indicates that surgical reconstruction is the best method of treatment for ACL tears in this age group. However, there is no consensus on the best surgical technique because of a deficiency in basic science studies on physeal injury and the methodologic limitations of clinical studies documenting the results of different surgical techniques. Until better evidence is available, the surgical techniques used to reconstruct the ACL in this age group should be modified to reduce the consequences of possible growth disturbance. A high-risk prepubescent patient should be treated with a physis-sparing technique. The treatment of intermediate-risk patients is controversial; they can be treated with a physis-sparing or a transphyseal technique. A lower risk patient should be treated with a transphyseal technique using a soft-tissue graft.

Annotated References

1. Kocher MS, Garg S, Micheli LJ: Physeal sparing reconstruction of the anterior cruciate ligament in skeletally immature prepubescent children and adolescents. *J Bone Joint Surg Am* 2005;87(11):2371-2379.

   Forty-four skeletally immature patients in Tanner stage I or II underwent a physis-sparing combined intra-articular and extra-articular reconstruction of the ACL with an autogenous iliotibial band graft. Two patients underwent revision for graft failure. The mean International Knee Documentation Committee score was 96.7. The Lachman test was normal in 23 patients, almost normal in 18 patients, and abnormal in 1 patient. Four of the 23 patients had repeat meniscal repair. The mean growth from surgery to final evaluation was 21.5 cm. There was no growth disturbance.

2. Kocher MS, Smith JT, Zoric BJ, Lee B, Micheli LJ: Transphyseal anterior cruciate ligament reconstruction in skeletally immature pubescent adolescents. *J Bone Joint Surg Am* 2007;89(12):2632-2639.

   Fifty-nine patients (61 knees) who were in Tanner stage III and had a mean chronologic age of 14.7 years underwent transphyseal ACL reconstruction with the use of a quadruple hamstring graft. Two patients had graft failure. The mean International Knee Documentation Committee score was 89.5. The pivot shift was normal in 56 patients and nearly normal in 3. The growth from surgery to follow-up was 8.2 cm, with no growth disturbance.

3. Aichroth PM, Patel DV, Zorrilla P: The natural history and treatment of rupture of the anterior cruciate ligament in children and adolescents: A prospective review. *J Bone Joint Surg Br* 2002;84(1):38-41.

4. Stanitski CL, Harvell JC, Fu F: Observations on acute knee hemarthrosis in children and adolescents. *J Pediatr Orthop* 1993;13(4):506-510.

5. Engebretsen L, Svenningsen S, Benum P: Poor results of anterior cruciate ligament repair in adolescence. *Acta Orthop Scand* 1988;59(6):684-686.

6. Parker AW, Drez D Jr, Cooper JL: Anterior cruciate ligament injuries in patients with open physes. *Am J Sports Med* 1994;22(1):44-47.

7. Micheli LJ, Rask B, Gerberg L: Anterior cruciate ligament reconstruction in patients who are prepubescent. *Clin Orthop Relat Res* 1999;364(364):40-47.

8. Lipscomb AB, Anderson AF: Tears of the anterior cruciate ligament in adolescents. *J Bone Joint Surg Am* 1986;68(1):19-28.

9. Kocher MS, Saxon HS, Hovis WD, Hawkins RJ: Management and complications of anterior cruciate ligament injuries in skeletally immature patients: Survey of the Herodicus Society and the ACL Study Group. *J Pediatr Orthop* 2002;22(4):452-457.

10. Pressman AE, Letts RM, Jarvis JG: Anterior cruciate ligament tears in children: An analysis of operative versus nonoperative treatment. *J Pediatr Orthop* 1997;17(4):505-511.

11. Andrews M, Noyes FR, Barber-Westin SD: Anterior cruciate ligament allograft reconstruction in the skeletally immature athlete. *Am J Sports Med* 1994;22(1):48-54.

12. McCarroll JR, Shelbourne KD, Porter DA, Rettig AC, Murray S: Patellar tendon graft reconstruction for midsubstance anterior cruciate ligament rupture in junior high school athletes: An algorithm for management. *Am J Sports Med* 1994;22(4):478-484.

13. Anderson AF: Transepiphyseal replacement of the anterior cruciate ligament in skeletally immature patients: A preliminary report. *J Bone Joint Surg Am* 2003;85(7):1255-1263.

14. Kannus P, Järvinen M: Knee ligament injuries in adolescents: Eight year follow-up of conservative management. *J Bone Joint Surg Br* 1988;70(5):772-776.

15. Angel KR, Hall DJ: Anterior cruciate ligament injury in children and adolescents. *Arthroscopy* 1989;5(3):197-200.

16. Graf BK, Lange RH, Fujisaki CK, Landry GL, Saluja RK: Anterior cruciate ligament tears in skeletally immature patients: Meniscal pathology at presentation and after attempted conservative treatment. *Arthroscopy* 1992;8(2):229-233.

17. McCarroll JR, Rettig AC, Shelbourne KD: Anterior cruciate ligament injuries in the young athlete with open physes. *Am J Sports Med* 1988;16(1):44-47.

18. Millett PJ, Willis AA, Warren RF: Associated injuries in pediatric and adolescent anterior cruciate ligament tears: Does a delay in treatment increase the risk of meniscal tear? *Arthroscopy* 2002;18(9):955-959.

19. Mizuta H, Kubota K, Shiraishi M, Otsuka Y, Nagamoto N, Takagi K: The conservative treatment of complete tears of the anterior cruciate ligament in skeletally immature patients. *J Bone Joint Surg Br* 1995;77(6):890-894.

20. Kellenberger R, von Laer L: Nonosseous lesions of the anterior cruciate ligaments in childhood and adolescence. *Prog Pediatr Surg* 1990;25:123-131.

21. Greulich WW, Pyle SL: *Radiographic Atlas of Skeletal Development of the Hand and Wrist,* ed 2. Stanford, CA, Stanford University Press, 1959.

22. Tanner JM, Whitehouse RH: Clinical longitudinal standards for height, weight, height velocity, weight velocity, and stages of puberty. *Arch Dis Child* 1976;51(3):170-179.

23. Pritchett JW: Longitudinal growth and growth-plate activity in the lower extremity. *Clin Orthop Relat Res* 1992;275(275):274-279.

24. Anderson M, Green WT, Messner MB: Growth and predictions of growth in the lower extremities. *Am J Orthop* 1963;45:1-14.

25. Wester W, Canale ST, Dutkowsky JP, Warner WC, Beaty JH: Prediction of angular deformity and leg-length discrepancy after anterior cruciate ligament reconstruction in skeletally immature patients. *J Pediatr Orthop* 1994;14(4):516-521.

26. Mäkelä EA, Vainionpää S, Vihtonen K, Mero M, Rokkanen P: The effect of trauma to the lower femoral epiphyseal plate: An experimental study in rabbits. *J Bone Joint Surg Br* 1988;70(2):187-191.

27. Guzzanti V, Falciglia F, Gigante A, Fabbriciani C: The effect of intra-articular ACL reconstruction on the growth plates of rabbits. *J Bone Joint Surg Br* 1994;76(6):960-963.

28. Houle JB, Letts M, Yang J: Effects of a tensioned tendon graft in a bone tunnel across the rabbit physis. *Clin Orthop Relat Res* 2001;391:275-281.

29. Babb JR, Ahn JI, Azar FM, Canale ST, Beaty JH: Transphyseal anterior cruciate ligament reconstruction using mesenchymal stem cells. *Am J Sports Med* 2008;36(6):1164-1170.

    Fifteen immature rabbits were divided into three surgical groups. Group 1 had drilling through the distal femoral and proximal tibial physis; group 2 had drilling and reconstruction with an extensor tendon autograft; and group 3 had drilling, reconstruction with an extensor tendon autograft, and seeding with mesenchymal stem cells. Bony bridges and angular deformity occurred in groups 1 and 2, but not in group 3. The soft-tissue graft did not prevent growth disturbance, but the addition of mesenchymal stem cells prevented or minimized growth disturbance.

30. Janarv PM, Wikström B, Hirsch G: The influence of transphyseal drilling and tendon grafting on bone growth: An experimental study in the rabbit. *J Pediatr Orthop* 1998;18(2):149-154.

31. Stadelmaier D, Arnoczky S, Dodds J, Ross H: The effects of drilling and soft tissue grafting across open growth plates: A histologic study. *Am J Sports Med* 1995;23(4):431-435.

32. Chudik S, Beasley L, Potter H, Wickiewicz T, Warren R, Rodeo S: The influence of femoral technique for graft placement on anterior cruciate ligament reconstruction using a skeletally immature canine model with a rapidly growing physis. *Arthroscopy* 2007;23(12):1309-1319, e1.

    Three different femoral techniques for ACL reconstruction were performed in immature canines. Achilles tendon autografts were tensioned at 80 N using transepiphyseal, over-the-top, or transphyseal technique. Angular and rotational deformities were noted. The transepiphyseal technique resulted in less angular deformity and was more anatomic, but it carried a risk of rotational deformity.

33. Edwards TB, Greene CC, Baratta RV, Zieske A, Willis RB: The effect of placing a tensioned graft across open growth plates: A gross and histologic analysis. *J Bone Joint Surg Am* 2001;83(5):725-734.

34. Odensten M, Gillquist J: Functional anatomy of the anterior cruciate ligament and a rationale for reconstruction. *J Bone Joint Surg Am* 1985;67(2):257-262.

Chapter 37

Meniscal Injuries and the Discoid Lateral Meniscus

Dennis E. Kramer, MD   Mininder S. Kocher, MD, MPH

Introduction

Meniscal injuries in children are increasing in incidence. These injuries are believed to have greater healing potential than adult meniscal tears. Prompt diagnosis and meniscal repair have led to excellent clinical results. A discoid meniscus most commonly occurs in the lateral meniscus, and it represents a spectrum of morphologic abnormalities resulting in meniscal enlargement with varying instability. A highly unstable discoid meniscus often appears in a younger child as a so-called snapping knee. More stable discoid variants often are asymptomatic but in adolescents are likely to tear. An asymptomatic discoid meniscus should be observed, but a symptomatic, unstable discoid meniscus should be treated with saucerization and repair.

Meniscal Injuries

The exact incidence of injuries to the meniscus in children and adolescents is unknown, but it appears to be increasing because of widespread athletic participation, greater physician familiarity with the injury, and the availability and use of MRI and arthroscopy.[1] The healing potential of the pediatric meniscus and the consequences of meniscectomy in a young, active patient (including increased contact forces and early osteoarthritic changes) underscore the importance of properly diagnosing and treating pediatric meniscal injuries.

Neither Dr. Kramer nor any immediate family member has received anything of value from or owns stock in a commercial company or institution related directly or indirectly to the subject of this chapter. Dr. Kocher or an immediate family member serves as a board member, owner, officer, or committee member of the American Academy of Orthopaedic Surgeons, the ACL Study Group, the American Orthopaedic Society for Sports Medicine, the Herodicus Society, the Pediatric Orthopaedic Society of North America, and the Steadman Hawkins Research Foundation; has received royalties from Biomet; serves as a paid consultant to or is an employee of Biomet, OrthoPediatrics, PediPed, and Smith & Nephew; and owns stock or stock options in Fixes 4 Kids and Pivot Medical.

New surgical techniques have facilitated arthroscopic meniscal repair, which has become the standard of care for repairable tears.

Anatomy and Function

The C-shaped medial meniscus covers 50% of the medial tibial plateau and has ligamentous attachments to the tibia through the coronary ligament and to the deep medial collateral ligament through the meniscotibial ligament. These attachments prevent the medial meniscus from translating more than 2 to 5 mm with knee motion. The circular lateral meniscus covers 70% of the lateral tibial plateau and lacks attachments to the fibular collateral ligament or the popliteal hiatus. This lack of attachment allows increased mobility of the lateral meniscus, which normally translates 9 to 11 mm during knee motion. The meniscal blood supply arises from the geniculate arteries, which form a peripheral perimeniscal synovial plexus. The developing meniscus is fully vascularized at birth, but its vascularity gradually diminishes to the peripheral 10% to 30% of the meniscus (the so-called red-red zone); by age 10 years, it resembles the adult meniscus.[2,3] Synovial diffusion is responsible for the nutrition of the central portion of the meniscus. The medial and lateral menisci share the load and reduce the contact stresses across the knee joint, transmitting 50% to 70% of the load in extension and 85% of the load in 90° of flexion.[4]

Diagnosis

Nondiscoid meniscal tears usually occur in older children and adolescents as the result of a twisting knee injury.[3,5-7] Concurrent ligament injuries, such as a tear of the anterior cruciate ligament (ACL), are common.[7] Meniscal injuries in children generally appear as joint line pain and swelling. A pediatric medial or lateral meniscal tear can be reliably diagnosed by an experienced examiner; one study found 62% sensitivity and 80% specificity for a medial tear and 50% sensitivity and 89% specificity for a lateral tear.[8] The modified McMurray test (40° of knee flexion with rotational varus or valgus stress) can be used for children who resist the traditional McMurray test. The Lachman test is reliable in children, although comparison to the contralateral

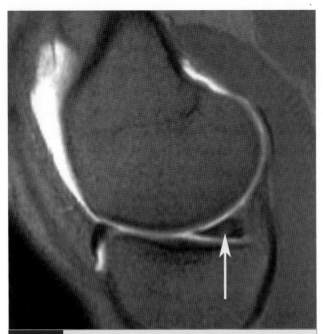

Figure 1 Sagittal T2-weighted MRI showing a high intrameniscal signal *(arrow)* in the posterior horn of the developing meniscus of an adolescent patient.

knee is necessary.[9] Knee radiographs, including the tunnel and sunrise views, can rule out alternative diagnoses, including patellar subluxation, osteochondritis dissecans, and osteochondral loose bodies.[10]

MRI can be helpful in diagnosing and characterizing meniscal disorders in children and adolescents. In skeletally immature children, MRI is 79% sensitive and 92% specific for medial meniscal tears, and it is 67% sensitive and 83% specific for lateral meniscal tears.[11] MRI may not be necessary for the diagnosis, however. Normal variant signal abnormalities seen on MRI in younger children can be mistaken for a meniscal tear. MRI is less sensitive or specific for diagnosing a meniscal tear in children younger than 12 years than in children age 12 to 16 years (62% sensitive and 90% specific in younger children, 78% sensitive and 95.5% specific in older children).[11] The high vascularity of the developing meniscus is believed to cause an intrameniscal signal change that can be misinterpreted as a tear[12] (**Figure 1**).

Management

Fifty percent to 90% of meniscal tears in children are peripheral longitudinal tears, which have a great healing potential.[13] A bucket-handle tear is not uncommon, often involving a large portion of the meniscus. A small (less than 10-mm) longitudinal tear in the peripheral red-red zone that can be manually displaced less than 3 mm often heals on its own.[14] However, surgery is indicated for most symptomatic meniscal tears in children. Given the consequences of partial meniscectomy and

the healing potential in children, meniscal repair should be attempted for most middle- and peripheral-third tears, especially if ACL reconstruction is being done concurrently. Meniscal repair is preferable to meniscectomy for a larger, unstable tear because of the high risk of osteoarthritis 10 to 20 years after meniscectomy.[15] A judicious partial meniscectomy may be required for a degenerative pattern such as a horizontal cleavage, radial, or complex tear. Contact forces increase in proportion to the volume of meniscal tissue removed.[16]

The meniscus is arthroscopically repaired using an outside-in, inside-out, or all-inside technique. The common surgical principles include repair site preparation with abrasion or trephination, anatomic reduction, and stable fixation. Recent advances have expanded the role of the all-inside repair. Second-generation suture-based systems limit chondral wear and provide suture compression across the tear. In a relatively small knee, an all-inside repair places the posterior neurovascular structures at risk because of instrument size and overpenetration of the posterior capsule. A standard inside-out approach is safest to use for a smaller knee. An anterior horn tear is best repaired using an outside-in approach.

Results

Few studies have specifically analyzed the results of meniscal repair in children. At 5-year follow-up, one study found 100% clinical healing in 26 patients (mean age, 15.3 years; range, 11 to 17 years). Of the 29 meniscal repairs, 25 used an inside-out technique, and 4 used an all-inside technique.[17] Another study analyzed arthroscopic repairs in which an inside-out technique was used on meniscal tears extending into the central avascular zone in 71 children (mean age, 16 years; range, 9 to 19 years; skeletal immaturity, 88%). At a mean 51-month follow-up, 53 patients (75%) were clinically healed, including 39 of 45 patients (87%) who underwent simultaneous ACL reconstruction.[18] A retrospective study of meniscal repair in 12 children (mean age, 13 years; range, 8 to 16 years) found that 7 were asymptomatic, 2 had occasional pain, and 3 (25%) had required partial meniscectomy at 3-year follow-up.[19] Long-term data are lacking, and it is unknown whether meniscal repair lowers the rate of future osteoarthritis. The complications of meniscal repair in children include neurovascular injury, arthrofibrosis, and infection. Only two incidences of arthrofibrosis and one painful neuroma of the infrapatellar branch of the saphenous nerve were reported.[17]

Discoid Menisci

A discoid meniscus is block shaped, thickened, and enlarged, and it occupies a larger-than-normal portion of the tibial plateau (**Figure 2**). Ninety-seven percent of discoid menisci occur in the lateral meniscus. The prevalence is greatest in children of Asian descent (15% of incidences). The true prevalence is unknown, however, because many discoid menisci are asymptomatic.[20,21] A normal meniscus is never discoid during development, and a discoid meniscus probably represents a congenital variant.[2,22]

Anatomy and Classification

Discoid menisci represent a spectrum of abnormalities of meniscal size, shape, and peripheral rim stability. The classic Watanabe description identified three variants. Types I and II are stable, uniformly thick (8 to 10 mm), and block shaped; tibial plateau coverage by the discoid meniscus is complete in type I and less than 80% in type II. A type III discoid meniscus is unstable, has a variable appearance, and lacks peripheral posterior attachments except for the ligament of Wrisberg.[23] A recent study of 128 discoid lateral menisci (62% complete, 38% incomplete) found peripheral rim instability in 28%; 47% had instability at the anterior horn, 40% in the posterior third, and 11% in the middle third (2% had complete detachment at all three sites).[24] Rim instability was associated with a young age (mean, 8.2 years) and a complete discoid meniscus.[24]

Discoid menisci have fewer collagen fibers and a more disorganized arrangement than normal menisci, and these characteristics may be responsible for their higher rates of tearing.[25] Horizontal cleavage tearing accounts for 58% to 98% of tears in discoid menisci; it probably is caused by repetitive microtrauma leading to delamination.[10,26-29] Mucoid fibrinous degeneration often occurs.[29]

Diagnosis

Most discoid menisci are asymptomatic. Some unstable variants appear as the snapping-knee syndrome, in which painless snapping occurs as the knee moves from flexion to extension and the unstable meniscus reduces to its normal position. Physical examination may reveal a lateral joint line bulge with knee flexion, and the McMurray test may elicit a clunk. The contralateral knee is involved in as many as 20% of children. A stable discoid meniscus is asymptomatic but prone to tearing. Often a stable discoid meniscus is diagnosed in an older adolescent with signs of meniscal injury including joint line pain, effusion, and a positive McMurray test.[2]

Radiographic findings usually are normal; the classic findings of squaring of the lateral femoral condyle, cupping of the lateral tibial plateau, widening of the joint line, and meniscal calcification are uncommon.[10] MRI has low sensitivity (39%) in comparison with physical examination (89%) for the diagnosis of discoid lateral meniscus in children.[11] Sagittal MRI may show the bow-tie sign (continuity between the anterior and posterior horns, as seen in three or more 5-mm MRI slices), and coronal MRI may show a meniscal diameter of more than 15 mm or 20% of the total tibial width[10,30] (Figure 3). Many discoid menisci are incomplete and appear normal.[8] On T2-weighted MRI, the Wrisberg variant (Watanabe type III) may have subtle

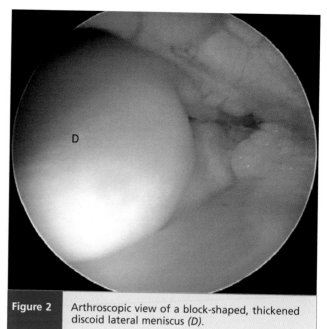

anterior subluxation of the posterior horn with a high signal interposed between the posterior horn and capsule.[31]

Management

An asymptomatic discoid meniscus usually is left untreated, as the knee may have adapted to the discoid anatomy.[8,27] Such a meniscus may be incidentally discovered during arthroscopy. A symptomatic discoid meniscus is best treated with arthroscopic saucerization, which preserves meniscal tissue, rather than total meniscectomy.

The goal of arthroscopic saucerization of a discoid lateral meniscus is to create a stable and functioning meniscus that will provide adequate shock absorption without retearing.[1] Most authors recommend leaving intact a 6- to 8-mm peripheral rim of tissue because larger remnants are associated with higher rates of retearing.[27,29,32] The indentation on the lateral femoral condyle and the size of the medial meniscus also can guide the amount of resection.[10,33] Saucerization is accomplished using a combination of low-profile arthroscopic baskets, shavers, and a meniscal knife (Figure 4). Cleavage tears within the zone of saucerization are excised. After saucerization, peripheral rim stability is carefully assessed with a probe. If necessary, unstable areas of the saucerized meniscus are repaired to the capsule.

Results

Total meniscectomy is still preferred by a few authors who believe residual discoid tissue is abnormal and will not function properly.[34,35] Many studies have reported significantly high rates of osteoarthritis after total meniscectomy, however.[6,15,28,36,37] At 19.8-year follow-up,

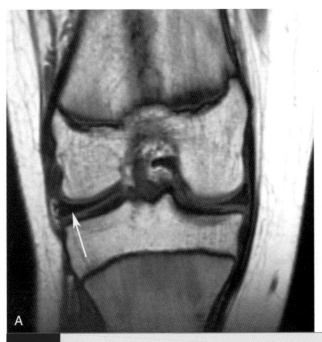
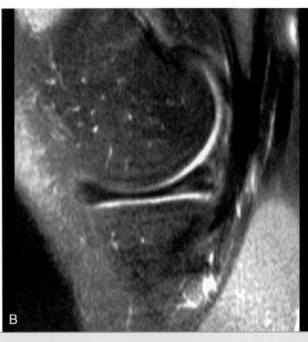

Figure 3 A, Coronal T1-weighted MRI showing a discoid lateral meniscus *(arrow)* occupying the entire lateral tibial plateau. B, Sagittal T2-weighted MRI showing continuity between the anterior and posterior horns (the bow-tie sign).

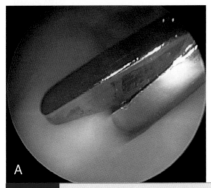
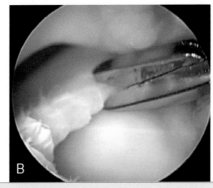
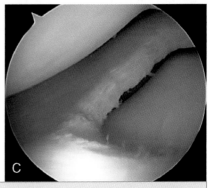

Figure 4 Arthroscopic views showing saucerization of a discoid lateral meniscus A, A low-profile basket was used to begin the procedure. B, Gradual progression of the saucerization. C, The final appearance, with preservation of a 6- to 8-mm rim of meniscal tissue.

10 of 17 children treated with total meniscectomy had clinical and radiographic changes consistent with lateral compartment arthritis.[28] An analysis of 125 discoid menisci found that partial meniscectomy had better results than total meniscectomy after more than 5 years; the long-term prognosis was related to the amount of meniscal tissue removed.[36] Multiple studies reported that osteochondritis dissecans of the lateral femoral condyle can develop after a total meniscectomy to treat discoid lateral meniscus.[38,39] Another study found an association between osteochondritis dissecans of the lateral femoral condyle and the presence of a complete or incomplete discoid lateral meniscus.[40]

Recent studies found that arthroscopic saucerization has favorable short-term results. At 4.5-year follow-up, a good or excellent clinical result and an absence of de-generative radiographic changes were reported in 11 children treated with arthroscopic saucerization.[41] A study of 27 consecutive children (mean age, 10.1 years) who underwent arthroscopic saucerization found that 77% of the discoid menisci had peripheral instability that required repair.[26] All patients had an excellent clinical result at 3.1-year follow-up. Long-term studies are lacking to determine the efficacy of saucerization in preventing lateral compartment knee arthritis. Meniscal allograft transplantation may be an option for a symptomatic patient who has undergone an earlier total meniscectomy to treat discoid lateral meniscus. At a mean 4.8-year follow-up after meniscal allograft transplantation in 14 patients, Lysholm knee scores had improved from 71.4 to 91.4, and six second-look arthroscopies revealed only one retear.[42]

Annotated References

1. Kramer DE, Micheli LJ: Meniscal tears and discoid meniscus in children: Diagnosis and treatment. *J Am Acad Orthop Surg* 2009;17(11):698-707.

   Anatomy, diagnosis, management, results, and complications associated with meniscal tears and discoid menisci in children are comprehensively reviewed.

2. Clark CR, Ogden JA: Development of the menisci of the human knee joint: Morphological changes and their potential role in childhood meniscal injury. *J Bone Joint Surg Am* 1983;65(4):538-547.

3. Greis PE, Bardana DD, Holmstrom MC, Burks RT: Meniscal injury: I. Basic science and evaluation. *J Am Acad Orthop Surg* 2002;10(3):168-176.

4. Ahmed AM, Burke DL: In-vitro measurement of static pressure distribution in synovial joints: Part I. Tibial surface of the knee. *J Biomech Eng* 1983;105(3):216-225.

5. Busch MT: Meniscal injuries in children and adolescents. *Clin Sports Med* 1990;9(3):661-680.

6. Manzione M, Pizzutillo PD, Peoples AB, Schweizer PA: Meniscectomy in children: A long-term follow-up study. *Am J Sports Med* 1983;11(3):111-115.

7. Stanitski CL, Harvell JC, Fu F: Observations on acute knee hemarthrosis in children and adolescents. *J Pediatr Orthop* 1993;13(4):506-510.

8. Kocher MS, Micheli LJ: The pediatric knee: Evaluation and treatment, in Insall JN, ed: *Surgery of the Knee*, ed 3. Philadelphia, PA, Churchill-Livingstone, 2001, pp 1374-1376.

9. Flynn JM, Mackenzie W, Kolstad K, Sandifer E, Jawad AF, Galinat B: Objective evaluation of knee laxity in children. *J Pediatr Orthop* 2000;20(2):259-263.

10. Kocher MS, Klingele K, Rassman SO: Meniscal disorders: Normal, discoid, and cysts. *Orthop Clin North Am* 2003;34(3):329-340.

11. Kocher MS, DiCanzio J, Zurakowski D, Micheli LJ: Diagnostic performance of clinical examination and selective magnetic resonance imaging in the evaluation of intraarticular knee disorders in children and adolescents. *Am J Sports Med* 2001;29(3):292-296.

12. Takeda Y, Ikata T, Yoshida S, Takai H, Kashiwaguchi S: MRI high-signal intensity in the menisci of asymptomatic children. *J Bone Joint Surg Br* 1998;80(3):463-467.

13. Fu F, Baratz ME: Meniscal injuries, in DeLee J, Drez D, eds: *Orthopaedic Sports Medicine: Principles and Practice*. Philadelphia, PA, WB Saunders, 1994, pp 1146-1162.

14. Weiss CB, Lundberg M, Hamberg P, DeHaven KE, Gillquist J: Non-operative treatment of meniscal tears. *J Bone Joint Surg Am* 1989;71(6):811-822.

15. Lohmander LS, Englund PM, Dahl LL, Roos EM: The long-term consequence of anterior cruciate ligament and meniscus injuries: Osteoarthritis. *Am J Sports Med* 2007;35(10):1756-1769.

    Poor-quality studies were found to limit meta-analysis in a review of the literature on long-term consequences of ACL and meniscal injuries. An approximately 50% rate of osteoarthritis was noted at 10- to 20-year follow-up.

16. Baratz ME, Fu FH, Mengato R: Meniscal tears: The effect of meniscectomy and of repair on intraarticular contact areas and stress in the human knee: A preliminary report. *Am J Sports Med* 1986;14(4):270-275.

17. Mintzer CM, Richmond JC, Taylor J: Meniscal repair in the young athlete. *Am J Sports Med* 1998;26(5):630-633.

18. Noyes FR, Barber-Westin SD: Arthroscopic repair of meniscal tears extending into the avascular zone in patients younger than twenty years of age. *Am J Sports Med* 2002;30(4):589-600.

19. Accadbled F, Cassard X, Sales de Gauzy J, Cahuzac JP: Meniscal tears in children and adolescents: Results of operative treatment. *J Pediatr Orthop B* 2007;16(1):56-60.

    A retrospective study of 12 arthroscopic meniscal repairs of nondiscoid tears in children younger than 17 years found that 7 patients were asymptomatic, 2 had minor pain, and 3 had undergone revision partial meniscectomy at 3-year follow-up.

20. Jordan MR: Lateral meniscal variants: Evaluation and treatment. *J Am Acad Orthop Surg* 1996;4(4):191-200.

21. Young R: The external semilunar cartilage as a complete disc, in Cleland J, Mackey JY, Young RB, eds: *Memoirs and Memoranda in Anatomy*. London, England, Williams and Norgate, 1887, pp 179-187.

22. Kaplan EB: Discoid lateral meniscus of the knee joint: Nature, mechanism, and operative treatment. *J Bone Joint Surg Am* 1957;39(1):77-87.

23. Watanabe M, Takeda S, Ikeuchi H: *Atlas of Arthroscopy*, ed 3. Tokyo, Japan, Igaku-Shoin, 1979.

24. Klingele KE, Kocher MS, Hresko MT, Gerbino P, Micheli LJ: Discoid lateral meniscus: Prevalence of peripheral rim instability. *J Pediatr Orthop* 2004;24(1):79-82.

25. Atay OA, Pekmezci M, Doral MN, Sargon MF, Ayvaz M, Johnson DL: Discoid meniscus: An ultrastructural study with transmission electron microscopy. *Am J Sports Med* 2007;35(3):475-478.

    The ultrastructure of the discoid meniscus was compared to that of a normal meniscus using transmission

7: Sports-Related Topics

electron microscopy. Discoid menisci had fewer collagen fibers and a more disorganized arrangement.

26. Good CR, Green DW, Griffith MH, Valen AW, Widmann RF, Rodeo SA: Arthroscopic treatment of symptomatic discoid meniscus in children: Classification, technique, and results. *Arthroscopy* 2007;23(2):157-163.

    In a retrospective study of 30 knees treated with saucerization, 77% of menisci had tears and 77% had peripheral rim instability (predominantly at the anterior horn). Most patients had a good result at 37.4-month follow-up. An arthroscopic classification system is proposed.

27. Hayashi LK, Yamaga H, Ida K, Miura T: Arthroscopic meniscectomy for discoid lateral meniscus in children. *J Bone Joint Surg Am* 1988;70(10):1495-1500.

28. Räber DA, Friederich NF, Hefti F: Discoid lateral meniscus in children: Long-term follow-up after total meniscectomy. *J Bone Joint Surg Am* 1998;80(11):1579-1586.

29. Smith CF, Van Dyk GE, Jurgutis J, Vangsness CT Jr: Cautious surgery for discoid menisci. *Am J Knee Surg* 1999;12(1):25-28.

30. Silverman JM, Mink JH, Deutsch AL: Discoid menisci of the knee: MR imaging appearance. *Radiology* 1989;173(2):351-354.

31. Singh K, Helms CA, Jacobs MT, Higgins LD: MRI appearance of Wrisberg variant of discoid lateral meniscus. *AJR Am J Roentgenol* 2006;187(2):384-387.

    The MRI appearance of the Wrisberg-variant discoid meniscus is described. Subtle anterior subluxation of the posterior horn can be seen, with high T2-weighted signal interposed between the posterior horn and capsule.

32. Atay OA, Doral MN, Leblebicioğlu G, Tetik O, Aydingöz U: Management of discoid lateral meniscus tears: Observations in 34 knees. *Arthroscopy* 2003;19(4):346-352.

33. Kocher MS: Discoid lateral meniscus saucerization and repair, in Micheli LJ, Kocher MS, eds: *The Pediatric and Adolescent Knee.* Philadelphia, PA, Elsevier, 2006, pp 264-271.

    A detailed, comprehensive description of the surgical technique for lateral meniscus saucerization and repair is presented.

34. Habata T, Uematsu K, Kasanami R, et al: Long-term clinical and radiographic follow-up of total resection for discoid lateral meniscus. *Arthroscopy* 2006;22(12):1339-1343.

    A retrospective study of 37 knees (mean patient age, 31.2 years) found that at a mean 14.5-year follow-up after total meniscectomy for discoid lateral meniscus, most patients had excellent functional scores and mild radiographic changes consistent with osteoarthritis.

35. Okazaki K, Miura H, Matsuda S, Hashizume M, Iwamoto Y: Arthroscopic resection of the discoid lateral meniscus: Long-term follow-up for 16 years. *Arthroscopy* 2006;22(9):967-971.

    A retrospective study of 29 knees found good clinical results and few radiographic changes of osteoarthritis at an average 16-year follow-up after total meniscectomy for a torn discoid meniscus. Results were best for patients younger than 25 years.

36. Kim SJ, Chun YM, Jeong JH, Ryu SW, Oh KS, Lubis AM: Effects of arthroscopic meniscectomy on the long-term prognosis for the discoid lateral meniscus. *Knee Surg Sports Traumatol Arthrosc* 2007;15(11):1315-1320.

    A retrospective study of 125 complete and incomplete discoid menisci treated with partial or total meniscectomy found that partial meniscectomy had better radiographic results after 5 years. The long-term prognosis was related to the volume of removed meniscus.

37. Wroble RR, Henderson RC, Campion ER, el-Khoury GY, Albright JP: Meniscectomy in children and adolescents: A long-term follow-up study. *Clin Orthop Relat Res* 1992;279:180-189.

38. Hashimoto Y, Yoshida G, Tomihara T, et al: Bilateral osteochondritis dissecans of the lateral femoral condyle following bilateral total removal of lateral discoid meniscus: A case report. *Arch Orthop Trauma Surg* 2008;128(11):1265-1268.

    A 12-year-old boy developed bilateral osteochondritis dissecans of the lateral femoral condyle after bilateral total meniscectomy for discoid lateral meniscus.

39. Mizuta H, Nakamura E, Otsuka Y, Kudo S, Takagi K: Osteochondritis dissecans of the lateral femoral condyle following total resection of the discoid lateral meniscus. *Arthroscopy* 2001;17(6):608-612.

40. Deie M, Ochi M, Sumen Y, et al: Relationship between osteochondritis dissecans of the lateral femoral condyle and lateral menisci types. *J Pediatr Orthop* 2006;26(1):79-82.

    The relationship between osteochondritis dissecans of the lateral femoral condyle and the presence of a discoid meniscus was retrospectively analyzed in 38 knees. The lateral meniscus was completely discoid in 19 knees, partially discoid in 15, and normal in 4.

41. Oğüt T, Kesmezacar H, Akgün I, Cansü E: Arthroscopic meniscectomy for discoid lateral meniscus in children and adolescents: 4.5 year follow-up. *J Pediatr Orthop B* 2003;12(6):390-397.

42. Kim JM, Bin SI: Meniscal allograft transplantation after total meniscectomy of torn discoid lateral meniscus. *Arthroscopy* 2006;22(12):1344-1350.e1.

    A retrospective study of clinical results in 14 patients who had meniscal allograft transplantation after total meniscectomy for torn discoid meniscus found improved Lysholm knee scores and one retear at a mean 4.8-year follow-up.

Chapter 38

Juvenile Osteochondritis Dissecans

Theodore J. Ganley, MD   Christopher R. Hydorn, MD

7: Sports-Related Topics

Introduction

Osteochondritis dissecans (OCD) is an acquired, potentially reversible disorder of the subchondral bone and overlying articular cartilage. Its etiology and pathogenesis remain an enigma, as does its treatment in some patients. The initial softening of the overlying articular cartilage with an intact articular surface (**Figure 1**) can progress to early articular cartilage separation, partial detachment of an articular lesion, and eventually osteochondral separation with loose bodies. OCD in its juvenile form is a relatively common cause of knee pain and dysfunction in children and adolescents.

Juvenile OCD (JOCD) has a much better prognosis than its adult counterpart. JOCD is a lesion of the articular cartilage and subchondral bone that occurs before closure of the physis, particularly in the distal femoral physis. The etiology of JOCD is unknown, but repetitive microtrauma often is implicated. Boys are more commonly affected than girls, by a 61:39 ratio.[1] Increased sport participation by girls and by younger children of both sexes has led to an increased incidence of JOCD. Although JOCD lesions can be found in most joints, those in the knee and elbow are the focus of this chapter; JOCD in the ankle is discussed in chapter 41.

History and Etiology

OCD originally was described as quiet necrosis. The exact etiology of the condition is unknown but probably is multifactorial. Inflammation, genetic predisposition, ischemia, accessory centers of ossification, and repetitive trauma have been implicated in the etiology of JOCD. Most studies of etiology do not differentiate between JOCD and adult OCD, however. Adult OCD is believed to develop during adolescence and to persist during adulthood. The etiology originally was believed to be inflammatory (hence the name osteochondritis dissecans), but later research has not supported inflam-

mation as a primary cause of OCD. JOCD has been ascribed to an ossification abnormality of the distal femoral epiphysis. Abnormalities in ossification do not account for most incidences of OCD, but an ossification variant may account for some lateral femoral condyle lesions that are incidentally found in younger children and resolve spontaneously. Ischemia also was implicated in OCD lesions. However, later studies have not found osteonecrosis of the OCD fragment or a relative ischemic watershed of the lateral aspect of the medial femoral condyle.[2,3] A genetic predisposition to OCD has been suggested. One researcher found OCD only in one of 86 first-degree relatives, but others found as many as 12 family members with OCD over the course of four generations.[4,5] It is widely believed that the common form of OCD is not familial.

A "violent rotation inwards of the tibia, driving the tibial spine against the inner condyle" was suggested as the cause of OCD.[6] Although anterior tibial spine impingement may not account for OCD lesions in their most common location (the posterolateral aspect of the medial femoral condyle), a repetitive traumatic etiology

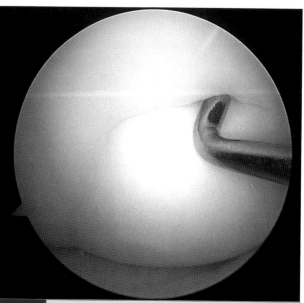

Figure 1 Arthroscopic view of the medial femoral condyle, with the arthroscopic probe pointing to the partially fissured and softened articular cartilage overlying an OCD lesion.

is suggested by the common occurrence of OCD in patients who are involved in sports with repetitive impact.[7] OCD may begin when repetitive trauma causes a stress reaction, which progresses to a stress fracture of the underlying subchondral bone. As the repetitive loading continues, the ability of the subchondral bone to heal is exceeded, necrosis of the fragment occurs, and eventually fragment dissection and separation develop.

OCD of the humeral capitellum is an acquired lesion that is increasing in incidence among young athletes who experience excessive loading of the radiocapitellar joint. Although the etiology of this condition is unknown, its high prevalence among throwing athletes, gymnasts, weight lifters, and cheerleaders suggests a role for microtrauma and overuse of the joint, leading to fatigue fracture of the subchondral bone at the site of repetitive lateral compression.[8]

In histologic studies on core samples from OCD lesions, the changes in the dissecate (the loose osteochondral fragment of the OCD lesion) were found to be unstable at the level of the macroscopic separation of the lesion from the bone.[9] There also is variability in the matrix of the articular cartilage, with evidence of disorganization of the cartilage homeostasis and an increase in embryologic processes and markers. The embryologic processes, combined with the viability of cells within the dissecate, suggest preservation of an intrinsic repair capacity within the tissue.[10] Biopsy specimens taken at the time of surgery were compared with specimens taken an average of 7.8 months later in 10 patients who had undergone fixation of an unstable OCD knee lesion. The cartilage of the dissecates was found to be improved in terms of histologic grading scores and regeneration.[11]

An OCD lesion may resemble acute osteochondral fracture, chondral injury, or osteonecrosis. Thirty years ago, the estimated incidence of OCD lesions in the knee ranged from 15 to 29 per 100,000 patients of all ages.[12,13] Since then, the mean age of patients with OCD appears to have decreased, and an increasing proportion of patients are girls.[14] The widespread use of MRI and arthroscopy in pediatric patients probably has led to greater recognition of OCD lesions. Trends in youth sports such as the loss of free play, early sport specialization, multiple-team participation in a single sport, and intensive training may be contributing factors.

The true natural history of OCD is not known, but a large multicenter European study has provided clues.[1] Patients with knee JOCD had a better outcome than adults with knee OCD; 22% had an abnormal knee at follow-up, compared with 42% of adults with OCD. The outcome of JOCD is significantly better if the lesion is stable at diagnosis and in the classic location on the medial femoral condyle and if the patient is relatively inactive. Patients with a stable lesion at diagnosis had a better outcome after nonsurgical rather than surgical treatment, regardless of the type of nonsurgical

treatment. Conversely, patients with an unstable lesion had a better outcome after surgical rather than nonsurgical treatment.[1] Adult and juvenile OCD lesions that do not heal have the potential for later sequelae, including osteoarthritis.

Diagnosis

Clinical Evaluation

Knee

Most children and adolescents with JOCD have a stable lesion. The symptoms are nonspecific and most commonly consist of aching and activity-related pain in the anterior aspect of the knee. The symptoms resemble those of chondromalacia patella and subtle forms of patellofemoral malalignment. In both OCD and patellofemoral pain, symptoms may be produced by climbing hills or stairs. A multicenter study found that 32% of patients initially had little or no pain.[1] Children with JOCD usually do not report knee instability. With progression of the disease, the patient may report that the knee gives way, locks, catches, or swells.

The physical examination findings often are subtle. The knee examination is neither sensitive nor specific in a patient with JOCD. Children and adolescents with a stable knee lesion may walk with a slight antalgic gait. With careful palpation through varying amounts of knee flexion, a point of maximum tenderness corresponding to the lesion can be located over the lateral aspect of the distal medial femoral condyle. Knee effusion, crepitus, and extreme pain through a normal range of motion are rarely observed with a stable lesion. Mechanical symptoms are more pronounced if the lesion is unstable. The Wilson sign may be helpful but often is not present.[15] The Wilson test begins with the knee flexed to 90°; the tibia is internally rotated as the knee is extended toward full extension. A positive test elicits pain over the anterior aspect of the medial femoral condyle at approximately 30° of knee flexion. This pain is believed to result from contact of the medial tibial eminence with the OCD lesion.

Elbow

The symptoms in the elbow often are similarly vague. Patients may report mechanical pain and dysfunction, such as grinding, clicking, locking, and motion restriction of the elbow joint. Patients with a capitellar JOCD lesion are likely to have a history of elbow sprain, instability, or trauma. Examination of the elbow joint for a capitellar OCD lesion often reveals range-of-motion deficits in flexion and/or extension. Palpation of the radiocapitellar joint may cause pain. There may be an effusion, synovitis, or crepitus in a chronic lesion.

Imaging Studies

The primary goals of imaging are to characterize the lesion, determine the prognosis with nonsurgical management, and monitor the healing of the lesion. Imaging protocols have received close attention because imaging findings have been linked to the probability of successful nonsurgical treatment.

Knee

Imaging of the knee should begin with AP, lateral, and tunnel radiographs (**Figure 2**). The typical location of a JOCD lesion on the lateral portion of the medial femoral condyle and often on the posterior portion means that the tunnel view is particularly useful (**Figure 3**). A Merchant or skyline view radiograph should be included to detect a patellar lesion. Plain radiographs usually are sufficient to characterize the lesion and rule out other bony pathology, such as acute fracture or subluxation of the knee. In children age 6 years or younger, the distal femoral epiphyseal ossification center may exhibit irregularities that simulate the appearance of JOCD. In older children, the status of the physis (open, closing, or closed) should be assessed, as it has major implications for the prognosis for healing.

Elbow

Imaging of the elbow begins with an AP radiograph in extension and a lateral view in flexion. The capitellum is the most common location for a JOCD lesion of the elbow. The AP and lateral views have low sensitivity for identifying capitellar JOCD. It may be beneficial to obtain a radiocapitellar view to reveal a lesion on the anterior portion of the capitellum. In a study of 15 patients in whom the presence of JOCD was proved surgically or with MRI, a lesion initially was identified on radiographs only in 7 patients and was identified retrospectively on radiographs in 10 patients.[16] In children younger than 10 years, the irregular ossification center seen in Panner disease must not be confused with a JOCD lesion. Panner disease appears as irregularity throughout the epiphysis, whereas JOCD usually is a well-defined subchondral bone lesion. Panner disease often heals after several weeks of rest.

MRI is most useful for determining the size of the lesion and the status of the cartilage in the subchondral bone (**Figure 4**). The extent of bony edema, the presence of a high signal zone beneath the fragment, and

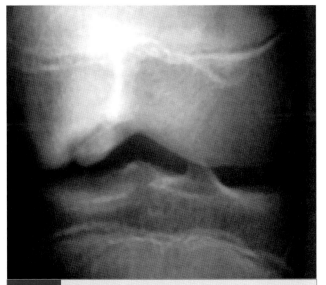

Figure 2 AP radiograph showing OCD of the lateral aspect of the medial femoral condyle.

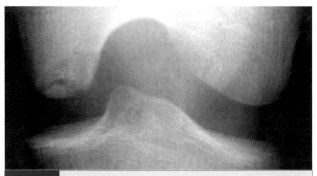

Figure 3 Tunnel radiograph showing OCD of the medial femoral condyle.

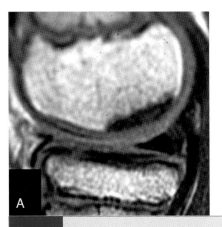 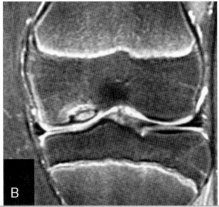 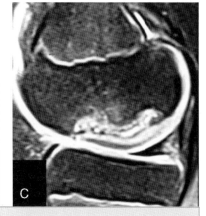

A

B

C

Figure 4 MRI of three OCD lesions. **A**, The articular surface is intact and not marginated. **B**, The articular surface is intact but marginated. **C**, The articular surface is disrupted and marginated.

the presence of loose bodies are additional important findings on the initial MRI. Routine imaging studies during the course of nonsurgical treatment are useful for determining whether a skeletally immature patient is at risk of treatment failure. A high-signal line on T2-weighted studies represents healing vascular granulation tissue or articular fluid beneath the subchondral bone, and it is a predictor of instability.[17-19] A breach in the cartilage, as seen on T1-weighted studies, also can be useful in determining the risk of treatment failure, particularly in conjunction with a high-signal line on T2-weighted studies.[18] Investigations of the relationship between gadolinium enhancement and healing have been inconclusive.[17] A recent study of the healing potential of stable JOCD found that 16 of 47 stable lesions (34%) had not progressed to healing after 6 months of nonsurgical treatment. The size of the lesion as determined on MRI was the strongest prognostic variable.[20] On MRI, the appearance of an OCD lesion of the capitellum is similar to that of an OCD lesion of the femoral condyle. MRI and arthroscopic findings are closely correlated.[21]

Some researchers have found that serial technetium Tc 99m bone scanning can be used to reveal the extent of JOCD healing. This imaging technique has not been widely accepted, however, probably because of the time required, the need for intravenous access, and the perceived risk of the radiotracer injection.

Treatment

The prognosis for JOCD is considerably better than the prognosis for adult OCD. More than 50% of patients have healing within 6 to 18 months of nonsurgical treatment.[1,22] The goals of treatment in JOCD are to preserve the articular cartilage and maintain stability of the lesion. Healing potential can be affected by factors that include lesion size, extent of skeletal maturity, and radiographic findings.[19]

Nonsurgical Treatment

Skeletally immature children with an intact JOCD lesion initially should be treated nonsurgically. The methods commonly include activity restriction and bracing or casting. A wide range of weight-bearing restrictions and immobilization has been recommended, and no algorithm has been proved superior over others. All programs encompass a structured therapy regimen for strength and flexibility, but the value of therapy has not been proved. It is advisable for the patient to refrain from sports participation for as long as 6 months to allow lesions to heal.

Nonsurgical treatment often is recommended for a small, stable lesion in a skeletally immature patient. High-impact activities are limited by instituting short-term immobilization and protected weight bearing. In a large European multicenter study, all nonsurgical treatment methods, including cast immobilization, bracing,

physical therapy, and no weight bearing, had equivocal results (level IV evidence).[1] The type of nonsurgical treatment is less important than its consistent use. A study of the healing potential of stable JOCD found that 31 of 47 stable lesions (66%) healed after 6 months of nonsurgical treatment.[20] The size of the lesion, as determined on MRI, was the strongest prognostic variable for successful healing. JOCD lesions that had progressed toward healing had a significantly smaller surface area (208 mm^2) than JOCD lesions that did not heal (288 mm^2). Larger JOCD lesions with associated swelling or mechanical symptoms at presentation were less likely to heal than those without these symptoms.[20]

Nonsurgical treatment of capitellar OCD is effective in young patients and those with intact cartilage. As determined clinically and radiographically, 90.5% of lesions with intact cartilage healed, but only 52.9% of lesions with fractured articular cartilage healed.[23] Whether the physis is open or closed also is significant; there is a dramatic decrease in healing rate once the physes are closed.[24,25] A level IV retrospective study of baseball pitchers who had a JOCD lesion found that 16 of 17 with open physes healed with nonsurgical measures, but only 11 of 22 with closed physes healed.[25] There is little evidence in the literature to guide specific nonsurgical treatment protocols.

Although immobilization often is successful for treating JOCD, it may not be the ideal option for young athletes. Patients and their parents should be informed of the risks and benefits of nonsurgical treatment compared with surgical treatment.

Surgical Treatment

An algorithm for the treatment of JOCD is provided in **Figure 5**.

Knee

It is widely accepted that surgical treatment should be considered if the patient has an unstable or detached lesion, is approaching skeletal maturity, or has undergone an unsuccessful course of nonsurgical treatment that was approved by the patient, family, and physician. The goals of surgical treatment are to promote the healing of subchondral bone, maintain joint congruity, rigidly fix unstable fragments, and replace osteochondral defects with cells that can replace and grow cartilage. The optimal surgical treatment should provide a stable construct of subchondral bone, a calcified tidemark, and repair cartilage that has viability and biomechanical properties similar to those of native hyaline cartilage.

Arthroscopic drilling is used for a stable lesion with an intact articular surface. Arthroscopic drilling differs from microfracturing in that the cartilage surface often is left intact, subchondral bone exposure is not required, and a drill is used (rather than the pick used for microfracture). Drilling has been used in both antegrade and retrograde fashion.[26,27] Radiographic resolu-

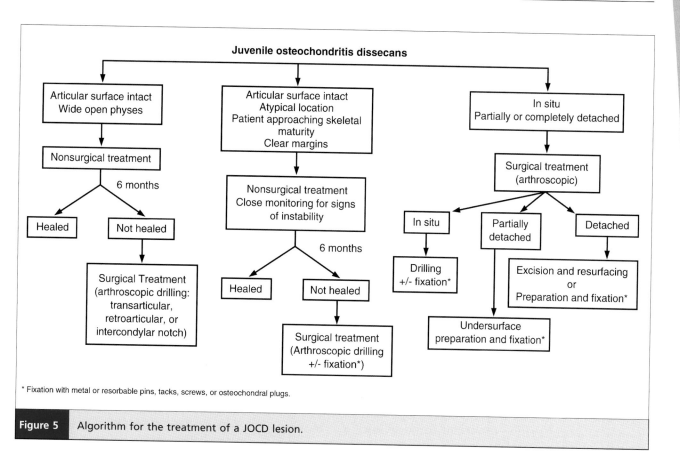

Figure 5 Algorithm for the treatment of a JOCD lesion.

tion and improved Lysholm knee scores have been reported throughout postoperative follow-up.[27,28] Transarticular drilling led to successful healing in 19 of 20 stable lesions in 12 skeletally immature patients (mean age, 12 years).[28] The treatment is much more likely to succeed in children with open physes than in skeletally mature patients. Another study found that 18 of 20 lesions healed in skeletally immature patients but that only 2 of 4 lesions healed in skeletally mature patients at an average 5-year follow-up.[27] Younger age was found to be a predictor of a more favorable post-treatment score on the Lysholm knee scale.[29] However, a multicenter study had comparatively discouraging results; little healing or other benefit was found after transarticular drilling in 58 juvenile and adult patients with marked sclerosis.[1] The factors associated with inadequate healing after drilling included an atypical lesion location, the presence of multiple lesions, and an underlying medical condition.

The goal of surgical treatment of an unstable JOCD lesion is to remove the fibrous tissue between the fragments and underlying bone without disrupting the underlying bone from the fragment or the subchondral bone at the base of the lesion. Open or arthroscopic fixation can be performed if the patient has an unstable or partially unstable lesion with adequate subchondral bone in the defect and fragment. If subchondral bone loss has occurred, autogenous bone graft can be packed into the crater before reduction and fixation. The rapid relief of discomfort upon reduction has led some au-

thors to suspect that the pain is the result of increased pressure at the line of separation between the fragment and the epiphysis.[30,31]

The poor long-term results of excising a loose OCD fragment in skeletally mature patients have led to more aggressive attempts to preserve the articular cartilage and avoid excision. Herbert screws and cannulated screws have been used successfully,[32] but a second surgery may be required to remove them. At 50-month follow-up, a review of Herbert screw fixation found that 14 of 15 knees in 14 patients (age 12 to 35 years) had a stable fragment at second-look arthroscopy.[32] Screw fixation also is reported to have a successful functional outcome. At an average 9 years after loose bodies were treated with screw fixation in 12 patients with JOCD, there were no incidences of osteoarthritis pain, and all patients reported normal knee function.[33]

Good results have been reported with bioabsorbable pin fixation as an alternative to metal fixation.[10,34] Union was found on MRI in all 12 knees (11 patients) treated with bioabsorbable pin fixation; one incidence of early synovitis was successfully treated with non-steroidal anti-inflammatory drugs.[34] Ten unstable JOCD knee lesions in 10 patients (mean age, 15 years) were histologically evaluated before and after treatment with bioabsorbable pins alone or with pins and grafting. The postsurgical specimens had significantly better grading scores as well as signs of regeneration in the articular cartilage.[11] In a retrospective analysis of JOCD knee lesions treated with a bioabsorbable implant, 22 of 24 patients had good or excellent healing of the lesion. One patient had no radiographic improvement, and one patient developed a loose body.[35]

The goal for an unsalvageable fragment is to replace the defect with subchondral bone, calcified tidemark, and overlying cartilage. Drilling, abrasion arthroplasty, and microfracturing are used to recruit pluripotent cells from the bone marrow that will preferentially differentiate into fibrocartilage. These techniques are primarily used for smaller lesions because fibrocartilage does not respond to shear stress as effectively as native hyaline cartilage, and deterioration of the repaired site over time has been reported.[36] Fragment removal with simple débridement of the crater is an alternative. However, weight-bearing AP radiographs at long-term follow-up after fragment removal showed progression of arthritic changes and suggest a poor prognosis for a lesion larger than 2 cm.[37]

A cartilaginous extracellular matrix can be generated in the defect by using periosteum and transplant of the cambium layer. Studies with long-term follow-up suggest that this technique is not ideal because of the high rates of reoperation and persistent knee pain.[19,38] Concerns about the durability of repair fibrocartilage have provided the impetus for developing alternative techniques. Autologous osteochondral plugs obtained from non–weight-bearing regions of the knee, such as the edge of the intercondylar notch or the upper outer trochlea, have been transplanted to replace defects, with good results reported in both skeletally immature and mature patients. A recent prospective randomized study of 47 patients compared treatment with microfracture or autologous osteochondral plugs. Both microfracture and osteochondral autograft had encouraging clinical results, but the lesions treated with osteochondral plugs had better outcomes at 4.2-year follow-up.[39] The potential disadvantages of osteochondral grafting, including donor site morbidity, are balanced by the advantages of biologic internal fixation. Secondary reconstruction with bone–articular surface allograft has been successful in patients with a significant OCD surface defect. No long-term results are available for skeletally immature patients.[40]

Autologous chondrocyte implantation has been used in adolescent patients to repair large, isolated femoral defects, with high success rates. However, information about the long-term outcome is not yet available.[41,42] Autologous chondrocyte transplantation for large defects in the articular cartilage of the distal femur had slightly better outcomes in adolescent patients than in adult patients, probably because of the adolescents' superior articular substance in adjacent regions of the knee.[43,44]

Elbow

Capitellar JOCD lesions can be surgically treated using any of the procedures described for OCD of the knee. The patients who most benefit from fixation of an unstable capitellar lesion have closed physes, fragmentation of the lesion, or a range-of-motion restriction of at least 20°. A recent study evaluated the results of arthroscopic microfracture or osteochondral transfer.[8] At 4-year follow-up, the 25 patients had gained an average of 17° of extension and 10° of flexion. Eighty-six percent had returned to their preinjury level of athletic competition. Some patients required a larger incision for removal of large loose bodies or the addition of bone plugs in deep defects.[8]

Mosaicplasty or osteochondral transfer often is indicated for a relatively large OCD lesion of the capitellum. The results after fragment removal are dependent on lesion size, with defects larger than 50% of the capitellar width having a relatively poor prognosis.[25] Pain and range of motion are significantly better after fragment fixation or reconstruction than after fragment excision alone.[25] A recent outcome study of mosaicplasty in JOCD of the capitellum found a pain-free elbow in 18 of 19 patients and mild pain in 1 patient. Range of motion improved, with 17 patients returning to their preinjury level of athletic activity.[45]

Donor site morbidity is a concern with the use of mosaicplasty or autologous osteochondral transplantation. The donor site usually is over a non–weight-bearing portion of the trochlea or intercondylar notch, and there is the potential for morbidity to an otherwise asymptomatic knee. A review of 11 patients who underwent mosaicplasty of a capitellar lesion with osteochondral plugs from the knee found that all patients had a good or excellent outcome and returned to full athletic activity.[45] However, anterior knee symptoms affecting activities of daily living developed in 6 of 11 patients who underwent osteochondral harvesting from an asymptomatic knee for use in the ankle; 4 of these patients had an unsatisfactory outcome, and 1 patient required additional knee surgery.[46] Cylinder size, number of grafts, and patient age did not affect the outcome of 112 patients after osteochondral plug harvesting from the knee for use elsewhere. However, a high body mass index and low patient satisfaction did lead to knee pain and a relatively low functional outcome.[47]

Summary

The prevalence of OCD of the knee is increasing among children. Careful attention to symptoms and appropriate imaging studies are integral to the diagnosis. Timely recognition is essential because a stable lesion with an intact articular surface usually can be successfully treated nonsurgically. If a stable lesion does not show signs of resolution after 6 months of nonsurgical treatment, arthroscopic drilling should be considered to prevent progression to an unstable lesion. The excision of a large lesion generally has a poor result, but chondral resurfacing techniques may decrease the risk of subsequent arthrosis. Fixation and bone grafting of an unstable lesion and cartilage resurfacing of a full-thickness defect have evolved and have had encouraging results, although further study is required before definitive statements can be made as to the long-term prognosis in children and adolescents. In general, early recognition and treatment of these lesions helps to minimize the extent of intervention for healing.

Annotated References

1. Hefti F, Beguiristain J, Krauspe R, et al: Osteochondritis dissecans: A multicenter study of the European Pediatric Orthopedic Society. *J Pediatr Orthop B* 1999;8(4):231-245.

2. Koch S, Kampen WU, Laprell H: Cartilage and bone morphology in osteochondritis dissecans. *Knee Surg Sports Traumatol Arthrosc* 1997;5(1):42-45.

3. Reddy AS, Frederick RW: Evaluation of the intraosseous and extraosseous blood supply to the distal femoral condyles. *Am J Sports Med* 1998;26(3):415-419.

4. Petrie PW: Aetiology of osteochondritis dissecans: Failure to establish a familial background. *J Bone Joint Surg Br* 1977;59(3):366-367.

5. Mubarak SJ, Carroll NC: Familial osteochondritis dissecans of the knee. *Clin Orthop Relat Res* 1979;140:131-136.

6. Fairbank HA: Osteochondritis dissecans. *Br J Surg* 1933;21(21):67-82.

7. Flynn JM, Kocher MS, Ganley TJ: Osteochondritis dissecans of the knee. *J Pediatr Orthop* 2004;24(4):434-443.

8. Jones KJ, Wiesel BB, Sankar WN, Ganley TJ: Arthroscopic management of osteochondritis dissecans of the capitellum: Mid-term results in adolescent athletes. *J Pediatr Orthop* 2010;30(1):8-13.

   At 4-year follow-up of arthroscopic treatment for an OCD lesion, 25 patients were evaluated for range of motion and outcome.

9. Yonetani Y, Nakamura N, Natsuume T, Shiozaki Y, Tanaka Y, Horibe S: Histological evaluation of juvenile osteochondritis dissecans of the knee: A case series. *Knee Surg Sports Traumatol Arthrosc* 2010;18(6):723-730.

   Histologic findings and cartilage changes were evaluated in eight patients with JOCD lesions.

10. Aurich M, Anders J, Trommer T, et al: Histological and cell biological characterization of dissected cartilage fragments in human osteochondritis dissecans of the femoral condyle. *Arch Orthop Trauma Surg* 2006;126(9):606-614.

    In a histologic and biologic marker evaluation of biopsies from OCD lesions in 14 patients, the authors concluded that the presence of viable cells within the cartilage matrix suggests an intrinsic repair capacity.

11. Adachi N, Motoyama M, Deie M, Ishikawa M, Arihiro K, Ochi M: Histological evaluation of internally-fixed osteochondral lesions of the knee. *J Bone Joint Surg Br* 2009;91(6):823-829.

    A needle biopsy of 10 patients' JOCD lesions revealed significant improvement in histologic grade at follow-up arthroscopy.

12. Hughston JC, Hergenroeder PT, Courtenay BG: Osteochondritis dissecans of the femoral condyles. *J Bone Joint Surg Am* 1984;66(9):1340-1348.

13. Lindén B: The incidence of osteochondritis dissecans in the condyles of the femur. *Acta Orthop Scand* 1976; 47(6):664-667.

14. Cahill BR: Osteochondritis dissecans of the knee: Treatment of juvenile and adult forms. *J Am Acad Orthop Surg* 1995;3(4):237-247.

15. Conrad JM, Stanitski CL: Osteochondritis dissecans: Wilson's sign revisited. *Am J Sports Med* 2003;31(5): 777-778.

16. Kijowski R, De Smet AA: Radiography of the elbow for evaluation of patients with osteochondritis dissecans of the capitellum. *Skeletal Radiol* 2005;34(5):266-271.

    Elbow radiographs were reviewed for 15 patients who were confirmed to have an OCD lesion on MRI or arthroscopy. Seven lesions were prospectively identified, and 10 were retrospectively identified. These results illustrate the difficulty of making an OCD diagnosis from elbow radiographs.

17. Bohndorf K: Osteochondritis (osteochondrosis) dissecans: A review and new MRI classification. *Eur Radiol* 1998;8(1):103-112.

18. O'Connor MA, Palaniappan M, Khan N, Bruce CE: Osteochondritis dissecans of the knee in children: A comparison of MRI and arthroscopic findings. *J Bone Joint Surg Br* 2002;84(2):258-262.

19. Pill SG, Ganley TJ, Milam RA, Lou JE, Meyer JS, Flynn JM: Role of magnetic resonance imaging and clinical criteria in predicting successful nonoperative treatment of osteochondritis dissecans in children. *J Pediatr Orthop* 2003;23(1):102-108.

20. Wall EJ, Vourazeris J, Myer GD, et al: The healing potential of stable juvenile osteochondritis dissecans knee lesions. *J Bone Joint Surg Am* 2008;90(12):2655-2664.

    Multiple variables, including age, lesion size, location, symptoms, and sex, were evaluated for their effect on healing with nonsurgical treatment of JOCD lesions. Level of evidence: II.

21. Kijowski R, De Smet AA: MRI findings of osteochondritis dissecans of the capitellum with surgical correlation. *AJR Am J Roentgenol* 2005;185(6):1453-1459.

7: Sports-Related Topics

The characteristics of OCD lesions in the capitellum are described. OCD lesions in the knee and talus have similar characteristics.

22. Cahill BR, Phillips MR, Navarro R: The results of conservative management of juvenile osteochondritis dissecans using joint scintigraphy: A prospective study. *Am J Sports Med* 1989;17(5):601-606.

23. Matsuura T, Kashiwaguchi S, Iwase T, Takeda Y, Yasui N: Conservative treatment for osteochondrosis of the humeral capitellum. *Am J Sports Med* 2008;36(5):868-872.

   A review of the nonsurgical management of OCD lesions found healing in 90.5% of stage I lesions and 52.9% of stage II lesions. The mean time to healing was 14.9 months or 12.3 months, respectively.

24. Mihara K, Tsutsui H, Nishinaka N, Yamaguchi K: Nonoperative treatment for osteochondritis dissecans of the capitellum. *Am J Sports Med* 2009;37(2):298-304.

   A retrospective review of 39 baseball players at a mean 14.4-month follow-up found a higher rate of healing in patients with open physes.

25. Takahara M, Ogino T, Sasaki I, Kato H, Minami A, Kaneda K: Long term outcome of osteochondritis dissecans of the humeral capitellum. *Clin Orthop Relat Res* 1999;363:108-115.

26. Donaldson LD, Wojtys EM: Extraarticular drilling for stable osteochondritis dissecans in the skeletally immature knee. *J Pediatr Orthop* 2008;28(8):831-835.

   Twelve of 13 knees with a stable JOCD lesion healed after extra-articular drilling.

27. Anderson AF, Richards DB, Pagnani MJ, Hovis WD: Antegrade drilling for osteochondritis dissecans of the knee. *Arthroscopy* 1997;13(3):319-324.

28. Adachi N, Deie M, Nakamae A, Ishikawa M, Motoyama M, Ochi M: Functional and radiographic outcome of stable juvenile osteochondritis dissecans of the knee treated with retroarticular drilling without bone grafting. *Arthroscopy* 2009;25(2):145-152.

   Lysholm scores were used to evaluate radiologic and functional outcomes after retrograde drilling of intact JOCD lesions in 12 patients.

29. Kocher MS, Micheli LJ, Yaniv M, Zurakowski D, Ames A, Adrignolo AA: Functional and radiographic outcome of juvenile osteochondritis dissecans of the knee treated with transarticular arthroscopic drilling. *Am J Sports Med* 2001;29(5):562-566.

30. Johnson LL, Uitvlugt G, Austin MD, Detrisac DA, Johnson C: Osteochondritis dissecans of the knee: Arthroscopic compression screw fixation. *Arthroscopy* 1990;6(3):179-189.

31. Thomson NL: Osteochondritis dissecans and osteochondral fragments managed by Herbert compression screw fixation. *Clin Orthop Relat Res* 1987;224:71-78.

32. Makino A, Muscolo DL, Puigdevall M, Costa-Paz M, Ayerza M: Arthroscopic fixation of osteochondritis dissecans of the knee: Clinical, magnetic resonance imaging, and arthroscopic follow-up. *Am J Sports Med* 2005;33(10):1499-1504.

   Fifteen knees underwent OCD fixation with compression screws into the fragment. MRI and second-look arthroscopy revealed good healing of the lesions.

33. Magnussen RA, Carey JL, Spindler KP: Does operative fixation of an osteochondritis dissecans loose body result in healing and long-term maintenance of knee function? *Am J Sports Med* 2009;37(4):754-759.

   Eleven of 12 patients who underwent fixation of OCD loose bodies had healing and good results with respect to knee function and lack of osteoarthritis at an average 9-year follow-up.

34. Din R, Annear P, Scaddan J: Internal fixation of undisplaced lesions of osteochondritis dissecans in the knee. *J Bone Joint Surg Br* 2006;88(7):900-904.

   Eleven patients (12 knees) underwent bioabsorbable fixation of JOCD fragments. One patient developed a transient synovitis. All patients had achieved union at follow-up.

35. Tabaddor RR, Banffy MB, Andersen JS, et al: Fixation of juvenile osteochondritis dissecans lesions of the knee using poly 96L/4D-lactide copolymer bioabsorbable implants. *J Pediatr Orthop* 2010;30(1):14-20.

   A retrospective review of unstable JOCD lesions treated with bioabsorbable implants found healing in 22 of 24 knees, with no reactions to the degradation products.

36. Mandelbaum BR, Browne JE, Fu F, et al : Articular cartilage lesions of the knee. *Am J Sports Med* 1998;26(6):853-861.

37. Anderson AF, Pagnani MJ: Osteochondritis dissecans of the femoral condyles: Long-term results of excision of the fragment. *Am J Sports Med* 1997;25(6):830-834.

38. Madsen BL, Noer HH, Carstensen JP, Nørmark F: Long-term results of periosteal transplantation in osteochondritis dissecans of the knee. *Orthopedics* 2000;23(3):223-226.

39. Gudas R, Simonaityte R, Cekanauskas E, Tamosiūnas R: A prospective, randomized clinical study of osteochondral autologous transplantation versus microfracture for the treatment of osteochondritis dissecans in the knee joint in children. *J Pediatr Orthop* 2009;29(7):741-748.

   A prospective randomized study of JOCD lesions compared microfracture and osteochondral autologous transfer. The results of both procedures were encouraging, but patients had significantly better results after an osteochondral autologous transfer.

40. Garrett JC: Osteochondritis dissecans. *Clin Sports Med* 1991;10(3):569-593.

41. Bentley G, Biant LC, Carrington RW, et al: A prospective, randomised comparison of autologous chondrocyte implantation versus mosaicplasty for osteochondral defects in the knee. *J Bone Joint Surg Br* 2003;85(2):223-230.

42. Peterson L, Minas T, Brittberg M, Lindahl A: Treatment of osteochondritis dissecans of the knee with autologous chondrocyte transplantation: Results at two to ten years. *J Bone Joint Surg Am* 2003;85(suppl 2):17-24.

43. King PJ, Ganley TJ, Lou JE, Gregg JR: Autologous chondrocyte transplantation for the treatment of large defects in the articular cartilage of the distal femur in adolescent patients. *70th Annual Meetings Proceedings.* Rosemont, IL, American Academy of Orthopaedic Surgeons, 2003.

44. Micheli LJ, Moseley JB, Anderson AF, et al: Articular cartilage defects of the distal femur in children and adolescents: Treatment with autologous chondrocyte implantation. *J Pediatr Orthop* 2006;26(4):455-460.

     The outcomes of 37 patients who underwent autogenous chondrocyte implantation were assessed at 1- to 2-year follow-up using patient questionnaires and scoring systems.

45. Iwasaki N, Kato H, Ishikawa J, Masuko T, Funakoshi T, Minami A: Autologous osteochondral mosaicplasty for osteochondritis dissecans of the elbow in teenage athletes. *J Bone Joint Surg Am* 2009;91(10):2359-2366.

     Retrospective review of capitellar JOCD lesions treated with mosaicplasty found good results in 18 of 19 elbows and no significant donor site complications or morbidity.

46. Reddy S, Pedowitz DI, Parekh SG, Sennett BJ, Okereke E: The morbidity associated with osteochondral harvest from asymptomatic knees for the treatment of osteochondral lesions of the talus. *Am J Sports Med* 2007; 35(1):80-85.

     After osteochondral harvest from an asymptomatic knee for transfer to the talus, 4 of 11 patients had a poor score on the Lysholm knee scale. Level of evidence: IV.

47. Paul J, Sagstetter A, Kriner M, Imhoff AB, Spang J, Hinterwimmer S: Donor-site morbidity after osteochondral autologous transplantation for lesions of the talus. *J Bone Joint Surg Am* 2009;91(7):1683-1688.

     The knee scores and functional outcomes of 112 patients were retrospectively evaluated at 2-year follow-up after osteochondral harvest from an asymptomatic knee. Higher body mass index and satisfaction with the initial procedure were most predictive of the final knee outcome.

Chapter 39

Shoulder Injuries in the Pediatric Athlete

Jeremy S. Frank, MD   Dennis E. Kramer, MD   Mininder S. Kocher, MD, MPH

Introduction

Shoulder injury has become more common in skeletally immature athletes as participation in high-demand overhead sports has become more widespread. The injury patterns are unique to the developing musculoskeletal system and specific to the involved sport. Prompt recognition, meticulous treatment, and effective prevention strategies are critical to forestall long-term functional disability and allow a timely return to play.

Shoulder Anatomy and Maturation

The proximal humeral physis contributes approximately 80% of the longitudinal growth of the upper extremity; it typically fuses at age 14 to 22 years. The hypertrophic zone is particularly vulnerable to the acute macrotraumatic and chronic repetitive microtraumatic forces that often are present in sports activities.[1-5] The capsuloligamentous and muscular structures of the shoulder serve as static and dynamic stabilizers. The dynamic stabilizers are the rotator cuff, deltoid, and scapulothoracic tendons and muscles, which exert a concavity compression force during the midrange of motion to compress the humeral head against the relatively flat glenoid. The static stabilizers (the glenohumeral ligaments, the capsule, the labrum, and the glenoid) function at the terminal range of motion to limit abnormal humeral head translation. Injury to these dynamic and static restraints creates a unique pattern of disability that can limit normal shoulder function in the young athlete.[1-3,6]

A young athlete's maturational stage is a unique factor contributing to injury patterns. A skeletally immature athlete has less muscular development than an adult, and during periods of rapid growth there is a predisposition to repetitive overuse injury in the developing physis.[5] Changes in soft-tissue laxity also have an important role. In a newborn, the predominantly synthesized collagen is of the elastic type III; as the child grows, the ratio of type III to the less elastic type I collagen decreases with each passing year. Individual variations in this ratio may predispose a young athlete to multidirectional instability (MDI) secondary to laxity of the capsuloligamentous structures.[7]

Epidemiology

Injury patterns in the skeletally immature shoulder generally are specific to the sport. Acute traumatic injuries including glenohumeral dislocation, acromioclavicular (AC) separation, and clavicle fracture are common in contact sports.[8] In amateur wrestling, 30% of injuries occur in the upper extremity, most commonly in the shoulder, and AC separations occur as a result of direct blows to the mat.[9] In skiers, 40% of upper extremity injuries occur in the shoulder.[10] Chronic overuse injuries also are common in overhead sports. In baseball pitchers, high-volume repetitive motions and large rotational forces on the proximal humeral physis can lead to chronic physeal stress fractures (known as little league shoulder).[11,12] Internal impingement and MDI are common among tennis players and swimmers. The generally poor training of coaches is a contributing factor to the increasing incidence of shoulder injuries in pediatric athletes. Fewer than 10% of volunteer coaches and 33% of interscholastic coaches have had any type of formal education in sports coaching.[13-15]

Neither of the following authors nor any immediate family members have received anything of value from or owns stock in a commercial company or institution related directly or indirectly to the subject of this chapter: Dr. Frank, Dr. Kramer. Dr. Kocher or an immediate family member has received royalties from Biomet; serves as a paid consultant for or an employee of Biomet, CONMED Linvatec, Covidian, OrthoPediatrics, PediPed, Regen Biologics, and Smith & Nephew; owns stock or stock options in Pivot Medical; has received research or institutional support from CONMED Linvatec; and serves as a board member, owner, officer, or committee member of the American Academy of Orthopaedic Surgeons, the ACL Study Group, the American Orthopaedic Society for Sports Medicine, the Herodicus Society, the Pediatric Orthopaedic Society of North America, and the Steadman Hawkins Research Foundation.

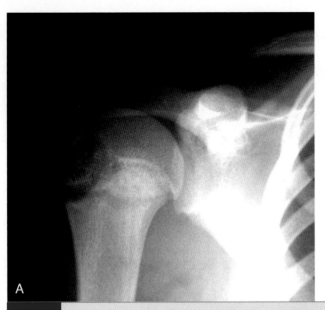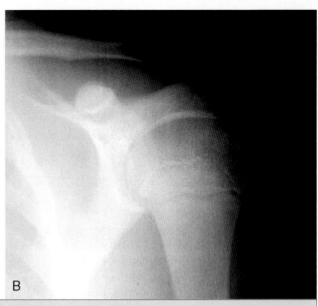

Figure 1   **A,** AP radiograph showing proximal physeal widening with irregularity in a patient with little league shoulder. **B,** AP radiograph of the normal contralateral shoulder.

Injury Patterns

Distal Clavicle

In adults, a direct blow to the shoulder typically results in an AC separation, but a physeal fracture of the distal clavicle is more common in skeletally immature athletes. The proximal fragment usually displaces superiorly through a rent in the clavicular periosteum. The lateral epiphysis remains congruent with the AC joint through the intact AC and coracoclavicular ligaments, as well as the remaining periosteal sleeve.[16,17] Patients have point tenderness and localized deformity over the lateral clavicle. AP and 15° cephalic tilt radiographs are commonly obtained, and comparison views can be helpful. The Rockwood classification of AC injuries is based on the position of the lateral clavicle and the integrity of the periosteal sleeve.[18] A type I injury is a mild sprain of the AC ligament with an intact periosteum; a type II injury involves slight AC joint widening and partial dorsal disruption of the periosteal sleeve; and a type III injury includes a large dorsal disruption of the periosteum, with malalignment of the lateral clavicle. In a type IV, V, or VI injury, the periosteum is completely disrupted, and there is posterior, 100% superior, or inferior (subcoracoid) displacement of the lateral clavicle, respectively. Nonsurgical management is the mainstay for a type I, II, or III injury in a child. The potential for healing and remodeling is great because the periosteal sleeve remains attached to the lateral epiphyseal fragment, and the AC and coracoclavicular ligaments serve as a bridge for osseous union. A type IV, V, or VI injury with significant displacement requires surgical stabilization. Repair of the disrupted periosteal sleeve, with or without internal fixation, is typically performed. In an older adolescent or a young adult, the choice of surgical or nonsurgical treatment for a type III AC separation is controversial.[19,20]

Little League Shoulder

Little league shoulder is an epiphysiolysis of the proximal humerus secondary to repetitive microtrauma, large rotational torques, and chronic stress overload in a skeletally immature overhead athlete. This condition is most common in boys age 12 to 14 years who are high-performance baseball pitchers. Large rotational forces about the physis are produced by an imbalance between the rotator cuff muscles (which attach proximally to the proximal humeral physis), and the pectoralis major, deltoid, and triceps muscles (which attach distally to this physis). In addition, poor throwing mechanics and excessive pitch counts can create a predisposition to physeal injury.[21-25] Patients typically have anterolateral shoulder pain and loss of velocity after an increase in their throwing regimen. Weakness with resisted shoulder abduction and internal rotation may be noted on examination. Bilateral AP radiographs in internal and external rotation may reveal proximal physeal widening or irregularity with metaphyseal demineralization, which is best seen by comparison with the contralateral shoulder (**Figure 1**). The treatment typically includes a 2- to 3-month period of rest, followed by a gradual return to throwing. This interval protocol has excellent results, with 91% of patients remaining asymptomatic.[3] Because of the great remodeling potential of the proximal humerus, growth disturbances resulting in arm length discrepancy or angular deformity are rare. However, repetitive stress to the proximal humeral physis may account for the increased humeral retroversion noted in many adult pitchers. The American Academy of Orthopaedic Surgeons recommends

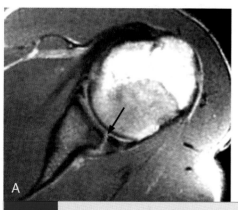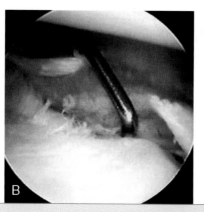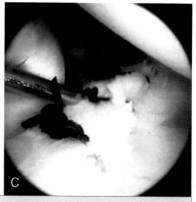

Figure 2 **A,** T1-weighted axial MRI showing a Bankart tear of the anteroinferior labrum *(arrow)*. **B,** Arthroscopic view of the glenohumeral joint showing detachment of the anteroinferior labrum from the glenoid (a Bankart tear). **C,** Arthroscopic view showing repair of the anteroinferior labrum with suture anchors.

specific pitch count limits for young pitchers.[26] Proper throwing mechanics, limits on the number of pitches, and coach, player, and parent education all are crucial to preventing little league shoulder.[12,27]

Glenohumeral Instability

The glenohumeral joint allows a greater arc of motion than any other joint and is the most commonly dislocated joint in adolescents and adults. Shoulder dislocations are rare in skeletally immature patients.[1-3,28] The three instability patterns are anterior, posterior, and multidirectional. Anterior shoulder dislocation is the most common and typically follows a traumatic injury. The affected arm is held in abduction and external rotation, with the humeral head palpable anteriorly. Posterior dislocation is much less common and initially may be missed. The arm typically is held in adduction and internal rotation. AP, Y-scapular, and axillary radiographs help in determining the location of the humeral head in relation to the glenoid. The West Point axillary and Stryker notch views may be necessary to identify a fracture of the glenoid rim (a bony Bankart lesion) or the humeral head (a Hill-Sachs lesion).[29] Gentle reduction should be performed promptly, using one of several reduction maneuvers. Postreduction MRI may be obtained to assess for capsulolabral injuries such as a Bankart tear (a tear of the anteroinferior labrum off the glenoid).

Conservative management of an anterior dislocation begins with a 1- to 3-week period of sling immobilization. There is controversy as to whether the optimal position for immobilization is in internal or external rotation.[30,31] A randomized controlled study found a 40% lower recurrence rate after 3 weeks of immobilization in external rotation, compared with internal rotation.[31] The results of this study have not yet been duplicated, and another randomized controlled study suggested that the two positions offer similar outcomes.[32] After immobilization, a course of physical therapy focuses on periscapular and rotator cuff strengthening exercises. High rates of recurrent insta-

bility (50% to 100%) have been reported after a first dislocation in patients younger than 20 years.[33-36] The cause probably is multifactorial and involves the patients' high-demand activities, a relatively high ratio of type III to type I collagen, and greater ligamentous laxity.[37] Whether surgical or nonsurgical management is preferable for a first adolescent dislocation is controversial.[33,35,36,38] A meta-analysis concluded that for boys who perform high-demand activities, early surgical stabilization reduces the risk of recurrence and may be preferable. No significant outcome differences were noted among any of the other patient populations, and no definite conclusions could be drawn.[33] In a randomized study of first dislocations, patients treated with arthroscopic repair had a 76% lower risk of redislocation than patients treated with arthroscopic lavage, with better functional scores, return to previous activity level, and satisfaction, as well as lower cost of treatment.[38]

The surgical treatment of glenohumeral instability involves repair of the capsulolabral injury, with or without additional capsulorrhaphy. Both arthroscopic and open methods have been described. Recurrence rates after arthroscopic repair with suture anchors have declined to equal those of the classic open Bankart procedure, probably as the result of newer methods, equipment, and implants (**Figure 2**).[39-41] A meta-analysis that included studies of older arthroscopic techniques and studies of both adults and children found that open procedures were more reliable for restoring stability and allowing the patient to return to work or sports. However, patients had better Rowe scores after arthroscopic repair, probably because they had less stiffness and better function.[42] There are few adolescents-only studies of arthroscopic repair. A retrospective study of 32 shoulders in patients age 11 to 18 years found five redislocations (a 15% rate) 2 years after arthroscopic repair, with two of the redislocations occurring in one patient with familial hyperlaxity.[43] All of the patients returned to sports and had high scores on the Single Assessment Numeric Evaluation. Other studies

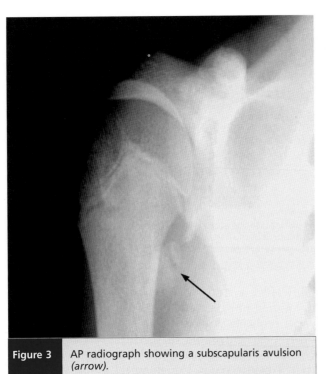

Figure 3 AP radiograph showing a subscapularis avulsion (*arrow*).

Rotator Cuff

A rotator cuff tear is rare in adolescent athletes but is most likely to occur with a shoulder dislocation. An avulsion of the lesser tuberosity signifies a subscapularis avulsion that may require surgical repair if the displacement is significant (**Figure 3**). Rotator cuff tendinitis caused by repetitive overuse is relatively common among overhead athletes. The initial treatment consists of rest, activity modification, and physical therapy that emphasizes periscapular stabilization and rotator cuff strengthening. A gradual return to activities is allowed as the symptoms abate.

Internal Impingement and Superior Labrum Anterior and Posterior Tears

Shoulder pain in the overhead athlete often results from internal impingement that occurs because of a combination of scapular malpositioning, muscle imbalance, and capsular contracture. Patients have anterolateral shoulder pain with overhead activities. The physical examination often reveals rotator cuff weakness, scapular protraction, and limited internal rotation. Limited internal rotation indicates a tight posterior capsule, which causes a posterosuperior shift in the glenohumeral rotation point during abduction and external rotation and leads to internal impingement of the greater tuberosity onto the posterosuperior labrum and the infraspinatus undersurface. MRI may be normal or reveal a posterior capsular contracture, a superior labrum anterior and posterior (SLAP) tear, or fraying of the undersurface of the infraspinatus tendon.[51,52] Magnetic resonance arthrography is more likely than MRI to reveal a SLAP tear. Many types of SLAP tears have been described. A type II tear is a separation of the superior biceps-labrum complex from the underlying glenoid; it is the most common type in the adolescent and young adult population and the most amenable to arthroscopic repair (**Figure 4**).

The initial treatment of internal impingement consists of physical therapy for posterior capsular stretching, scapular stabilization, and rotator cuff strengthening. Impingement that is not resolved with physical therapy often involves a SLAP tear, and surgical treatment should be considered. Shoulder arthroscopy can be beneficial for débridement of a partial thickness rotator cuff tear or for repair or débridement of a SLAP tear.[53,54] Anterior capsulorrhaphy can be considered, as failure to address a subtle instability pattern may compromise the functional result. Good or excellent short-term results were recently reported after type II SLAP lesions were repaired in a mostly adult population.[55]

Scapulothoracic Dysfunction

The scapulothoracic disorders include scapular dyskinesis, scapulothoracic crepitus, and bursitis. Scapular dyskinesis consists of an alteration in the position and motion of the scapula and can lead to shoulder pain through worsening internal impingement, weakness, and susceptibility to fatigue. Scapular dyskinesis is clas-

reported good results in adolescents who were included with adult patients.[39,40,44-46]

Symptoms of subluxation in more than one direction (anterior, posterior, inferior) are characteristic of MDI, in the absence of a major traumatic event.[47-49] MDI typically affects an overhead athlete who participates in a sports activity that requires repetitive shoulder abduction and external rotation, such as gymnastics or the butterfly swimming stroke. Underlying glenohumeral laxity coupled with repetitive microtrauma can lead to painful MDI. Asymptomatic patients may experience painless episodes of shoulder subluxation with spontaneous reduction. Evaluation for a hyperlaxity syndrome such as Ehlers-Danlos syndrome may be necessary. It is critical to determine the one or more directions of glenohumeral instability that replicate the patient's symptoms, as laxity does not indicate instability. Radiographs and MRI usually are normal, except that a patulous capsule with increased volume may be seen. Nonsurgical management is the mainstay for MDI. A vigorous physical therapy program focusing on rotator cuff and periscapular strengthening is necessary. Surgery is indicated for a patient with symptoms that affect activities after at least 6 months of unsuccessful rehabilitation. Arthroscopic or open capsulorrhaphy should focus on the symptomatic direction of instability. Newer arthroscopic techniques have had encouraging results in groups that included both adults and adolescents, including a return to sports in 85% and a satisfactory outcome in more than 90%.[50]

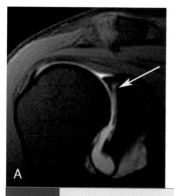
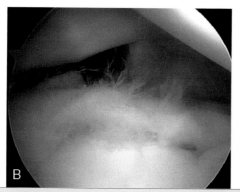
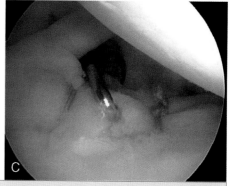

Figure 4 **A,** T1-weighted coronal magnetic resonance arthrogram showing a type II SLAP tear *(arrow).* **B,** Arthroscopic view showing a type II SLAP tear. **C,** Arthroscopic view showing repair of the superior labrum with suture anchors.

sified into three types based on the position of the scapula at rest. In type I, the inferior scapular border is prominent; in type II, the medial border is prominent; and in type III, scapular protraction, superior translation, and a prominent superior border are present. The treatment consists of exercises for periscapular strengthening, posture, and scapular positioning.[56] Patients with scapulothoracic bursitis and crepitus have pain or crepitus during coordinated scapulothoracic motion. A variety of bursa are present around the scapula, most prominently along its inferomedial border. Associated pathologies including scapular osteochondromas must be ruled out. Symptomatic crepitus that is refractory to anti-inflammatory drugs and physical therapy can be treated with scapulothoracic bursoscopy or open excision of the superomedial scapular angle.

Summary

The incidence of shoulder injuries in pediatric athletes is increasing along with greater participation in high-demand overhead sports at younger ages. Injury patterns in skeletally immature patients are unique to the developing musculoskeletal system and specific to the involved sport. A prompt and accurate diagnosis coupled with proper treatment can prevent long-term sequelae and expedite return to play. Although most injuries respond well to a nonsurgical regimen of rest and rehabilitation, surgical management is necessary in certain circumstances. Injury prevention strategies, including pitch count limits and education of coaches and parents, should be used to decrease the incidence and severity of shoulder injuries in pediatric athletes.

Annotated References

1. Chen FS, Diaz VA, Loebenberg M, Rosen JE: Shoulder and elbow injuries in the skeletally immature athlete. *J Am Acad Orthop Surg* 2005;13(3):172-185.
   Shoulder and elbow functional anatomy, biomechanics, and pathophysiology in the skeletally immature athlete are comprehensively reviewed.

2. Ireland ML, Hutchinson MR: Upper extremity injuries in young athletes. *Clin Sports Med* 1995;14(3):533-569.

3. Kocher MS, Waters PM, Micheli LJ: Upper extremity injuries in the paediatric athlete. *Sports Med* 2000; 30(2):117-135.

4. Patel PR, Warner JJ: Shoulder injuries in the skeletally immature athlete. *Sports Med Arthrosc Rev* 1996;4:99-113.

5. Tibone JE: Shoulder problems of adolescents: How they differ from those of adults. *Clin Sports Med* 1983;2(2): 423-427.

6. Bigliani LU, Kelkar R, Flatow EL, Pollock RG, Mow VC: Glenohumeral stability: Biomechanical properties of passive and active stabilizers. *Clin Orthop Relat Res* 1996;330:13-30.

7. Finsterbush A, Pogrund H: The hypermobility syndrome: Musculoskeletal complaints in 100 consecutive cases of generalized joint hypermobility. *Clin Orthop Relat Res* 1982;168:124-127.

8. Culpepper MI, Niemann KM: High school football injuries in Birmingham, Alabama. *South Med J* 1983; 76(7):873-875, 878.

9. Requa R, Garrick JG: Injuries in interscholastic wrestling. *Phys Sportsmed* 1981;9:44-51.

10. Kocher MS, Feagin JA Jr: Shoulder injuries during alpine skiing. *Am J Sports Med* 1996;24(5):665-669.

11. Albright JA, Jokl P, Shaw R, Albright JP: Clinical study of baseball pitchers: Correlation of injury to the throwing arm with method of delivery. *Am J Sports Med* 1978;6(1):15-21.

12. Andrews JR, Fleisig GS: Preventing throwing injuries. *J Orthop Sports Phys Ther* 1998;27(3):187-188.

7: Sports-Related Topics

13. Zaricznyj B, Shattuck LJ, Mast TA, Robertson RV, D'Elia G: Sports-related injuries in school-aged children. *Am J Sports Med* 1980;8(5):318-324.

14. Lyman S, Fleisig GS, Waterbor JW, et al: Longitudinal study of elbow and shoulder pain in youth baseball pitchers. *Med Sci Sports Exerc* 2001;33(11):1803-1810.

15. Oberlander MA, Chisar MA, Campbell B: Epidemiology of shoulder injuries in throwing and overhead athletes. *Sports Med Arthrosc Rev* 2000;8:115-123.

16. Havránek P: Injuries of distal clavicular physis in children. *J Pediatr Orthop* 1989;9(2):213-215.

17. Black GB, McPherson JA, Reed MH: Traumatic pseudodislocation of the acromioclavicular joint in children: A fifteen year review. *Am J Sports Med* 1991; 19(6):644-646.

18. Rockwood CA: Fractures of outer clavicle in children and adults. *J Bone Joint Surg Br* 1982;64:642-649.

19. Galpin RD, Hawkins RJ, Grainger RW: A comparative analysis of operative versus nonoperative treatment of grade III acromioclavicular separations. *Clin Orthop Relat Res* 1985;193:150-155.

20. Larsen E, Bjerg-Nielsen A, Christensen P: Conservative or surgical treatment of acromioclavicular dislocation: A prospective, controlled, randomized study. *J Bone Joint Surg Am* 1986;68(4):552-555.

21. Torg JS, Pollack H, Sweterlitsch P: The effect of competitive pitching on the shoulders and elbows of preadolescent baseball players. *Pediatrics* 1972;49(2):267-272.

22. Carson WG Jr, Gasser SI: Little Leaguer's shoulder: A report of 23 cases. *Am J Sports Med* 1998;26(4):575-580.

23. Keeley DW, Hackett T, Keirns M, Sabick MB, Torry MR: A biomechanical analysis of youth pitching mechanics. *J Pediatr Orthop* 2008;28(4):452-459.

    A biomechanical analysis of 16 healthy right hand–dominant youth baseball pitchers found that initiation of trunk rotation early in the pitching cycle leads to shoulder hyperangulation and increased torque on the proximal humeral physis.

24. Mair SD, Uhl TL, Robbe RG, Brindle KA: Physeal changes and range-of-motion differences in the dominant shoulders of skeletally immature baseball players. *J Shoulder Elbow Surg* 2004;13(5):487-491.

25. Sabick MB, Kim YK, Torry MR, Keirns MA, Hawkins RJ: Biomechanics of the shoulder in youth baseball pitchers: Implications for the development of proximal humeral epiphysiolysis and humeral retrotorsion. *Am J Sports Med* 2005;33(11):1716-1722.

    A motion analysis of youth baseball pitchers found increased proximal humeral physeal shear stress arising from high torque late in the arm-cocking phase. Over time, this shear stress results in humeral retrotorsion and proximal humeral epiphysiolysis.

26. American Academy of Orthopaedic Surgeons: Your Orthopaedic Connection: Baseball injury prevention. http://orthoinfo.aaos.org/topic.cfm?topic=A00185. Updated August 2009. Accessed August 10, 2010.

27. American Academy of Pediatrics Committee on Sports Medicine: Risk of injury from baseball and softball in children 5 to 14 years of age. *Pediatrics* 1994;93(4): 690-692.

28. Allen AA, Warner JJ: Shoulder instability in the athlete. *Orthop Clin North Am* 1995;26(3):487-504.

29. Bankart AS: The pathology and treatment of recurrent dislocation of the shoulder joint. *Br J Surg* 1938;26: 23-28.

30. Itoi E, Sashi R, Minagawa H, Shimizu T, Wakabayashi I, Sato K: Position of immobilization after dislocation of the glenohumeral joint: A study with use of magnetic resonance imaging. *J Bone Joint Surg Am* 2001;83(5): 661-667.

31. Itoi E, Hatakeyama Y, Sato T, et al: Immobilization in external rotation after shoulder dislocation reduces the risk of recurrence: A randomized controlled trial. *J Bone Joint Surg Am* 2007;89(10):2124-2131.

    A prospective study of 198 first anterior shoulder dislocations found statistically significant data to indicate that external rotation bracing reduces the rate of recurrent dislocation in comparison with traditional internal rotation bracing.

32. Finestone A, Milgrom C, Radeva-Petrova DR, et al: Bracing in external rotation for traumatic anterior dislocation of the shoulder. *J Bone Joint Surg Br* 2009;91(7): 918-921.

    In a randomized prospective study, 51 young men (age 17 to 27 years) were braced in external or internal rotation after a primary traumatic anterior shoulder dislocation to ascertain which method produces the lower recurrence of glenohumeral dislocation. No statistically significant difference was detected.

33. Handoll HH, Almaiyah MA, Rangan A: Surgical versus non-surgical treatment for acute anterior shoulder dislocation. *Cochrane Database Syst Rev* 2004;1: CD004325.

34. Hovelius L, Augustini BG, Fredin H, Johansson O, Norlin R, Thorling J: Primary anterior dislocation of the shoulder in young patients: A ten-year prospective study. *J Bone Joint Surg Am* 1996;78(11):1677-1684.

35. Kirkley A, Griffin S, Richards C, Miniaci A, Mohtadi N: Prospective randomized clinical trial comparing the effectiveness of immediate arthroscopic stabilization versus immobilization and rehabilitation in first traumatic anterior dislocations of the shoulder. *Arthroscopy* 1999;15(5):507-514.

36. Jakobsen BW, Johannsen HV, Suder P, Søjbjerg JO: Primary repair versus conservative treatment of first-time traumatic anterior dislocation of the shoulder: A randomized study with 10-year follow-up. *Arthroscopy* 2007;23(2):118-123.

    In a randomized controlled study of 76 patients with an arthroscopically diagnosed first anterior glenohumeral dislocation, 39 patients were treated with sling immobilization, and 37 were treated with open repair. At 10-year follow-up, the patients treated with open repair had a statistically significant lower rate of instability recurrence, compared with the conservatively treated patients.

37. Sachs RA, Lin D, Stone ML, Paxton E, Kuney M: Can the need for future surgery for acute traumatic anterior shoulder dislocation be predicted? *J Bone Joint Surg Am* 2007;89(8):1665-1674.

    In a prospective review of 131 patients after a first shoulder dislocation, younger patients involved in a contact or collision sport or requiring occupational overhead use of the arm were more likely to have recurrent dislocation than less active or older patients. The average follow-up time was 4 years.

38. Robinson CM, Jenkins PJ, White TO, Ker A, Will E: Primary arthroscopic stabilization for a first-time anterior dislocation of the shoulder: A randomized, double-blind trial. *J Bone Joint Surg Am* 2008;90(4):708-721.

    Arthroscopic stabilization was compared with arthroscopy without stabilization in 88 adults with a first anterior glenohumeral dislocation. A marked treatment benefit was found from arthroscopic repair of a Bankart lesion in comparison with arthroscopy and joint lavage alone, as measured using functional scores, treatment costs, patient satisfaction, and recurrent dislocation and instability episodes.

39. Cole BJ, L'Insalata J, Irrgang J, Warner JJ: Comparison of arthroscopic and open anterior shoulder stabilization: A two to six-year follow-up study. *J Bone Joint Surg Am* 2000;82:(8):1108-1114.

40. Guanche CA, Quick DC, Sodergren KM, Buss DD: Arthroscopic versus open reconstruction of the shoulder in patients with isolated Bankart lesions. *Am J Sports Med* 1996;24(2):144-148.

41. Bottoni CR, Smith EL, Berkowitz MJ, Towle RB, Moore JH: Arthroscopic versus open shoulder stabilization for recurrent anterior instability: A prospective randomized clinical trial. *Am J Sports Med* 2006;34(11):1730-1737.

    In a prospective randomized controlled study of 64 patients, all major clinical outcomes were found to be comparable after arthroscopic or open stabilization for recurrent anterior shoulder instability.

42. Lenters TR, Franta AK, Wolf FM, Leopold SS, Matsen FA III: Arthroscopic compared with open repairs for recurrent anterior shoulder instability: A systematic review and meta-analysis of the literature. *J Bone Joint Surg Am* 2007;89(2):244-254.

    A systematic analysis of 18 studies comparing arthroscopic and open repair of recurrent anterior shoulder instability found that arthroscopic repair was less effective than open repair. The study was limited by the small number of randomized controlled studies and differing study designs.

43. Jones KJ, Wiesel B, Ganley TJ, Wells L: Functional outcomes of early arthroscopic bankart repair in adolescents aged 11 to 18 years. *J Pediatr Orthop* 2007;27(2):209-213.

    A retrospective review of 32 arthroscopic Bankart repairs after anterior shoulder dislocation (30 patients, age 11 to 18 years) found primary arthroscopic Bankart repair to be effective for treating traumatically induced shoulder instability and limiting recurrent shoulder dislocation and instability.

44. DeBerardino TM, Arciero RA, Taylor DC: Arthroscopic stabilization of acute initial anterior shoulder dislocation: The West Point experience. *J South Orthop Assoc* 1996;5(4):263-271.

45. Gartsman GM, Roddey TS, Hammerman SM: Arthroscopic treatment of anterior-inferior glenohumeral instability: Two to five-year follow-up. *J Bone Joint Surg Am* 2000;82(7):991-1003.

46. Gill TJ, Micheli LJ, Gebhard F, Binder C: Bankart repair for anterior instability of the shoulder: Long-term outcome. *J Bone Joint Surg Am* 1997;79(6):850-857.

47. Neer CS II, Foster CR: Inferior capsular shift for involuntary inferior and multidirectional instability of the shoulder: A preliminary report. *J Bone Joint Surg Am* 1980;62(6):897-908.

48. Paxinos A, Walton J, Tzannes A, Callanan M, Hayes K, Murrell GA: Advances in the management of traumatic anterior and atraumatic multidirectional shoulder instability. *Sports Med* 2001;31(11):819-828.

49. Pollock RG, Owens JM, Flatow EL, Bigliani LU: Operative results of the inferior capsular shift procedure for multidirectional instability of the shoulder. *J Bone Joint Surg Am* 2000;82(7):919-928.

50. Baker CL III, Mascarenhas R, Kline AJ, Chhabra A, Pombo MW, Bradley JP: Arthroscopic treatment of multidirectional shoulder instability in athletes: A retrospective analysis of 2- to 5-year clinical outcomes. *Am J Sports Med* 2009;37(9):1712-1720.

    A retrospective evaluation of 43 shoulders with MDI (40 patients; mean age, 19.1 years) at an average 33.5 months after arthroscopic stabilization found that the treatment was effective, maintained satisfactory range of motion and strength, and allowed a successful, timely return to sports.

51. Bigliani LU, D'Alessandro DF, Duralde XA, McIlveen SJ: Anterior acromioplasty for subacromial impingement in patients younger than 40 years of age. *Clin Orthop Relat Res* 1989;246(246):111-116.

7: Sports-Related Topics

52. Hawkins RJ, Kennedy JC: Impingement syndrome in athletes. *Am J Sports Med* 1980;8(3):151-158.

53. Tibone JE, Elrod B, Jobe FW, et al: Surgical treatment of tears of the rotator cuff in athletes. *J Bone Joint Surg Am* 1986;68(6):887-891.

54. Payne LZ, Altchek DW, Craig EV, Warren RF: Arthroscopic treatment of partial rotator cuff tears in young athletes: A preliminary report. *Am J Sports Med* 1997;25(3):299-305.

55. Brockmeier SF, Voos JE, Williams RJ III, Altchek DW, Cordasco FA, Allen AA; Hospital for Special Surgery Sports Medicine and Shoulder Service: Outcomes after arthroscopic repair of type-II SLAP lesions. *J Bone Joint Surg Am* 2009;91(7):1595-1603.

A prospective analysis of arthroscopic repair of a symptomatic type II SLAP tear in 47 patients found that 75% returned to their earlier level of competition. Favorable outcomes can be anticipated after arthroscopic SLAP lesion repair, and a traumatic etiology affords a greater likelihood of successful return to sports.

56. Kibler WB, McMullen J: Scapular dyskinesis and its relation to shoulder pain. *J Am Acad Orthop Surg* 2003;11(2):142-151.

Chapter 40
Overuse Syndromes of the Knee

Jennifer M. Weiss, MD

Introduction

An overuse injury is brought on by repetitive trauma that inflicts multiple small stresses too frequently to allow recovery. The patient typically reports an insidious onset of pain and does not recall an acute traumatic incident. The avoidance of overuse injury from sports participation has not been well studied. However, the American Academy of Pediatrics Council on Sports Medicine and Fitness recommends that young athletes rest from a sport at least 1 to 2 days per week and 2 to 3 months per year.[1] Athletes who specialize in a sport before puberty are more likely to experience an overuse injury than those whose sports regimen is more well rounded.[2] To decrease risk of overuse injury, young athletes should be taught to improve their sports-related strength, flexibility, biomechanics, and alignment.[3]

Iliotibial Band Friction Syndrome

Iliotibial band friction syndrome is caused by repetitive friction of the distal iliotibial band on the lateral femoral epicondyle. Runners, bikers, and dancers are most frequently affected because their sport requires repetitive knee-bending motions. Abductor weakness probably contributes to the etiology of this syndrome, as does poor form in executing sports movements. The patient typically reports a painful snapping on the lateral aspect of the knee. The pain can be reproduced on physical examination by compressing the iliotibial band onto the lateral femoral epicondyle with the knee flexed to 30°.[4] The diagnosis should be made by history and physical examination, and imaging is not recommended.

Iliotibial band friction syndrome is treated with activity modification, icing of the injured area, stretching exercises, and anti-inflammatory medications. A steroid injection into the bursa over the lateral femoral epicondyle can be both diagnostic and therapeutic.[5] Surgery is rarely needed for a recalcitrant injury. The iliotibial band can be surgically lengthened by release of the posterior fibers or by Z-lengthening, with good results.[6,7] Bursectomy also is an effective surgical option.[8]

Osgood-Schlatter Disease

Osgood-Schlatter disease is a traction apophysitis (irritation) caused by the pull of the patellar tendon on the tibial tubercle apophysis.[9-11] This injury occurs in a growing child or adolescent, with a peak incidence at age 10 to 15 years.[12] It is more common in boys than in girls. The patient reports pain and swelling, with the pain primarily occurring during or after sports activity. Physical examination reveals point tenderness over the tibial tubercle. The tibial tubercle may be prominent, even after the symptoms resolve at skeletal maturity. Radiographs show prominence and fragmentation of the tibial tubercle (**Figure 1**). If the disease is unilateral, radiographs are recommended to rule out another pathology. Radiographs typically are not necessary if there is bilateral involvement.

The symptoms of Osgood-Schlatter disease usually can be managed by reassuring the patient and using activity modification, hamstring stretching, and anti-inflammatory medications. Bracing or cast immobilization occasionally is needed. An orthosis can be considered if the patient has a lower extremity malalignment.

Although Osgood-Schlatter disease almost always resolves spontaneously with the closure of the tibial tubercle physis,[13] surgical treatment should be considered for a patient whose pain persists after skeletal maturity. The available procedures include epiphysiodesis (drilling) of the tibial tubercle apophysis, ossicle excision, and tibial tubercleplasty.[14-16] Arthroscopic tubercleplasty has had good results.[17]

Validated knee scales were used to evaluate 15 patients (16 knees) after tibial tubercleplasty and ossicle resection.[18] Twelve patients (80%) and 13 knees (81%) had a return to full preoperative activity; 2 patients (13%) had a partial return to activity, and 1 patient (7%) had not returned to activity. The patients' pain frequency and severity were graded as mild (within the lowest one third to one quarter on a pain scale and a questionnaire).

Neither Dr. Weiss nor any immediate family member has received anything of value from or owns stock in a commercial company or institution related directly or indirectly to the subject of this chapter.

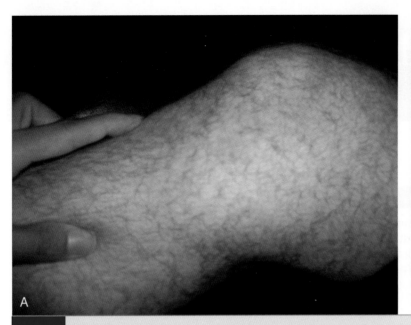
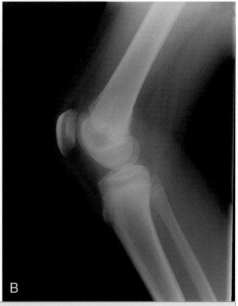

Figure 1 Osgood-Schlatter disease. **A,** Photograph showing the prominent tibial tubercle. **B,** Lateral radiograph showing a tibial tubercle that is prominent but not fragmented.

Sinding-Larsen-Johansson Disease

Sinding-Larsen-Johansson disease is a traction apophysitis of the inferior pole of the patella. The bone sometimes fragments, the patellar tendon may thicken, and the infrapatellar bursa may become inflamed.[19] Most patients are age 10 to 12 years. The patient typically reports pain and swelling at the bottom of the kneecap, especially after activity. Physical examination reveals point tenderness over the inferior pole of the patella. Radiographs show a fragmentation or elongation of the inferior pole of the patella, although ultrasonography may be more reliable than plain radiography.[19] Sinding-Larsen-Johansson disease is treated with icing, stretching, anti-inflammatory medications, and activity modification. No surgical interventions have been described.

Jumper's Knee

Jumper's knee is an inflammation of the patellar tendon just inferior to the patella. In its severe form, the posterior aspect of the tendon becomes necrotic, and the anterior aspect of the tendon may become hypertrophic.[20] The patient reports pain below the kneecap, especially during and after running or jumping. Physical examination reveals tenderness along the patellar tendon and pain on resisted extension of the knee (**Figure 2**). Although the diagnosis should be based on the patient's history and physical examination, it can be confirmed on MRI and ultrasonographs.[21]

The treatment consists of activity modification, stretching, and the use of anti-inflammatory medications. Ultrasonographically guided steroid injections

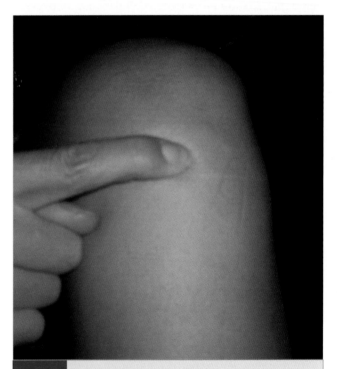

Figure 2 Photograph showing the area of point tenderness over the patellar tendon in a patient with jumper's knee.

have been used in adults with good results.[22] Of 16 high-level athletes who underwent surgical patellar tendon débridement followed by rigorous physical therapy, 14 were able to return to their preoperative sports level, with good pain relief.[20] In another study, 15 athletes underwent arthroscopic débridement for recalcitrant patellar tendinosis; ultrasonography revealed decreased edema 3 weeks after surgery.[23]

Plica

A plica (an infolding of synovial tissue) is a normal finding in the knee joint. A medial plica, which is present in approximately one of three knees, can become irritated and symptomatic after trauma or overuse.[24] The patient reports snapping or popping that sometimes is painful. Pain associated with a plica may account for so-called anterior knee pain in as many as 40% of patients.[25] The condition is treated with activity modification, icing, and anti-inflammatory medications. The patient's symptoms almost always respond to these nonsurgical measures, but steroid injections and arthroscopic resection may be offered if necessary.[26-28]

Summary

Overuse syndromes of the knee usually are self-limited, and surgical intervention is rarely required. Nonsurgical management largely consists of stretching, strengthening, and activity modification. It is important to teach athletes, their families, and their coaches that cross-training and rest are important for the prevention and treatment of overuse syndromes of the knee.

Annotated References

1. Brenner JS; American Academy of Pediatrics Council on Sports Medicine and Fitness: Overuse injuries, overtraining, and burnout in child and adolescent athletes. *Pediatrics* 2007;119(6):1242-1245.

   Nine recommendations are described for prevention of overuse injuries, including rest 1 to 2 days per week, 2 to 3 months away from each sport per year, participation on only one team at a time, and avoidance of multigame tournaments. Level of evidence: V.

2. American Academy of Pediatrics. Committee on Sports Medicine and Fitness: Intensive training and sports specialization in young athletes. *Pediatrics* 2000;106(1, pt 1):154-157.

3. Kidd PS, McCoy C, Steenbergen L: Repetitive strain injuries in youth. *J Am Acad Nurse Pract* 2000;12(10):413-426.

4. Noble CA: The treatment of iliotibial band friction syndrome. *Br J Sports Med* 1979;13(2):51-54.

5. Gunter P, Schwellnus MP: Local corticosteroid injection in iliotibial band friction syndrome in runners: A randomised controlled trial. *Br J Sports Med* 2004;38(3):269-272.

6. Barber FA, Boothby MH, Troop RL: Z-plasty lengthening for iliotibial band friction syndrome. *J Knee Surg* 2007;20(4):281-284.

   This is a retrospective review of eight patients who underwent Z-lengthening of the iliotibial band. At an average 6-year follow-up, outcomes scores revealed no complications. Level of evidence: IV.

7. Drogset JO, Rossvoll I, Grøntvedt T: Surgical treatment of iliotibial band friction syndrome: A retrospective study of 45 patients. *Scand J Med Sci Sports* 1999;9(5):296-298.

8. Hariri S, Savidge ET, Reinold MM, Zachazewski J, Gill TJ: Treatment of recalcitrant iliotibial band friction syndrome with open iliotibial band bursectomy: Indications, technique, and clinical outcomes. *Am J Sports Med* 2009;37(7):1417-1424.

   A retrospective review of 12 patients who underwent bursectomy for iliotibial band friction syndrome reports results using outcomes scores and pain scales. Nine of 11 patients were completely or mostly satisfied with the surgical outcome. Level of evidence: IV.

9. Cohen B, Wilkinson RW: The Osgood-Schlatter lesion: A radiological and histological study. *Am J Surg* 1958;95(5):731-742.

10. Mital MA, Matza RA, Cohen J: The so-called unresolved Osgood-Schlatter lesion: A concept based on fifteen surgically treated lesions. *J Bone Joint Surg Am* 1980;62(5):732-739.

11. Osgood RB: Lesions of the tibial tubercle occurring during adolescence: 1903. *Clin Orthop Relat Res* 1993;286:4-9.

12. Yashar A, Loder RT, Hensinger RN: Determination of skeletal age in children with Osgood-Schlatter disease by using radiographs of the knee. *J Pediatr Orthop* 1995;15(3):298-301.

13. Krause BL, Williams JP, Catterall A: Natural history of Osgood-Schlatter disease. *J Pediatr Orthop* 1990;10(1):65-68.

14. Glynn MK, Regan BF: Surgical treatment of Osgood-Schlatter's disease. *J Pediatr Orthop* 1983;3(2):216-219.

15. Flowers MJ, Bhadreshwar DR: Tibial tuberosity excision for symptomatic Osgood-Schlatter disease. *J Pediatr Orthop* 1995;15(3):292-297.

16. Binazzi R, Felli L, Vaccari V, Borelli P: Surgical treatment of unresolved Osgood-Schlatter lesion. *Clin Orthop Relat Res* 1993;289(289):202-204.

17. DeBerardino TM, Branstetter JG, Owens BD: Arthroscopic treatment of unresolved Osgood-Schlatter lesions. *Arthroscopy* 2007;23(10):1127, e1-e3.

    An arthroscopic technique is described in which ossicles are shaved and a tubercleplasty is performed to avoid a patella-splitting approach. Postoperative weight bearing and range of motion were not restricted. Level of evidence: IV.

18. Weiss JM, Jordan SS, Andersen JS, Lee BM, Kocher M: Surgical treatment of unresolved Osgood-Schlatter disease: Ossicle resection with tibial tubercleplasty. *J Pediatr Orthop* 2007;27(7):844-847.

Surgery is recommended after skeletal maturity if extensive nonsurgical treatment of Osgood-Schlatter disease is unsuccessful. Both ossicle excision and tibial tubercleplasty should be performed.

19. De Flaviis L, Nessi R, Scaglione P, Balconi G, Albisetti W, Derchi LE: Ultrasonic diagnosis of Osgood-Schlatter and Sinding-Larsen-Johansson diseases of the knee. *Skeletal Radiol* 1989;18(3):193-197.

20. Shelbourne KD, Henne TD, Gray T: Recalcitrant patellar tendinosis in elite athletes: Surgical treatment in conjunction with aggressive postoperative rehabilitation. *Am J Sports Med* 2006;34(7):1141-1146.

In a retrospective review of 16 athletes (22 knees) who underwent surgical débridement of patellar tendinosis refractory to nonsurgical management, all patients felt subjective improvement, and 87% returned to their preoperative sport. Level of evidence: IV.

21. Warden SJ, Kiss ZS, Malara FA, Ooi AB, Cook JL, Crossley KM: Comparative accuracy of magnetic resonance imaging and ultrasonography in confirming clinically diagnosed patellar tendinopathy. *Am J Sports Med* 2007;35(3):427-436.

When 30 patients with a clinical diagnosis of patellar tendinosis were compared with 33 activity- and age-matched individuals, ultrasonography (gray scale and color Doppler) was found more accurate and sensitive than MRI for confirming the diagnosis. Level of evidence: II.

22. Fredberg U, Bolvig L, Pfeiffer-Jensen M, Clemmensen D, Jakobsen BW, Stengaard-Pedersen K: Ultrasonography as a tool for diagnosis, guidance of local steroid injection and, together with pressure algometry, monitoring of the treatment of athletes with chronic jumper's knee and Achilles tendinitis: A randomized, double-blind, placebo-controlled study. *Scand J Rheumatol* 2004;33(2):94-101.

23. Ogon P, Maier D, Jaeger A, Suedkamp NP: Arthroscopic patellar release for the treatment of chronic patellar tendinopathy. *Arthroscopy* 2006;22(4):462, e1-e5.

In a retrospective review of 15 athletes who underwent arthroscopic débridement of synovitis related to patellar tendinitis, tendon edema was evaluated by ultrasonography 3 weeks after surgery. A decrease in edema was found. Level of evidence: IV.

24. Dupont JY: Synovial plicae of the knee: Controversies and review. *Clin Sports Med* 1997;16(1):87-122.

25. Brushøj C, Hölmich P, Nielsen MB, Albrecht-Beste E: Acute patellofemoral pain: Aggravating activities, clinical examination, MRI and ultrasound findings. *Br J Sports Med* 2008;42(1):64-67.

Anterior knee pain can occur in the peripatellar area, Hoffa fat pad, medial plica, or joint line. The patellofemoral compression test was positive in less than one third of knees. Level of evidence: IV.

26. Griffith CJ, LaPrade RF: Medial plica irritation: Diagnosis and treatment. *Curr Rev Musculoskelet Med* 2008;1(1):53-60.

Treatment for medial plica should begin with hamstring strengthening and only rarely progresses to steroid injection and surgery. Level of evidence: V.

27. Rovere GD, Adair DM: Medial synovial shelf plica syndrome: Treatment by intraplical steroid injection. *Am J Sports Med* 1985;13(6):382-386.

28. Weckström M, Niva MH, Lamminen A, Mattila VM, Pihlajamäki HK: Arthroscopic resection of medial plica of the knee in young adults. *Knee* 2010;17(2):103-107.

MRI and arthroscopic findings were poorly correlated in 33 patients who underwent arthroscopic plica resection. Patients did well after surgery. Level of evidence: IV.

Chapter 41

Ankle Injuries in Young Athletes

Drew E. Warnick, MD   Michael T. Busch, MD

Introduction

Pediatric ankle injuries are occurring more frequently as the number of children participating in sports increases and as the intensity of sports participation appears to increase. Almost 8 million students participate in high school athletic activities.[1] Nationally from 2005 to 2007, high school athletes sustained an estimated 446,715 severe injuries resulting in a loss of more than 21 days of sports participation.[2] More than 12% of these severe injuries occurred in the ankle. The sport with the highest incidence of severe ankle injury was girls' volleyball, followed by girls' basketball, girls' softball, girls' soccer, and boys' soccer.[2]

Ankle Sprains

Ankle sprains are among the most common sports injuries, occurring most frequently during jumping and cutting sports such as basketball, football, soccer, and volleyball. Skeletally immature athletes tend to injure the distal fibular physis. Skeletally mature athletes usually sustain an ankle ligament sprain. Ankle sprain occurs in approximately 6% of all high school sports participants every year and in as many as 70% of all high school basketball players over 4 years of participation.[3] Most ankle sprains involve the lateral ligaments, but approximately 3% are medial.[3] Although most ankle sprains are minor, one third of these injuries result in more than 2 weeks of disability.[4] Minimal intervention is not always sufficient for severe ankle sprains, and treatment does have a positive impact.

Anatomy and Etiology

The trapezoidal shape of the talus provides significant stability to the ankle when the foot is in full dorsiflexion. The wider portion of the anterior talus locks into the mortise and adds bony restraint to lateral displacement and inversion stress. In plantar flexion, the narrow posterior portion of the talus articulates with the mortise, with most of the stability provided by the lig-

amentous complexes. The lateral ligamentous complex of the ankle joint is composed of the anterior talofibular ligament, the calcaneofibular ligament, and the posterior talofibular ligament. The anterior talofibular ligament is the weakest of the lateral ligaments; it is the primary restraint to inversion in plantar flexion and resists anterolateral translation of the talus in the mortise. When the ankle is in the neutral or dorsiflexed position, the calcaneofibular ligament is the primary restraint to inversion. The calcaneofibular ligament is extra-articular and spans both the tibiotalar and subtalar joints, thereby restraining subtalar inversion. The posterior talofibular ligament is the strongest of the collateral ligaments; it connects the posterolateral tubercle of the talus to the posterior aspect of the lateral malleolus.[3,5]

Mechanism and Classification of Injury

Injury to the lateral ligament complex usually occurs with plantar flexion and inversion, whereas an anterior tibiofibular sprain typically results from a dorsiflexion injury. An inversion and supination injury sequentially tears the anterior ankle capsule, the anterior talofibular ligament, and the calcaneofibular ligament. These injuries typically are classified into three grades for treatment decision making. A grade I injury is a mild sprain involving stretching and interstitial tearing of the ligament, with little swelling and disability. A grade II injury is a moderate sprain involving partial disruption of the ligaments, with modest swelling, diffuse tenderness, and difficulty in bearing weight. A grade III injury is a severe sprain with complete ligament disruption, often with extensive bleeding, swelling, instability, and disability.

Clinical Evaluation

Examination of an acute injury should be directed toward identifying the most tender structures. The entire length of the tibia and fibula should be inspected, with specific attention to the area of the physeal plates. Gentle fingertip percussion of the physis and epiphysis is useful for differentiating a nondisplaced Salter-Harris type I physeal fracture from an ankle sprain. The anterior drawer maneuver is used to assess the stability of the anterior talofibular ligament complex. This test is performed by securing the distal leg with one hand and applying an anterior pull on the heel, with the foot held in 20° to 30° of plantar flexion. Alternatively, with the patient supine on a table and the knees flexed 90°, a posterior force is applied to the lower leg while the foot is held flat on the table. The calcaneofibular ligament is tested by applying an inversion stress while the ankle is in neutral or slight dorsiflexion. A more reliable assessment of tenderness and stability often can be achieved after the acute swelling has resolved. It is also important to assess hindfoot alignment for the presence of a plantar-flexed first ray.

The primary differential diagnoses include physeal fracture of the tibia and fibula, osteochondral lesion of the talus, peroneal tendon subluxation, fracture of the base of the fifth metatarsal, midfoot ligament sprain, and Maisonneuve fracture.

Diagnostic Imaging

In adult patients, tenderness over the malleoli and inability to bear weight are indicators that diagnostic imaging is needed. Similar criteria can be used for children and adolescents, although the topic has not been studied.[6] The routine diagnostic radiographs of the ankle include the AP, lateral, and mortise views. Talar tilt or anterior drawer stress radiographs also can be useful. If subtalar motion is limited after resolution of the acute injury, radiographs or CT of the foot should be obtained to look for tarsal coalition. An athlete's risk of recurrent ankle sprain is increased by the presence of a coalition. The os subtibiale and os subfibulare are accessory ossification centers at the tip of the medial and lateral malleoli, respectively. Particularly in children and adolescents, injury to these structures can be confused with avulsion fracture.[7] MRI occasionally is helpful for identifying acute edema surrounding the bony fragment, which suggests recent bony trauma rather than a developmentally incomplete union.

Prevention

Taping and bracing are effective in reducing the incidence of ankle injuries. A recent study of collegiate female volleyball players found that prophylactic use of a double-upright ankle brace led to a rate of ankle injury significantly lower than the overall rate of injury to unbraced ankles (as reported by the National Collegiate Athletic Association).[8] In sports that do not involve shoes, such as gymnastics and dance, the stabilizing effect of a stirrup ankle brace is minimal, and soft braces may be more effective for restricting the passive range of motion of the foot and ankle complex.[8]

Balance-training programs can play an important role in preventing ankle sprain in an athlete, regardless of whether there was an earlier sprain. A randomized controlled study of 765 high school soccer and basketball players found that a balance-training program decreased the rate of ankle sprain compared with standard conditioning exercises. The decrease in the rate of ankle sprains was very small, however; in the intervention-group athletes, there were 1.13 sprains per 1,000 exposures, and in the control-group athletes, the rate was 1.87 sprains per 1,000 exposures.[9] Studies finding that a proactive proprioceptive training regimen leads to a lower rate of ankle sprain are supported by evidence that patients with chronic ankle instability have an altered muscle activation pattern.[10] Patients with chronic ankle instability have delayed recruitment of the ankle, knee, and hip muscles during the transition from a double-leg stance to a single-leg stance.[10,11] This finding may lead to therapeutic and prevention techniques focused on the entire lower extremity rather than the ankle alone.[10] A multidisciplinary approach to prevention may include bracing, balance training, rehabilitation, and evaluation of muscle recruitment in the entire lower extremity.

Treatment

Although the treatment of ankle sprain varies considerably, a few sound principles have evolved. A sprain initially is treated with rest, ice, compression, and elevation. The goal is to limit bleeding, edema, and any further soft-tissue injury. After the severity of injury is determined, an appropriate course of treatment is planned.

In a grade I sprain, the pain usually resolves and motion typically returns in less than 1 week. An athlete should have minimal pain and be able to run, cut, and perform sport-specific tasks before returning to sports activities. This level of recovery sometimes is achieved almost immediately. Supporting the ankle with tape, a laced stabilizer, or a semirigid orthosis facilitates early return and diminishes the risk of recurrent injury. A randomized controlled study found that patients treated with a combination of an ankle-stirrup brace and an elastic wrap returned to normal walking and stair climbing in half the time required for patients treated with an ankle-stirrup brace or elastic wrap alone.[12] A laced stabilizer or an orthosis may offer an advantage over tape, which loosens after a short period of exercise.

A grade II sprain results in an average of 2 weeks of disability. An ankle support offers similar treatment advantages for grade I and grade II sprains. Crutches can be used for a few days as weight bearing is progressively increased. Supervised rehabilitation to decrease swelling and regain motion can facilitate an early return to sports. Ice packs and compression boots are useful initial modalities. Isometric exercises are started immediately, and progressive resistance and proprioceptive training exercises are subsequently introduced. Satisfactory strength must be restored in all muscle groups, especially the peroneal muscles, to ensure dynamic protection from the risk of repeat injury. The athlete can continue aerobic conditioning during rehabilitation by swimming, using an upper body ergometer, running in a pool, or cycling.

Treatment of a grade III sprain is more controversial. The options include bracing, casting, and surgical repair. Treatment with a dorsiflexion cast reduces the talus into the mortise and theoretically relaxes the torn ligament fibers to their premorbid location, but it has not been found to have better results than bracing. A randomized controlled study found that the use of a walking cast for 10 days, followed by ankle-stirrup bracing, or the use of an ankle-stirrup brace alone returned patients to normal walking and stair climbing in the same amount of time.[12] At 6-month follow-up, no difference was found in terms of frequency of reinjury, ankle motion, or function. Advocates of surgical treatment believe that anatomic reduction of the torn ligament fibers may be prevented by interposed edematous soft tissues, especially if there is a bony fragment. However, studies reported no difference between the outcomes of surgery and nonsurgical care; other studies included an inadequate number of control subjects for determining a clear superiority of one treatment over another.[13] A Cochrane systematic review found that both surgery and functional treatment have a good or excellent outcome after an acute ankle sprain but that functional treatment offers a more rapid return to full range of motion, work, and physical activity.[13] The initial nonsurgical treatment of most ankle sprains is further supported by the finding that the results of delayed reconstruction are comparable to those of primary surgical repair.[14]

Sequelae of Acute Ankle Sprain

Residual disability, including swelling, pain, instability, or a combination of these symptoms, occurs after 32% to 76% of ankle sprains.[15] Elucidating the cause of disability in pediatric patients can be a complex and challenging process requiring history, physical examination, and some combination of stress radiography, CT, MRI, and ankle arthroscopy.

Multiple diagnoses need to be considered in a pediatric athlete with dysfunction after a lateral ankle sprain. The alternative diagnoses include, but are not limited to, missed physeal fracture of the ankle, fracture of the fifth metatarsal, fracture of the lateral or posterior process of the talus, calcaneus injury, syndesmotic injury, subtalar instability, osteochondral lesion of the talus or plafond, osseous or soft-tissue impingement, symptomatic ossicles, peroneal tendon injury, avulsion fracture of the fibula, or tarsal coalition. A nerve entrapment syndrome is possible but uncommon in pediatric patients.

Physical examination and imaging studies are critical for evaluating the etiology of the injury. Tenderness at the physis differentiates a physeal fracture from an ankle sprain. CT is helpful for diagnosing tarsal coalitions, fracture of the lateral posterior process of the talus, injury of the anterior process of the calcaneus, or other foot fractures. Stress radiography can diagnose a syndesmotic injury or ligamentous instability. MRI is the modality of choice for evaluating soft-tissue injury of the ligaments and tendons, although many injuries, such as anterolateral soft-tissue impingement and osteochondral injury, can be missed on MRI. Ankle arthroscopy should be considered to detect such an in-

jury, if the cause of residual ankle pain and instability is not determined using standard clinical examination and imaging techniques.[16] The treatment depends on the etiology of the residual disability after a lateral ankle sprain.

Chronic Lateral Ankle Instability

Chronic lateral ankle instability should be suspected in an adolescent with a history of recurrent ankle sprains. Chronic dysfunction associated with laxity of the medial or lateral ligamentous structures of the ankle is termed mechanical instability. The pain or sensation of instability that results from intra-articular or periarticular changes without ligamentous laxity is known as functional instability. These two conditions can occur in combination.[10]

The generally accepted definition of mechanical instability is the presence of 10 mm of anterior translation of the talus on the tibia or more than 3 mm of difference from the contralateral ankle, as seen using the anterior drawer test.[10] Mechanical instability is suggested by more than 9° of talar tilt or more than 3° of difference from the contralateral ankle on a radiograph taken with the foot in plantar flexion and the ankle subjected to an inversion stress.[10] Magnetic resonance arthrography can allow direct visualization of injured ligaments and indirect observation of instability.

A functional rehabilitation program with peroneal muscle strengthening and proprioceptive training, combined with the use of a brace during high-risk activities, is successful in treating chronic instability and pain in 90% of patients.[10] A variety of reconstructive procedures are available if nonsurgical treatment is unsuccessful, but they are not often needed. Numerous studies have investigated the biomechanics and long-term outcomes of different repair procedures in adults, but there are only a few studies of the surgical repair of chronic ankle instability in adolescents. Twenty patients with an average age of 15.4 years were treated using an anatomic repair. At an average 12.6-year follow-up, 19 patients (95%) had a good functional result, with stability and no pain. The patients were happy with the result and had returned to full activities.[17] Another study evaluated the results of four different nonanatomic procedures for chronic lateral ankle instability in 12 adolescent girls (average age, 14.3 years). At an average 3-year follow-up, nonanatomic reconstruction procedures were determined to be effective in restoring ankle instability in adolescents with chronic lateral ankle instability.[18]

Ankle Impingement

Ankle impingement is a common cause of chronic ankle pain in young athletes. The ankle impingement syndromes are pathologic conditions caused by hypertrophic soft tissue, a thickened ligament, or osseous obstruction that causes impingement and results in pain and restriction of movement at the tibiotalar joint. Impingement can be diagnosed through the patient history, a thorough physical examination, and the response to nonsurgical management. Diagnostic imaging studies often are most helpful for ruling out other sources of symptoms, such as a chondral or osteochondral lesion. The syndromes are classified by their relation to the tibiotalar joint. In young athletes, surgical treatment usually is reserved for pain recalcitrant to nonsurgical measures.

Soft-Tissue Impingement

Anterolateral soft-tissue impingement in young athletes frequently is a cause of chronic ankle pain after an inversion ankle sprain. This syndrome most often is caused by thickening of the accessory fascicle of the distal anteroinferior tibiofibular ligament and occasionally by injury to the anterior talofibular ligament. Thickening of the distal fascicle of the anteroinferior tibiofibular ligament causes talar impingement, abrasion of the talar articular cartilage, and pain in the anterolateral ankle.[19] Partial healing of the anterior talofibular ligament occurs with repetitive motion and causes ligament inflammation that leads to hypertrophic synovium and scar tissue in the lateral gutter. This condition, classically referred to as a meniscoid lesion, can cause impingement and chronic anterolateral ankle pain.[20]

Medial soft-tissue impingement is caused by an injury to the deltoid ligament or capsule. The resultant scarring and hypertrophy of the synovium can cause ankle pain similar to the pain caused by anterolateral impingement. Osteophytes may form if the condition becomes chronic.

Posterior soft-tissue impingement can cause chronic posterior ankle pain in young athletes. Fibrosis, capsulitis, and synovial swelling in the posterior capsuloligamentous structures can cause generalized posterior impingement. Hypertrophy or tearing in the posteroinferior tibiofibular ligament, transverse tibiofibular ligament, or tibial slip can cause localized posterior impingement.

Clinical Presentation

Soft-tissue ankle impingement is diagnosed by careful palpation and stress testing of the ankle joint. Tenderness during palpation over the anterior talofibular ligament, with increased tenderness during dorsiflexion, is 95% sensitive and 88% specific for anterolateral impingement.[21] Medial soft-tissue impingement is diagnosed if there is tenderness over the anteromedial ankle. Patients with posterior soft-tissue ankle impingement report chronic posterior ankle joint pain that is aggravated with plantar flexion. The tenderness is along the posterior ankle joint. Diagnostic injection can be used to confirm the diagnosis. The differential diagnosis of most soft-tissue impingements should include ankle instability, subtalar instability, tarsal coalition, symptomatic ossicles, and chondral or osteochondral lesions, especially of the talus.

Diagnostic Imaging

Conventional radiography is the only study required to diagnose soft-tissue impingement in most patients. The plain radiographs usually are normal and primarily serve to exclude bony pathology. Calcification or heterotopic bone in the interosseous space indicates a previous injury to the distal tibiofibular syndesmosis. Ossicles along the tip of the fibula and the lateral talar dome are consistent with anterior talofibular ligament injury. In a patient with ankle instability, stress radiographs may show medial joint space widening or avulsion fracture. Posterior osteophytes or loose bodies may be present with posterior impingement.

MRI can be used to confirm the diagnosis of soft-tissue impingement. However, the reported sensitivity and specificity of conventional MRI are less than 50% for anterolateral soft-tissue impingement of the ankle.[22,23] Magnetic resonance arthrography can increase the diagnostic accuracy by allowing capsular distention and separating the adjacent anatomic structures.[22] MRI can show hypertrophy or tears of the posterior ligaments of the ankle with posterior impingement. With medial impingement, inflammatory changes and scar tissue are found in the medial gutter. Edema or soft tissue causing anterior displacement of the subcutaneous fat adjacent to the anterior fibula is diagnostic of anterolateral impingement. MRI primarily serves to rule out other sources of pain, such as chondral or osteochondral injury.

Treatment

Rest, immobilization, nonsteroidal anti-inflammatory drugs, and physical therapy may reduce the severity of symptoms.[20] Injection of a local anesthetic and a steroid can be both diagnostic and therapeutic. If the pain persists, arthroscopic inspection, débridement of the reactive synovium, and resection of scar tissue and inflamed ligaments may be needed. The use of coaxial portals is safe, effective, and reproducible for posterior lesions[24] (**Figure 1**). The postsurgical treatment involves a brief period of immobilization, followed by nonimpact exercises at 2 weeks and impact exercises at 4 weeks. A good or excellent result can be expected in 80% to 95% of patients.[25]

Posterior Bony Ankle Impingement

The most common cause of posterior ankle bony impingement in a young athlete is a symptomatic os trigonum or Stieda process. In some children, a secondary ossification center mineralizes at age 7 to 13 years and fuses to the posterolateral body of the talus to form the Stieda process.[26] The secondary ossification center fails to unite with the main body of the talus in 7% to 14% of these children, and an os trigonum is thus formed.[27] Pain can develop in the young athlete during plantar flexion or a push-off maneuver and is most common in sports such as dancing, gymnastics, tumbling, kicking, martial arts, and downhill running. Symptoms occur when the os trigonum or Stieda process is pinched between the posterior tibia and the calcaneus after trauma or repetitive use.

Clinical Evaluation

The diagnosis of posterior ankle bony impingement is primarily based on the patient's clinical history and physical examination, as supported by imaging studies. The patient reports posterior ankle pain with forced plantar flexion during activity. In a ballet dancer, pain occurs in the en pointe position. The tenderness is between the Achilles and peroneal tendons and is exacer-

bated with plantar flexion. An associated inflammation of the peritenon of the flexor hallucis longus tendon is common in ballet dancers, giving rise to posteromedial pain and pain with passive dorsiflexion of the great toe. The differential diagnosis includes chronic synovitis, Achilles tendinitis, flexor hallucis tenosynovitis, retrocalcaneal bursitis, ankle and subtalar instability, fracture, anterior ankle impingement, posterior soft-tissue impingement, and osteochondritis dissecans.

Diagnostic Imaging

The os trigonum or Stieda process usually can be seen on a lateral radiograph(Figure 2). In a skeletally immature patient, the ossicle or process may be cartilaginous or only partially ossified, and it may not be easily visible on radiographs. Bone scanning can be used to identify the increased bony metabolic activity associated with posterior impingement caused by a Stieda process or os trigonum. MRI is more commonly used to show a cartilaginous process, and it can reveal fluid or edema in the symptomatic ossicle or Stieda process. MRI also is used to exclude other causes of posterior ankle pain.

Treatment

A trial of nonsurgical management is warranted in most patients. Rest, ice, anti-inflammatory medication, and avoidance of forceful plantar flexion are successful in as many as 60% of patients.[28] If an acute fracture or rupture of the synchondrosis is suspected in a skeletally immature patient, a period of immobilization in a cast

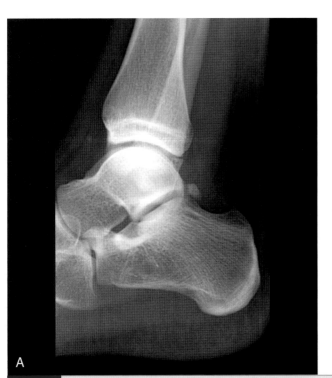

Figure 1	Schematic drawing showing an axial view of coaxial portals used in posterior ankle arthroscopy.

Flexor hallucis longus
Posterior tibial artery/nerve
Achilles tendon
Peroneal tendons
Flexor digitorum longus
Lateral portal
Posterior tibial tendon
Medial portal
Posterior transverse portal

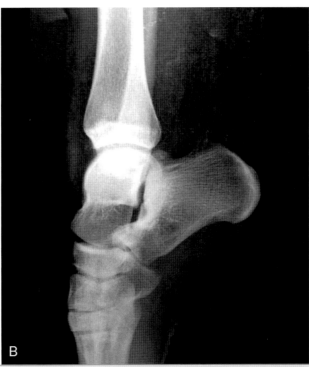

A

B

Figure 2	**A,** Lateral radiograph showing an os trigonum. **B,** Plantar flexion lateral radiograph showing impingement of an os trigonum against the posterior tibia.

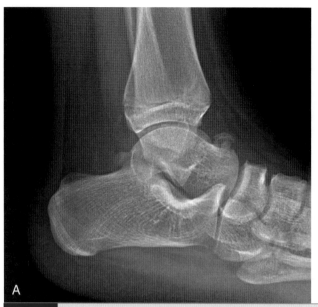
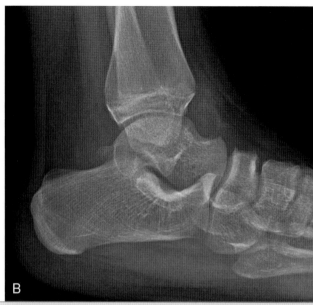

Figure 3 Lateral radiographs showing an anterior bony impingement lesion on the talus before (**A**) and after (**B**) arthroscopic resection of the lesion. A posterior prominent Stieda process can be seen.

or boot walker may allow the area to heal.[29] Corticosteroid injections often provide at least temporary relief of pain and may aid in the diagnosis.

Surgery is warranted if nonsurgical management is not successful. A symptomatic os trigonum or Stieda process can be treated using open or arthroscopic excision. Associated flexor hallucis longus tendinitis that does not respond to nonsurgical treatment sometimes requires release of the constrictive flexor retinaculum. Rehabilitation may proceed more rapidly after arthroscopic excision of the os trigonum.[30] Coaxial portals are used in posterior ankle arthroscopy to provide good visualization and ease of excision.[24]

Anterior Bony Ankle Impingement

Acute trauma or repetitive overuse injury to the ankle during sports, particularly tumbling or gymnastics, can lead to anterior bone spurs that result in bony impingement and ankle pain. These bony spurs originally were believed to represent a response to capsular traction during extreme plantar flexion. However, anatomic study found that the spurs are formed within the capsule rather than its site of insertion.[31] The bony spurs are believed to develop from repetitive trauma to the anterior articular cartilage rim, either from impaction between the tibia and talus during repeated dorsiflexion or from external direct trauma to the anterior ankle joint.[31]

Clinical Evaluation and Classification

Patients have localized anterior ankle tenderness, swelling, and limited ankle dorsiflexion. The pain is exacerbated by dorsiflexion and occasionally by plantar flexion. The classification system used to guide treatment is based on the size and location of the lesion.[32] A grade I lesion is a tibial spur with a diameter of less than 3 mm in diameter. A grade II lesion is at least 3 mm in diameter. A grade III lesion has significant tibial exostosis, with or without fragmentation, with secondary spur formation on the dorsum of the talus. A grade IV lesion has pantalocrural arthritic destruction.[32] Even a small spur causes cartilage lesions, and the extent of cartilage lesions increases as spurs become larger.[33]

Diagnostic Imaging

AP, lateral, and oblique radiographs should be obtained. A lateral radiograph will show bone spurs on the talar neck or distal tibia. Oblique radiographs were found to increase the sensitivity of detection.[34] CT provides more detail on the impingement lesion, if necessary (**Figure 3**).

Treatment

The nonsurgical treatment includes limitation of the symptom-provoking activity. Surgical treatment of anterior bony ankle impingement usually is reserved for a patient with symptoms recalcitrant to nonsurgical management. The typical procedure is arthroscopic débridement of the lesion on the distal tibia or dorsum of the talus. Adequate visualization of the lesion is essential for avoiding injury to the dorsal neurovascular structures.

Osteochondral Lesions of the Talus

An osteochondral lesion of the talus (OLT) is uncommon in young athletes. This lesion represents a disorder

7: Sports-Related Topics

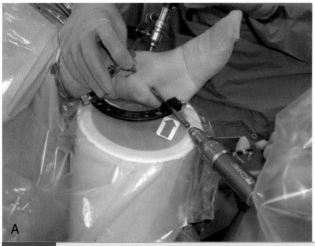
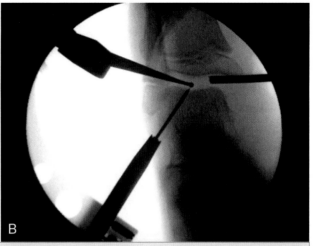

Figure 4 **A,** Intraoperative photograph showing extra-articular drilling of an osteochondral lesion of the talus. **B,** Fluoroscopic view showing retrograde drilling of the lesion using the Micro Vector (Smith & Nephew, Memphis, TN) drill guiding device.

of the subchondral bone leading to separation and fragmentation of the overlying cartilage. Medial lesions reportedly are more common in children than lateral lesions.[18,35,36] Approximately 50% to 80% of children with OLT have a history of acute trauma or repetitive microtrauma.[18,35,36] Ninety-three percent of patients with a lateral talar lesion and 61% of those with a medial lesion report a history of trauma.[37] Lateral lesions tend to be shallower and more anterior than medial lesions.[37] The trauma mechanism in lateral lesions usually is a combination of inversion and dorsiflexion. In medial lesions, the combination is inversion, plantar flexion, and rotation.[38]

The lesions are classified as primary and secondary based on their etiology. Primary OLT is nontraumatic and most likely results from a deficiency of the talar blood supply. These lesions have an insidious onset of subchondral bone necrosis. Genetic, metabolic, repetitive overload, and endocrine factors also can be a primary cause. Secondary OLT usually occurs after a traumatic event such as ankle sprain, fracture, or instability. OLT also can be classified based on radiographic, CT, MRI, or arthroscopic findings.[39-41]

Clinical Evaluation

A patient with primary OLT usually has persistent ankle pain without any recognized traumatic event. A young athlete with secondary OLT usually has a history of traumatic or chronic ankle sprain. Children and young adults usually report ankle swelling, pain, limp, tenderness, and reduced range of motion.[36] Some patients have locking or instability. A careful examination can identify limitations in the range of motion as well as the location of tenderness. The anterior drawer test should be performed with the ankle in dorsiflexion and plantar flexion. Inversion and eversion stress testing should also be performed.

Diagnostic Imaging

Weight-bearing AP, lateral, and mortise radiographs of the ankle should be obtained for the initial evaluation. However, plain radiographs usually do not show low-grade lesions.[42] A stress-view radiograph can be used to detect ligamentous instability. CT and MRI have been used for diagnosing and evaluating osteochondral defects of the talus, but CT may not show some cartilaginous or nondisplaced lesions. MRI shows the surface of the articular cartilage, subchondral bone, and surrounding soft tissue for defining the pathology, location, and extent of involvement of the lesion.[42]

Treatment

The appropriate treatment of OLT in young athletes remains controversial. Nonsurgical treatment can be attempted but often is unsuccessful in young athletes with a nondisplaced lesion. Successful nonsurgical management was reported in 40% of children with OLT.[18] In another study, only 5 of 31 patients with OLT (16%; mean age, 11.9 years) had complete clinical and radiographic healing with 6 months of nonsurgical treatment.[36] Nonsurgical treatment is a viable option, but the patient and family must be aware of the relatively low healing rate.

Surgical management is indicated if the pain persists or the patient is not willing to modify activity. Ankle arthroscopy and extra-articular drilling usually are the treatment of choice if the articular cartilage of the talus remains intact (Figure 4). Extra-articular percutaneous autografting has been used for larger subchondral lesions.[36] If the articular surface is disrupted, the available surgical methods include fragment fixation, débridement, microfracture, drilling, autologous chondrocyte implant, bone grafting followed by autologous chondrocyte implantation, mosaicplasty, or fresh allografting[43-46] (Figure 5). In theory, the hyaline cartilage produced by cartilage restoration techniques can

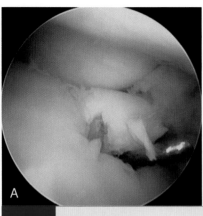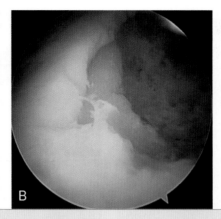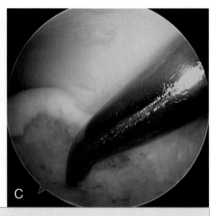

A   B   C

Figure 5   Arthroscopic views showing treatment of an osteochondral lesion of the talus. **A,** Complete avulsion of the fragment without displacement. **B,** Débridement of the lesion. **C,** Microfracture of the lesion.

provide a better weight-bearing surface than the fibrocartilage formed after microfracture. In practice, however, no studies have shown a clear benefit of one treatment method over the others. Long-term comparison studies are needed to clearly define the roles of these techniques. Coaxial portals provide good access to lesions in the posterior talus.[24]

Ossicles

Accessory ossicles are common in skeletally immature individuals. The lateral ossicle is called the os subfibulare, and the medial ossicle is the os subtibiale. These accessory centers appear when the child is age 7 to 10 years, and they fuse with the secondary center of the malleolus at approximately age 15 to 17 years. Ossicles that appear later are considered avulsion fragments associated with acute or recurrent injury to the ankle. Os subtibiale may be present in as many as 20% of individuals, and os subfibulare in approximately 1%.[47] The accessory ossicles can become symptomatic in young athletes and may require surgical treatment.

The accessory ossicles are not anatomically separate entities but contiguous secondary centers of the malleoli. Usually these ossicles are asymptomatic, but they may become symptomatic if acutely or chronically injured. If the cartilaginous continuity of an accessory ossicle is disrupted, fracture or fibrous union can result. In addition, the ossicle may be avulsed as a ligament failure analogue (similar to a patellar sleeve fracture). This avulsion is more common in the lateral than in the medial malleolus, and it can progress to delayed union, nonunion, or a chronically painful ankle.

Clinical Evaluation
Patients have point tenderness at the site of the ossicle at the tip of the malleolus. The anterior drawer test should be performed with the ankle in dorsiflexion and plantar flexion. Inversion and eversion stress testing also should be performed.

Diagnostic Imaging
Radiographs of the ankle are obtained during the initial evaluation. An ossicle of the medial or lateral malleolus is classified as small (less than 5 mm), medium (5 to 10 mm), or large (more than 10 mm)[48] (**Figure 6**). The shape is angular or round to oval, and sometimes there is an osteosclerotic rim. Three-dimensional, contrast-enhanced, fat-suppressed, fast-gradient-recalled MRI can show linear and nodular enhancement of symptomatic ossicles and is well correlated with arthroscopic findings (91% sensitivity).[48] Technetium Tc 99m bone scanning can support a diagnosis of injury.

Treatment
If an accessory center is associated with an acute ankle injury or if the patient has chronic symptoms, it is appropriate to immobilize the ankle for 3 to 4 weeks and then encourage mobilization and weight bearing. Open or arthroscopic excision of the ossicle is reserved for a patient with recurrent symptoms recalcitrant to nonsurgical measures. In 24 patients with chronic symptomatic ossicles who underwent arthroscopic excision, the average American Orthopaedic Foot and Ankle Society score had improved from 74.5 to 93 points at a mean 30.5-month follow-up; 21 patients (88%) were satisfied.[48]

Summary

A thorough history and focused physical examination are essential to diagnosing pathology specific to the ankle in children and adolescents. Most ankle sprains can be treated with a multidisciplinary approach that includes bracing, balance training, and physical therapy. Persistent conditions must be identified and appropriately treated. Soft-tissue or bony ankle impingement causes chronic ankle pain; these lesions can be successfully treated with arthroscopic débridement if nonsurgical treatment is unsuccessful. The choice among the many methods for treating OLT depends on the integ-

7: Sports-Related Topics

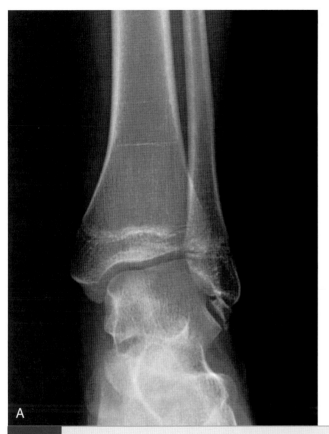
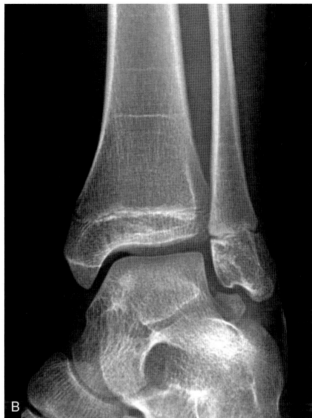

Figure 6 AP (**A**) and oblique (**B**) radiographs showing a symptomatic os subfibulare.

rity of the cartilage surface and the size of the lesion; no studies have shown a clear benefit of one method over the others. Accessory ossicles are common in skeletally immature patients. These ossicles may become symptomatic in an athlete, and they may require open or arthroscopic excision. Most pediatric patients with ankle pathology recover full function with appropriate treatment.

Annotated References

1. National Federation of State High School Associations: 2009-2010 high school athletics participation summary. http://www.nfhs.org. Accessed January 10, 2011.

   Athletic participation in high schools throughout the United States is summarized.

2. Darrow CJ, Collins CL, Yard EE, Comstock RD: Epidemiology of severe injuries among United States high school athletes: 2005-2007. *Am J Sports Med* 2009; 37(9):1798-1805.

   Sports injury data were collected from 100 US high schools during the academic years from 2005 to 2007. Rates of severe injury (resulting in a loss of more than 21 days of sports participation) varied by sport, sex, and type of exposure.

3. Garrick JG: The frequency of injury, mechanism of injury, and the epidemiology of ankle sprains. *Am J Sports Med* 1985;9:241.

4. Smith RW, Reischl SF: Treatment of ankle sprains in young athletes. *Am J Sports Med* 1986;14(6):465-471.

5. Amendola A, Najibi S, Wasserman L: Athletic ankle injuries, in Garrick JG, ed: *Orthopaedic Knowledge Update: Sports Medicine 3*. Rosemont, IL, American Academy of Orthopaedic Surgeons, 2004, pp 233-248.

6. Stiell IG, Greenberg GH, McKnight RD, et al: Decision rules for the use of radiography in acute ankle injuries: Refinement and prospective validation. *JAMA* 1993; 269(9):1127-1132.

7. Ogden JA, Lee J: Accessory ossification patterns and injuries of the malleoli. *J Pediatr Orthop* 1990;10(3):306-316.

8. Pedowitz DI, Reddy S, Parekh SG, Huffman GR, Sennett BJ: Prophylactic bracing decreases ankle injuries in collegiate female volleyball players. *Am J Sports Med* 2008;36(2):324-327.

   Prophylactic use of a double-upright ankle brace in collegiate female volleyball players reduced the ankle injury rate from 0.98 to 0.07 per 1,000 exposures.

9. McGuine TA, Keene JS: The effect of a balance training program on the risk of ankle sprains in high school athletes. *Am J Sports Med* 2006;34(7):1103-1111.

In a randomized controlled clinical study, 765 high school soccer and basketball players were assigned to a balance training program or standard conditioning exercises. The balance training program reduced the risk of ankle sprains. Level of evidence: I.

10. Reed ME, Feibel JB, Donley BG, Gaza E. Athletic ankle injuries, in Kibler WB, ed: *Orthopaedic Knowledge Update: Sports Medicine 4*. Rosemont, IL, American Academy of Orthopaedic Surgeons, 2009, pp 200-201.

11. Van Deun S, Staes FF, Stappaerts KH, Janssens L, Levin O, Peers KK: Relationship of chronic ankle instability to muscle activation patterns during the transition from double-leg to single-leg stance. *Am J Sports Med* 2007; 35(2):274-281.

A descriptive epidemiologic study reviewed sports-related injury data from 100 US high schools during the academic years from 2005 to 2007. Severe injury rates and patterns varied by sport, sex, and type of exposure. The highest rate of severe injury was in football players.

12. Beynnon BD, Renström PA, Haugh L, Uh BS, Barker H: A prospective, randomized clinical investigation of the treatment of first-time ankle sprains. *Am J Sports Med* 2006;34(9):1401-1412.

Treatment of first-time grade I and II ankle sprains with the combination of an ankle-stirrup brace and an elastic wrap led to an earlier return to preinjury function than treatment with an ankle-stirrup brace alone, an elastic wrap alone, or a walking cast for 10 days. Level of evidence: I.

13. Kerkhoffs GM, Struijs PA, Marti RK, Assendelft WJ, Blankevoort L, van Dijk CN: Different functional treatment strategies for acute lateral ankle ligament injuries in adults. *Cochrane Database Syst Rev* 2002;3(3): CD002938.

14. Cass JR, Morrey BF, Katoh Y, Chao EY: Ankle instability: Comparison of primary repair and delayed reconstruction after long-term follow-up study. *Clin Orthop Relat Res* 1985;198(198):110-117.

15. Gerber JP, Williams GN, Scoville CR, Arciero RA, Taylor DC: Persistent disability associated with ankle sprains: A prospective examination of an athletic population. *Foot Ankle Int* 1998;19(10):653-660.

16. Takao M, Uchio Y, Naito K, Fukazawa I, Ochi M: Arthroscopic assessment for intra-articular disorders in residual ankle disability after sprain. *Am J Sports Med* 2005;33(5):686-692.

Arthroscopy can be used to diagnose the cause of residual pain after an ankle sprain if the cause was not diagnosed by clinical examination and imaging. Level of evidence: II.

17. Barnum MJ, Ehrlich MG, Zaleske DJ: Long-term patient-oriented outcome study of a modified Evans procedure. *J Pediatr Orthop* 1998;18(6):783-788.

18. Letts M, Davidson D, Mukhtar I: Surgical management of chronic lateral ankle instability in adolescents. *J Pediatr Orthop* 2003;23(3):392-397.

19. Bassett FH III, Gates HS III, Billys JB, Morris HB, Nikolaou PK: Talar impingement by the anteroinferior tibiofibular ligament: A cause of chronic pain in the ankle after inversion sprain. *J Bone Joint Surg Am* 1990;72(1): 55-59.

20. McCarroll JR, Schrader JW, Shelbourne KD, Rettig AC, Bisesi MA: Meniscoid lesions of the ankle in soccer players. *Am J Sports Med* 1987;15(3):255-257.

21. Molloy S, Solan MC, Bendall SP: Synovial impingement in the ankle: A new physical sign. *J Bone Joint Surg Br* 2003;85(3):330-333.

22. Robinson P, White LM, Salonen DC, Daniels TR, Ogilvie-Harris D: Anterolateral ankle impingement: MR arthrographic assessment of the anterolateral recess. *Radiology* 2001;221(1):186-190.

23. Liu SH, Nuccion SL, Finerman G: Diagnosis of anterolateral ankle impingement: Comparison between magnetic resonance imaging and clinical examination. *Am J Sports Med* 1997;25(3):389-393.

24. Acevedo JI, Busch MT, Ganey TM, Hutton WC, Ogden JA: Coaxial portals for posterior ankle arthroscopy: An anatomic study with clinical correlation on 29 patients. *Arthroscopy* 2000;16(8):836-842.

25. Kim SH, Ha KI: Arthroscopic treatment for impingement of the anterolateral soft tissues of the ankle. *J Bone Joint Surg Br* 2000;82(7):1019-1021.

26. Maquirriain J: Posterior ankle impingement syndrome. *J Am Acad Orthop Surg* 2005;13(6):365-371.

Posterior bony and soft-tissue impingement syndrome is reviewed.

27. Lawson JP: Symptomatic radiographic variants in extremities. *Radiology* 1985;157(3):625-631.

28. Hedrick MR, McBryde AM: Posterior ankle impingement. *Foot Ankle Int* 1994;15(1):2-8.

29. Sammarco VJ: Common dance and ballet injuries of the foot and ankle. *Orthopaedic Knowledge Online*. http://www5.aaos.org/oko/description.cfm?topic=FOO028&referringPage=/oko/mainmenu.cfm. Accessed November 22, 2010.

30. Marumoto JM, Ferkel RD: Arthroscopic excision of the os trigonum: A new technique with preliminary clinical results. *Foot Ankle Int* 1997;18(12):777-784.

31. Tol JL, van Dijk CN: Etiology of the anterior ankle impingement syndrome: A descriptive anatomical study. *Foot Ankle Int* 2004;25(6):382-386.

32. Scranton PE Jr, McDermott JE: Anterior tibiotalar spurs: A comparison of open versus arthroscopic debridement. *Foot Ankle* 1992;13(3):125-129.

33. Moon JS, Lee K, Lee HS, Lee WC: Cartilage lesions in anterior bony impingement of the ankle. *Arthroscopy* 2010;26(7):984-989.

    Investigation of the correlation between spur severity, clinical characteristics, and articular cartilage lesions found that cartilage lesions were present even in ankles with small spurs. The extent of cartilage lesions increased as spurs became larger. Level of evidence: IV.

34. Tol JL, Verhagen RA, Krips R, et al: The anterior ankle impingement syndrome: Diagnostic value of oblique radiographs. *Foot Ankle Int* 2004;25(2):63-68.

35. Higuera J, Laguna R, Peral M, Aranda E, Soleto J: Osteochondritis dissecans of the talus during childhood and adolescence. *J Pediatr Orthop* 1998;18(3):328-332.

36. Perumal V, Wall E, Babekir N: Juvenile osteochondritis dissecans of the talus. *J Pediatr Orthop* 2007;27(7):821-825.

    Retrospective review found a low healing rate after 6 months of nonsurgical treatment of osteochondritis dissecans of the talus in skeletally immature patients. Level of evidence: IV

37. Verhagen RA, Struijs PA, Bossuyt PM, van Dijk CN: Systematic review of treatment strategies for osteochondral defects of the talar dome. *Foot Ankle Clin* 2003; 8(2):233-242.

38. van Dijk CN, Bossuyt PM, Marti RK: Medial ankle pain after lateral ligament rupture. *J Bone Joint Surg Br* 1996;78(4):562-567.

39. Berndt AL, Harty M: Transchondral fractures (osteochondritis dissecans) of the talus. *J Bone Joint Surg Am* 1959;41:988-1020.

40. Hepple S, Winson IG, Glew D: Osteochondral lesions of the talus: A revised classification. *Foot Ankle Int* 1999; 20(12):789-793.

41. Pritsch M, Horoshovski H, Farine I: Arthroscopic treatment of osteochondral lesions of the talus. *J Bone Joint Surg Am* 1986;68(6):862-865.

42. Anderson IF, Crichton KJ, Grattan-Smith T, Cooper RA, Brazier D: Osteochondral fractures of the dome of the talus. *J Bone Joint Surg Am* 1989;71(8):1143-1152.

43. Hangody L, Kish G, Kárpáti Z, Szerb I, Eberhardt R: Treatment of osteochondritis dissecans of the talus: Use of the mosaicplasty technique. A preliminary report. *Foot Ankle Int* 1997;18(10):628-634.

44. Giannini S, Vannini F: Operative treatment of osteochondral lesions of the talar dome: Current concepts review. *Foot Ankle Int* 2004;25(3):168-175.

45. Gross AE, Agnidis Z, Hutchison CR: Osteochondral defects of the talus treated with fresh osteochondral allograft transplantation. *Foot Ankle Int* 2001;22(5):385-391.

46. Lahm A, Erggelet C, Steinwachs M, Reichelt A: Arthroscopic management of osteochondral lesions of the talus: Results of drilling and usefulness of magnetic resonance imaging before and after treatment. *Arthroscopy* 2000;16(3):299-304.

47. Powell HD: Extra centre of ossification for the medial malleolus in children: Incidence and significance. *J Bone Joint Surg Br* 1961;43:107-113.

48. Han SH, Choi WJ, Kim S, Kim SJ, Lee JW: Ossicles associated with chronic pain around the malleoli of the ankle. *J Bone Joint Surg Br* 2008;90(8):1049-1054.

    In a retrospective review of 24 arthroscopic procedures in patients with symptomatic ossicles, arthroscopic and MRI findings were found to be well correlated. The overall rate of patient satisfaction was 88%.

7: Sports-Related Topics

Chapter 42
Back Pain in the Pediatric Athlete

Lyle Micheli, MD   Peter L. Gambacorta, DO

Introduction

Back pain among pediatric patients formerly was believed to be relatively uncommon. Research increasingly suggests that its prevalence has been underestimated, particularly among children participating in sports; a prevalence of 24% to 36% was found in patients younger than 15 years.[1] The true prevalence may be higher, as many adolescents do not seek care for back pain. Adolescent athletes represent a separate at-risk population. Those involved in a sport such as gymnastics, wrestling, or football are twice as likely as the general pediatric population to develop acute back pain.[2,3]

Back pain may be associated with significant pathology, such as neoplasm, osteomyelitis, or diskitis, but in most pediatric patients the pain has a nonspecific cause. No definitive diagnosis was found for 57 of 73 pediatric patients (78%) evaluated for back pain over 2 years.[4] This rate is similar to that of the adult population, which has a high prevalence of mechanical back pain. Pain in pediatric athletes usually has a specific etiology, however.[5] Athletes may experience injury to the soft-tissue or osseous structures of the spine, often associated with trauma, overuse, or fatigue, in which anthropomorphic, sport-specific, hormonal, and nutritional factors coalesce to create unique pathophysiologic conditions.

Anatomy

The vertebral body has two epiphyseal growth plates with an associated ring apophysis located on the superior and inferior margins. Latitudinal growth occurs through perichondral and periosteal apposition, and longitudinal growth occurs through endochondral ossification. The vertebral end plates develop from these epiphyses and function to nourish the intervertebral disk through hydrostatic motion. The posterior arch has three primary growth centers, which are located in both pedicles and the spinous process. The posterior epiphysis closes during the first 5 to 8 years of life, but the anterior column continues to grow until age 16 to 18 years.[6]

The intervertebral disk is a fibrocartilaginous structure composed of two layers: the anulus fibrosus and the nucleus pulposus. The outer layer, the anulus fibrosus, is an arrangement of obliquely oriented bundles of type I collagen fibers. This dense 10- to 20-layer ring contains the neural and vascular tissues of the disk. It surrounds the inner two thirds of the disk, called the nucleus pulposus. The nucleus pulposus has high polysaccharide content, and its composition is approximately 88% water. The cartilaginous end plate separates the anulus fibrosus and the nucleus pulposus from the vertebral body. The anulus fibrosus attaches to the ring apophysis and the end plate at the periphery. When intradiskal pressures are increased through a compressive force, the nucleus pulposus absorbs the load by expanding, thus transmitting the force to the anulus fibrosus. In the immature spine, the point of weakness during compressive force is at the connection of the epiphyseal end plate and the anulus fibrosus (Figure 1).

The sacrum attaches to the pelvis through the sacroiliac joints, which are true diarthrodial joints. The sacroiliac joint is flat until puberty, when it develops furrows, and it fuses later in life. This joint compresses with the ipsilateral posterior pelvic rotation of hip flexion and distracts with hip extension.

Lumbar flexion and extension involve a constantly moving axis of rotation. In flexion, the axis of rotation is in the disk, with a posterior distraction force. In extension, the compression is transferred to the posterior anulus fibrosus and the facet joints. Axial rotation also involves a simultaneous compressive force at the facet joint and a shear force at the posterolateral disk.

Risk Factors

Growth Factors

Approximately 30 million preadolescents and adolescents participate in organized sports each year in the United States.[7] Intense training can place the developing athlete at risk for injury. The physis is a weak link

Neither Dr. Micheli nor any immediate family member has received anything of value from or owns stock in a commercial company or institution related directly or indirectly to the subject of this chapter. Dr. Gambacorta or an immediate family member owns stock or stock options in Amgen Co, Pfizer, Sanofi-Aventis, Smith & Nephew, Stryker, and Zimmer.

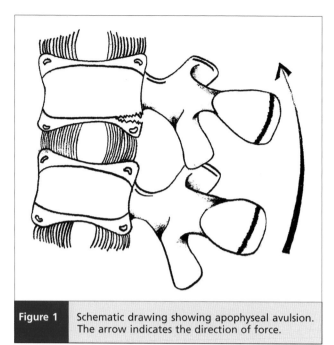

Figure 1 Schematic drawing showing apophyseal avulsion. The arrow indicates the direction of force.

in the spine of the young athlete and a common site of injury, which occurs through the zone of provisional calcification. Compressive forces can rupture the cartilaginous end plate, causing Schmorl nodes to form or the ring apophysis to produce limbus vertebrae. Tensile stresses can result in apophysitis or apophyseal avulsion. Incomplete ossification of the posterior neural arch combined with repetitive loading in a hyperextension sport such as ballet or gymnastics can predispose a child to stress fracture.

Anthropomorphic Factors

Malalignment of the lower extremities can result in improper transfer of ground forces to the lower trunk. The lack of flexibility and a lack of conditioning contribute to this biomechanical problem, along with limb-length inequality. In a study of 98 pediatric patients, boys who participated in sports requiring excessive lower lumbar flexion and girls who had above-normal body weight and participated in sports requiring excessive lower lumbar flexion were found to be at risk for low back pain.[8] Weak lower abdominal muscles and tight hip flexors are postulated to contribute to increased lumbar lordosis, resulting in a compressive load to the posterior elements and a tensile force to the disk.

Sex-Specific Factors

The comparative risk in girls and boys varies by pathologic entity and by sport. Limited objective data are available. Spondylolysis was found to be two to three times more prevalent in boys than in girls,[9] but a more recent study found an equal risk for male and female patients.[10] Spondylolisthesis may occur more frequently in girls.[11-13] The rate of scoliosis also is greater in girls than in boys.[14]

Sport-Specific Factors

The motion and force exerted on the lumbar spine are unique to each sport. The cause of injury in a specific sport may be linked to direct macrotrauma or repetitive microtrauma. Repetitive hyperextension, as in gymnastics or football, places the athlete's posterior spine elements at risk of injury. Most soccer players with spondylolysis recall an episode of acute pain following a high-velocity kick.[15] Baseball players, bowlers, and swimmers are susceptible to disk pathology secondary to repetitive rotational motions. Participation in collision sports, weight lifting, snowboarding, or another sport that involves flexion and axial loading has been linked to herniated nucleus pulposus (HNP) and fracture.[16,17]

Clinical Evaluation

History

Obtaining a thorough history is paramount for determining the cause of a young athlete's back pain, including a traumatic or atraumatic etiology. The sport-specific questions should include the patient's playing position, level of conditioning, and amount of training. Pain location, duration, quality, and radicular symptoms should be noted, as well as any functional changes (including changes related to bowel and bladder function) and any history of back injury or surgery. Movements that alleviate or aggravate the pain should be identified. Pain that is aggravated by extension movements suggests posterior element involvement; pain aggravated by flexion movements or the Valsalva maneuver suggests discogenic involvement. Mechanical back pain is most likely to be experienced in the low back; nerve compression pain is often felt in the legs. The use and effect of medications such as acetaminophen and nonsteroidal anti-inflammatory drugs (NSAIDs) must be included. Night pain, recent weight loss, or fever often is associated with a serious pathologic condition, as is a history of immunocompromise, cancer, or inflammatory arthropathy. Obtaining a nutritional history is important for any young athlete and especially for a female athlete. A history of an eating disorder, menstrual irregularity, and osteoporosis (called the female athlete triad) places the patient at increased risk for certain injuries, including stress fracture.[11]

Physical Examination

The examination begins by observing the patient's body habitus, attitude, and gait pattern. A patient who is severely underweight and appears lethargic may have a different pathology than a patient who is overweight and appears anxious. Gait observation can be used to identify a waddling gait pattern or positions of avoidance or muscular weakness. It is important to assess the patient's ability to heel-and-toe walk. With the patient sufficiently unclothed, the posture is evaluated for the presence of scoliosis, kyphosis, or a flat back. The presence of cutaneous markings and hair tufts may signify an underlying anomaly.

Palpation of the lumbar spine can reveal clues as to the pathology. Spinous process tenderness may coincide with ligamentous injury, fracture, or apophysitis. An acute paraspinal muscular spasm feels warm and boggy to the touch, but a chronic injury feels cool and ropy. A palpable step-off deformity may indicate a spondylolisthesis. A complete palpatory examination should include the sacroiliac joints, piriformis fossa, and greater trochanters.

Testing for lumbar range of motion includes flexion, extension, side bending, and rotation. Any of these movements may elicit a provocative response implicating specific spinal elements. The stork test (a one-leg stance with lumbar hyperextension) can elicit pain from the posterior elements.

A detailed neurologic examination is crucial. The tested dermatomes and myotomes should include hip flexion with sensation to the anterior thigh (L2), knee extension (L3), ankle dorsiflexion with sensation to the dorsum of the foot (L4), great toe extension with sensation to the web space between the first and second toes (L5), and ankle plantar flexion with sensation to the plantar surface of the foot (S1). The presence of deep tendon reflexes at the patellar tendon (L4) and Achilles tendon (S1) also should be recorded.

Tension tests, including the Lasègue straight leg raise and the femoral nerve stretch, can implicate nerve compression from an HNP or a fracture. A positive flexion-abduction–external rotation test may be associated with sacroiliac joint involvement. A Thomas test indicates tightness of the hip flexors. Tight hamstrings may suggest spondylolysis. Abnormal Babinski and abdominal reflexes often are associated with upper motor neuron pathology.

Acute Injuries

Fractures

Pediatric thoracolumbar trauma is estimated to account for 0.6% to 0.9% of all spine fractures.[18] These rare fractures most commonly occur in adolescents, among whom sports-related causes may account for 21% to 53%.[19,20] Contact sports such as hockey and wrestling place the athlete at increased risk for blunt trauma injury. Thoracolumbar fractures have been found among participants in sports involving axial loading, such as diving and snowboarding.

The evaluation of a patient with a suspected fracture begins with strict spine precautions and the use of Advanced Trauma Life Support protocols, including proper immobilization with a spine board. A full secondary survey and a spine survey should be undertaken after the primary assessment. Inspection of the spine for bruising, swelling, tenderness, and widening of

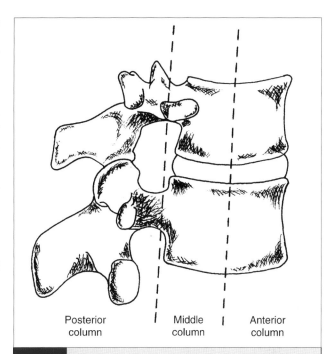

Posterior column   Middle column   Anterior column

Figure 2   Schematic drawing showing the posterior, middle, and anterior spine columns, as used to assess stability.

spinous processes is essential, along with a detailed neurologic examination. However, the physical indicators of thoracolumbar fracture are not always present in a pediatric patient. Clinical evaluation was found to be 81% sensitive and 68% specific for diagnosing thoracolumbar fracture; 19% of patients with a fracture had a normal examination.[21]

Radiography is important for identifying spinal column injury. Screening radiographs should be obtained for a pediatric patient with a history of thoracolumbar trauma. In the presence of fracture, radiographs can be used to evaluate spine stability, based on the three-column classification system (Figure 2). Involvement of two or more columns suggests instability, which may be associated with neurologic compromise. CT is recommended if an unstable fracture is suspected. CT is helpful in assessing canal compromise and the integrity of the surrounding osseous structures. If a neurologic deficit is present, MRI can provide additional information about the cord and surrounding soft tissues.

Spinal cord injury without radiographic abnormality (SCIWORA) is more common in pediatric patients than in adults because of the physiologic characteristics of children. The pediatric spine is inherently more elastic than the adult spine, and it can accommodate more motion and displacement before a fracture or ligamentous rupture occurs. The spinal cord cannot stretch without causing injury, however. Approximately 30% to 40% of spinal cord injuries in pediatric patients do not have radiographic abnormalities.[22] SCIWORA is considered an unstable spine injury.

Most thoracolumbar fractures in athletically active

children are stable fractures that are not associated with neurologic deficit and can be treated nonsurgically. The stable fractures include a fracture of the spinous process or the transverse process and a compression fracture with less than 30° of angulation. A compression fracture is the most common thoracolumbar fracture in the pediatric population. Healing of a compression fracture with less than 30° of angulation typically is not associated with cessation of growth. Restoration of vertebral body height can be expected in a patient with open physes. Burst fractures usually occur at the thoracolumbar junction and often involve the disk and ring apophysis. A burst fracture can be treated nonsurgically as a stable fracture if the posterior elements are intact, with less than 40% to 50% loss of height, 40% to 50% canal compromise, or 20% to 25% of kyphotic deformity.[8] Premature fusion of the growth plates often occurs with this pattern, however, and close monitoring is required to detect any progressive deformity. The nonsurgical treatment of a stable fracture consists of bed rest followed by activity restriction, application of ice, and often the use of a brace. A thoracolumbosacral orthosis is used until the pain subsides, usually after 4 to 12 weeks. Sports activity is prohibited during this period, and physical therapy is begun when tolerated. Surgical treatment is reserved for a patient who has instability after nonsurgical treatment. However, progressive neurologic deterioration, cord compression, subluxation, or dislocation requires immediate surgical attention.

Acute Disk Herniation

The true prevalence of lumbar disk herniation in pediatric athletes is unknown. A discogenic cause, including herniation, was found in 11% of pediatric athletes with lumbar pain.[5] Athletes involved in a collision sport or weight lifting are at increased risk for lumbar disk herniation. The HNP can be located at any level but is in the L4-5 or L5-S1 disk space in 92% of patients.[23] Most herniations are centrolateral and remain subligamentous. In both adult and pediatric patients, the pain is located in the low back, buttock, posterior thigh, and/or leg. Overt neurologic deficits are rare in pediatric patients. Herniation often is associated with a traumatic event, and the symptoms can be provoked by coughing, sneezing, or forward flexion. In contrast to adults, the dramatic physical findings in adolescents may be accompanied by a low pain level.

The physical evaluation includes analysis of the gait as well as the lumbar range of motion, which often is abnormal. The patient may be apprehensive about lumbar flexion and the Valsalva maneuver. A straight leg raise test was positive in 67% of patients who had MRI evidence of lumbar nerve root compression.[24] If there is any evidence of saddle paresthesia or bowel or bladder dysfunction, a rectal examination should be performed to rule out cauda equina syndrome. Standard radiographs should be used to rule out other pathology, although MRI is the diagnostic imaging study of choice.

Most young athletes with HNP initially are treated nonsurgically. Bed rest, lumbar spine icing, and NSAIDs may be accompanied by lumbar brace use. The use of a rigid hyperlordotic brace over a 3- to 4-month period can alleviate the symptoms and help prevent a recurrence. Epidural steroid injections have been used, but no prospective studies have been done to determine the efficacy of this treatment. Surgical intervention is rarely needed to treat disk herniation in pediatric patients. The surgical indications include cauda equina syndrome, persistent pain despite more than 3 months of nonsurgical treatment, and progressive neurologic deficit. The outcome of surgery is promising. Only 20% of 72 pediatric patients required additional surgery within the first 10 years after lumbar diskectomy for HNP, and only 26% required surgery within the first 20 years.[25]

After nonsurgical or surgical treatment, physical therapy and rehabilitation are needed before the patient returns to sports. The therapy programs should be tailored to lumbar stretching as well as sport-specific and core-strengthening exercises. A return to play can be expected 3 to 6 months after nonsurgical treatment and 6 to 12 months after surgical treatment.

Apophyseal Injuries

An apophyseal ring fracture, often referred to as a limbus fracture, is exclusive to skeletally immature athletes. Spine growth can be divided into the cartilaginous, apophyseal, and epiphyseal stages. Injury most frequently occurs during the apophyseal stage, usually after a compressive or traction force. Most such injuries occur after acute trauma, although some result from overuse microtrauma. The site of injury is the junction between the vertebral body and apophysis, where the anulus fibrosus attaches. The ring can be avulsed and posteriorly displaced into the spinal canal, most commonly at the L4 vertebra. Athletes younger than 18 years who are involved in a sport such as weight lifting or gymnastics are particularly at risk.

On examination, the patient may have tenderness and spasm of the paraspinal musculature. The physical findings may be similar to those of HNP, including pain with coughing, sneezing, or flexion. The straight leg raise and nerve tension sign usually are positive. A bony avulsion sometimes can be seen on a lateral radiograph. CT is the diagnostic imaging study of choice. Diagnosis with MRI is challenging because of poor visualization of the bone.[26]

The treatment protocol is similar to that of HNP, with nonsurgical measures including bed rest, icing, and NSAIDs. Surgery is reserved for patients with cauda equina syndrome or neurologic deficit.

Strains, Sprains, and Contusions

Sprains occur when ligaments are stretched beyond the normal range. Strains are muscle tearing that can occur during concentric or eccentric loading. Contusions are caused by direct impact to the soft tissue, resulting in hematoma formation. Sprains, strains, and contusions are common among athletes. The diagnosis is made by exclusion. The pain associated with these injuries is correlated with inflammation and muscle spasm. Patients often have pain in the low back 1 to 2 days after injury. Examination may reveal muscle spasm and palpatory tenderness. Diagnostic studies usually are negative. The main forms of treatment are icing and rest from activity for a period of days to weeks, depending on the severity of the injury. NSAIDs can be used during the acute phases of recovery. A physical therapy program focused on stretching and core strengthening can help decrease the risk of recurrent injury.

Spondylolysis and Spondylolisthesis

The term spondylolysis refers to a defect or dissolution of the pars interarticularis, which is the narrow part of the lamina located between the superior and inferior articular processes of the vertebra. In the pediatric athlete, spondylolysis often occurs as a result of overuse associated with repetitive hyperextension. Bilateral involvement is most common, and L5 is the most commonly involved vertebra. Spondylolisthesis refers to the slipping of a vertebra onto the adjacent vertebra. The five types of spondylolisthesis are dysplastic, isthmic, degenerative, traumatic, and pathologic. Isthmic spondylolisthesis is the most common type in children. The isthmic type is subdivided into spondylolisthesis that is caused by stress fracture, caused by an acute fracture, or associated with elongation of the pars interarticularis. Spondylolisthesis can occur in the presence of bilateral spondylolysis. The treatment of these conditions is centered on pain control and prevention of slip progression.

Several etiologies have been proposed for spondylolysis. The nutcracker hypothesis involves spine extension, in which the inferior articular process of the superior vertebra affects the pars interarticularis of the inferior vertebra.[27] However, some studies suggest that the pars interarticularis fails through traction forces.[28] Abnormalities of the sacral growth plate also have been implicated as a possible cause.[29]

The risk factors for developing spondylolysis include a positive family history, a developmental spine defect, and Inuit ancestry.[30-32] Spondylolysis is two to three times more likely to occur in boys than in girls, but spondylolisthesis occurs more frequently in girls.[33] The rates are two to three times higher in children of European descent than in those of African descent.[34]

Most lesions are asymptomatic. In a prospective study of 500 children followed for 45 years beginning in first grade, the prevalence of pars interarticularis lesion was 4.4% among 6-year-olds and 6% among adults.[35] Fifteen percent of those with a spondylolysis had progression to spondylolisthesis. Slippage is associated with a bilateral spondylolysis, which most often occurs during adolescence. No association was found between pain and the development of spondylolysis or progression of the slip.

Pediatric athletes are subject to more severe and more repetitive forces than most children and adolescents. When 100 adolescent athletes were evaluated for back pain, spondylolysis was found to be the cause in 47%.[5] Unlike the general pediatric population, many athletes have low back pain, and 40% can associate its inception with a specific event.[15] A sport that causes lumbar spine hyperextension places the posterior elements at risk. Consequently, spondylolysis is most common in sports such as gymnastics, ballet, figure skating, crew, weight lifting, soccer, and football (particularly among linemen).

The athlete's back pain becomes worse with activity, especially lumbar hyperextension. The pain often is severe if there is an associated high-grade slip. Physical evaluation may reveal a palpable step-off. Bilateral hamstring tightness is common, and hyperextension with a one-leg stance exacerbates the pain. The gait is usually normal, however. Paresthesia, neurologic deficit, and tension signs can occur in the presence of a slip.

Standard AP and lateral radiographs are followed by an oblique lateral radiograph, if necessary for confirming the diagnosis. Lucency or irregularity of the pars interarticularis may be identified. With the scotty dog sign, which can be seen in the oblique view, a break in the neck of the dog outline signifies a defect in the pars interarticularis. However, only 32% of lesions were detected on an oblique lateral radiograph, and CT was recommended for diagnosis.[36] Some clinicians omit the relatively insensitive oblique lateral radiograph to minimize the patient's exposure to ionizing radiation.

Single-photon emission computed tomography (SPECT) is used if plain radiographs are normal. SPECT can reveal a stress reaction or fracture of the pars interarticularis with greater sensitivity than plain radiographs or a planar bone scan.[37] The intensity of SPECT corresponds to the amount of radiotracer uptake in the metabolically active bone. There appears to be a correlation between increased signal intensity and osseous healing potential.[38] CT can be used after positive SPECT because it is more specific for diagnosing a complete spondylolysis (as opposed to a stress reaction). However, the use of CT is limited to reduce the patient's radiation exposure. Limited fine-cut CT images and three-dimensional sagittal CT reconstruction can be used to confirm the presence and stage of a pars interarticularis defect. CT has been used to classify lesions as early, progressive, or terminal (chronic).[39] CT also can be used to monitor the healing of lesions and to rule out the presence of another lesion such as osteoid osteoma, facet fracture, or stenosis.

The indications for using MRI to detect a pars interarticularis lesion are evolving. MRI is useful for detecting bone marrow edema in a prelysis lesion. A thinslice, fat-saturated T2-weighted MRI study can detect spondylolysis in the early stage. A grading scheme using MRI was found to have high interrater reliability for the diagnosis of spondylolysis.[40] MRI can be used to monitor healing during treatment and offers the advantage of showing other spine elements, including the cord and disk, without the need to subject the patient to additional radiation.[41] Although MRI is an effective and reliable first-line modality for detecting spondylolysis, localized CT also may be needed.[42,43]

The initial nonsurgical treatment consists of activity modification, including sports restriction as well as physical therapy and often a spine orthosis. Activity restriction for 3 to 6 months has been recommended, with physical therapy focused on reducing the lumbar lordosis, strengthening the core musculature, and stretching the hamstring contracture. The use of an orthosis to treat symptomatic spondylolysis (with or without low-grade spondylolisthesis) has been successful in reducing lumbar lordosis but remains controversial. The brace is molded in 0° to 15° of flexion; it is worn 24 hours a day for 3 months and during sports activity for an additional 3 months. The patient can return to play when a pain-free range of motion is achieved. Of 67 adolescents with spondylolysis who were treated for 6 months with a modified Boston brace, 78% had a good or excellent result.[44] In other studies, 72% to 89% of patients had a successful return to sports.[43,45] Bracing is controversial, however, because similar results have been reported without spinal orthotic treatment.[46] In most patients, formation of a fibrous union appears to offer acceptable stability in the short term. Healing is believed to occur in most unilateral lesions, half of bilateral lesions, and no chronic lesions.[43]

Surgical treatment is appropriate for patients with painful nonunion, slipping spondylolisthesis (grade III or higher), neurologic deficit, or persistent back pain despite nonsurgical treatment. The gold standard for surgically treating a lesion at L5 is in situ fusion of L5-S1 using autogenous bone graft. Surgical repair of the pars interarticularis can be considered if nonsurgical treatment is unsuccessful after 6 months, there is no evidence of a degenerative disk, the lesion is in the terminal phase, or the defect is larger than 7 mm. Direct repair usually is done if the lesion is at L4 or more cephalad. Union can be achieved using Scott wiring (posterior wiring of the transverse process and spinous processes), pedicle screw-and-hook techniques, or Buck translaminar interfragmentary screws.

Degenerative Disk Disease

It is estimated that 11% of adolescent athletes with back pain have a discogenic etiology, compared with 48% of adults with back pain.[5] The main functions of the intervertebral disk are to distribute loads, permit motion, and dissipate force. Pain can occur as the disk dehydrates and desiccates from overuse with aging. In the pediatric athlete, the force from the disk can overcome the strength of the vertebral end plate. The result

can be end plate irregularities and the formation of Schmorl nodes; this condition is referred to as lumbar Scheuermann disease or juvenile disk disorder. The athlete's pain may be associated with annular tearing, disk protrusion, end plate fracturing, or Schmorl nodes.

Although the etiology of lumbar disk degeneration is multifactorial, several studies have associated it with participation in competitive athletic activities.[3,47] Repetitive hyperflexion-extension and axial loading in gymnastics have been correlated with an increased incidence of lumbar disk degeneration. An epidemiologic study to compare the prevalence of disk abnormalities in elite swimmers and gymnasts found lumbar pathology in 5 of 8 gymnasts and in 2 of 11 swimmers.[3] When MRI was used to compare 24 elite male gymnasts with back pain and 16 male nonathletes, a reduction in disk signal intensity was found in 75% of the gymnasts and 31% of the nonathletes.[17] An MRI comparison of 308 college athletes from six different sports with 71 nonathletes found a higher incidence of degenerative disk disease throughout the athletic population, most significantly in the baseball players and swimmers.[47] It was suggested that sports with more frequent trunk rotation may create a predisposition to degenerative disk disease. In adults, a predisposition to degenerative disk disease can be created by past experience of severe low back pain. A 15-year follow-up study of 71 athletes and 21 nonathletes found that 90% of the athletes had disk degeneration, with the greatest prevalence among weight lifters and ice hockey players.[17] The study concluded that athletes with high physical demands on their back are at increased risk for developing degenerative disk disease and back pain. Most of the spine abnormalities in athletes appeared to occur during the growth spurt, and most abnormalities observed on the follow-up MRI also were present on the baseline MRI.

Degenerative disk disease often has a nonspecific appearance. The patient may report aching low back pain, with or without referred pain. Pain associated with disk pathology often is experienced with forward flexion. Loss of flexibility in the lumbar spine and hamstrings often occurs before the onset of pain. One unique characteristic of adolescent disk disease is that a physical finding such as sciatic scoliosis often is accompanied by a low level of pain. In the presence of juvenile disk disorder, a thoracic hypokyphosis and a lumbar hypolordosis (a flat back) may be present. Disk space height, end plate spurring, and sclerosis can be assessed with plain radiographs. T2-weighted MRI can show signal change correlated with disk dehydration. T1-weighting has potential for diagnosing the early stages of disk degeneration.[48]

The symptoms of most young patients with degenerative disk disease resolve with nonsurgical treatment. An initial short period of bed rest and restriction from sports are recommended, along with the use of NSAIDs. It is important to instruct the patient about the disease process and ways to prevent reinjury. A corset brace can be used to alleviate symptoms. Approximately 50% of patients benefit from using a brace for discogenic pain, although long-term brace use in adults is associated with muscle wasting.[49] In pediatric athletes, physical therapy aimed at increasing trunk strength and a sport-specific interval program can help to prevent recurrence and facilitate a return to sports. The rehabilitation should be divided into phases: pain control and stretching, core musculature training, strength training, and, finally, sport-specific training.

Surgery, usually in the form of microdiskectomy, may be necessary if nonsurgical treatment is unsuccessful. Intradiskal electrothermal techniques have been used with some success. The role of disk replacement has not been studied in pediatric patients.

Lordotic Low Back Pain

Lordotic low back pain is the second most common type of low back pain in pediatric athletes.[5] During the adolescent growth spurt, the bones may develop more rapidly than the surrounding soft tissue can accommodate. Flexibility is lost with tightening of the thoracolumbar fascia, interspinous ligaments, and tendinous attachments on the spine. This tightness can lead to traction apophysitis, impingement of spinous processes, and occasionally, pseudarthrosis of the transitional vertebrae.

Sports activity with repetitive hyperextension can create a predisposition to lordotic low back pain. The patient has low back pain associated with activity, often mimicking the pain of spondylolysis. Pain may be elicited with provocative hyperextension testing of the low back. The patient usually has tight hamstrings. Radiographs may show apophyseal avulsion or incomplete segmentation of a vertebra at the transitional zone, consistent with pseudarthrosis or Bertolotti syndrome. Although the diagnosis often is made by exclusion, a bone scan may reveal increased uptake in the spinous process apophyses.

The treatment consists of physical therapy emphasizing antilordotic, hamstring, and peripelvic stretching. A brief period of rest from sports may be indicated. Antilordotic bracing can be beneficial if necessary. The patient can return to sports when the symptoms have resolved.

Scheuermann Kyphosis

Scheuermann disease, also known as juvenile kyphosis, is the most common cause of kyphotic deformity in adolescents. The thoracic form of Scheuermann disease is defined by hyperkyphosis of more than 40° or wedging of 5° or more in at least three consecutive vertebrae, as seen on a lateral radiograph. The associated findings include irregular vertebral end plates, Schmorl nodes, and apophyseal ring fractures. Scheuermann disease

most frequently is diagnosed between age 13 and 17 years. Hereditary genetic factors have been linked to the etiology, but height, weight, and sex have not been linked. Sports activity usually is not believed to be a cause of Scheuermann disease, but there is an increased prevalence among participants in sports requiring repetitive hyperflexion and axial loading.

Scheuermann disease typically appears as a cosmetic deformity, and in the general pediatric population it often is painless. An athlete with high physical demands on the back, as in gymnastics, water skiing, and wrestling, often has pain. The pain may be exacerbated by physical activity. On examination, the patient is found to have a fixed thoracic kyphosis. In contrast, postural kyphosis is corrected with overhead arm extension. The thoracic kyphosis may be accompanied by a compensatory hyperlumbar lordosis, which is associated with an increased incidence of spondylolysis. Other physical findings include hamstring and thoracolumbar fascia tightness.

Treatment is considered for a skeletally immature patient with a kyphotic deformity of 45° to 50°. Intensive physical therapy is initiated, with a focus on postural improvement and stretching. Participation in sports that involve extension, such as gymnastics, aerobics, and swimming, is encouraged, but sports that involve axial loading are discouraged. Braces such as the Milwaukee brace can be used if the curve is greater than 50° to 60°. Full-time brace use for 12 to 18 months is suggested. Bracing does not resolve the pain but can treat the deformity. Surgery is reserved for patients with a curve greater than 70° to 80°, and often it is done in two stages (anterior release and posterior fusion). Sports activity usually is prohibited for 1 year after surgery, and contact sports are prohibited.

Atypical Scheuermann Kyphosis

Atypical Scheuermann disease is a relatively uncommon cause of back pain in pediatric patients. In this condition, the vertebral body changes typical of thoracic Scheuermann disease occur at the thoracolumbar junction and in the upper lumbar spine. The patient invariably has so-called flat back syndrome, with thoracic hypokyphosis and lumbar hypolordosis. This condition is believed to be caused by a repetitive flexion injury of the thoracolumbar vertebrae. The treatment is rest from aggravating activity and extension-based physical therapy. Lordotic bracing sometimes is needed.

Summary

Back pain is less common in young athletes than pain in other anatomic sites, such as the knee or shoulder, but it can occur at a debilitating level inconsistent with sports participation for an extended period of time. An exact diagnosis is important, with reference to the

7: Sports-Related Topics

differential diagnosis. It is important to remember that infection, a neoplasm, or a rheumatologic condition in a young athlete may be mistaken for a sports injury.

Annotated References

1. Olsen TL, Anderson RL, Dearwater SR, et al: The epidemiology of low back pain in an adolescent population. *Am J Public Health* 1992;82(4):606-608.

2. Soler T, Calderón C: The prevalence of spondylolysis in the Spanish elite athlete. *Am J Sports Med* 2000;28(1):57-62.

    Spondylolysis is prevalent in participants in specific sports, which are classified by risk.

3. Goldstein JD, Berger PE, Windler GE, Jackson DW: Spine injuries in gymnasts and swimmers: An epidemiologic investigation. *Am J Sports Med* 1991;19(5):463-468.

4. Bhatia NN, Chow G, Timon SJ, Watts HG: Diagnostic modalities for the evaluation of pediatric back pain: A prospective study. *J Pediatr Orthop* 2008;28(2):230-233.

    The rate of diagnosis for pediatric back pain and the value of several diagnostic studies are prospectively examined. Level of evidence: II.

5. Micheli LJ, Wood R: Back pain in young athletes: Significant differences from adults in causes and patterns. *Arch Pediatr Adolesc Med* 1995;149(1):15-18.

6. Labrom RD: Growth and maturation of the spine from birth to adolescence. *J Bone Joint Surg Am* 2007;89(suppl 1):3-7.

    The normal development of the spine and some consequences of spine deformity are reviewed.

7. Powell JW, Barber-Foss KD: Injury patterns in selected high school sports: A review of the 1995-1997 seasons. *J Athl Train* 1999;34(3):277-284.

8. Kujala UM, Taimela S, Oksanen A, Salminen JJ: Lumbar mobility and low back pain during adolescence: A longitudinal three-year follow-up study in athletes and controls. *Am J Sports Med* 1997;25(3):363-368.

9. Roche MB, Rowe GG: The incidence of separate neural arch and coincident bone variations: A summary. *J Bone Joint Surg Am* 1952;34(2):491-494.

10. d'Hemecourt PA, Gerbino PG II, Micheli LJ: Back injuries in the young athlete. *Clin Sports Med* 2000;19(4):663-679.

11. Loud KJ, Micheli LJ: Common athletic injuries in adolescent girls. *Curr Opin Pediatr* 2001;13(4):317-322.

12. McTimoney CA, Micheli LJ: Managing back pain in young athletes. *J Musc Med* 2004;21(2):63-69.

13. Wiltse LL, Jackson DW: Treatment of spondylolisthesis and spondylolysis in children. *Clin Orthop Relat Res* 1976;117:92-100.

14. Omey ML, Micheli LJ, Gerbino PG II: Idiopathic scoliosis and spondylolysis in the female athlete: Tips for treatment. *Clin Orthop Relat Res* 2000;372:74-84.

15. El Rassi G, Takemitsu M, Woratanarat P, Shah SA: Lumbar spondylolysis in pediatric and adolescent soccer players. *Am J Sports Med* 2005;33(11):1688-1693.

    The treatment of spondylolysis in adolescent soccer players is described.

16. Watkins RG: Lumbar disc injury in the athlete. *Clin Sports Med* 2002;21(1):147-165.

17. Baranto A, Hellström M, Cederlund CG, Nyman R, Swärd L: Back pain and MRI changes in the thoraco-lumbar spine of top athletes in four different sports: A 15-year follow-up study. *Knee Surg Sports Traumatol Arthrosc* 2009;17(9):1125-1134.

    MRI was used to compare changes associated with degenerative disk disease in the spines of athletes and nonathletes.

18. Herkowitz HN, Garfin SR, Eismont FJ, Bell GR, Balderston RA: Thoracic and lumbar spinal trauma in the immature spine, in *Rothman-Simeone The Spine*, ed 5. Philadelphia, PA, Sanders Elsevier, 2006, pp 603-612.

    Thoracolumbar trauma in the pediatric spine is discussed.

19. Dogan S, Safavi-Abbasi S, Theodore N, et al: Thoracolumbar and sacral spinal injuries in children and adolescents: A review of 89 cases. *J Neurosurg* 2007;106(6, suppl):426-433.

    The mechanism of injury, management, and outcomes of pediatric thoracolumbar fractures are reviewed.

20. Hamilton MG, Myles ST: Pediatric spinal injury: Review of 61 deaths. *J Neurosurg* 1992;77(5):705-708.

21. Junkins EP Jr, Stotts A, Santiago R, Guenther E: The clinical presentation of pediatric thoracolumbar fractures: A prospective study. *J Trauma* 2008;65(5):1066-1071.

    Physical examination findings are described in pediatric patients with a lumbar spine fracture.

22. Slotkin JR, Lu Y, Wood KB: Thoracolumbar spinal trauma in children. *Neurosurg Clin N Am* 2007;18(4):621-630.

    This review of thoracolumbar trauma discusses spine development, injury patterns, and treatment options.

23. Epstein JA, Lavine LS: Herniated lumbar intervertebral discs in teen-age children. *J Neurosurg* 1964;21:1070-1075.

24. Rabin A, Gerszten PC, Karausky P, Bunker CH, Potter DM, Welch WC: The sensitivity of the seated straight-

leg raise test compared with the supine straight-leg raise test in patients presenting with magnetic resonance imaging evidence of lumbar nerve root compression. *Arch Phys Med Rehabil* 2007;88(7):840-843.

A cohort study compared the sensitivity of the straight leg raise test in the supine and seated positions in patients with signs and symptoms consistent with lumbar radiculopathy.

25. Papagelopoulos PJ, Shaughnessy WJ, Ebersold MJ, Bianco AJ Jr, Quast LM: Long-term outcome of lumbar discectomy in children and adolescents sixteen years of age or younger. *J Bone Joint Surg Am* 1998;80(5):689-698.

26. Peh WC, Griffith JF, Yip DK, Leong JC: Magnetic resonance imaging of lumbar vertebral apophyseal ring fractures: Magnetic resonance imaging of lumbar vertebral apophyseal ring fractures. *Australas Radiol* 1998;42(1):34-37.

27. Labelle H, Roussouly P, Berthonnaud E, Dimnet J, O'Brien M: The importance of spino-pelvic balance in L5-S1 developmental spondylolisthesis: A review of pertinent radiologic measurements. *Spine (Phila Pa 1976)* 2005;30(6, suppl):S27-S34.

28. Labelle H, Roussouly P, Berthonnaud E, et al: Spondylolisthesis, pelvic incidence, and spinopelvic balance: A correlation study. *Spine (Phila Pa 1976)* 2004;29(18):2049-2054.

29. Yue WM, Brodner W, Gaines RW: Abnormal spinal anatomy in 27 cases of surgically corrected spondyloptosis: Proximal sacral endplate damage as a possible cause of spondyloptosis. *Spine (Phila Pa 1976)* 2005;30(6, suppl):S22-S26.

30. Albanese M, Pizzutillo PD: Family study of spondylolysis and spondylolisthesis. *J Pediatr Orthop* 1982;2(5):496-499.

31. Wynne-Davies R, Scott JH: Inheritance and spondylolisthesis: A radiographic family survey. *J Bone Joint Surg Br* 1979;61(3):301-305.

32. Stewart TD: The age incidence of neural-arch defects in Alaskan natives, considered from the standpoint of etiology. *J Bone Joint Surg Am* 1953;35(4):937-950.

33. Roche MB, Rowe GG: The incidence of separate neural arch and coincident bone variations: A summary. *J Bone Joint Surg Am* 1952;34(2):491-494.

34. Fredrickson BE, Baker D, McHolick WJ, Yuan HA, Lubicky JP: The natural history of spondylolysis and spondylolisthesis. *J Bone Joint Surg Am* 1984;66(5):699-707.

35. Beutler WJ, Fredrickson BE, Murtland A, Sweeney CA, Grant WD, Baker D: The natural history of spondylolysis and spondylolisthesis: 45-year follow-up evaluation. *Spine (Phila Pa 1976)* 2003;28(10):1027-1035.

36. Saifuddin A, White J, Tucker S, Taylor BA: Orientation of lumbar pars defects: Implications for radiological detection and surgical management. *J Bone Joint Surg Br* 1998;80(2):208-211.

37. Bellah RD, Summerville DA, Treves ST, Micheli LJ: Low-back pain in adolescent athletes: Detection of stress injury to the pars interarticularis with SPECT. *Radiology* 1991;180(2):509-512.

38. van den Oever M, Merrick MV, Scott JH: Bone scintigraphy in symptomatic spondylolysis. *J Bone Joint Surg Br* 1987;69(3):453-456.

39. Morita T, Ikata T, Katoh S, Miyake R: Lumbar spondylolysis in children and adolescents: Lumbar spondylolysis in children and adolescents. *J Bone Joint Surg Br* 1995;77(4):620-625.

40. Hollenberg GM, Beattie PF, Meyers SP, Weinberg EP, Adams MJ: Stress reactions of the lumbar pars interarticularis: The development of a new MRI classification system. *Spine (Phila Pa 1976)* 2002;27(2):181-186.

MRI criteria were developed for staging spondylolytic lesions.

41. Cohen E, Stuecker RD: Magnetic resonance imaging in diagnosis and follow-up of impending spondylolysis in children and adolescents: Early treatment may prevent pars defects. *J Pediatr Orthop B* 2005;14(2):63-67.

MRI has potential for detecting and monitoring the healing of spondylolysis.

42. Campbell RS, Grainger AJ, Hide IG, Papastefanou S, Greenough CG: Juvenile spondylolysis: A comparative analysis of CT, SPECT and MRI. *Skeletal Radiol* 2005;34(2):63-73.

MRI was found to be an effective, reliable first-line modality for the diagnosis of juvenile spondylolysis.

43. Sys J, Michielsen J, Bracke P, Martens M, Verstreken J: Nonoperative treatment of active spondylolysis in elite athletes with normal X-ray findings: Literature review and results of conservative treatment. *Eur Spine J* 2001;10(6):498-504.

44. Steiner ME, Micheli LJ: Treatment of symptomatic spondylolysis and spondylolisthesis with the modified Boston brace. *Spine (Phila Pa 1976)* 1985;10(10):937-943.

45. McCleary MD, Congeni JA: Current concepts in the diagnosis and treatment of spondylolysis in young athletes. *Curr Sports Med Rep* 2007;6(1):62-66.

A current-concept review describes management and treatment protocols for spondylolysis.

46. Standaert CJ: Spondylolysis in the adolescent athlete. *Clin J Sport Med* 2002;12(2):119-122.

47. Hangai M, Kaneoka K, Hinotsu S, et al: Lumbar intervertebral disk degeneration in athletes. *Am J Sports Med* 2009;37(1):149-155.

Degenerative disk disease was found to be more prevalent in athletes than in nonathletes.

48. Nguyen AM, Johannessen W, Yoder JH, et al: Noninvasive quantification of human nucleus pulposus pressure with use of T1rho-weighted magnetic resonance imaging. *J Bone Joint Surg Am* 2008;90(4):796-802.

A cadaver study found that MRI T1-rho weighting has strong potential as a quantitative biomarker of the mechanical function of the nucleus pulposus and disk degeneration.

49. Yancey RA, Micheli LJ: Thoracolumbar spine injuries in pediatric sports, in Stanitiski DL, DeLee JC, Drez DD Jr, eds: *Pediatric Adolescent Sports Medicine*. Toronto, ON, WB Saunders, 1994, vol 3, pp 162-174.

Chapter 43

Issues Related to Adolescent Athletes

Jordan D. Metzl, MD

Introduction

Adolescence is a 7- to 9-year period characterized by tremendous flux in body anthropomorphic measurements, physiologic potential, and athletic prowess. The challenging care of an adolescent athlete is based on the patient's age, stage of skeletal maturity, and sport type.

Shifting Participant Demographics

Adolescent sports participation changed dramatically between 1970 and 2010 (Figure 1). After the 1972 enactment of the US law commonly known as Title IX, the number of female athletes grew significantly, and this law has been largely responsible for the overall increase in the number of adolescent athletes. In 1972 there were approximately 4 million high school sport participants, of whom approximately 300,000 were girls. In 2009, there were almost 8 million high school athletes, of whom more than 3 million were girls.[1]

Sports participation by girls is believed to encourage a lifetime pattern of healthy behavior and has been linked to favorable changes in self-esteem, health profiles, and obesity incidence extending into adulthood.[2] However, there has been an epidemic of devastating knee injuries among adolescent girls, most notably injuries to the anterior cruciate ligament (ACL). ACL injury is approximately four to five times more common among female adolescent athletes than their male counterparts.[3] The worrisome prognosis of ACL injury includes an almost-doubled risk of knee pain and arthritis symptoms within 15 years. The rapid deterioration of the injured knee seems to occur regardless of whether the ACL was reconstructed.[4]

Adolescent sports participation formerly was characterized by a specific sport for each season of the year. During the past 10 to 15 years, however, adolescents who wish to excel have tended to concentrate on one

sport year-round. It is now common for a baseball, soccer, gymnastic, lacrosse, basketball, or swimming program to threaten to disqualify a team member who also participates in another sport. There are two primary reasons the trend to intensive participation in one sport is potentially harmful for almost all adolescent athletes. The rate of sports injury at any age is significantly increased if the athlete exclusively participates in one sport.[5] Overuse injury to the developing skeleton carries a greater risk than a similar injury to the adult skeleton. Adolescent sport-specific injuries such as little leaguer's elbow and gymnast's wrist often result from a combination of repetitive use and a developing musculoskeletal system. The injury sometimes leads to life-long impairment. In addition, it is important to recognize the psychological effect on an adolescent of exclusively focusing on one activity. The psychological trauma of an injury is magnified in a specialized adolescent athlete because participation in the sport has been a basis of identity formation. If the athlete's sport becomes the focus of the family dynamic, time and financial resources can be strained, with attention diverted from the needs of other family members. The burnout rate from sport specialization at a young age has been well documented.[6] For these and other reasons, sport specialization is discouraged for most developing ath-

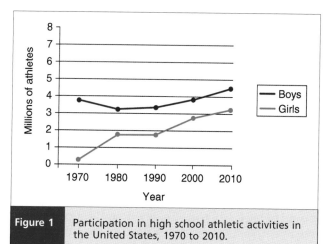

Figure 1   Participation in high school athletic activities in the United States, 1970 to 2010.

Dr. Metzl or an immediate family member is a member of a speakers' bureau or has made paid presentations on behalf of Ferring Pharmaceuticals and Gatorade; and owns stock or stock options in Merck.

letes. Sport specialization is considered acceptable only if the athlete is emotionally mature, the athlete and the family understand the relative advantages and disadvantages of sport specialization, the athlete possesses the talent and skill to truly excel in the sport, and the effects of sport specialization appear to be balanced within the family dynamic.

Healthy Competition in Youth Sports

As sports participation has changed to include more specialization in a particular sport, the type of competition also has changed. A "win at all costs" attitude to competition has become an aspect of the changed climate in youth sports. Although competition can be beneficial for developing a higher level of athletic performance, the increasingly intense competition in youth sports has created an environment in which violent incidents are more common, sometimes involving parents, a parent and a coach, or a referee and a coach.[7]

The health practitioner should consider the suitability of a young patient's sport and competition level based on several questions: Is the child having fun in the sport? Are there any signs of emotional burnout? Are the child's frequency and severity of injury typical of the sport? If the answers to these questions are not reassuring, the health practitioner is encouraged to initiate a discussion with the patient and the family. For example, a discussion of the appropriateness of the sport and the level of competition is warranted for a baseball pitcher who has torn the medial collateral ligament by age 14 years, a gymnast who has sustained several stress fractures by age 13 years, or a swimmer who appears disdainful of the sport and unenthusiastic about continued participation.

Medical Conditions Affecting the Adolescent Athlete

Concussion

Adolescent concussion is a focus of increasing attention. Concussion is defined as a complex pathophysiologic process affecting the brain and brought on by biomechanical forces.[8] Adolescents who sustain a concussion recover more slowly than adults.[9] The implementation of neurocognitive testing for athletes participating in contact sports has provided important data on recovery rates after concussion. Neurologic deficits were found to remain after a concussion is considered healed on the basis of clinical examination.[10] This surprising finding is especially important for adolescent athletes, who are at the highest risk from a traumatic blow that occurs before the brain has fully recovered from a previous concussion. Head injury in this second-impact syndrome is significant and potentially fatal. Although concussion-related fatality in sports is less common than cardiac-related fatality, it occurs approximately two to three times per year, almost always as a result of second-impact syndrome.[11] Therefore, any adolescent athlete who has a clinical symptom of postconcussive syndrome (headache, dizziness, irritability, or photophobia) should be considered at high risk for second-impact syndrome.[11]

The risk of head injury in a sport is correlated with the extent of contact or collision in the sport.[12] Athletes who sustained a previous concussion are at higher risk for a repeat concussion compared with their teammates. This predisposition is especially important to consider during screening for athletic participation. No data are available to correlate an adolescent athlete's cumulative number of concussions with long-term outcome. However, recent data from professional athletes found an increased incidence of neurologic damage and impaired function in those who sustained multiple concussions over the course of their contact sports career.[13] An adolescent athlete who has sustained several concussions should consider switching to a sport that involves less risk of neurologic trauma.

Every effort should be made to protect pediatric athletes from concussion, and especially from repeated concussion. Return-to-activity guidelines should be followed with caution and safety in mind. As computer-based neurocognitive testing has become more widely accessible during the past decade, it is being used for the care and prevention of adolescent concussion. Neurocognitive testing is used in determining an athlete's recovery from mild traumatic brain injury. Testing now can be performed at the start of the sports season for all potential participants.

The use of computerized neurocognitive testing is widespread in high- or medium-contact professional and collegiate sports, and it is increasingly used at the high school and middle school levels. The growth of this technology has led to several questions: Should testing be required for all high school and middle school athletes? If not, which athletes should be tested? How are brain-function changes revealed by neurocognitive testing reflected in an athlete's scholastic performance, and should the school be notified if the athlete sustains a concussion? These important questions should be answerable as information on the short- and long-term effects of adolescent concussions becomes available.

It is essential to recognize that neurocognitive testing data alone should not determine whether an athlete is ready for a healthy return to competition. Any adolescent athlete who has sustained a concussion should be cleared for return to competition only after undergoing a clinical examination, with consideration of available neurocognitive testing data. Both the patient and the family must consider the patient's symptoms and behavior patterns. It is important for them to understand that the consequences of concussion are more severe in teen athletes than in other athletes. Extreme caution always is required in determining whether an adolescent athlete with a history of concussion should return to competition.

Asthma

Reactive airway disease, including asthma and exercise-induced bronchospasm (EIB), is common among adolescent athletes. Asthma is the most common chronic disease among adolescent athletes. EIB, a relatively indolent and often-unrecognized variant of asthma, was found to affect almost 15% of all adolescent athletes; the rate was even higher among African American athletes, who also have a higher rate of asthma.[14] The hallmarks of both asthma and EIB include shortness of breath that worsens during and after exercise, as well as a restrictive breathing pattern that worsens during periods of extreme exertion. Classic asthma is characterized by a long history of wheezing and restrictive airway symptoms. An athlete with asthma usually has a good working knowledge of his or her symptoms, symptom triggers, and current disease status, based on many years' experience, and is able to recognize the symptoms during exercise. An asthma episode can occur at any time but is most likely if the weather is hot and humid, the athlete has an underlying viral illness, or the air contains a high concentration of allergens such as pollens or pollutants.

Unlike the symptoms of classic asthma, the symptoms of EIB occur only with exercise. Athletes with asthma also have EIB. In addition, approximately 15% of the athletic population have EIB without an asthma diagnosis.[15] The diagnosis in these athletes often is difficult to make because they may otherwise be healthy. Unlike athletes with asthma, athletes with EIB often do not recognize shortness of breath, especially after exercise, as a symptom of restrictive airway disease. As with asthma, the symptoms of EIB are most likely to occur in the presence of certain environmental conditions or an underlying viral illness. EIB often prevents athletes from reaching their full athletic potential.

Asthma and suspected EIB should be treated by a physician who is particularly knowledgeable about these conditions. Testing for EIB often includes the use of a peak expiratory flow meter to compare forced expiratory volume before and after exertion. The treatment of asthma and EIB involves medication and awareness of measures to prevent symptoms from developing. These measures can include proper hydration before exercise as well as the use of a respiratory warm-up period, during which the respiratory system is taxed in a heated, controlled environment before cold-weather exercise.

Performance-Enhancing Drugs

Some adolescent athletes experiment with the use of performance-enhancing drugs in emulation of professional athletes who have been implicated in the use of such drugs. The spectrum of performance-enhancing drugs ranges from common, probably benign agents such as creatine (a protein supplement promoted as a means of increasing muscle mass) to dangerous compounds such as anabolic steroids. During the past decade, the annual revenue of the supplement industry has grown from between $1.2 and $3 billion to approximately $20 billion.[16] This increase is directly correlated with the increasing prevalence of supplement use among college, high school, and even middle school athletes. The medical implications of performance-enhancing drug use by professional and adolescent athletes are very different.

Creatine is by far the most popular of the many over-the-counter nutritional supplements used by adolescent athletes. A survey of middle and high school students (in grades 6 through 12) found that 5.6% had used the drug.[17] Creatine is a complex amino acid made up of arginine, glycine, and methionine. Dietary creatine can be found in protein-rich foods such as meat and fish.[18] Most endogenous creatine is produced by the liver, kidneys, and pancreas; it is primarily stored in skeletal muscle in an amount that varies from 90 to 160 mmol/kg depending on the size of the person. The function of creatine as related to exercise is in the rapid synthesis of adenosine triphosphate once it is hydrolyzed. Adenosine triphosphate is the first form of free energy used for muscle contraction. The normal stores of adenosine triphosphate are exhausted after 5 to 10 seconds of exertion, and the second round of energy stores, in the form of creatine phosphate, is depleted after an additional 5 to 15 seconds. Because the supply of creatine phosphate is a limiting factor in aerobic exercise, creatine supplementation may be beneficial, especially in a short-duration, high-intensity repetitive activity such as weight training.[19] Creatine use may lead to desirable weight gain, improved performance, and increased strength. However, no studies have examined its short- or long-term effects on children and adolescents. The American College of Sports Medicine and the American Academy of Pediatrics recommend against the use of creatine by people younger than 18 years.[20,21]

Anabolic steroids are testosterone derivatives used to enhance anabolic muscle-building properties. These drugs have important medical uses for patients with severe osteoporosis, acquired immunodeficiency syndrome–wasting syndrome, or another chronic medical disease, such as hypogonadism. More commonly, these compounds are used by athletes who hope to gain a competitive benefit. The use of steroids was first described in the medical literature during the 1960s. Since then, the realization has slowly developed that significant medical issues are associated with steroid use, including impotence, cardiovascular disease, mood instability, and hepatic cancer.[22] The medical implications of anabolic steroid use in a developing body are not fully known; in adolescents, whose minds as well as bodies are in a state of flux, mood instability appears to be an especially acute issue. Endocrine conditions including hypogonadism and gynecomastia have been well documented in adolescent athletes who use anabolic steroids.[23]

Approximately 3% to 9% of high school students were found to have used anabolic steroids.[24] Many young athletes continue to use anabolic steroids despite being fully informed of the danger because these drugs are effective in making the body stronger and faster. More needs to be done to actively discourage steroid use by young athletes. The US Anabolic Steroid Control Act of 2004 banned the sale of over-the-counter steroid precursor supplements. However, momentum toward controlling the use of anabolic steroids must arise from a concerted grassroots effort by those who work with young athletes at the team and community level. Medical professionals can help by presenting educational seminars for parents and coaches on the topic of performance-enhancing drugs.

Preseason Clearance for Adolescent Athletes

Preseason clearance for athletic competition can contribute to a healthy sports experience for young athletes. Although there is no standard clearance form for adolescent athletes, a consensus has emerged with the publication of a joint position statement approved by major organizations, including the American Academy of Pediatrics, the American Orthopaedic Society for Sports Medicine, and the American College of Sports Medicine.[25] This document provides guidelines on the medical and orthopaedic aspects of clearance for sport participation.

In general, preparticipation screening of adolescents is expensive and time consuming. An apparently healthy adolescent rarely seeks medical attention, however, and many of the medical conditions affecting adolescents are silent. The general belief, therefore, is that screening adolescents before sports participation is imperfect but can be helpful.

Summary

Adolescents should be encouraged to participate in sports. Several health concerns require particular attention in adolescent athletes, although current trends and policies are designed to make their sports participation safer. Adolescents should be counseled as to the best choice of sports and ways to prevent injury. Those who care for young athletes can further health and safety by taking a more active role with respect to issues such as sport specialization, concussion, and performance-enhancing drug use.

Annotated References

1. National Federation of State High School Associations: 2009-2010 high school athletics participation survey. http://www.nfhs.org/content.aspx?id=3282&linkidentifier=id&itemid=3282. Accessed January 10, 2011.

2. Wake M, Canterford L, Patton GC, et al: Comorbidities of overweight/obesity experienced in adolescence: Longitudinal study. *Arch Dis Child* 2010;95(3):162-168.

   Obesity in adolescents was studied.

3. Ford KR, Myer GD, Hewett TE: Valgus knee motion during landing in high school female and male basketball players. *Med Sci Sports Exerc* 2003;35(10):1745-1750.

4. Amin S, Guermazi A, Lavalley MP, et al: Complete anterior cruciate ligament tear and the risk for cartilage loss and progression of symptoms in men and women with knee osteoarthritis. *Osteoarthritis Cartilage* 2008;16(8):897-902.

   The correlation between ACL injury and the development of arthritis was examined.

5. American Academy of Pediatrics, Committee on Sports Medicine and Fitness: Intensive training and sports specialization in young athletes. *Pediatrics* 2000;106(1, pt 1):154-157.

6. Brenner JS, American Academy of Pediatrics Council on Sports Medicine and Fitness: Overuse injuries, overtraining, and burnout in child and adolescent athletes. *Pediatrics* 2007;119(6):1242-1245.

   The American Academy of Pediatrics issued a position statement on sports specialization by young athletes.

7. Fields SK, Collins CL, Comstock RD: Violence in youth sports: Hazing, brawling and foul play. *Br J Sports Med* 2010;44(1):32-37.

   Issues related to violence in youth sports were reviewed.

8. McCrory P, Johnston K, Meeuwisse W, et al: Summary and agreement statement of the 2nd International Conference on Concussion in Sport, Prague 2004. *Br J Sports Med* 2005;39(4):196-204.

   The long-term effects of concussion in sports participants are examined.

9. Sim A, Terryberry-Spohr L, Wilson KR: Prolonged recovery of memory functioning after mild traumatic brain injury in adolescent athletes. *J Neurosurg* 2008;108(3):511-516.

   This study examined recovery time of adolescents after a concussion.

10. Collins MW, Field M, Lovell MR, et al: Relationship between postconcussion headache and neuropsychological test performance in high school athletes. *Am J Sports Med* 2003;31(2):168-173.

11. Halstead ME, Walter KD: Council on Sports Medicine and Fitness, American Academy of Pediatrics: Clinical report: Sport-related concussion in children and adolescents. *Pediatrics* 2010;126(3):597-615.

    This is an excellent, detailed review of adolescent concussion from the American Academy of Pediatrics.

12. Guskiewicz KM, Weaver NL, Padua DA, Garrett WE Jr: Epidemiology of concussion in collegiate and high

school football players. *Am J Sports Med* 2000;28(5): 643-650.

13. Makdissi M, Darby D, Maruff P, Ugoni A, Brukner P, McCrory PR: Natural history of concussion in sport: Markers of severity and implications for management. *Am J Sports Med* 2010;38(3):464-471.

    The long-term consequences of sports-related concussions were examined.

14. Parsons JP, Mastronarde JG: Exercise-induced bronchoconstriction in athletes. *Chest* 2005;128(6):3966-3974.

    This is a review of exercised-induced asthma in athletes.

15. Billen A, Dupont L: Exercise induced bronchoconstriction and sports. *Postgrad Med J* 2008;84(996):512-517.

    This is a review of exercised-induced bronchospasm in athletes.

16. Tscholl P, Alonso JM, Dollé G, Junge A, Dvorak J: The use of drugs and nutritional supplements in top-level track and field athletes. *Am J Sports Med* 2010;38(1): 133-140.

    The epidemiology of supplement use among athletes was examined.

17. Metzl JD, Small E, Levine SR, Gershel JC: Creatine use among young athletes. *Pediatrics* 2001;108(2):421-425.

18. Rodriguez NR, Di Marco NM, Langley S, American Dietetic Association; Dietitians of Canada, American College of Sports Medicine: American College of Sports Medicine position stand: Nutrition and athletic performance. *Med Sci Sports Exerc* 2009;41(3):709-731.

    The American College of Sports Medicine issued a position statement on the use of nutritional supplements by athletes.

19. Kendall KL, Smith AE, Graef JL, et al: Effects of four weeks of high-intensity interval training and creatine supplementation on critical power and anaerobic work-

ing capacity in college-aged men. *J Strength Cond Res* 2009;23(6):1663-1669.

    A prospective study examined the role of creatine in the development of muscle strength.

20. American College of Sports Medicine: The physiological and health effects of oral creatine supplementation. 2000. http://www.acsm.org/AM/Template.cfm?Section= Past_Roundtables&Template=/CM/ContentDisplay.cfm &ContentID=2832. Accessed January 10, 2011.

21. Gomez J, American Academy of Pediatrics Committee on Sports Medicine and Fitness: Use of performance-enhancing substances. *Pediatrics* 2005;115(4):1103-1106.

    A functional definition of performance-enhancing substances is provided. The American Academy of Pediatrics strongly condemns their use.

22. Kuehn BM: Teen steroid, supplement use targeted: Officials look to prevention and better oversight. *JAMA* 2009;302(21):2301-2303.

    An editorial evaluated methods for discouraging anabolic steroid use by teenagers.

23. Hartgens F, Kuipers H: Effects of androgenic-anabolic steroids in athletes. *Sports Med* 2004;34(8):513-554.

24. Faigenbaum AD, Zaichkowsky LD, Gardner DE, Micheli LJ: Anabolic steroid use by male and female middle school students. *Pediatrics* 1998;101(5):E6.

25. American Academy of Family Physicians, American Academy of Pediatrics, American College of Sports Medicine, American Medical Society for Sports Medicine, American Orthopedic Society for Sports Medicine, American Osteopathic Academy of Sports Medicine: *Preparticipation Physical Examination*, ed 3. Minneapolis, MN, McGraw-Hill, 2004.

7: Sports-Related Topics

Chapter 44

Rehabilitation for the Pediatric Athlete

Angela D. Smith, MD

Introduction

The traditional assumption is that children do not require formal rehabilitation after an injury but instead rehabilitate themselves during the course of their usual activities. Recent research has challenged this belief, however. An unrehabilitated ankle or foot injury may create a predisposition to subsequent ankle injury; an adolescent or young adult athlete who rehabilitates an ankle sprain has a lower risk of recurrence.[1] The rate of injury among previously injured high school athletes was found to be almost twice that of other athletes.[2]

Today's children rarely climb trees, ride a bicycle to school, engage in long periods of free play, or participate in other unstructured activities that strengthen multiple muscle groups. Their typical physical activities are more likely to involve short continuous episodes, often with movements repeated many times, as in year-round soccer or basketball. If a child or adolescent athlete resumes a sport after injury without adequate musculoskeletal and cardiovascular rehabilitation, altered biomechanics (especially with fatigue) may lead to a recurrent or new injury, possibly related to increased loads on the musculoskeletal tissues.[3]

Few randomized clinical studies have evaluated injury prevention, and very few studies have focused on children or adolescents. Recommendations regarding the training and rehabilitation of skeletally immature athletes must be largely based on experience and opinion. The primary focus of rehabilitation for youth athletes is on therapeutic exercise. In addition, heat and cold therapy, in the form of warm or cold packs or baths, is used as needed. Other rehabilitation modalities have not been adequately studied in children and adolescents, and their use should be questioned. The goal for a young athlete is to return to sport as rapidly as is safely possible.

Dr. Smith or an immediate family member serves as a board member, owner, officer, or committee member of the American College of Sports Medicine and the International Federation of Sports Medicine.

Principles of Pediatric Sports Rehabilitation

Exercise programs for pediatric athletes should focus on building adequate muscle and bone strength, soft-tissue flexibility, dynamic body alignment, cardiovascular readiness, and sport-specific skills for both prevention and rehabilitation of injury. The causes of an overuse injury (resulting from repeated microtrauma) must be determined to avoid a recurrence. Some pediatric athletes develop chronic pain, which may be diagnosed as amplified pain syndrome or reflex neuropathic dystrophy. Treatment of these patients is a multidisciplinary effort.

Optimal biomechanics require not only strength and flexibility but also sport-specific learned skills. In general, young athletes should have bilaterally symmetric muscle development at the level required for the activity. A safe level of flexibility is desirable for all sports, but sports such as gymnastics, diving, and dance require an unusually great soft-tissue range of motion. Cardiovascular and muscle metabolic requirements vary from short bursts of sprint activity to endurance activity. In activities requiring running, single-leg squatting, or hopping, lower extremity functional rotational and angular alignment appears to be related to injuries along the entire lower extremity kinetic chain. Anterior cruciate ligament (ACL) injury related to dynamic malalignment has been more studied than other injuries in young athletes.[4]

Core strength provides the ability to stabilize the torso and solidly connect the actions of the upper and lower extremities. Adolescents undergoing a rapid spine growth spurt have relatively poor core strength, and this factor probably contributes to the peak incidence of spondylolysis symptoms at this stage of growth and development. Young athletes may temporarily lose flexibility during rapid growth spurts, especially in muscles that cross two joints such as the hamstrings, rectus femoris, and gastrocnemius. Young athletes who routinely practice stretching exercises can mitigate growth-related flexibility loss. Athletes may report significantly altered balance and kinesthetic sense during rapid growth spurts. These difficulties may be caused by altered proprioception related to changes in

Table 1

Muscle Tightness Related to Common Lower Body Injuries in Pediatric Athletes

Muscle Group	Test	Normal Test Finding	Associated Disorder(s)
Hip flexors	Thomas	No contracture	Anteroinferior iliac spine avulsion Back pain
Hamstrings	Popliteal angle	≤10° from vertical	Patellofemoral pain
Rectus femoris	Ely	Knee flexion with hip extended is the same as knee flexion with hip flexed	Osgood-Schlatter disease Sinding-Larsen-Johansson disease Patellar tendinitis
Gastrocnemius	Maximal ankle dorsiflexion, with hindfoot inverted and knee extended	≥10°	Calcaneal apophysitis (Sever disease) Anterior ankle joint line pain

(Adapted with permission from Smith AD: Sport injuries of children and adolescents, in Nicholas JA and Hershman E, eds: *Sports Medicine: Spine and Lower Extremity*. Philadelphia, PA, Mosby, 1995.)

the athlete's muscle flexibility, center of gravity, and/or relative muscle strength. Young athletes and their parents can observe changes in the limbs as they become long and gangly and then fill out. Changes in torso muscle size and strength during the rapid spine growth beginning at puberty are less visible.

Many musculoskeletal conditions are associated with a phase of normal growth and development. For example, spondylolysis most frequently occurs in midadolescence, near the end of the period of rapid spine growth. Often spondylolysis is associated with tight hip flexor muscles and weak lower abdominal muscles, which lead to hyperlordotic posture and back pain. Patellofemoral pain syndrome, one of the most common orthopaedic conditions in 14-year-old girls, often is associated with the stage of growth and development that includes widening of the pelvis, alteration of the Q angle, and decreased hip external rotation strength. The result is poor functional angular and rotational alignment during athletic activities. Calcaneal apophysitis (Sever disease) often is associated with a tight gastrocnemius-soleus complex, usually in a child between age 6 and 10 years (Table 1).[5]

The history of a young athlete with an overuse injury may include a recent significant illness such as mononucleosis or Lyme disease that required several weeks of bed rest or a long absence from sport training. A too-rapid resumption of the previous level of activity may result in injury to the musculoskeletal system.

Recurrent injury is believed to be uncommon if a young athlete's injury is completely rehabilitated to the point of symmetric muscle development, balance, and functional sport-specific movements. The use of a prescribed exercise program was found to decrease the incidence of injury recurrence in patients age 12 to 70 years; however, this study relied on self-reported diagnoses and exercise compliance.[1] A study of the strength and range of motion of adolescent pitchers with or without shoulder or elbow pain found that those who

were symptomatic during the previous year but pain free at the time of study had weaker posterior shoulder muscles.[6] Cause and effect were not determined in this cross-sectional study.

Sudden alterations in athletic training, including changes in session length or intensity, techniques, coaching, equipment, playing surface, or shoes, often are related to the occurrence of injury, especially overuse injury. Sport-specific considerations should be included in the patient history whenever a repetitive microtrauma injury is being evaluated.

The so-called female athlete triad (an eating disorder, menstrual irregularity, osteoporosis) has been associated with stress fracture.[7] Menstrual irregularity can be regarded as an indicator of energy imbalance in an otherwise normal postmenarcheal young athlete. Unless the athlete's nutritional status is improved, restoring the menstrual period by using oral contraceptives is unlikely to decrease the risk of stress fracture. The focus should be on adequate nutrition throughout the day, so that energy taken in as food is matched relatively closely to energy expenditure. Nutritional improvement can lead not only to better performance but also to improved injury prevention and rehabilitation. Young female athletes may be convinced to maintain a closer energy balance throughout the day by learning that gymnasts and runners with a large daily energy deficit were found to have a greater percentage of body fat than those who better matched their energy intake and expenditure.[8] Boys who participate in sports in which weight or appearance is important, such as running, wrestling, or ski jumping, may have a similar energy imbalance. Questions about weight change during the past year can be used to trigger a discussion of nutritional status.

During the past 10 years, decreased free play, a lack of daily physical education in schools, and inattention to torso strength and overall coordination in many youth sports appear to have led to increased adiposity

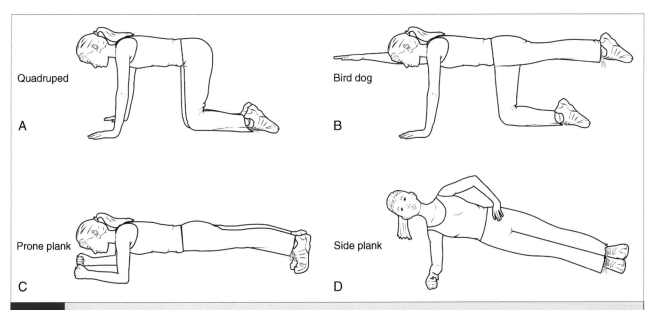

Quadruped

A

Bird dog

B

Prone plank

C

Side plank

D

Figure 1 Pain-free positions for rehabilitation exercises. **A,** In the quadruped position, the patient balances on all four extremities. The pelvis and rib cage are in a neutral position achieved by cocontracting the torso muscles rather than arching the back or tucking the pelvis under (anterior or posterior pelvic tilt). The quadruped position is the basis for the following exercises. **B,** In the bird dog position, one arm or leg first is brought into alignment with the torso. When this position can be held with good form using each of the four extremities, the patient reaches forward with one arm and reaches back with the opposite leg, maintaining a straight line without arching. **C,** In the prone forearm plank position, the elbows are directly under the shoulders, the weight is held by the forearms, and the dorsiflexed feet are balanced on the pads of the toes. **D,** In the side forearm plank position, the patient lies on one side with the arm partially under the body and the legs and torso aligned, then lifts the hips to achieve a plank position.

among children as well as decreased muscle development of the abdomen and back. Back, neck, or shoulder pain is no longer unusual among children. However, even pain of several years' duration almost always is resolved within 2 to 3 months with the use of a simple torso strengthening program. An initial focus on lumbopelvic stabilization enables young throwing athletes, tennis players, and swimmers to improve their postural awareness and subsequently to enhance scapulothoracic stabilization and resolve the head-forward posture causing the neck and shoulder pain. An attempt to decrease upper back or shoulder pain or instability without improving lumbopelvic position and strength is unlikely to be successful.[9]

A child or adolescent who participates in organized sports needs significantly greater strength than a sedentary adult. A physical therapist who primarily treats older adults may tell an adolescent athlete with back pain or other symptoms related to torso weakness that a strengthening program is not needed. However, the symptoms should rapidly resolve when the young athlete begins a challenging therapeutic exercise program that is appropriate for the athlete's age and sport. Even a patient with significant pain should be able to progress relatively rapidly through a sequence of exercises in pain-free positions held with good alignment (**Figure 1**).

Clinically observed side-to-side muscle symmetry is an inexpensive and reasonably reliable indicator that muscle strength and endurance have returned to an injured limb (unless the injury was bilateral or the opposite side had an earlier, incompletely rehabilitated injury). Specific mechanical testing can be used to determine parameters such as peak torque and the total work that a muscle can generate. These numeric values can be particularly helpful as the athlete follows a graduated return to sport-specific activities, as is done, for example, after ACL reconstruction. The soft-tissue flexibility parameters associated with a decreased incidence of common lower body injuries are listed in **Table 1**.[10]

The deconditioning associated with a musculoskeletal injury affects not only musculoskeletal mechanical properties but also muscle metabolic status and cardiovascular readiness to meet the aerobic and anaerobic needs of the sport. Most sports require quickness and agility. Readiness to meet these requirements often requires physical therapy focusing on sport-specific technique and overall biomechanics.

Return to Sports

Depending on the injury and the sport, it may be possible to begin training the uninjured areas of the body long before the injured area can safely be targeted. Such a program can provide a psychological boost and speed the athlete's return to sport. For example, a gymnast who has sustained an ankle injury can return to working out on the parallel bars before weight bearing

7: Sports-Related Topics

Playing With Pain

It's OK to participate in your sports activities as long as you stay in the happy-face range on the 10-point pain scale. You are in the happy-face range (1, 2, or 3) when you feel like laughing, telling a joke, or singing a silly song.

If you begin to wonder whether your symptoms are out of the happy-face range, your pain probably is at least 4 on the 10-point scale. You should stop the activity as soon as you can safely do so. If the symptoms decrease and you try out your skills on the sidelines without causing more pain, you may resume activity for as long as symptoms remain in the happy-face range.

If your pain is greater than 4 on the 10-point scale it's best not to even start to play that day. However, your physician or physical therapist may tell you that stretching or conditioning exercises are OK.

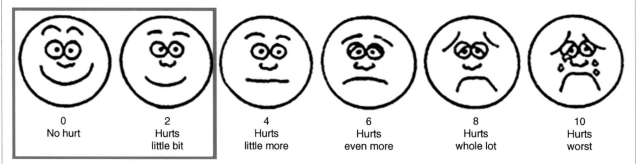

| 0 | 2 | 4 | 6 | 8 | 10 |
| No hurt | Hurts little bit | Hurts little more | Hurts even more | Hurts whole lot | Hurts worst |

Figure 2   Sample instructions for evaluating pain status, for use by a pediatric athlete who is being allowed to play with mild discomfort.

is allowed. It is critically important to determine the cause of a repetitive microtrauma injury. The young athlete may need to decide whether to leave one of several teams or to leave a coach whose demands are unrealistic for the athlete's developmental or ability level.

Most young athletes want to immediately return to their previous level of sport. The result may be rapid reinjury or a different injury resulting from inadequate strength or endurance. A physical therapist or certified athletic trainer can provide a specific program for incremental resumption of practice and play. The orthopaedic surgeon should reinforce the need for a gradual progression of activity, with careful attention to the body's signals of pain or lack of readiness. The surgeon should emphasize that activity should not be continued if the athlete has pain exceeding a predetermined level, limping or other favoring of the injured limb, or a nonspecific impression that the activity is "not quite right." A pain scale, such as the Wong-Baker scale, can be used in this process (**Figure 2**).

A general strategy that works in most sports is to gradually increase both the length and number of playing intervals until the activity is continuous. For example, a running athlete may jog a quarter of the way around a 0.25-mile track, walk around to the starting point, and repeat that pattern for a specific number of minutes. The progression may include increasing the percentage of the lap that is jogged and thereby decreasing the amount that is walked, while increasing the total number of laps. Typically, the athlete should focus either on speed or total distance during each session and should avoid increasing both speed and distance on the same day. Similarly, more difficult work (such as hill running or soccer skills) should be added on days when no other change is introduced. Useful return-to-activity guidelines developed by sports medicine groups and national sports governing bodies are available in sport-specific publications and on relevant Websites.

Core Exercise Programs

Although most sports-related injuries in children involve the extremities, core and proximal muscle strength is important. Young athletes with back, shoulder, or hip pain can undergo a therapeutic exercise program that is initially similar to a program for adults, including exercises such as the quadruped and pelvic tilt. However, young athletes need to rapidly advance to a much higher level to avoid becoming bored and frustrated by lack of progress (as sometimes happens when a physical therapist is working with several clients simultaneously or has little experience with pediatric clients).

Prepubertal children with back pain frequently have strength deficits. Young adolescents with low back pain are likely to have tight hip flexors and possibly tight hamstrings. If both the hip flexors and hamstrings are tight, the athlete has excessive lumbopelvic motion and a short stride while running. A stable lumbopelvic base is established by restoring strength, alignment, and flexibility to this area before the athlete strengthens the chest, upper back, scapular stabilizer, and cervical muscles. Alternatively, the upper torso muscles can be strengthened from a sitting position to avoid poor alignment caused by the lack of a stable lumbopelvic base.

Baseball pitchers, throwers, tennis players, gymnasts, and wrestlers especially need strong, symmetrically functioning scapulothoracic stabilizers. Dyskinetic patterns should be resolved by strengthening and

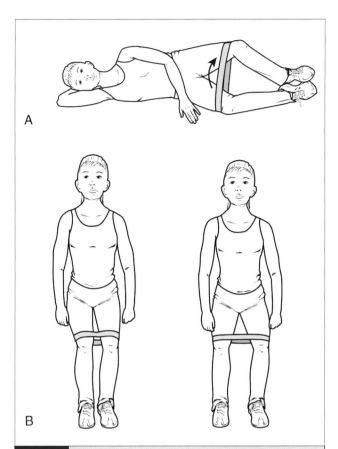

Figure 3 **A,** The clam position is a functional athletic position used to strengthen the hip external rotators with the hips and knees flexed. The athlete lies on one side, without letting the torso roll in either direction, and brings the knee of the upper leg upward with maximal external rotation of the upper hip. The difficulty of the exercise can be increased by using an elastic band to add resistance around the distal thighs. **B,** Side stepping from a functional athletic stance *(left)* not only strengthens the hip external rotators and abductors in position but also works the hips symmetrically and simultaneously. With an elastic band around the lower thighs, the athlete maintains a knees-over-toes alignment while side stepping in the functional athletic positions of moderate hip and knee flexion *(right).*

stretching the anterior shoulder and pectoral muscles in swimmers or the posterior shoulder capsule in throwing athletes, in conjunction with lumbopelvic stabilization.[9] Both the hip abductors and the hip external rotators must be strong to maintain angular and rotational alignment in running, squatting, and jump landing. These muscles should be strengthened in athletically functional positions and not solely in a seated position (**Figure 3**). Programs designed to decrease the incidence of ACL injury in young female athletes focus on avoiding knee valgus with extension; instead, landing jumps and cutting or pivoting should be done with the knee and hip flexed, the knees over the toes, and the torso adequately aligned over the primary weight-bearing ex-

tremity.[4,11] It is unclear whether programs focusing on such techniques are successful in decreasing the incidence of ACL injury.

Resistance training for children and adolescents recently has been emphasized.[12] As the exercises become more difficult, they are done on less stable surfaces and require the simultaneous use of more muscle groups.

Psychological Considerations

An orthopaedic surgeon caring for a young athlete often must consider the athlete's psychological needs. Much of the athlete's identity may be related to sports, and often the parents and siblings also are focused on sports. The emotional difficulty of separation from the sports peer group may compound the physical difficulties the athlete is facing. The orthopaedist should be sensitive to these difficulties and attempt to help the family deal with them. It is also necessary to be aware that some young athletes consciously or subconsciously use an injury as a way of gracefully leaving a sport. This possibility should be sensitively explored if the situation seems atypical. Psychologists who specialize in sports are not readily available in most regions, and therefore the orthopaedist may need to deal with psychological as well as musculoskeletal issues.

Summary

Young athletes who have been injured typically follow a gradually progressive course of therapeutic exercises, with a careful resumption of sports activity as soon as is safely possible. Rehabilitation includes therapeutic exercises to attain or restore core stability. Lumbopelvic and scapulothoracic work are included, as well as hip and shoulder strengthening. A solid athletic stance should be achieved, with flexed knees generally over the toes and the torso well balanced. Additional sport-specific strength and flexibility may be required. Fitness components such as aerobic and anaerobic capacity, quickness, agility, and balance should be restored. Sport-specific skills should be tested in the therapeutic environment to allow the young athlete a rapid, safe stepwise reentry into sport.

Annotated References

1. Hupperets MD, Verhagen EA, van Mechelen W: Effect of unsupervised home based proprioceptive training on recurrences of ankle sprain: Randomised controlled trial. *BMJ* 2009;339:b2684.

   Adolescent and adult athletes who rehabilitated an ankle sprain decreased the likelihood of a recurrence. The study patients were age 12 to 70 years; the number of adolescent patients was not indicated.

2. Knowles SB, Marshall SW, Bowling JM, et al: A prospective study of injury incidence among North Carolina high school athletes. *Am J Epidemiol* 2006; 164(12):1209-1221.

   In a prospective cohort study, the incidence of injury among previously injured high school athletes was almost twice that of previously uninjured athletes.

3. Davis JT, Limpisvasti O, Fluhme D, et al: The effect of pitching biomechanics on the upper extremity in youth and adolescent baseball pitchers. *Am J Sports Med* 2009;37(8):1484-1491.

   A cross-sectional laboratory study of pitchers age 9 to 18 years found that those with better pitching mechanics had lower loads on the shoulder and elbow as well as greater pitching efficiency.

4. Renstrom P, Ljungqvist A, Arendt E, et al: Non-contact ACL injuries in female athletes: An International Olympic Committee current concepts statement. *Br J Sports Med* 2008;42(6):394-412.

   This consensus statement provides a thorough review of the topic.

5. Micheli LJ, Ireland ML: Prevention and management of calcaneal apophysitis in children: An overuse syndrome. *J Pediatr Orthop* 1987;7(1):34-38.

6. Trakis JE, McHugh MP, Caracciolo PA, Busciacco L, Mullaney M, Nicholas SJ: Muscle strength and range of motion in adolescent pitchers with throwing-related pain: Implications for injury prevention. *Am J Sports Med* 2008;36(11):2173-2178.

   In a laboratory study of adolescent male pitchers, the authors compared those who did and did not have shoulder or elbow pain during the preceding season. Those with pain had more posterior shoulder weakness, but only an association was possible, not a determination of cause and effect, in this cross-sectional study.

7. Nattiv A, Loucks AB, Manore MM, et al: American College of Sports Medicine position stand: The female athlete triad. *Med Sci Sports Exerc* 2007;39(10):1867-1882.

   This updated review discusses the relationship of eating disorders, menstrual irregularity, and bone health.

8. Deutz RC, Benardot D, Martin DE, Cody MM: Relationship between energy deficits and body composition in elite female gymnasts and runners. *Med Sci Sports Exerc* 2000;32(3):659-668.

9. Kibler WB, Sciasia A: Throwing injuries in young athletes, in Kibler WB, ed: *OKU: Sports Medicine 4.* Rosemont, IL, American Academy of Orthopaedic Surgeons, 2009, pp 425-431.

   Normal scapulothoracic function is necessary for young overhead athletes, such as tennis and baseball players. Not only the shoulder but the entire kinetic chain should be strong, flexible, and engaged in a coordinated fashion.

10. Smith AD: Sport injuries of children and adolescents, in Nicholas JA, Hershman E, eds: *Sports Medicine: Spine and Lower Extremity.* Philadelphia, PA, Mosby, 1995.

11. Santa Monica Sports Medicine Foundation: PEP Program 2010. http://www.aclprevent.com/pep-program.htm Accessed November 23, 2010.

    A stepwise ACL injury prevention program is provided.

12. Faigenbaum AD, Myer GD: Pediatric resistance training: Benefits, concerns, and program design considerations. *Curr Sports Med Rep* 2010;9(3):161-168.

    Current data and practical considerations in pediatric strength training are reviewed.

Index

Index

Index

Index